Emergency Department Resuscitation of the Critically Ill

2nd Edition

Michael E. Winters, MD, FACEP, FAAEM
Editor-in-Chief
Associate Professor
Director, Critical Care Education
Co-Director, Combined Emergency Medicine/Internal Medicine/Critical Care Residency
Departments of Emergency Medicine and Medicine
University of Maryland School of Medicine
Baltimore, Maryland

Peter DeBlieux, MD, FACEP
Associate Editor
Professor of Clinical Medicine
Louisiana State University School of Medicine
Chief Medical Officer and Director of Quality
University Medical Center
New Orleans, Louisiana

Michael C. Bond, MD, FACEP, FAAEM
Associate Editor
Associate Professor
Director, Emergency Medicine Residency
Department of Emergency Medicine
University of Maryland School of Medicine
Baltimore, Maryland

Evie G. Marcolini, MD, FAAEM
Associate Editor
Assistant Professor of Emergency Medicine and Neurocritical Care
Department of Emergency Medicine
Yale University School of Medicine
New Haven, Connecticut

Dale P. Woolridge, MD, PhD, FACEP
Associate Editor
Professor of Pediatrics and Emergency Medicine
Director, Combined Pediatrics/Emergency Medicine Residency
University of Arizona
Tucson, Arizona

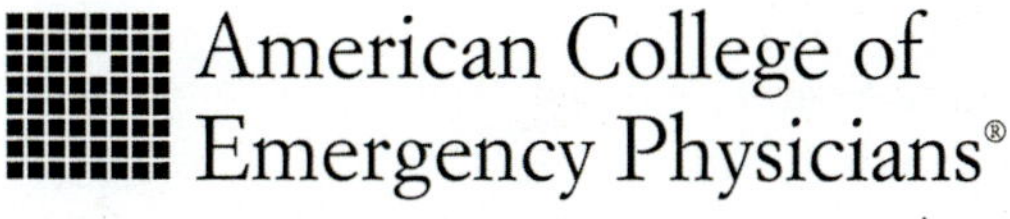

DISCLAIMER AND COPYRIGHT NOTICE

First printing April 2017
ISBN 978-0-9889973-9-4

ACEP BOOKSTORE
PO Box 619911, Dallas, TX 75261-9911
800-798-1822, 972-550-0911
bookstore.acep.org

SENIOR EDITOR Rachel Donihoo
PUBLICATIONS ASSISTANT Jessica Hamilton
EDUCATIONAL PRODUCTS DIRECTOR Marta Foster
DESIGN AND PRODUCTION Susan McReynolds
INDEXING Sharon Hughes

About the Editors

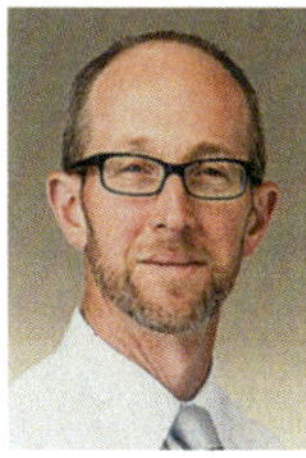

Michael E. Winters, MD, FACEP, FAAEM. Dr. Winters is an associate professor of emergency medicine and medicine at the University of Maryland School of Medicine. He is the Director of the Combined Emergency Medicine/Internal Medicine Residency Program and the founder and Co-Director of the Combined Emergency Medicine/Internal Medicine/Critical Care Residency Program. Dr. Winters has received numerous teaching awards, including the National Emergency Medicine Faculty Teaching Award from the American College of Emergency Physicians (ACEP), the Young Educators Award from the American Academy of Emergency Physicians, and the 2014-2015 Honorable Mention Outstanding Speaker of the Year from ACEP. He has lectured nationally and internationally, authored numerous articles and textbook chapters, and hosts a monthly podcast on the management of the critically ill emergency department patient, Critical Care Perspectives in Emergency Medicine. Dr. Winters completed a combined emergency medicine/internal medicine residency at the University of Maryland, after which he completed a teaching fellowship with a special focus on emergency critical care.

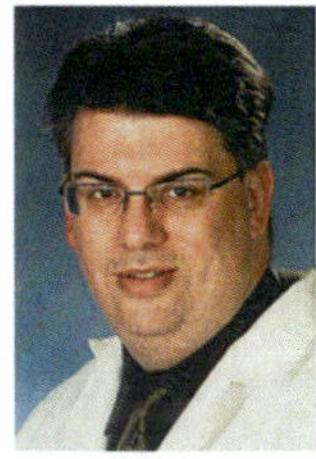

Michael C. Bond, MD, FACEP, FAAEM. Dr. Bond is an associate professor and the Residency Program Director in the Department of Emergency Medicine at the University of Maryland. He was guest editor of an *Emergency Medicine Clinics of North America* edition on orthopedic emergencies; has written several book chapters on cardiology emergencies, specifically pericarditis, myocarditis, Wolff-Parkinson-White syndrome, and temporary pacing; and has coauthored multiple orthopedic and cardiology literature summaries. In June 2005, Dr. Bond completed the combined Emergency Medicine/Internal Medicine Residency Program at Allegheny General Hospital, where he found it particularly rewarding to care for the most critical of patients while teaching new interns to do the same.

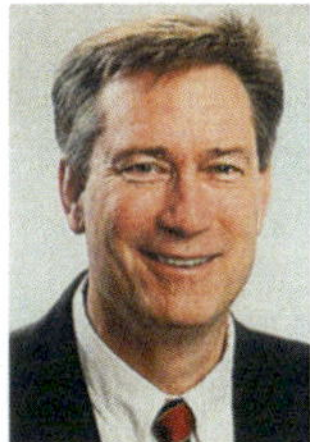

Peter DeBlieux, MD, FACEP. Dr. DeBlieux is a professor of clinical medicine and an attending physician in emergency medicine and the medical intensive care unit of Louisiana State University Health Sciences Center (LSUHSC) Charity Hospital, where has served for 25 years. He also is the Chief Medical Officer and Director of Quality at University Medical Center and a clinical professor of surgery at Tulane University Medical School, both in New Orleans. He is the former Program Director of the LSUHSC Charity Hospital Emergency Medicine Residency and former Director of Resident and Faculty Development—positions he held for a decade each. Dr. DeBlieux earned his medical degree from LSUHSC, where he later completed an internship in internal medicine. He has remained at his alma mater, where he completed an emergency medicine residency followed by a pulmonary critical care fellowship.

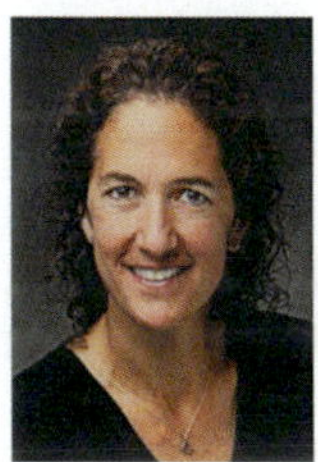

Evie G. Marcolini, MD, FAAEM. Dr. Marcolini is an assistant professor in emergency medicine and neurocritical care at Yale University School of Medicine. She completed a fellowship in surgical critical care at the R. Adams Cowley Shock Trauma Center at the University of Maryland, where she was an attending physician in emergency medicine and surgical critical care. She divides her time at Yale between the emergency department and the neuroscience intensive care unit. Dr. Marcolini lectures on neurocritical care and critical care issues in medical forums in Egypt, India, Vietnam, and Argentina. An avid mountaineer, she also teaches for Wilderness Medical Associates and has been an invited lecturer for the Wilderness Medical Society.

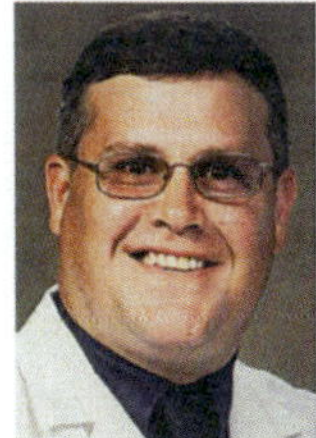

Dale P. Woolridge, MD, PhD, FACEP. Dr. Woolridge is a professor of emergency medicine and pediatrics at the University of Arizona, where he serves as the Director of the Pediatric and Emergency Medicine Combined Residency Training Program. He has received multiple awards for his teaching efforts, and is the Medical Director of the Southern Arizona Children's Advocacy Center, the primary referral center for all children in the region subjected to abuse and neglect. He also serves as Committee Chair for the Arizona State Health Department's Pediatric Advisory Council for Emergency Services (PACES), and is the pediatric representative on the Arizona State EMS Advisory Council. Dr. Woolridge lectures nationally and has published multiple books and chapters on pediatric emergency medicine, and serves as an associate editor for the *Journal of Emergency Medicine.*

DEDICATIONS

To Erika, Hayden, Emma, Taylor, and Olivia for your endless love and support; you are my world and my inspiration for everything. I love you dearly. To the emergency medicine residents and faculty at the University of Maryland, it is a privilege to be your colleague and friend. — MW

I would like to thank my wife, Ginger, and my three children, Gabbi, Emily, and Zachary, for their continued support, which enables me to participate in great projects like this book, and for keeping life fun and interesting. — MB

To Karen, Joshua, and Zachary for patience, love, and understanding. You are the joy in my life. To my emergency medicine and critical care colleagues at LSUHSC New Orleans, thanks for your inspiration, education, and support. — PD

To my husband, Paul, whose support made my participation possible and whose love and inspiration help me accomplish my dreams. To my past, present, and future residents, who constantly teach and inspire me. — EM

To my family, Michelle, Anna, and Garrett, for being there; my parents, Brenda and Joe, for not giving up on me; and my residents, who continue to teach me daily. Many thanks! — DW

ACKNOWLEDGMENTS

We wish to acknowledge all those who care for critically ill emergency department patients. Your tireless efforts are an inspiration. We also wish to acknowledge and thank Linda J. Kesselring, ELS, MS, the technical editor/writer for the Department of Emergency Medicine at the University of Maryland, for her outstanding contributions and assistance in preparing this textbook.

— The Editors

Contributors

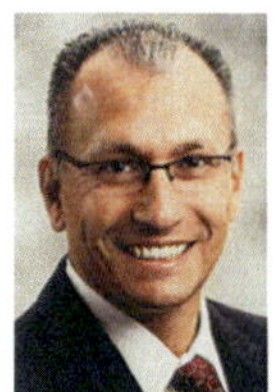

Fermin Barrueto, Jr., MD, FACEP
Senior Vice President, Medical Affairs
Chief Medical Officer
University of Maryland Upper Chesapeake Health
Bel Air, MD

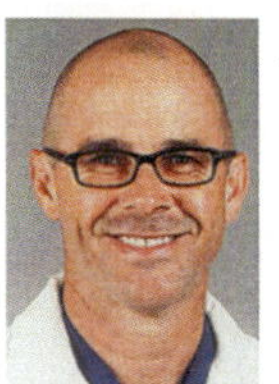

Joe Bellezzo, MD
Chair, Department of Emergency Medicine
Co-Director, ED ECMO
Director, Ultrasound
Sharp Memorial Hospital
San Diego, CA

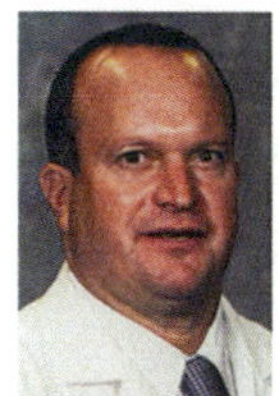

Dale S. Birenbaum, MD, FACEP
Associate Professor of Emergency Medicine
University of Central Florida
Orlando, FL

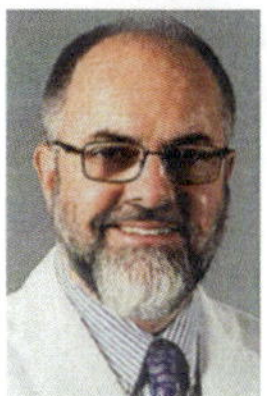

William J. Brady, MD, FACEP
Professor of Emergency Medicine
David A. Harrison Distinguished Educator
University of Virginia School of Medicine
Charlottesville, VA

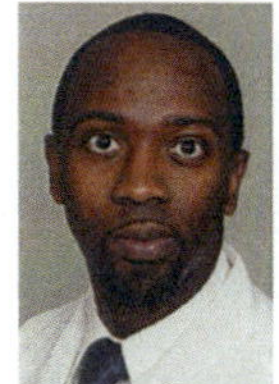

Justin D. Britton, MD
Emergency Medicine Physician
Kaiser Permanente
Fontana, CA

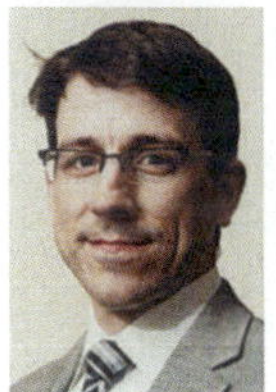

David Callaway, MD, FACEP
Director, Division of Operational and Disaster Medicine
Department of Emergency Medicine
Carolinas Medical Center
Charlotte, NC

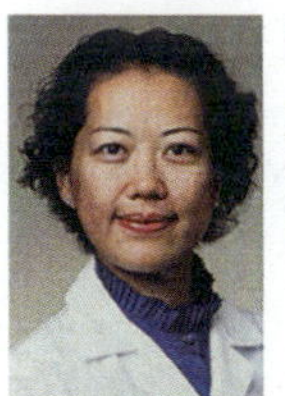

Wan-Tsu W. Chang, MD
Assistant Professor of Emergency Medicine
University of Maryland School of Medicine
Baltimore, MD

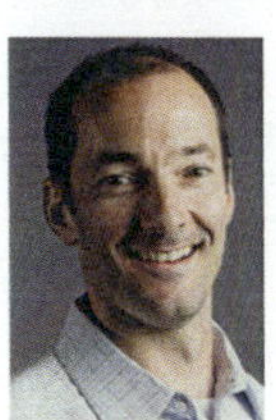

Justin O. Cook, MD, FACEP
Emergency Physician
Legacy Emanuel Health Center
Northwest Acute Care Specialists
Portland, OR

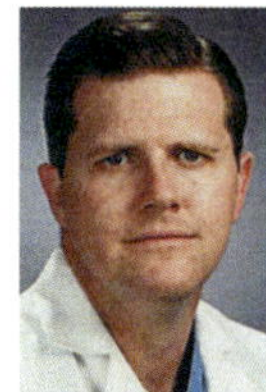

James M. Dargin, MD
Assistant Clinical Professor of Medicine
Tufts University School of Medicine
Director, Medical Intensive Care Unit
Lahey Hospital and Medical Center
Burlington, MA

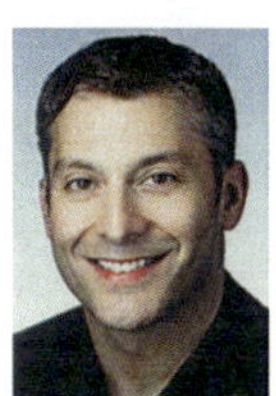

Jonathan E. Davis, MD, FACEP
Professor, Academic Chair, and Program Director, Department of Emergency Medicine
MedStar Georgetown University Hospital/ MedStar Washington Hospital Center
Georgetown University School of Medicine
Washington, DC

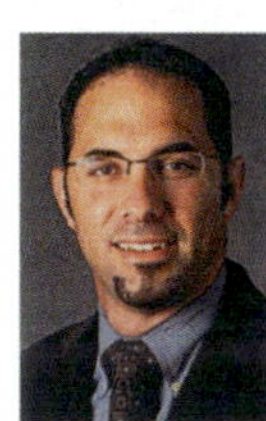

Timothy J. Ellender, MD
Assistant Professor
Co-Director, Critical Care Fellowship Track
Departments of Emergency Medicine and Critical Care
Indiana University Health-Methodist Hospital
Indianapolis, IN

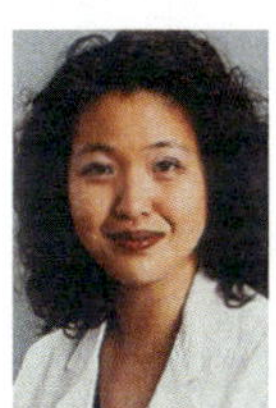

Lillian Emlet, MD, FACEP
Assistant Professor of Critical Care Medicine and Emergency Medicine
Associate Program Director, Internal Medicine Critical Care Fellowship of the Multidisciplinary Critical Care Training Program
University of Pittsburgh Medical Center
Pittsburgh, PA

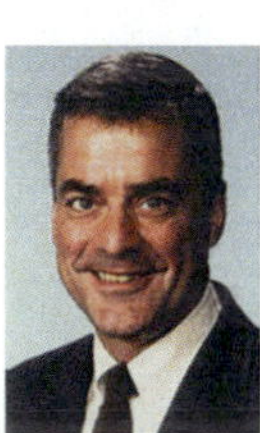

Michael A. Gibbs, MD, FACEP
Chair, Department of Emergency Medicine
Carolinas Medical Center
Charlotte, NC

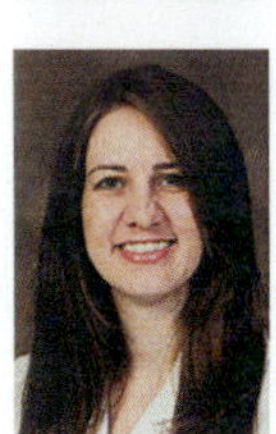

Lisa Greenfield, MD, PGY-4
Resident
Departments of Emergency Medicine and Pediatrics
University of Arizona College of Medicine
Tucson, AZ

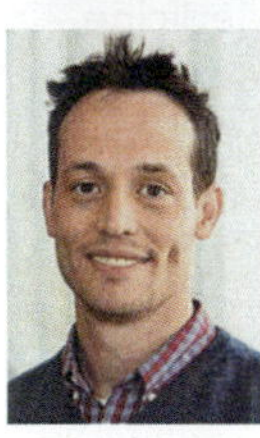

John C. Greenwood, MD
Assistant Professor
Departments of Emergency Medicine, Anesthesiology, and Critical Care
Hospital of the University of Pennsylvania
Perelman School of Medicine
Philadelphia, PA

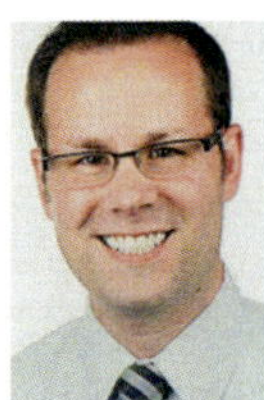

Bryan D. Hayes, PharmD, FAACT
Assistant Professor of Emergency Medicine
Harvard Medical School
Clinical Pharmacist, Emergency Medicine and Toxicology
Massachusetts General Hospital
Boston, MA

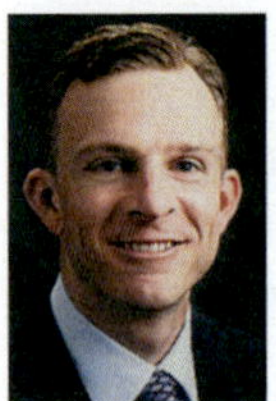

Alan C. Heffner, MD
Co-Director, Critical Care
Director, ECMO Services
Medical Director, Sepsis Initiative
Departments of Internal Medicine and Emergency Medicine
Carolinas Healthcare System
Charlotte, NC

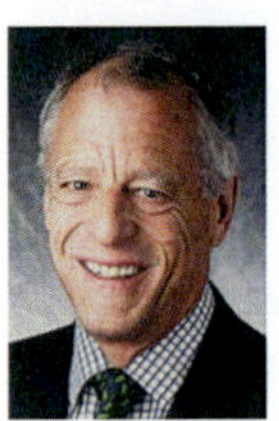

Daniel L. Herr, MD
Associate Professor of Medicine and Surgery
Chief, Surgical Critical Care
Director, Cardiac Surgery and Heart-Lung Transplant ICU
University of Maryland Medical Center
Baltimore, MD

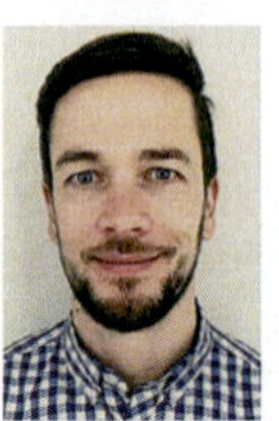

Nicholas J. Hiivala, BME
Artificial Heart Engineer
University of Maryland
Baltimore, MD

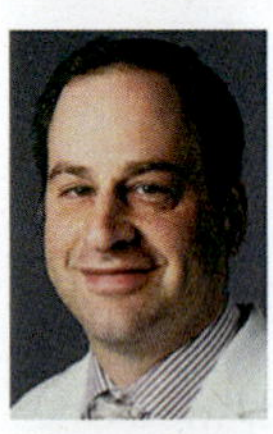

Benjamin J. Lawner, DO, FACEP
Medical Director, Prehospital Services
LifeFlight and EMS
Allegheny General Hospital
Pittsburgh, PA

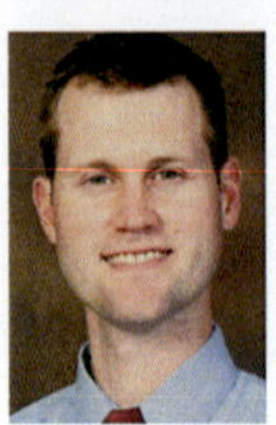

Aaron N. Leetch, MD, FACEP
Assistant Professor of Emergency Medicine and Pediatrics
Director, Combined Emergency Medicine/ Pediatrics Residency
University of Arizona College of Medicine
Tucson, AZ

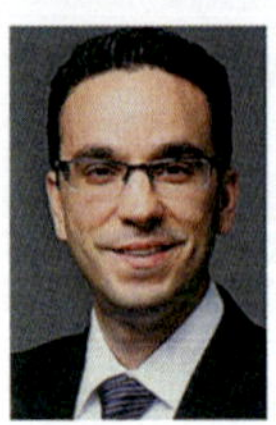

Daniel M. Lugassy, MD
Assistant Professor of Emergency Medicine
Division of Medical Toxicology
New York University School of Medicine
Assistant Medical Director, Undergraduate Medical Education
New York Simulation Center for the Health Sciences
New York, NY

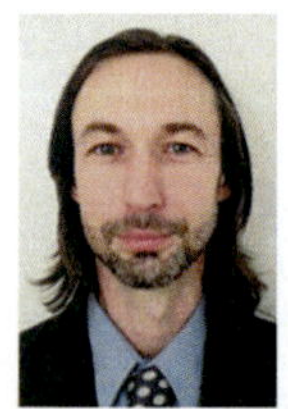

Daniel Mantuani, MD, MPH
Emergency Physician
Assistant Director, Emergency Ultrasound
Alameda Health System
Highland Hospital
Oakland, CA

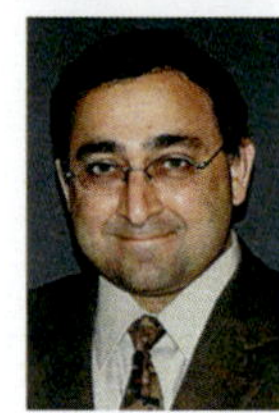

Amal Mattu, MD, FACEP
Professor of Emergency Medicine
Vice Chair, Education
Director, Faculty Development Fellowship
Co-Director, Emergency Cardiology Fellowship
University of Maryland School of Medicine
Baltimore, MD

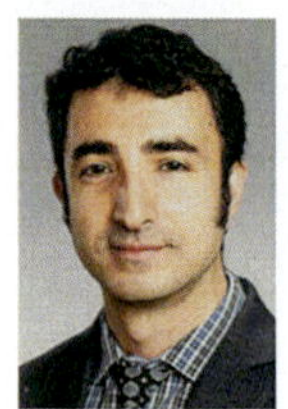

Jehangir Meer, MD, FACEP
Assistant Professor of Emergency Medicine
Director, Emergency Ultrasound Services
Emory University School of Medicine
Atlanta, GA

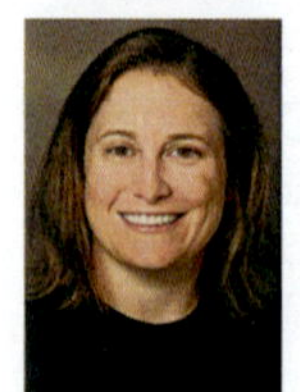

Jenny S. Mendelson, MD
Assistant Professor of Pediatrics and Emergency Medicine
Division of Pediatric Critical Care Medicine
University of Arizona College of Medicine
Tucson, AZ

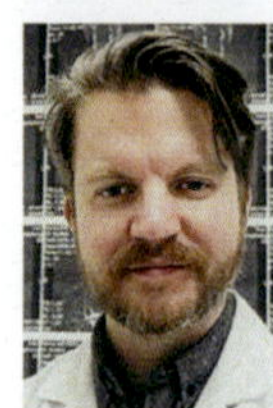

Chad M. Meyers, MD
Director, Emergency Critical Care
Assistant Professor of Clinical Emergency Medicine and Surgical Critical Care
Icahn School of Medicine at Mount Sinai
New York, NY

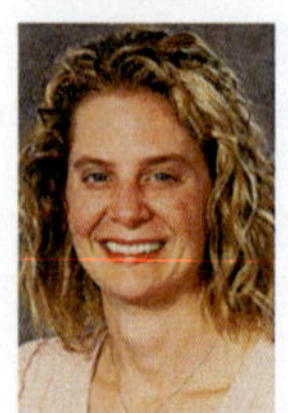

Lisa D. Mills, MD, FAAEM
Clinical Professor
Department of Emergency Medicine
UC Davis School of Medicine
Sacramento, CA

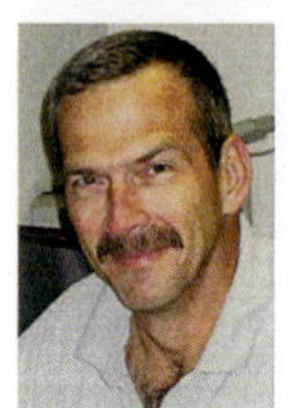

Robert L. Norris, Jr., MD, FACEP
Professor Emeritus of Emergency Medicine
Stanford University School of Medicine
Stanford, CA

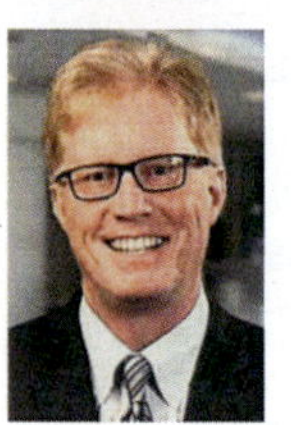

Robert E. O'Connor, MD, FACEP
Professor and Chair, Department of Emergency Medicine
University of Virginia School of Medicine
Charlottesville, VA

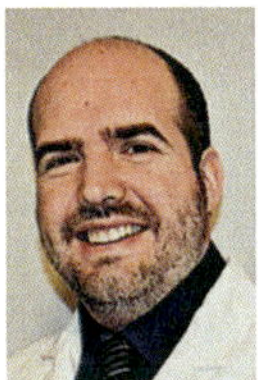
Brian Oloizia, MD
Attending Physician
Department of Emergency Medicine
Fellow, Neurocritical Care
University of Cincinnati College of Medicine
Cincinnati, OH

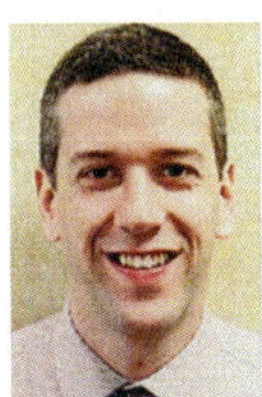
Joshua C. Reynolds, MD, MS
Assistant Professor of Emergency Medicine
Michigan State University College of Human Medicine
East Lansing, MI

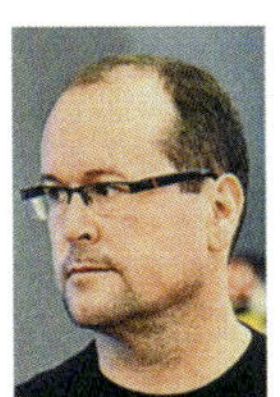
Robert L. Rogers, MD
Professor and Vice Chair for Faculty Development
University of Tennessee College of Medicine
Knoxville, TN

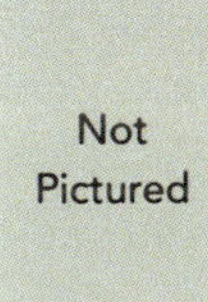
Gregory Ruppel, MD
Post-Doctoral Fellow, Critical Care
Department of Emergency Medicine
Indiana University
Indianapolis, IN

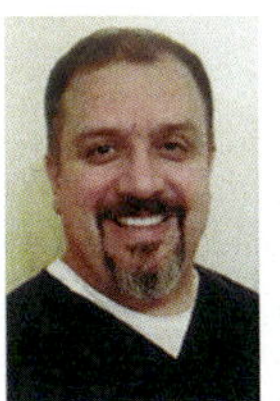
Jairo I. Santanilla, MD
Clinical Assistant Professor of Pulmonary/Critical Care
Louisiana State University School of Medicine
New Orleans, LA

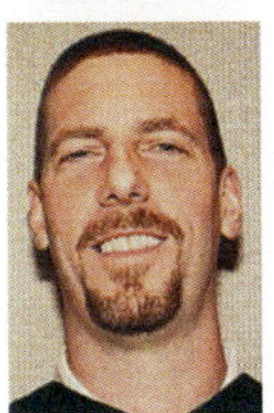
Joseph R. Shiber, MD, FACEP
Associate Professor of Medicine, Emergency Medicine, Neurology, and Surgery
Director, ECMO Service
Co-Director, Neurointensive Care Unit
University of Florida College of Medicine
Jacksonville, FL

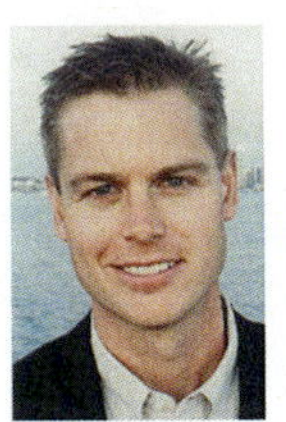
Zack Shinar, MD, FACEP
Vice Chair, Department of Emergency Medicine
Co-Director, ED ECMO
Sharp Memorial Hospital
San Diego, CA

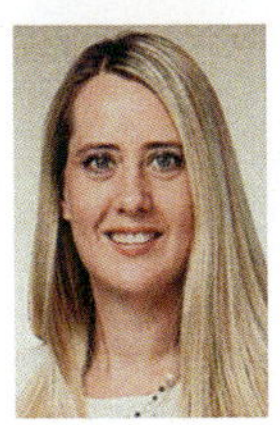
Sarah K. Sommerkamp, MD, RDMS
Assistant Professor of Emergency Medicine
Director, Emergency Ultrasound
University of Maryland School of Medicine
Baltimore, MD

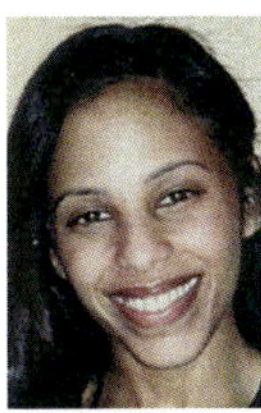
Semhar Z. Tewelde, MD, FAAEM
Assistant Professor of Emergency Medicine
University of Maryland School of Medicine
Baltimore, MD

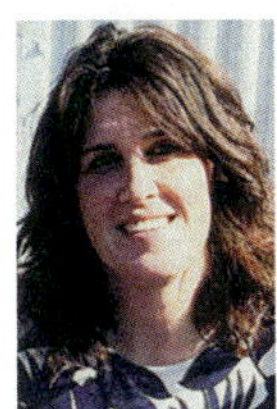
Carrie D. Tibbles, MD
Assistant Professor of Emergency Medicine
Associate Director, Graduate Medical Education
Associate Director, Emergency Medicine Residency
Beth Israel Deaconess Medical Center
Boston, MA

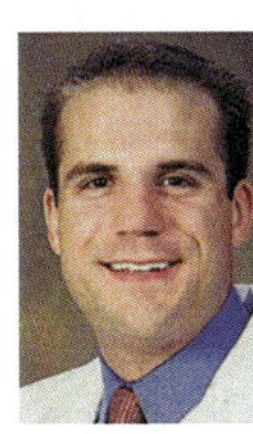
Chad D. Viscusi, MD, FACEP
Assistant Professor of Emergency Medicine and Pediatrics
University of Arizona College of Medicine
Associate Medical Director, Pediatric Emergency Medicine
Banner-University Medical Center/Diamond Children's Hospital
Tucson, AZ

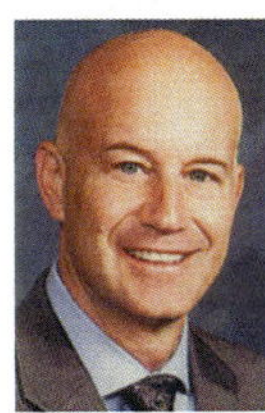
Robert J. Vissers, MD, MBA, FACEP
Chief Executive Officer and President
Boulder Community Health, Colorado
Adjunct Associate Professor
School of Management, Department of Emergency Medicine
Oregon Health & Science University
Portland, OR

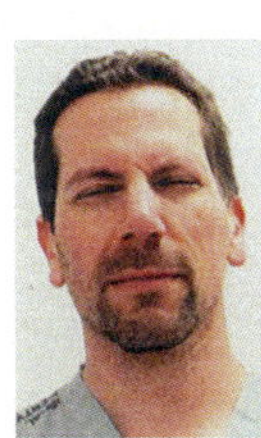
Scott D. Weingart, MD, FACEP
Clinical Associate Professor
Chief, Division of Emergency Critical Care
Director, Resuscitation and Acute Critical Care Unit
Stony Brook Hospital
Stony Brook, NY

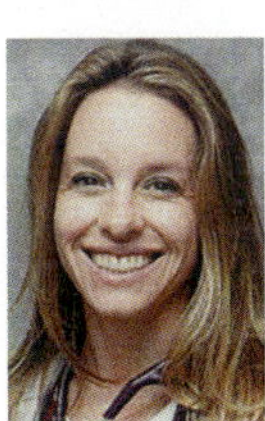
Kelly Williamson, MD
Clinical Assistant Professor of Emergency Medicine
University of Illinois Chicago
Assistant Program Director, Emergency Medicine Residency
Advocate Christ Medical Center
Oak Lawn, IL

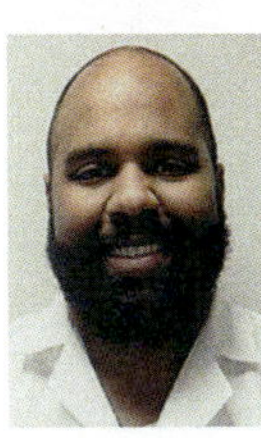
George C. Willis, MD, FACEP
Director, Undergraduate Medical Education
Department of Emergency Medicine
University of Maryland School of Medicine
Baltimore, MD

Foreword

Read this book!

The 2nd edition of *Emergency Department Resuscitation of the Critically Ill* is packed with essential information focused on the high-risk conditions that produce the greatest anxiety and concern in the daily practice of emergency medicine. From undifferentiated shock and difficult airways to critical poisonings and pediatric resuscitations, this comprehensive textbook gets to the heart of the presentations, diagnoses, and stabilization of a broad range of acute conditions that threaten our patients' lives.

The text is practical, evidenced based, and presents a synthesis of current knowledge in a format that is easy to read and to assimilate quickly. The expert authors of this updated edition take a refined approach to critical care, providing even more pearls, summaries, and practical clinical information than in the highly regarded first iteration. Simply put, it is the definitive text on the acutely ill patient, written *by* emergency physicians *for* emergency physicians. *Emergency Department Resuscitation of the Critically Ill* should be required reading for all emergency physicians, whether in practice or in training.

Jeffrey Tabas, MD, FACEP

Chair, ACEP Education Committee
Professor of Clinical Emergency Medicine
Director, Faculty Development
Zuckerberg San Francisco General Hospital
San Francisco, California

Preface

As emergency care providers, we rise to our professional best when evaluating, diagnosing, and providing life-sustaining therapies to critically ill patients. Whether performing rapid sequence intubation, initiating and adjusting mechanical ventilation, titrating vasoactive medications, administering intravenous fluids, or initiating extracorporeal membrane oxygenation, the emergency physician must be an expert at resuscitation. In recent years, it has become common for critically ill patients to remain in the acute setting for exceedingly long periods of time. In fact, the amount of critical care delivered in emergency departments across the United States has escalated more than 200% over the last decade!

During these crucial initial hours of critical illness, many pathological processes begin to take hold — processes that, if not recognized and reversed, will undoubtedly lead to poor outcomes. During this time, lives can be saved — or lost. With these critical scenarios in mind, we have prepared this textbook for the acute health care provider working in an emergency department, urgent care center, or intensive care unit. Rather than discuss general medical conditions, we have emphasized scenarios in which a patient is "crashing" before your eyes. We have focused on caring for the sickest of the sick: the unstable patient with undifferentiated shock; the crashing ventilated patient; the crashing patient with pulmonary hypertension, septic shock, or cardiogenic shock; the crashing obese patient; and the hypotensive patient with a left ventricular assist device. You'll also find imperative information about managing pediatric and neonatal resuscitation, intracerebral hemorrhage, and the difficult emergency delivery.

What physiological possibilities must you consider immediately? What steps should you take *now* to save the patient's life? The authors of these chapters were selected based on their expertise in critical care and emergency medicine. Within each chapter, essential information is emphasized in tables, figures, "key points," and "pearls." Many chapters also contain flow diagrams that can be referenced quickly during a shift.

It is our hope that acute health care providers will refer to this text frequently to broaden their knowledge base for the delivery of rapid, efficient, and appropriate critical care to the moribund patient. Quite simply, we believe this book will help you save lives.

Michael Winters, MD, FACEP, FAAEM

Editor-in-Chief

April 2017

Contents

Undifferentiated Shock

1

IN THIS CHAPTER

- Assessing and stabilizing the patient in shock
- Making a definitive diagnosis
- The expanded RUSH examination
- Vasoactive medications and push-dose pressors

Chad M. Meyers and Scott D. Weingart

The ability to adeptly manage patients who are in shock is among the defining skills of our specialty. In some cases, the cause of the shock state is immediately apparent. The hypotensive patient with a gunshot wound to the abdomen, for example, does not present a diagnostic dilemma. However, there are many other cases in which the diagnosis is neither quick nor simple. Emergency physicians frequently are forced to initiate resuscitation while simultaneously gathering the information needed to identify a patient's underlying etiology.

Reduced to the simplest description, shock is inadequate tissue perfusion. In its early stages, patients might have a benign physical examination and normal vital signs. This shock state is sometimes referred to as *cryptic shock* and is revealed only by examining biomarkers such as lactate, or by using tissue perfusion monitors. For many emergency care clinicians, shock is almost synonymous with hypotension — a conflation that usually delays recognition of the shock state and results in a more challenging treatment course.

Low blood pressure should be taken into consideration when assessing an otherwise well-looking patient. Although it is tempting to discount borderline or transient hypotension, even a single episode of systolic blood pressure lower than 100 mm Hg has been associated with increased mortality in emergency department patients.[1] The lower the blood pressure observed, the higher the risk of death.[1] In cases of severe sepsis, the patient may experience transient self-limited dips in blood pressure.

Initial Assessment

In addition to the standard history and physical examination obtained on every sick patient in the emergency department, the following simple evaluations should be immediately performed on a patient with undifferentiated shock:

- Blood glucose measurement to screen for hypoglycemia
- Pregnancy test in female patients of childbearing age for suspected ectopic pregnancy
- ECG to identify arrhythmia and ischemia
- Assessment of feet and hands for abnormal vasodilation
- Examination of the neck veins as an indicator of paradoxically increased central venous pressure
- Rectal examination for melena/gastrointestinal blood for occult bleeding
- Chest radiograph to evaluate for pneumonia, pneumothorax or hemothorax, and pulmonary edema

Initial Stabilization

After a patent airway and adequate oxygenation are ensured, it is crucial to establish access to the circulation. Short large-bore intravenous lines are the first option for venous access. If peripheral access is difficult, central venous catheterization, using a percutaneous introducer catheter or a dialysis catheter, provides a reliable means of fluid resuscitation. In addition, a variety of devices allow immediate cannulation of the intraosseous (IO) space and provide a reliable temporizing method in the unstable patient presenting without intravascular access. However, IO flow rates differ by anatomical site. While proximal tibial access quickly establishes a route for drug administration, the flow is not adequate for rapid volumes or blood products. When more aggressive resuscitation is required, proximal humeral and sternal IO cannulation combined with a pressurized bag or infusion pump can achieve flow rates comparable to those of an 18-gauge peripheral intravenous catheter.

Empiric fluid administration typically is the first consideration in the undifferentiated hypotensive patient. While overzealous volume resuscitation is associated with increased mortality, most unresuscitated hemodynamically unstable patients in the emergency department will benefit from a small bolus of crystalloid during the initial evaluation. The one exception is the patient with hemorrhagic shock, in whom crystalloid will further dilute hemoglobin, platelets, and clotting factors. Instead, blood products (eg, packed red blood cells, plasma, and platelets) should be used. After immediate priorities such as airway and respiratory compromise have been addressed, a rapid ultrasound survey (see below) can provide valuable information to more carefully guide further resuscitation and volume administration. After immediate priorities such as airway and respiratory compromise have been addressed, a rapid ultrasound survey (see below) can provide valuable information to more carefully guide further resuscitation and volume administration.

The goal of fluid loading is to achieve a mean arterial pressure (MAP) greater than 65 mm Hg. Values below this level can lead to poor organ perfusion and further worsen the cardiac output secondary to poor cardiac perfusion. Raising the MAP significantly above 65 mm Hg with exogenous medications or aggressive fluid loading predisposes the patient to complications with no added benefit.[2]

It is dangerous to await the effects of fluid loading in patients with MAP levels below 40 to 50 mm Hg. In such cases, vasopressors should be administered while fluid loading is underway. A continuous infusion of any of the agents in Table 1-1 will suffice for this purpose, and push-dose pressors *(Table 1-2)* can be used during the initial stages of patient evaluation/stabilization.[3]

PEARLS

- ✓ The Trendelenburg position will have only transient effects on blood pressure and should not be used as a resuscitation position during shock.[4-6]
- ✓ Hypocalcemia can cause decreased blood pressure. Administration of calcium chloride, 500 to 1,000 mg, preferably through a central line or into a large antecubital vein, will increase inotropy and vasoconstriction in any patient, but especially in patients with hypocalcemia.

Differential Diagnosis

The causes of shock can be conceptualized by analogy to a simple water-pumping system, which consists of a reservoir, a pump, and the pump's inflow and outflow pipes.[7] Shock results from an empty reservoir, pump failure, inflow obstruction, or leaky, enlarged pipes *(Figure 1-1)*.

Clues to the Diagnosis

The following concepts can hint at the cause of undifferentiated shock:

- In a patient with hypotension, warm extremities point to abnormal vasodilation from conditions such as sepsis, anaphylaxis, pancreatitis, and overdose or poisoning.[8]
- Conversely, cold extremities in a patient with hypotension can indicate hemorrhagic, hypovolemic, or cardiogenic causes, and are indicative of endogenous sympathetic compensation for the hypotension.

TABLE 1-1. Conventional Vasoactive Drugs

Drug	Dosing
Dopamine	Initial dose: 5 mcg/kg/min Titrate by: 5–10 mcg/kg/min Maximum dose: 20 mcg/kg/min
Norepinephrine	Initial dose: 0.5–1 mcg/min Titrate by: 1–2 mcg/min Maximum dose: 30 mcg/min
Dobutamine	Initial dose: 2.5 mcg/kg/min Titrate by: 2.5 mcg/kg/min Maximum dose: 20 mcg/kg/min
Epinephrine	Initial dose: 1 mcg/min Titrate by: 1 mcg/min Maximum dose: 10 mcg/min
Phenylephrine	Initial dose: 100–180 mcg/min Titrate by: 100 mcg/min Maximum dose: 10 mcg/kg/min
Vasopressin	Initial dose: 0.01 units/min Titrate by: 0.01 units/min Maximum dose: 0.04 units/min

TABLE 1-2. Push-Dose Pressors (may be administered through peripheral lines)

Phenylephrine
This drug is a pure alpha agent, so it has no intrinsic inotropy; it increases heart perfusion by normalizing the MAP and can improve cardiac output.
Onset: 1 minute
Duration: 20 minutes
Mixing instructions: Into a 3-mL syringe, draw up 1 mL from a vial of phenylephrine (10 mg/mL). Inject into a 100-mL bag of normal saline. This yields 100 mL of phenylephrine with a concentration of 100 mcg/mL. Draw some solution into a syringe; each milliliter contains 100 mcg.
Dose: 0.5 to 2 mL (50–200 mcg) every 2–5 minutes

Epinephrine
This drug is an inopressor with alpha-, beta1-, and beta2-effects.
Onset: 1 minute
Duration: 5–10 minutes
Mixing instructions: Draw 9 mL of normal saline into a 10-mL syringe. Into this syringe, draw up 1 mL from the cardiac epinephrine ampule. (A cardiac ampule contains 10 mL of the drug at a concentration of 100 mcg/mL or 1:10,000.) This yields 10 mL of epinephrine at a concentration of 10 mcg/mL (1:100,000).
Dose: 0.5–2 mL (5–20 mcg) every 2 to 5 minutes

FIGURE 1-1. Schematic of the Circulatory System (by analogy to a water pump)

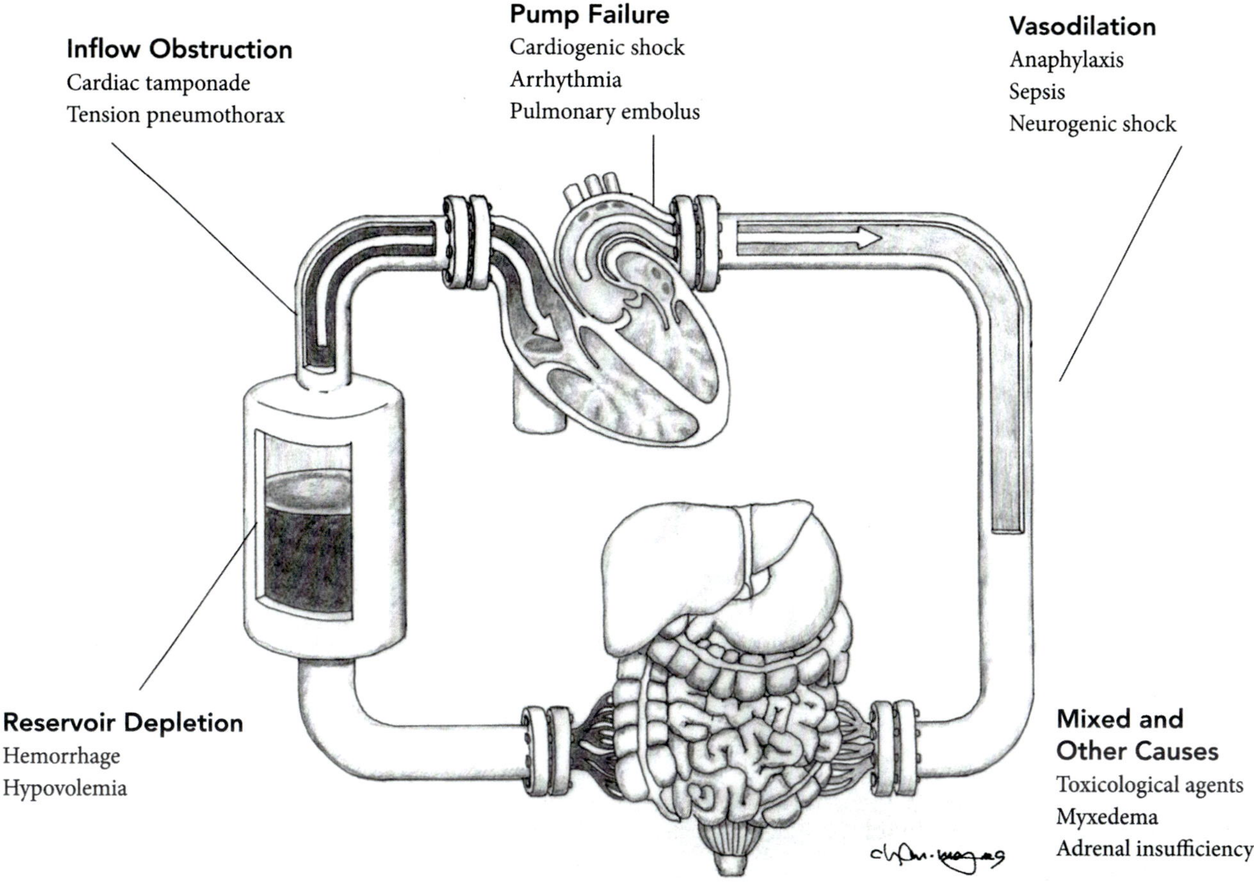

- Cardiogenic shock from myocardial infarction is extremely unlikely with an ECG that shows no signs of ischemia. It is virtually impossible to have cardiogenic shock with completely clear lungs unless a right ventricular infarction is the cause of the hypotension.
- In patients in anaphylactic shock, skin findings (urticaria, angioedema), facial swelling, and respiratory compromise might not accompany the hypotension.
- Undifferentiated shock in a female patient of child-bearing age should be assumed to be from a ruptured ectopic pregnancy until a negative pregnancy test is returned.
- Jugular vein distention in the setting of hypotension should prompt consideration of an obstruction (pulmonary embolism, tension pneumothorax, or pericardial tamponade) or pump failure.

Ultrasonography

Although a patient's history and physical examination offer clues about the cause of the shock state, ultrasonography can provide a more rapid, precise, and sensitive diagnosis of the underlying cause. Many protocols, including expanded Rapid Ultrasound for Shock and Hypotension and Rapid Ultrasound for SHock (RUSH), can help elucidate the extent of many hypotensive states.[9-14]

PEARLS

- ✓ Although patients with cirrhosis have abnormal vasodilation and therefore low baseline MAP, they are predisposed to infections. Septic shock should be considered in these patients.
- ✓ In suspected cardiogenic shock patients, carefully auscultate the heart for new murmurs. Valve rupture and ischemic pump failure require very different treatments.

The sequencing of the RUSH examination is shown in Figure 1-2, and a more detailed description with images and videos can be found at http://rush.emcrit.org. The entire examination can be completed in less than 2 minutes using readily available portable machines.

FIGURE 1-2. Expanded RUSH Examination

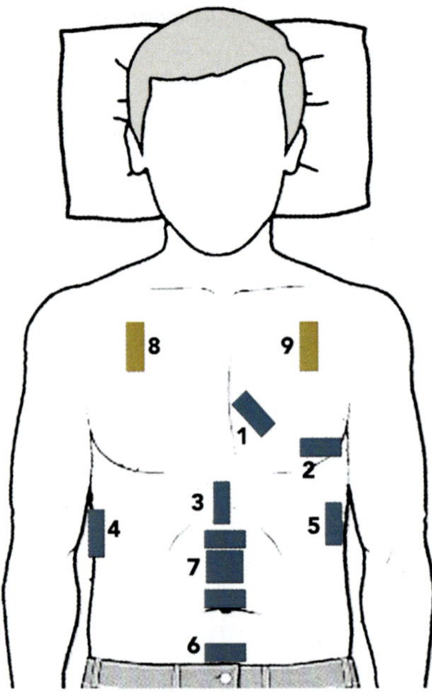

Sequencing

1. Parasternal long cardiac view
2. Apical four-chamber cardiac view
3. Inferior vena cava view
4. Morison with hemothorax view
5. Splenorenal with hemothorax view
6. Bladder view
7. Aortic slide view
8. Pulmonary view
9. Pulmonary view

Use curvilinear array for all views. Add search for ectopic pregnancy (curvilinear array) and DVT (high-frequency array) depending on the clinical circumstance.

The HI-MAP ED acronym indicates these steps, in order:

- **H** Examine the heart (parasternal long and then four-chamber cardiac views) with a general purpose or cardiac probe.
- **I** Obtain an inferior vena cava view with the same probe.
- **M** Scan the Morison pouch and splenorenal views with thorax. Then examine the bladder window using a general purpose abdominal probe.
- **A** Increase the depth, and find the aorta with four views, as follows: just below the xiphoid, above the renal artery, below the renal artery, and at the bifurcation of the aorta to the iliac arteries.
- **P** Scan both sides of the chest for pneumothorax and pulmonary findings. The phased-array probe is ideal for scanning for pulmonary abnormalities. To search for pneumothorax specifically, it might be beneficial to use a small parts, high-frequency transducer and markedly reduce the overall gain.

The following additional scans should be performed in the appropriate clinical situation:

- **E** In female patients of childbearing age, a transabdominal pelvic ultrasound using the general purpose abdominal probe may identify an ectopic pregnancy and/or the presence of pelvic free fluid.
- **D** In cases of dyspnea or right ventricular enlargement, perform a rapid three-point deep venous thrombosis (DVT) ultrasound survey. Using the small-parts probe, evaluate both lower extremities for compressibility of the common femoral, proximal deep and superficial femoral, and popliteal veins.

The expanded RUSH examination protocol provides:

- Identification or exclusion of pericardial tamponade (cardiac windows)
- Hints as to the presence of pulmonary embolism or right ventricular infarction (cardiac windows)
- A rough evaluation of cardiac output (cardiac windows)
- Assessment of whether the patient's cardiac output will increase with fluid administration (dynamic inferior vena cava assessment)
- Intraperitoneal bleeding or ascites (focused assessment with sonography for trauma [FAST] views)
- Pleural effusions or hemothoraces (FAST views)
- Abdominal aortic aneurysm (AAA views)
- Pneumothorax (lung windows)
- Extrauterine pregnancy (transabdominal pelvic)
- Pulmonary edema (lung windows)
- DVT (lower extremity ultrasound)

KEY POINTS

1. **Shock is a time-dependent disorder, and rapid, aggressive care is necessary.**
2. **Intermittent low blood pressures are concerning and should inspire a diligent search for a cause.**

Conclusion

Undifferentiated shock requires rapid recognition and aggressive empirical treatment to reestablish perfusion. Once the patient is stabilized, a search for the cause of the shock state can proceed with bedside assessments, laboratory testing, and ultrasonography. The underlying etiology will dictate specific treatments.

REFERENCES

1. Jones AE, Yiannibas V, Johnson C, et al. Emergency department hypotension predicts sudden unexpected in-hospital mortality: a prospective cohort study. *Chest.* 2006;130:941-946.
2. Bourgoin A, Leone M, Delmas A, et al. Increasing mean arterial pressure in patients with septic shock: effects on oxygen variables and renal function. *Crit Care Med.* 2005;33:780-786.
3. Weingart S. Push-dose pressors. *ACEP News.* 2010;29(3):4.
4. Bivins HG, Knopp R, dos Santos PA. Blood volume distribution in the Trendelenburg position. *Ann Emerg Med.* 1985;14:641-643.
5. Johnson S, Henderson SO. Myth: the Trendelenburg position improves circulation in cases of shock. *CJEM.* 2004;6:48-49.
6. Taylor J, Weil MH. Failure of the Trendelenburg position to improve circulation during clinical shock. *Surg Gynecol Obstet.* 1967;124:1005-1010.
7. Wood KE. Major pulmonary embolism: review of a pathophysiologic approach to the golden hour of hemodynamically significant pulmonary embolism. *Chest.* 2002;121:877-905.
8. Melo J, Peters JI. Low systemic vascular resistance: differential diagnosis and outcome. *Crit Care.* 1999;3:71-77.
9. Weingart SD, Duque D, Nelson B. Rapid ultrasound for shock and hypotension. Available at www.emedhome.com. 2009.
10. Perera P, Mailhot T, Riley D, et al. The RUSH exam: Rapid Ultrasound in SHock in the evaluation of the critically ill. *Emerg Med Clin North Am.* 2010;28:29-56.
11. Weekes AJ, Zapata RJ, Napolitano A. Symptomatic hypotension: ED stabilization and the emerging role of sonography. *Emerg Med Pract.* 2007;9:1-28.
12. Rose JS, Bair AE, Mandavia D, et al. The UHP ultrasound protocol: a novel ultrasound approach to the empiric evaluation of the undifferentiated hypotensive patient. *Am J Emerg Med.* 2001;19:299-302.
13. Jones AE, Tayal VS, Sullivan DM, et al. Randomized, controlled trial of immediate versus delayed goal-directed ultrasound to identify the cause of nontraumatic hypotension in emergency department patients. *Crit Care Med.* 2004;32:1703-1708.
14. Hernandez C, Shuler K, Hannan H, et al. C.A.U.S.E.: Cardiac arrest ultra-sound exam — a better approach to managing patients in primary non-arrhythmogenic cardiac arrest. *Resuscitation.* 2008;76:198-206.

The Difficult Airway

2

IN THIS CHAPTER

- Assessing and managing the difficult airway
- Predicting difficult laryngoscopy and intubation
- Pretreatment and induction agents
- Improving laryngoscopy
- Airway management tools and rescue devices

Robert J. Vissers and Michael A. Gibbs

Emergency airway management is one of the most challenging aspects of emergency care. When time is of the essence, this crucial task can take priority over complete patient assessment, diagnosis, and stabilization. By anticipating and managing potential airway problems, clinicians can reduce the risk of significant morbidity or death in critically ill patients, who are especially vulnerable to physiological insults. Airways that are at higher risk for failure or complications generally fall into three categories: the difficult airway, the failed airway, and the airway of the physiologically compromised patient.

A growing number of devices can assist with the identification, management, and rescue of the difficult airway. The optimal management strategy, which includes adequate preparation and pretreatment, is determined by the patient's underlying anatomical features and the amount of time oxygenation can be maintained.[1]

Airway Assessment

A difficult airway, as defined by the American Society of Anesthesiologists, is one that requires more than two attempts at intubation with the same laryngoscope blade, a change in blade, use of an intubation stylet, or an alternative intubation or rescue technique.[2] A preintubation assessment of anatomical characteristics can predict potential problems with bag-valve-mask (BVM) ventilation, laryngoscopy and intubation, cricothyrotomy, or placement of a rescue airway. Difficult BVM ventilation is defined as the inability to maintain oxygen saturation above 90% despite optimal positioning and airway adjuncts. If the cords are difficult to visualize (Cormack-Lehane grade 3 or 4 views) laryngoscopy and successful intubation will be challenging.[3]

The incidence of difficult airways in the emergent or critical care setting is less clearly defined than in the operating room.[4] The failure rate for the first laryngoscopic attempt during emergent rapid sequence intubation (RSI) ranges from 10% to 23%, and varies with the experience of the operator.[5-7] In 3% of patients, more than two attempts are needed, and 99% of patients are successfully intubated by the third attempt.[7-9] When more than three attempts at intubation are made by an experienced operator, a successful end is rare.[7,10] There is a significant increase in adverse events with each additional intubation attempt; therefore, success with the first intubation attempt is critical.[11,12] Higher first-pass success is associated with more experienced clinicians, trained emergency physicians, the use of RSI, the use of video laryngoscopy, and the absence of difficult airway predictors.[13,14]

PEARL

The need for multiple intubation attempts is associated with a significant increase in morbidity. When more than three attempts at intubation are made by an experienced operator, a successful end is rare.

The presence of a potentially difficult airway is not an absolute contraindication to RSI; however, early identification allows the clinician to plan appropriately and determine a rescue strategy. In some instances, the anticipated difficulty may present too great a risk for the administration of paralytics, requiring an awake or fiberoptic intubation to avoid the dangerous scenario of "cannot intubate/cannot ventilate" in a paralyzed patient.[15] If a difficult airway is predicted, optimal management can be determined based on airway difficulty and anatomy, the patient's physiology, the operator's experience, and the availability of alternative devices. The ability to maintain oxygenation determines the amount of time available, which plays an important role in choosing an appropriate intubation strategy. In cases of airway obstruction, the degree of obstruction, as well as how quickly it is progressing, will also factor into the treatment strategy.

PEARL

Plan for any anticipated difficulty or the failed airway. If special equipment might be needed, be sure it is immediately available and working.

Predicting Difficult BVM Ventilation

Although BVM ventilation should be the primary approach to rescue following a failed attempt, it is important to consider potential impediments before initiating RSI. It is imperative for emergency physicians to master this skill, be adept at anticipating potential difficulties, and understand which techniques can be used to overcome specific challenges. The presence of any two of the following five factors predicts difficult BVM ventilation: facial hair, obesity, lack of teeth, advanced age, and a history of snoring.[16]

When a BVM is unable to adequately ventilate, better positioning usually provides a solution. This can be done by aligning the oral and tracheal axes through the "sniff position" and placing a pad under the occiput if needed.[17] A jaw thrust and the use of oral and nasal airways can reduce obstruction caused by the tongue falling back into the posterior airway. A tighter seal can be obtained by using a two-person approach to bagging and applying a lubricant to any facial hair.

PEARL

If dentures are present, they should be left in place to facilitate BVM ventilation.

Predicting Difficult Laryngoscopy and Tracheal Intubation

Anatomical disruption from trauma or certain congenital syndromes are obvious predictors of difficult laryngoscopy and tracheal intubation. Several readily visible external features are also associated with challenges: facial hair, obesity, short neck, small or large chin, buckteeth, high-arched palate, and any airway deformity related to trauma, tumor, or inflammation.[4] A systematic and focused clinical examination of the airway anatomy, which can help identify subtler predictors of intubation difficulty, is required prior to the initiation of neuromuscular blockade. To be practical in the critical care environment, the approach must be rapid and reliable when performed on a potentially uncooperative or unresponsive patient. The results of the airway anatomy evaluation should guide the management plan.

The LEMON Airway Assessment

Rapid and practical, the LEMON mnemonic can be used to systematically evaluate any critically ill patient. The tool guides the assessment of five known independent predictors of difficult laryngoscopy and intubation: external features, geometry of the airway, the Mallampati score, obstruction, and neck mobility (*Table 2-1*).[18] The mnemonic has demonstrated predictive value in the emergent setting and is recommended in the most recent advanced trauma life-support guidelines.[19,20]

Visually apparent anatomical distortions and physical characteristics such as obesity; facial hair; a short, thick neck; or a receding mandible can be harbingers of trouble. With experience, the physician can usually predict difficulty through simple observation; however, a conscious effort is necessary to do so.

The patient's airway geometry can be evaluated using the 3-3-2 rule to predict the ability to align the oral, pharyngeal, and tracheal axes. The mandibular opening in an adult should be at least 4 cm (approximately three fingerbreadths). If it is less than this, visualization is reduced. A restricted oral opening can dictate the size of the device that may be employed. The distance between the mentum and the hyoid bone, which should be three to four fingerbreadths, can predict the ability of the mandible to accommodate the tongue during laryngoscopy. In a smaller mandible, the tongue is more likely to fill the oral cavity and obstruct visualization. An unusually large mandible can elongate the oral axis, making visual alignment more challenging. The anterior larynx can be high if the space between the mandible and the top of the thyroid cartilage is less than 2 fingerbreadths, increasing the likelihood of a Cormack-Lehane grade 3 or 4 view.

The Mallampati score is used to assess the degree to which the tongue obstructs the visualization of the posterior pharynx and is associated with the ability to visualize the glottis.[21] Four views are described, as follows:

- **Class I:** Faucial pillars, soft palate, and uvula can be visualized.
- **Class II:** Faucial pillars and soft palate can be visualized, but the uvula is masked by the base of the tongue.
- **Class III:** Only the base of the uvula can be visualized.
- **Class IV:** None of the three structures can be visualized.

Simply put, visualization of the posterior pharynx is correlated with visualization of the cords. Class III is associated with a 5% failure rate and class IV with up to 20% failure.

Obstruction presents unique, readily apparent challenges. To manage an airway obstruction, three aspects should be considered: the location of the obstruction, whether it is fixed (eg, tumor) or mobile (eg, epiglottis), and how rapidly it is progressing. The location can determine which approach or rescue device should be used. For example, nasal and surgical airways through the cricothyroid membrane may be the only options for oral airway obstruction from angioedema of the tongue. BVM ventilation is more likely to be successful with mobile, inflammatory obstructions such as croup, than with fixed obstructions from a hard foreign body. The speed of progression determines whether management can await patient transport to another facility or to the operating room, or whether it must occur immediately at the bedside.

Neck mobility can interfere with the alignment of the visual axes by preventing the desired "sniffing position." Most commonly, neck immobility is imposed by a cervical collar. To increase the chance of success during laryngoscopy, it is important to remove the anterior portion of the collar while maintaining cervical immobilization. If there are no signs of cervical injury, atlanto-occipital extension should be assessed even in the unconscious patient.

Predicting Difficult Airway Rescue

Alternative airway devices can be life-saving when laryngoscopy fails or is predicted to be difficult. In the rare patient who cannot be intubated or ventilated, surgical cricothyrotomy is the only option. It is therefore paramount to anticipate difficulties associated with rescue devices and be prepared to surgically create an airway if necessary.

Extraglottic airway devices, including the laryngeal mask airway (LMA) and the Combitube (Tyco-Kendall, Mansfield, MA), are commonly employed for rescue from failed intubation and can be a primary technique in selected circumstances. As with more commonly used techniques, patient characteristics can predict difficulty and potential failure.[1,4] Because adequate oral access and infraglottic patency are necessary for ventilation, extraglottic airway devices will not succeed in the presence of oral, laryngeal, or infraglottic obstruction. The seal above the glottis, which is necessary for ventilation, might not be achievable if there is significant disruption or abnormal anatomy of the upper airway. Ventilation can also be difficult in patients with high airway resistance such as those with asthma, and can fail at airway pressures exceeding 25 cm H_2O.

Video laryngoscopy is commonly used as a rescue technique for failed direct laryngoscopy intubation; however, it is fast becoming the primary technique for both routine and difficult airways in the emergency department. Video laryngoscopy improves glottic visualization and has first-pass and overall success rates that are superior to direct laryngoscopy in this setting.[14,22] Success rates when video laryngoscopy is used as a rescue device in patients who have failed direct laryngoscopy are greater than 90%.[23] These tools are particularly useful in difficult airways secondary to obesity and limited neck mobility.[24] Video laryngoscopy might require a longer time to intubation on the first attempt, particularly in children, where the technique lacks the advantages documented in the adult population.[25,26] In patients in whom the camera is obscured by blood or emesis, direct laryngoscopy might be superior. The expense and maintenance issues of video devices could preclude their use for some providers.

Flexible fiberoptic scopes are excellent tools for airway evaluation and intubation; however, the equipment requires adequate time to prepare — precious minutes that are not always available in the emergency department. Flexible fiberoptic scopes also require significantly more skill to operate than other rescue devices, and visibility can be obscured by excessive secretions or blood in the airway.[27] Several studies suggest that similar views can be obtained during awake intubation with video laryngoscopy, and achieved in a shorter period.[28,29]

A surgical airway is a potential rescue strategy when all other alternatives are predicted to be difficult. The biggest challenge to a surgical airway is the decision to proceed. Some anatomical variables make surgical cricothyrotomy more difficult. Obesity or a very short "bull" neck can present a challenge to landmark identification. Technical difficulties can arise in the presence of an overlying hematoma, abscess, tumor, or scarring from a previous surgery, radiation, or burns.[30]

The Failed Airway

In emergency management, the failed airway has been defined as an inability to maintain adequate oxygenation following a failed intubation attempt or three failed attempts by an experienced provider even if oxygenation can be maintained.[4] The rate of failed airways in emergent patients undergoing RSI is approximately 1%.[7,8] Despite a thorough assessment and appropriate patient selection for RSI, failed airways can still be expected, particularly in the emergent setting. Any clinician managing critically ill patients must possess a facility for operating rescue devices and applying surgical airway techniques. A plan for addressing a failed airway must be in

TABLE 2-1. The LEMON Mnemonic

Look externally	Look for external features predictive of airway difficulty.
Evaluate 3-3-2 (airway geometry)	The oral opening, the mentum to hyoid distance, and the mandible to thyroid cartilage distance are measured in fingerbreadths. Reduced distance may suggest difficulty aligning the oral, pharyngeal, and laryngeal axes.
Mallampati score	The degree of posterior pharynx visualization is associated with vocal cord visualization during laryngoscopy.
Obstruction and obesity	Identify where the obstruction is and how quickly it is progressing.
Neck mobility	An inability to flex or extend the neck could restrict visualization and the ability to reposition during BVM ventilation or laryngoscopy.

Adapted with permission from: "The Difficult Airway Course: Emergency," Airway Management Education Center, www.theairwaysite.com, and from: Murphy MF, Walls RM. Identification of the difficult and failed airway. In: Walls RM, Murphy MF, eds. *Manual of Emergency Airway Management.* 3rd ed. Philadelphia, PA: Lippincott Williams & Wilkins; 2008:81-93.

place before paralytic agents are initiated so the necessary equipment can be gathered. Ideally, this plan should be shared with the team managing the patient *(Table 2-2).*

The Difficult Airway

The most important aspect of airway management is thoughtful preparation, and this is particularly true for the critically ill patient. Ongoing physician education is necessary to maintain rarely performed airway and cricothyrotomy skills, and a well-stocked difficult-airway cart must be immediately available *(Table 2-3).* Steps such as preoxygenation and premedication should be taken to prepare the patient for RSI and mitigate the potential harm of intubation. Despite the urgency associated with emergent airway management, it is essential that the clinician take time to assess airway difficulty, optimize the physiological state of the patient, and develop a treatment plan. The use of a checklist and clear communication with the clinical team will facilitate decision making and prevent errors.[31]

Physiological Challenges

In patients with concomitant chronic or acute medical conditions, airway management poses an increased risk of hypoxia, hypotension, or exacerbation of the underlying disease state. Critically ill patients with preexisting respiratory or hemodynamic compromise are particularly at risk. RSI is the technique most commonly used to facilitate intubation in the emergency setting, and, in general, it is associated the highest first-pass success rate and lowest complication rate.[7] The drugs used to facilitate RSI and the physiological effects of the procedure may exacerbate certain conditions.[32] Many of these undesirable effects can be prevented or mitigated through recognition of the risk, adequate resuscitation, and attention to drug selection.

Preoxygenation

Preoxygenation should begin as soon as intubation is anticipated, regardless of the patient's oxygen saturation level.[33] Preoxygenation displaces nitrogen with oxygen in the alveolar space, creating a reservoir of oxygen that can prevent hypoxia for several minutes of apnea. Hypoxia develops more quickly in children, pregnant women, obese patients, and those who are physiologically compromised. The patient should be preoxygenated for at least 3 minutes using a nonrebreathing mask supplied with 15 L/min of oxygen, which will deliver approximately 60% to 70% oxygen. Nasal cannulas do not provide optimal preoxygenation. A decreased respiratory rate or hypoxia despite the use of a nonrebreathing mask may necessitate preoxygenation with BVM ventilation, which can deliver 90% to 97% oxygen. A tight mask-to-face seal is required and can be achieved either through active bagging or by providing enough inspiratory pressure to open the one-way valve.

Patients with oxygen saturation levels below 95% despite supplementation might benefit from a period of noninvasive positive-pressure ventilation to increase the oxygen reservoir. This strategy is particularly effective in obese patients.[34] Similarly, elevating the head of the bed 20 to 30 degrees can improve preoxygenation efforts. Finally, high-flow oxygen (15 L/min) through a nasal cannula throughout the apneic phase of RSI can significantly prolong the period of safe apnea during paralysis and is recommended for all critically ill patients undergoing the procedure.[34]

Pretreatment Agents

The direct physiological effects of laryngoscopy can exacerbate elevated intracranial pressure (ICP), reactive airway disease, and cardiovascular disease in critically ill patients. Theoretically, pretreatment agents *(Table 2-4)* attenuate adverse responses to laryngoscopy and intubation; however, there are no data demonstrating improved outcomes when used in the emergent setting.[35]

Laryngoscopy can increase heart rate and blood pressure secondary to a reflex sympathetic response, which might be harmful to patients with elevated ICP, myocardial ischemia, or aortic dissection. Patients who have lost cerebral autoregulation can also experience a centrally mediated increase in ICP. In children, the increased vagal response can result in significant bradycardia, particularly in the presence of succinylcholine.

TABLE 2-2. Verbal Checklist Prior to Initiating RSI

- ✓ Is this a difficult airway? What is the plan?
- ✓ Is the patient ready? Are preoxygenation, premedication, and blood pressure optimized?
- ✓ Is the support equipment ready (eg, IV, suction, and bag-valve-mask)?
- ✓ Is the correct equipment ready (eg, endotracheal tube, stylet, laryngoscope, and rescue devices)?
- ✓ Are the right drugs in the right doses ready?
- ✓ Is the team ready? Does everyone understand the plan if intubation fails?

TABLE 2-3. Contents of the Difficult Airway Cart

A surgical airway kit (open surgical, Seldinger wire-guided kit, or both)
A gum-elastic bougie (intubating stylet)
One of the blind insertion devices (eg, intubating LMA, Combitube [Tyco-Kendall, Mansfield, MA], King-LT [King Systems, Noblesville, IN])
One of the hand-held video laryngoscopes (eg, GlideScope [Verathon, Bothell, WA], McGrath [LMA North American, San Diego, CA], Storz [Storz, Tallinn, Estonia], Pentax [Pentax, Tokyo, Japan])
(Optional) Flexible fiberoptic scopes (nasopharyngoscope, intubating scope)
Medications to facilitate awake laryngoscopy

Laryngeal stimulation can have adverse respiratory effects (eg, laryngospasm, cough, and bronchospasm). Pretreatment agents should be administered 3 to 5 minutes before the initiation of RSI. Urgent airway management in a critically ill patient should not be delayed for the administration of pretreatment.

Lidocaine has been recommended as a pretreatment agent in patients with possible elevated ICP and in those with bronchospasm. Although evidence suggests that the drug mitigates the ICP response to laryngeal manipulation, studies demonstrating a favorable effect on outcomes are lacking.[36] Studies of lidocaine as a pretreatment agent in patients with severe asthma are also inconclusive.[37] Clinicians must balance the potential benefit of a relatively benign medication in a critically ill patient against the lack of clear outcome data.

Fentanyl is an opioid that attenuates the reflex sympathetic response to airway manipulation.[35,38] It can be used as a pretreatment agent when an increase in blood pressure and heart rate could be detrimental, as in patients with elevated ICP and certain cardiovascular diseases (eg, aortic dissection and ischemic heart disease). Although fentanyl is less likely than other opioids to produce hypotension in the suggested doses, it should not be given to patients who are dependent on their sympathetic drive (eg, those in compensated shock). Adverse reactions such as respiratory depression and chest rigidity, can occur but are minimized when fentanyl is given slowly.

Pretreatment with atropine does not consistently prevent bradycardia in pediatric patients and is no longer recommended for all children undergoing emergent intubation; however, it should be available at the bedside in the event that symptomatic bradycardia occurs.[39]

Induction Agents

Etomidate, a nonbarbiturate hypnotic, is a commonly used induction agent for RSI. Its advantages in critically ill patients include relative protection from myocardial and cerebral ischemia, minimal histamine release, a stable hemodynamic profile, and a short duration of action. There is no conclusive evidence that a single dose of etomidate affects outcomes through cortisol inhibition even for patients in septic shock.[40]

Propofol is another effective induction agent for emergent RSI. Compared with etomidate, it has a more rapid onset and a shorter duration of action. Some of the drug's pharmacological advantages include its anticonvulsant properties and ability to lower intracranial pressure. It does not cause histamine release but can cause hypotension through myocardial suppression and vasodilation. Because of its potential to cause hypotension, the drug should be avoided in patients with potential hemodynamic compromise.

Ketamine is a dissociative induction agent that provides analgesia and amnesia. In many ways, it is an ideal medication for critically ill patients. Because it increases blood pressure and heart rate through catecholamine release, the drug can be useful in hypotensive patients. Ketamine causes direct smooth muscle relaxation and bronchodilation and is the induction agent of choice for patients with refractory status asthmaticus. Its ability to preserve the respiratory drive makes it an ideal sedative during awake intubation and when using flexible fiberoptics. Despite its potential to increase heart rate and blood pressure, ketamine does not appear to cause an increase in ICP. Some studies suggest that it has possible cerebroprotective benefits.[41] Because of its inotropic

PEARL

Because it increases heart rate and blood pressure, ketamine might be the optimal induction agent in patients with hypotension requiring emergent intubation.

TABLE 2-4. RSI Drugs for the Critically Ill Patient

	Drugs	Dose	Indication	Dose in Shock States
Pretreatment agents	Lidocaine	1.5 mg/kg IV	Increased ICP Bronchospasm	Not indicated
	Fentanyl	3 mcg/kg IV	Increased ICP Cardiac ischemia Aortic dissection	Not indicated
	Atropine	0.02 mg/kg IV	Bradycardia from laryngoscopy or succinylcholine	0.02 mg/kg IV
Induction agents	Etomidate	0.3 mg/kg IV	RSI	0.1 mg/kg IV
	Propofol	0.5–1.5 mg/kg IV	RSI in hemodynamically stable patients	Not indicated
	Ketamine	1–2 mg/kg IV	Hypotension Status asthmaticus	0.5 mg/kg IV
Paralytic agents	Succinylcholine	1-1.5 mkg/kg	RSI	Consider higher dose range
	Rocuronium	0.6-1.2 mg/kg	RSI	Consider higher dose range
	Vecuronium	0.1-0.2 mg/kg	RSI	Consider higher dose range

and chronotropic cardiac effects, ketamine is not preferred in elderly patients or in those with a potential for cardiac ischemia. When ketamine is used with fiberoptics in awake patients, pretreatment with atropine can attenuate the increased secretion production associated with ketamine.

Paralytics

The neuromuscular blocking agents most commonly used during RSI are succinylcholine, rocuronium, and vecuronium. Succinylcholine has the most rapid onset and appears to provide the best intubating conditions at 60 seconds.[42,43] Its duration of action (8–10 minutes) is also much shorter, which is an advantage should difficulty with intubation occur. It is hydrolyzed rapidly by cholinesterase; therefore, its clearance is independent of hepatic or renal function. Succinylcholine is a depolarizing agent that will cause a transient increase (~0.5 mEq/L) in serum potassium; however, the drug can trigger a life-threatening hyperkalemic response in patients with receptor up-regulation. Critically ill patients who sustained a significant burn, crush injury, or denervation injury more than 5 days earlier are at risk, as are those with preexisting myopathies *(Table 2-5)*.

Rocuronium, an intermediate-duration, nondepolarizing agent, can be used in RSI for patients with potential contraindications to succinylcholine. Some clinicians prefer rocuronium as the primary neuromuscular blocking agent for RSI.[42] By increasing the dose to 1 mg/kg, the drug's onset of action approximates that of succinylcholine, but its duration of action is prolonged to approximately 45 minutes. Vecuronium can also be used in a higher dose (0.2 mg/kg) to achieve a more rapid onset (between 1 and 2 minutes); however, the duration of paralysis can be 60 to 120 minutes.

A new class of reversal drugs, selective relaxant binding agents, can reverse a long-acting nondepolarizing neuromuscular blocker prior to spontaneous recovery. Sugammadex, one such agent, reverses blockade within a few minutes. It is available in Europe but, at the time of this publication, has not been approved by the Food and Drug Administration for use in the United States.[44]

Patients in Shock

Critically ill patients who present in shock are, by definition, hemodynamically compromised and can have limited pulmonary reserve. Any procedure that exacerbates the underlying cardiopulmonary deficit can lead to significant morbidity or death. The clinician must weigh the potential detrimental effects of intubation and the time it could take to mitigate them against the urgency of airway protection, oxygenation, and ventilation.

Preoxygenation is paramount in the patient with compromised tissue perfusion. In the absence of significant airway difficulty, RSI remains the preferred method of intubation; however, appropriate drug selection is important. Pretreatment medications can exacerbate hypotension and are not indicated for patients in shock. Induction agents must be selected carefully to avoid further deterioration of cardiac output and perfusion. Though rare, some situations preclude the administration of any induction agent. In such cases, consider a reduced dose of etomidate or ketamine, or possibly an amnestic (noninduction) dose of midazolam. Propofol should not be used as an induction agent in patients with cardiogenic or septic shock because of its propensity to cause hypotension. The drug has been linked to cardiac failure and acidosis when used in critically ill patients. Referred to as the propofol infusion syndrome, the complication usually is described in the context of prolonged infusions or very high doses.[45]

Once the patient is intubated, positive-pressure ventilation can impair venous return and cardiac filling. This can reduce cardiac output and potentially exacerbate hypotension. If time allows, hypotension responsive to intravenous fluids should be managed aggressively prior to intubation. Rapid boluses of crystalloid should be considered as a possible pretreatment in all anticipated intubations in critically ill patients. Because these patients might also have associated metabolic acidosis, increased minute ventilation can be considered if cardiac output is not compromised. Even briefly impaired ventilation during an otherwise rapid and effective intubation will significantly worsen acidosis and further cardiovascular compromise. This can also occur in patients with severe metabolic acidosis secondary to causes other than shock (eg, acute aspirin overdose).

TABLE 2-5. Conditions Associated with Succinylcholine-Induced Hyperkalemia

Condition
More than 5 days after the following: • Burns • Denervation injury • Significant crush injuries • Severe infection
Preexisting myopathies
Preexisting hyperkalemia

Improving Laryngoscopy

The success rate of RSI approaches 99% when performed by an emergency physician or anesthesiologist. Success, however, can be largely dependent on each clinician's level of training. In the event of a failed intubation, a second immediate attempt can be made by a more experienced clinician.[8,9]

The most common reasons for intubation failures are inadequate equipment preparation and poor patient positioning. Before proceeding with RSI, it is critical that the clinician pause to run through a short checklist with the team, ensuring that all necessary equipment is working and at the bedside *(Table 2-2)*. Following a failed intubation attempt, the patient's position should be optimized. Improved visualization can be achieved with proper bed height; positioning the head of the patient at the end of the stretcher; and, in the absence of cervical spine precautions, extension at the atlanto-occipital joint. Elevation of the head with a pad under the occiput can help align the pharyngeal and tracheal visual axes, particularly in obese patients. Ideally, the ear canal should lie in a horizontal plane with the anterior shoulder.

The application of backward-upward-rightward pressure (BURP) on the thyroid cartilage (not the cricoid ring) can enhance visualization of an anterior glottis.[46] In a modification of this maneuver called bimanual laryngoscopy, the intubator manipulates the larynx with the right hand until ideal visualization is achieved, and then an assistant maintains this position.[46] Direct cricoid pressure, the Sellick maneuver, has been recommended to prevent the passive regurgitation of gastric contents during intubation of an unconscious or paralyzed patient. However, the effectiveness of the technique is questionable, and it has been shown to impair the laryngoscopic view and insertion of the endotracheal tube.[47] In a difficult laryngoscopy, cricoid pressure should be released.

When an intubation attempt fails, the first priority is to oxygenate through BVM ventilation. It is critical to change the technique, position, provider, or equipment between attempts to improve the likelihood of success. Preparation for a possible rescue airway must be considered. Persistence without altering the technique and attempts at blind passage are usually met with failure and anoxia and are therefore discouraged. It is important to recognize when further attempts at laryngoscopy are unlikely to succeed.

Rescue Devices

The number of airway rescue devices available in the emergent setting has increased dramatically, and the recent proliferation of video laryngoscopy is changing the approach to high-risk airway management in critically ill patients.[23] The drive toward lower-cost and durable or disposable tools, combined with rapid technological advances, suggests that the number of options will continue to grow.

Although the variety of choices is exciting, it can be intimidating as well. Given the relative infrequency of emergent difficult airways, emergency physicians cannot expect to be proficient in every technique, and it would be cost prohibitive to have every device on hand. Fortunately, most of these rescue tools fall into a few distinct categories based on their anatomical approach (supraglottic versus subglottic) and whether they provide direct glottic visualization (blind insertion) *(Table 2-6)*.[1]

TABLE 2-6. Airway Management Tools

BVM ventilation
Direct laryngoscopy
Intubating stylets (the bougie)
Supraglottic rescue devices: • Blind insertion devices (eg, double-balloon esophageal airways, laryngeal mask airways) • Direct visualization (eg, video laryngoscopy, flexible fiberoptics, fiberoptic stylets)
Subglottic rescue devices: • Open surgical cricothyrotomy • Percutaneous cricothyrotomy • Retrograde intubation • Transtracheal jet ventilation

Adapted from: Vissers RJ, Gibbs M. The high risk airway. *Emerg Med Clin North Am.* 2010:28;203-217. Copyright 2010. Adapted with permission.

The first failed airway should be followed by better laryngoscopic and BVM ventilation techniques. Clinicians also should be comfortable using an intubating stylet and have at least one supraglottic and one subglottic surgical airway technique in their armamentariums. With its wide availability, video laryngoscopy is rapidly becoming the preferred technique for primary emergent airway management. Facility with a flexible intubating scope, using either fiberoptic or microvideo technology, is also becoming more common among emergency physicians.

A mobile difficult-airway cart stocked with an appropriate variety of rescue devices should be available in all acute care settings, and the clinician should be familiar with these tools and proficient at employing them. Although critically ill patients with difficult airways present infrequently, the time to learn a new technique is not during an emergency. Expertise can be obtained in myriad ways outside the acute care setting. Medical educators traditionally have relied on the operating room to provide a controlled learning environment; however, high-fidelity simulation labs are increasingly being used to teach and practice difficult airway management skills.

KEY POINTS

1. A preintubation assessment of anatomical characteristics can predict potential difficulties with bag-valve-mask (BVM) ventilation, laryngoscopy and intubation, cricothyrotomy, or placement of a rescue airway.
2. The presence of any two of the following five factors predicts difficult BVM ventilation: facial hair, obesity, lack of teeth, advanced age, and a history of snoring.
3. The failed airway is defined as the inability to maintain adequate oxygenation following a failed intubation attempt or three failed attempts by an experienced provider.
4. Pretreatment with rapid boluses of crystalloid should be considered in all anticipated intubations of critically ill patients.
5. The evidence for the benefit of pretreatment drugs in rapid sequence intubation (RSI) is inconclusive. Greater benefit is obtained through adequate volume replacement and preoxygenation prior to RSI.

Choosing a Rescue Strategy

A thoughtful strategy that is based on patient characteristics, incorporates appropriate preparation, and employs the optimal technique is always more important than the tools themselves. Because these are low-frequency cases that can evolve rapidly, decision-making tools should be used to help frame a management strategy. Several algorithms have been proposed, including the American Society of Anesthesiologists' difficult airway algorithm, which works well in a controlled operating room but is difficult to apply in the emergency department or critical care setting.[2] Other algorithms designed specifically for acute care provide a logical framework for dealing with difficult and failed airways in critically ill patients.

It is essential to prepare the patient and equipment appropriately. All patients should be preoxygenated, and any physiological challenges should be addressed to mitigate the undesirable effects of emergent intubation. The "awake look" is an important technique that has become easier to perform with the increased availability of video-assisted airway devices. Recognizing the need for help from other consultants or colleagues is the key to success in some circumstances. Finally, the subglottic surgical airway is the last resort strategy in most difficult airway management situations.

It can be challenging to select the most appropriate airway device for a particular airway scenario — a choice that can be limited by availability and the clinician's skillset. One popular approach uses a four-box grid to help develop an appropriate plan and a rescue strategy (*Figure 2-1, Table 2-7*).[1] In the context of this framework, an "abnormal" anatomy implies one that has been disrupted or altered by complications such as trauma, hematoma, cancer, angioedema, a burn, abscess, or foreign body. "Normal" anatomical factors that may portend a difficult airway include obesity, a small mouth, and a high anterior larynx.

FIGURE 2-1. Difficult Airway Grid

Is oxygenation adequate? / Is anatomy normal or abnormal?		
	Normal anatomy Adequate oxygenation	Abnormal anatomy Adequate oxygenation
	Normal anatomy Inadequate oxygenation	Abnormal anatomy Inadequate oxygenation

From: Vissers RJ, Gibbs M. The high-risk airway. *Emerg Med Clin North Am.* 2010:28;203-217. Copyright 2010. Used with permission.

TABLE 2-7. Principles and Solutions for Clinical Scenarios in Figure 2-1

Principles	Solutions
Normal Anatomy + Adequate Oxygenation	
You have time. No need for a surgical airway. Blind-insertion devices (BID) are appropriate. Hand-held fiberoptic scopes are ideal. Cuffed tube is the goal.	**If a hand-held fiberoptic scope is available:** Any of these scopes should work. **If a hand-held fiberoptic scope is NOT available:** First choice: laryngeal mask airway Second choice: intubating stylet
Normal Anatomy + Inadequate Oxygenation	
You have no time. Multiple BID attempts are inappropriate. Use what you know best. Establish a surgical airway if first rescue plan fails.	**If a hand-held fiberoptic scope is available:** Limit attempts with scope. Establish a surgical airway if unsuccessful. **If a hand-held fiberoptic scope is NOT available:** Limit attempts with laryngeal mask airway. Establish a surgical airway if unsuccessful.
Abnormal Anatomy + Adequate Oxygenation	
BID is risky. Direct airway visualization is preferred. Fiberoptic scope is ok if view not obscured by blood. Surgical airway can be established as backup.	**If a hand-held fiberoptic scope is available:** Limit attempts with scope. Establish a surgical airway if unsuccessful. **If a hand-held fiberoptic scope is NOT available:** Establish a surgical airway.
Abnormal Anatomy + Inadequate Oxygenation	
You have no time. BIDs are contraindicated. Fiberoptic scope is ok if view not obscured by blood. Surgical airway often is the best first choice.	**If a hand-held fiberoptic scope is available:** Perform one attempt with scope. Establish a surgical airway if unsuccessful. **If a hand-held fiberoptic scope is NOT available:** Establish a surgical airway.

Based on: Vissers RJ, Gibbs M. The high-risk airway. *Emerg Med Clin North Am.* 2010:28;203-217. Copyright 2010. Used with permission.

Conclusion

Airway management is essential to the practice of emergency medicine. It is crucial to assess critically ill patients for the presence of a difficult airway, predict difficulty with BVM ventilation and intubation, and select appropriate rescue devices should direct laryngoscopy fail. Equally important in managing the difficult airway is the selection of appropriate pretreatment, induction, and paralytic medications for patients who are hemodynamically unstable.

REFERENCES

1. Vissers RJ, Gibbs M. The high-risk airway. *Emerg Med Clin North Am.* 2010;28:203-217.
2. Practice Guidelines for Management of the Difficult Airway: An Updated Report by the American Society of Anesthesiologists Task Force on Management of the Difficult Airway. *Anesthesiology.* 2013;118:251-270.
3. Cormack RS, Lehane J. Difficult trachea intubation in obstetrics. *Anaesthesia.* 1984;39:1105-1111.
4. Murphy MF, Walls RM. Identification of the difficult and failed airway. In: Walls RM, Murphy MF, eds. *Manual of Emergency Airway Management.* 4th ed. Philadelphia, PA: Lippincott Williams & Wilkins; 2012:8-21.
5. Sagarin MJ, Barton ED, Chang YM, et al. Airway management by U.S. and Canadian emergency medicine residents: a multicenter analysis of more than 6,000 endotracheal intubation attempts. *Ann Emerg Med.* 2005;46:328-336.
6. Levitan RM, Rosenblatt B, Meiner EM, et al. Alternating day emergency medicine and anesthesia resident responsibility for management of the trauma airway: a study of laryngoscopy performance and intubation success. *Ann Emerg Med.* 2004;43:48-53.
7. Walls RM, Brown CA, Bair AE, Pallin DJ. A multi-center report of 8937 emergency department intubations. *J Emerg Med.* 2011;41:347-354.
8. Bair AE, Filbin MR, Kulkami R, et al. Failed intubation in the emergency department: analysis of prevalence, rescue techniques, and personnel. *J Emerg Med.* 2002;23:131-140.
9. Tayal VS, Riggs RW, Marx JA, et al. Rapid-sequence intubation at an emergency medicine residency: success rate and adverse events during a two-year period. *Acad Emerg Med.* 1999;6:31-37.
10. Peterson GN. Management of the difficult airway: a closed claims analysis. *Anesthesiology.* 2005;103:33-39.
11. Sakles JC, Chiu S, Mosier J, et al. The importance of first pass success when performing orotracheal intubation in the emergency department. *Acad Emerg Med.* 2013;20:71-78.
12. Hasegawa K, Shigemitsu K, Hagiwara Y, et al. Association between repeated intubation attempts and adverse events in emergency departments: an analysis of a multicenter prospective observational study. *Ann Emerg Med.* 2012;60:749-54.
13. Kim C, Kang HG, Lim TH, et al. What factors affect the success rate of the first attempt at endotracheal intubation in emergency departments? *Emerg Med J.* 2013;30:888-892.
14. Sakles J. A comparison of the C-MAC video laryngoscopy to the Macintosh direct laryngoscope for intubation in the emergency department. *Ann Emerg Med.* 2012;60:739-748.
15. Murphy M, Hung O, Launcelott G, et al. Predicting the difficult laryngoscopic intubation: are we on the right track? *Can J Anaesth.* 2005;52:231-235.
16. Langeron O, Masso E, Huraux C, et al. Prediction of difficult mask ventilation. *Anesthesiology.* 2000;92:1229-1236.
17. Kheterpal S, Han R, Tremper KK, et al. Incidence and predictors of difficult and impossible mask ventilation. *Anesthesiology.* 2006;105:885-891.
18. Murphy MF, Walls RM. The difficult and failed airway. In: Walls RM, Luten RC, Murphy MF, et al, eds. *Manual of Emergency Airway Management.* Philadelphia, PA: Lippincott Williams & Wilkins; 2000:31-39.
19. Reed MJ, Dunn MJ, McKeown DW. Can an airway assessment score predict difficulty at intubation in the emergency department? *Emerg Med J.* 2005;22:99-102.
20. Kortbeck JB, Al Turki SA, Ali J, et al. Advanced trauma life support, 8th edition, the evidence for change. *J Trauma.* 2008;64:1638-1650.
21. Lee A, Fan LT, Gin T, et al. A systematic review (meta-analysis) of the accuracy of the Mallampati tests to predict the difficult airway. *Anesth Analg.* 2006;102:1867-1878.
22. Brown CA 3rd, Bair AE, Pallin DJ, et al. Improved glottis exposure with the video Macintosh laryngoscopy in adult emergency department tracheal intubations. *Ann Emerg Med.* 2010;56:83-88.
23. Jungbauer A, Schumann M, Brunkhorst V, et al. Expected difficult tracheal intubation: a prospective comparison of direct laryngoscopy and video laryngoscopy in 200 patients. *Br J Anaesth.* 2009;102:546-550.
24. Kill C, Risse J, Wallot P, et al. Videolaryngoscopy with Glidescope reduces cervical spine movement in patients with unsecured cervical spine. *J Emerg Med.* 2013;44:750-757.
25. Fiadjoe JE, Gurnaney H, Dalesio N, et al. A prospective randomized equivalence trial of the GlideScope Cobalt® video laryngoscope to traditional direct laryngoscopy in neonates and infants. *Anesthesiology.* 2012;116:622-628.
26. Riveros R, Sung W, Sessler DI, et al. Comparison of the Truview PCD™ and the GlideScope® video laryngoscopes with direct laryngoscopy in pediatric patients: a randomized trial. *Can J Anesth.* 2013;60:450-457.
27. Kovacs G, Law JA, Petrie D. Awake fiberoptic intubation using an optical stylet in an anticipated difficult airway. *Ann Emerg Med.* 2007;49:81-83.
28. Silverton NA, Youngquist ST, Mallin MP, et al. GlideScope versus flexible fiber optic for awake upright laryngoscopy. *Ann Emerg Med.* 2012;59:159-164.
29. Abdelmalak BB, Bernstein E, Egan C, et al. GlideScope® vs flexible fibreoptic scope for elective intubation in obese patients. *Anaesthesia.* 2011;66:550-555.
30. Vissers RJ, Bair AE. Surgical airway techniques. In: Walls RM, Murphy MF, eds. *Manual of Emergency Airway Management.* 4th ed. Philadelphia, PA: Lippincott Williams & Wilkins; 2012:193-219.
31. Weingart SD. EMCrit Intubation Checklist. http://emcrit.org/podcasts/emcrit-intubation-checklist. Accessed May 29, 2015.
32. Fox EJ, Sklar GS, Hill CH, et al. Complications related to the pressor response to endotracheal intubation. *Anaesthesiology.* 1977;47:524-525.
33. Benumof JL, Dagg R, Benumof R. Critical hemoglobin desaturation will occur before return to an unparalyzed state following 1 mg/kg of intravenous succinylcholine. *Anesthesiology.* 1997;87:979-982.
34. Weingart SD, Levitan RM. Preoxygenation and prevention of desaturation during emergency airway management. *Ann Emerg Med.* 2012;59:165-175.
35. Caro DA, Bush S. Pretreatment agents. In: Walls RM, Murphy MF, eds. *Manual of Emergency Airway Management.* 4th ed. Philadelphia, PA: Lippincott Williams & Wilkins; 2012:233-240.
36. Butler J, Jackson R. Towards evidence based emergency medicine: best BETS from Manchester Royal Infirmary. Lignocaine premedication before rapid sequence induction in head injuries. *Emerg Med J.* 2002;19:554.
37. Maslow A, Regan M, Israel E, et al. Inhaled albuterol, but not intravenous lidocaine, protects against intubation-induced bronchoconstriction in asthma. *Anesthesiology.* 2000;93:1198-1204.
38. Reynolds SF, Heffner J. Airway management of the critically ill patient: rapid sequence intubation. *Chest.* 2005;127:1397-1412.
39. Fleming B, McCollough M, Henderson SO. Myth: atropine should be administered before succinylcholine for neonatal and pediatric intubation. *Can J Emerg Med.* 2005;7:114-117.
40. Walls RM, Murphy MF. Clinical controversies: etomidate as an induction agent for endotracheal intubation in patients with sepsis: continue to use etomidate for intubation of patients with septic shock. *Ann Emerg Med.* 2008;52:13-14.
41. Sehdev RS, Symmons DA, Kindl K. Ketamine for rapid sequence induction in patients with head injury in the emergency department. *Emerg Med Australas.* 2006;18:37-44.
42. Mallon WK, Keim SM, Schoenberg JM, et al. Rocuronium vs succinylcholine in the emergency department: a critical appraisal. *J Emerg Med.* 2009;37:183-188.
43. Naguib M, Samarkandi AH, El-Din ME, et al. The dose of succinylcholine required for excellent endotracheal intubating conditions. *Anesth Analg.* 2006;102:151-155.
44. Sparr HJ, Vermeyen KM, Beaufort AM, et al. Early reversal of profound rocuronium-induced neuromuscular blockade by sugammadex in a randomized multicenter study: efficacy, safety, and pharmacokinetics. *Anesthesiology.* 2007;106:935-943.
45. Perrier ND, Baerga-Varela Y, Murray MJ. Death related to propofol use in an adult patient. *Crit Care Med.* 2000;28:3071-3074.
46. Levitan RM, Kinkle WC, Levin WJ, Everett WW. Laryngeal view during laryngoscopy: a randomized trial comparing cricoid pressure, backward-upward-rightward pressure, and bimanual laryngoscopy. *Ann Emerg Med.* 2006;47:548-555.
47. Hartsilver EL, Vanner RG. Airway obstruction with cricoid pressure. *Anaesthesia.* 2000;55:208-211.

The Crashing Ventilated Patient

3

IN THIS CHAPTER

- Evaluating and managing hemodynamically stable and unstable ventilated patients
- Assessing underlying etiologies
- Treating special populations, including children and tracheostomy patients
- Novel ventilation modes

Jairo I. Santanilla

Emergency physicians frequently are charged with managing ventilated patients, some of whom were intubated prior to arrival. These scenarios can be further complicated when a lack of critical care beds prevents a patient from being transferred. Although some hospitals employ a dedicated intensivist to take charge of such cases, this level of coverage is not always available. Therefore, emergency physicians must be adept at evaluating and managing acute complications and deteriorations in mechanically ventilated patients.

The information in this chapter will help the clinician differentiate between conditions related to underlying pathologies that necessitate ventilation and those caused by the procedure itself. This chapter does not fully address basic ventilator management, noninvasive positive-pressure ventilation, advanced trauma life support, or advanced cardiovascular life support (ACLS).

Hemodynamic Stability

The initial step in managing the crashing ventilated patient is to determine the patient's hemodynamic stability. The presence or absence of hypotension and hypoxia will dictate the amount of time available for implementing rescue strategies. It is equally important to anticipate the patient's clinical course. Managing a patient with pneumonia who requires mechanical ventilation to compensate for a gradually deteriorating cardiovascular status is dramatically different from managing one whose decline has occurred within a span of minutes *(Figure 3-1)*.

The following evaluation should be performed as soon as possible on intubated patients with new unexplained hypotension (systolic blood pressure [SBP] <90 mm Hg), new unexplained hypoxia (Sao_2 <90%), or a new marked change in vital signs (a drop in SBP >20 points, or a drop in Sao_2 >10%). Patients with *consistent* SBP measurements between 80 and 90 mm Hg and Sao_2 levels between 80% and 90% should be evaluated expeditiously, with the aim of halting the decline. Patients who are in rapid decline or have an SBP below 80 mm Hg or Sao_2 below 80% also should be evaluated expeditiously, with consideration given to entering the cardiac arrest/near arrest algorithm. These values are arbitrary demarcation points and do not take precedence over clinical judgment.

Cardiac Arrest/Near Arrest

Time is of the essence when managing the patient with cardiac arrest or near arrest. ACLS algorithms should be implemented quickly. Additionally, there are some key points to remember in the ventilated patient who has a cardiac arrest or becomes acutely hemodynamically unstable. The emergency department practitioner should follow a stepwise approach in which he "looks, listens, and feels" as he runs through the differential diagnosis.

During the stabilization phase, it is important to keep in mind the original pathology that necessitated intubation. The crashing ventilated patient could simply be growing worse as a result of the primary pathology. The multitrauma victim could have an intrathoracic or intraabdominal catastrophe, and the septic patient might be clinically deteriorating from a lack of source control.

It is important to determine and address special circumstances that the ventilator can precipitate, the most significant of which are tension pneumothorax and severe auto-positive end-expiratory pressure (auto-PEEP). Tension pneumothorax can lead to marked hypotension from decreased cardiac output and marked hypoxia from ventilation perfusion mismatch.[1] Auto-PEEP (also referred to as intrinsic PEEP, breath stacking, or dynamic hyperinflation) is caused by trapped volume in the pulmonary system. If severe enough, it will eventually lead to increased intrathoracic pressure. This can cause decreased venous return, resulting in hypotension and decreased organ perfusion complicated by marked hypoxia from ventilation perfusion mismatch.[2]

> **PEARL**
> Tension pneumothorax and severe auto-PEEP are important causes of ventilator-induced hemodynamic instability.

In critically ill ventilated patients who develop respiratory distress complicated by hemodynamic instability, the following steps will assist in pinpointing the cause of decompensation.

Step 1. Disconnect the patient from the ventilator.

This step can be both diagnostic and therapeutic. A quick rush of air or a prolonged expiration of trapped air from the endotracheal (ET) tube can be diagnostic of ventilator-induced auto-PEEP *(Table 3-1)*. A few seconds of observation can determine if this is the case. A rapid return of hemodynamic stability implies that the maneuver was successful.

Patients undergoing cardiopulmonary resuscitation should not be connected to a ventilator. The intrathoracic pressure variations caused by cardiopulmonary resuscitation will trigger ventilator breaths at high rates if the ventilator is set on assist control. Patients should not be removed from inhaled nitric oxide abruptly, and efforts should be made to quickly reestablish the supply through the bag-valve-mask system. In addition, care should be taken when disconnecting patients who are on high PEEP such as those with acute respiratory distress syndrome (ARDS). Although it is important to disconnect the patient from the ventilator to address the causes of auto-PEEP, doing so can cause derecruitment and worsen hypoxia. Once auto-PEEP has been ruled out, PEEP valves may be used to maintain the extrinsic PEEP levels, thus avoiding derecruitment. PEEP valves can be problematic in the markedly hypotensive patient by increasing intrathoracic pressures and decreasing venous return.

TABLE 3-1. Managing Auto-PEEP
Determine what caused the auto-PEEP (eg, high set respiratory rate, high patient respiratory rate, obstructive airway disease).
Consider decreasing the tidal volume in patients with obstructive or reactive airway disease.
Consider decreasing the set respiratory rate. (ineffective in assist-control mode with a high intrinsic rate).
Opioids can be used to control patient's respiratory rate.
Monitor ventilator flow-time waveform.
Consider changing to synchronized intermittent ventilation.
Consider chemical paralysis.

> **PEARL**
> Abrupt discontinuation of inhaled nitric oxide can cause rebound pulmonary hypertension and should be avoided. Administration should be reestablished quickly through the bag-valve-mask system.

Step 2. Hand ventilate with 100% oxygen.

Ensure that 100% oxygen is being delivered, and limit the respiratory rate to 8 to 10 breaths per minute. Particular attention should be given to the delivery of hand ventilation. Inadvertent rates as high as 40 breaths per minute are often present during codes.[3,4] Excessive rates will increase intrathoracic pressures, leading to decreases in venous return and cardiac output.[5] Visualize both sides of the chest to determine if the chest rise is unequal — a finding that can signify a main-stem intubation, pneumothorax, or mucus plug. Listen for air escaping from the mouth or nose (a sign of an air leak). Listen over the epigastric area and in both axilla. Decreased breath sounds can indicate main-stem intubation, pneumothorax, or atelectatic lung. Feel for subcutaneous crepitus (a sign of pneumothorax), and assess for difficulty in hand ventilating (a sign of low dynamic or static respiratory system compliance *[Table 3-2]*).

Step 3. Ensure the endotracheal tube is functioning and properly positioned.

The ET tube functions by providing a conduit to the lower trachea. Its cuff attempts to create a seal between it and the inner wall of the trachea. To determine if the device is functioning properly, pass the suction catheter through the lumen of the ET tube and listen for an air leak *(Figure 3-2)*. Easy passage of the suction catheter does not guarantee proper placement of the ET tube in the trachea; the catheter could be passing down the esophagus. If it is difficult or impossible to pass the suction catheter, the tube is dislodged, obstructed, or kinked or the patient is biting the tube. Attempt to correct a twisted or kinked ET tube by repositioning the patient's head; if the patient is biting on the tube, insert a bite block. Dislodged or obstructed tubes require reintubation. Patients with dislodged tubes should be treated as difficult intubations because unplanned extubations are notorious for causing trauma to the glottis, leading to vocal cord edema.[6]

In the cardiac arrest or near-arrest patient, the best method for ensuring proper positioning of the ET tube is direct visualization of the tube passing through the cords. This step is often omitted in the crashing ventilated patient because clinicians mistakenly assume the tube has not migrated. Unfortunately, unrecognized ET tube migration can occur during routine care. Patients are frequently moved in and out of emergency medical services vehicles, transferred to and from stretchers for imaging, and

FIGURE 3-1. The Crashing Ventilated Patient Algorithm

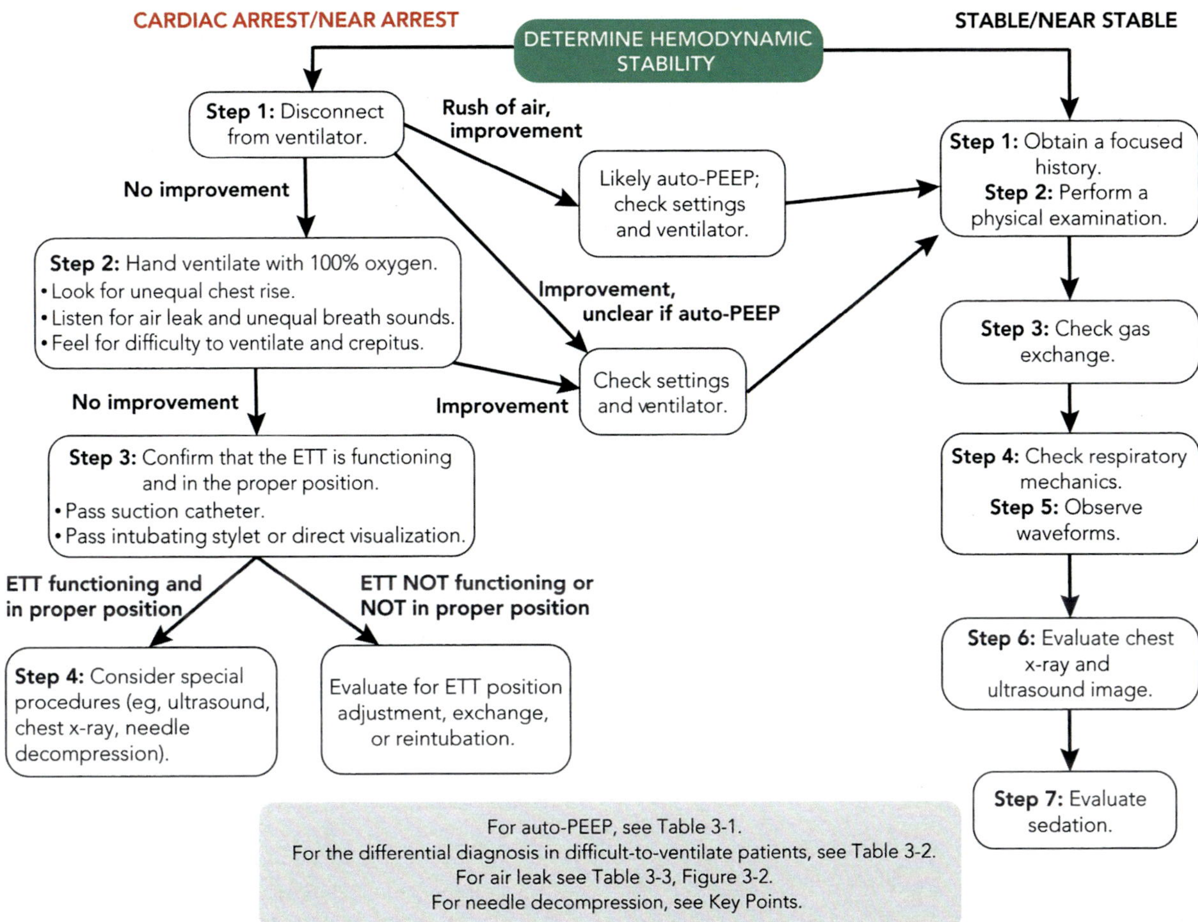

turned for procedures or bathing, increasing the risk of tube dislodgement. This visualization step can be performed while providing hand-bag ventilation.

Other simple techniques may be used to confirm placement of the ET tube in the trachea. Direct visualization of the carina with a fiberoptic scope is an option; however, this device typically is not available in the emergency department setting. Another quick technique is to pass an intubating stylet (gum elastic bougie or Eschmann introducer) gently through the ET tube.[7] If resistance is met at 30 cm, the ET tube is in the trachea. If the stylet passes beyond 35 cm without resistance, the tube is likely in the esophagus. If resistance is met too soon, the intubating stylet might be catching on the tube or lodged above the glottis.

At least one of these techniques to determine proper positioning should be employed early enough in the code to correct any airway issues. In addition, improper positioning should be confirmed before simply removing the tube and reintubating the patient, particularly if a difficult airway is suspected (unless it is glaringly evident that the patient is extubated).

PEARLS

Passage of an intubating stylet (gum elastic bougie or Eschmann introducer) is a quick, simple, and readily available technique for confirming placement of the ET tube in the trachea.

- Gently pass the intubating stylet through the ET tube — do not force it.
- Resistance should be encountered at approximately 30 cm.
- Passage of the stylet beyond 35 cm without resistance implies that the ET tube is in the esophagus.

Step 4. Consider special procedures.

If the patient remains in cardiac arrest or near arrest despite being disconnected from the ventilator, receiving a properly placed ET tube, and being hand ventilated with 100% oxygen, a clinical decision will be required regarding needle decompression of the chest. If time permits, a focused history from the bedside nurse, respiratory therapist, or paramedic and a focused

FIGURE 3-2. Approach to the Ventilated Patient with an Air Leak

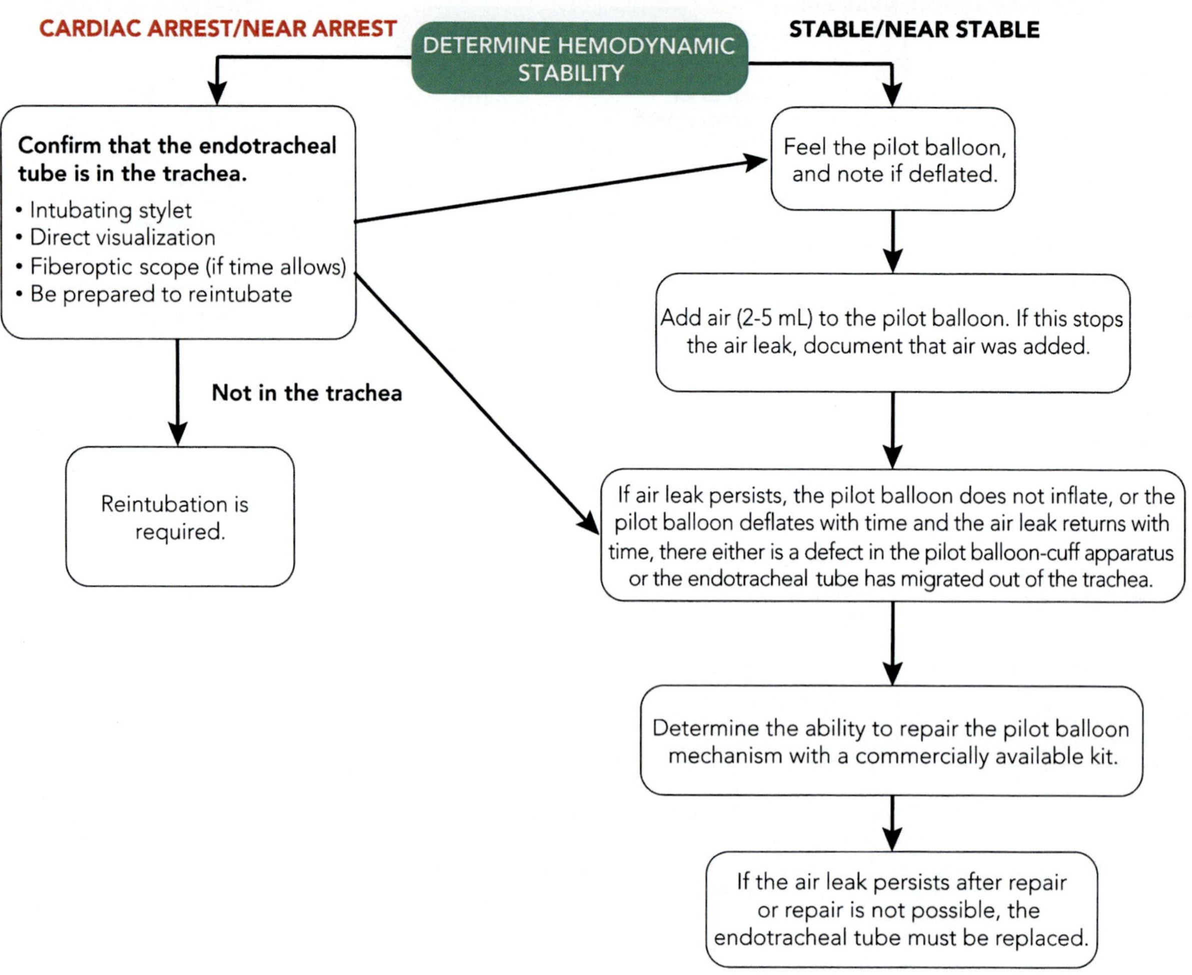

physical examination will indicate which side of the chest to decompress. Depending on the urgency of the situation, bedside ultrasonography and chest radiography also may be employed. The presence of a "lung-slide" artifact on bedside ultrasonography excludes pneumothorax. The "lung-slide" artifact appears in M-mode as the "seashore sign" *(Figure 3-3)*; its absence appears as the "stratosphere sign/bar-code sign" *(Figure 3-4)*.[8-10]

There are some clinical situations in which imaging studies and a focused history and physical examination may be unhelpful or even impossible. In these cases, needle decompression of both sides of the chest should be considered if likelier causes of acute decompensation are not found. It is important to remember that chest tube placement is required after needle decompression.[11-13]

PEARL

Use ultrasonography to quickly evaluate for pneumothorax.

The Stable/Near Stable Patient

If the patient is deemed stable or near stable, or quickly regains stability after disconnection from the ventilator and bag-valve-mask ventilation, the evaluation can be approached in a systematic manner *(Figure 3-1)*. The patient should be placed on 100% oxygen during this assessment.

Step 1. Obtain a focused history.

A focused history should be obtained from the practitioners most involved with the patient's care (eg, bedside nurse, respiratory therapist, resident, advanced practice provider, or paramedic). Valuable information includes the indication for intubation, difficulty of intubation, depth of the ET tube, ventilator settings, and recent procedures or moves (such as central line insertion, chest tube placement, removal or transition to water seal, thoracentesis, endotracheal tube manipulation, transport off stretcher, or rotation.

Step 2. Perform a focused physical examination.

Take a general survey of the patient. Observe for agitation, attempts to pull at the ET tube and lines, gasping for breath (the patient will have the mouth open and appear dyspneic), and tearing of the eyes.

Airway. Visualize the ET tube and determine if it has migrated from its previous position (eg, out of the trachea or into a main bronchus), and adjust if necessary. Listen for escaping air (an air leak) from the mouth or nose *(Figure 3-2)*. This finding, which typically signifies that the tube has lost its seal with the trachea, occurs in extubation or cuff failure. Feel the pilot balloon; if it is deflated, the cuff is deflated. Add air to the pilot balloon, and make note if this stops the air leak. If the pilot balloon does not inflate or deflates with time, there is a defect in the cuff apparatus and the ET tube will likely need to be exchanged. It occasionally is possible to repair the pilot balloon mechanism with a commercially available kit, which is a good option in patients who are difficult to intubate.

PEARL

If the pilot balloon does not inflate or deflates with time, there is a defect in the pilot balloon-cuff apparatus, and the ET tube will likely need to be exchanged.

Pass the suction catheter through the ET tube to confirm that it is functioning properly. If it is difficult or not possible to pass the suction catheter, the endotracheal tube is dislodged, obstructed, or kinked, or the patient is biting the tube. Attempt to correct any twists or kinks by repositioning the patient's head; insert a bite block if necessary. Dislodged or obstructed tubes require reintubation.

If extubation is suspected at any point in the evaluation, ensure that the ET tube is in proper position. Any of the techniques discussed in the previous section may be used.

Breathing. Look at both sides of the chest to determine if there is equal chest rise. Unequal chest rise can signify a main-stem intubation, pneumothorax, or mucus plug. Look at the ventilator tubing, and determine if there is an oscillating water collection. Listen for air escaping from the mouth or nose, which can signify an air leak. Listen over the epigastric area and in both axilla. Decreased breath sounds may provide clues regarding main-stem intubation, pneumothorax, or atelectatic lung. Feel for subcutaneous crepitus, which may indicate pneumothorax.

Circulation. Check for pulses, and cycle the blood pressure cuff frequently. If the patient has an arterial line, make sure the transducer is level. Determine the need for fluid administration or vasopressors.

Step 3. Assess gas exchange.

Hypoxia can be diagnosed based on pulse oximetry if the waveform is reliable. The waveform should not be highly variable, and its frequency should match the heart rate on the cardiac monitor. There are some presentations such as carbon monoxide poisoning, in which pulse oximetry is not reliable.[14] In such cases,

TABLE 3-2. Causes of Decreased Respiratory System Compliance

Causes of high peak pressures (increased airflow resistance, decreased dynamic compliance)	
Airway	Biting on the ET tube Bronchospasm Obstruction of the ET tube by secretions, mucus, blood Twisted ET tube
Pulmonary	Partial mucus plugging
Causes of high plateau pressures (low respiratory system compliance, decreased static compliance)	
Pulmonary	ARDS Atelectasis Auto-PEEP Mucus plugging Pneumonia Pneumothorax Pulmonary edema Unilateral intubation
Chest wall	Chest wall rigidity Circumferential chest wall burn Obesity
Other	Abdominal distention/pressure

FIGURE 3-3. Seashore Sign

The lung-slide artifact appears in ultrasound M-mode as the seashore sign, a finding that excludes pneumothorax.

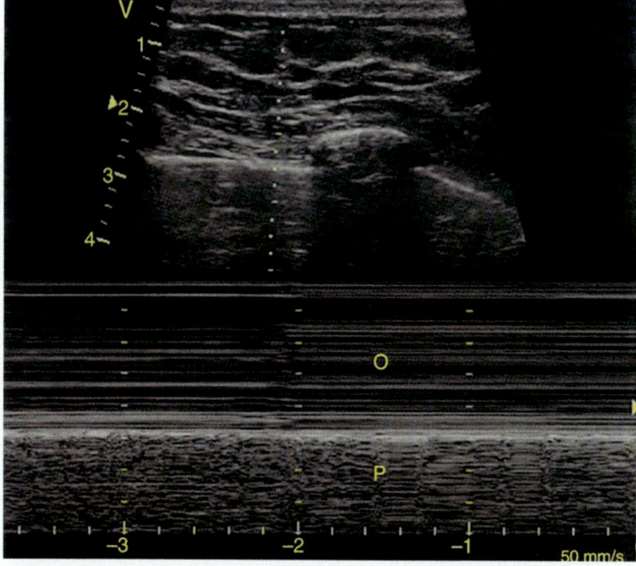

Image courtesy of Dr. Christine Butts and Dr. Matthew Bernard, Louisiana State University Health Sciences Center.

or if the pulse oximeter is not picking up, an arterial blood gas (ABG) sample should be obtained. Patients with a partial pressure of oxygen (PaO_2)/fraction of inspired oxygen (FiO_2) ratio less than 300 should be evaluated for ARDS; if the diagnosis is confirmed, a lung-protective strategy should be implemented *(Table 3-3)*.[16] Hypoventilation cannot be identified based on pulse oximetry measurements; continuous waveform capnography should be used in the intubated patient to monitor ventilation. If capnography is unavailable, ABG can be measured to evaluate hypoventilation.

PEARL

Hypoventilation cannot be identified based on pulse oximetry. Use capnography to monitor ventilation in the intubated patient.

Step 4. Check respiratory mechanics.

Determine if the peak pressures and plateau pressures have changed from their previous values. These values should be obtained on volume-targeted modes. Airway pressures are a function of volume and respiratory system compliance. The respiratory system incorporates the ventilator circuit, ET tube, trachea, bronchi, pulmonary parenchyma, and chest wall. A set volume with a set system compliance results in a specific pressure. Peak pressures are a function of the volume, resistance to airflow, and respiratory system compliance. The plateau pressure is obtained during an inspiratory pause. This eliminates airflow and reflects only the respiratory system compliance. An isolated increase in the peak pressure indicates increased resistance to airflow, while an isolated rise in the plateau pressure indicates decreased respiratory system compliance *(Table 3-2)*. Note that plateau pressure can never be higher than peak pressure, and they are directly related; if plateau pressure increases, so will the peak pressure. It is important to keep in mind the relationship of the change (delta = peak pressure – plateau pressure). Finally, these measurements assume a comfortable patient; peak pressures and plateau pressures are not reliable in the "bucking" patient.[17,18]

TABLE 3-3. Initial Ventilator Settings for ARDS

Volume-targeted, assist control
Tidal volume: 6–8 mL/kg ideal body weight (can start at 8 mL/kg ideal body weight and decrease to 6 mL/kg within 4 hours)
Respiratory rate: Set to approximate baseline minute ventilation (not to exceed 35 breaths/min)
PEEP: 5–8 cm H_2O (titrate based on protocol)
FiO_2: 100% (titrate based on protocol)
Flow rate: 60 L/min
Keep plateau pressures below 30 cm H_2O

FIGURE 3-4. Stratosphere/Barcode Sign

Absence of the lung-slide artifact is identified in ultrasound M-mode as the stratosphere/barcode sign. Pneumothorax cannot be excluded.

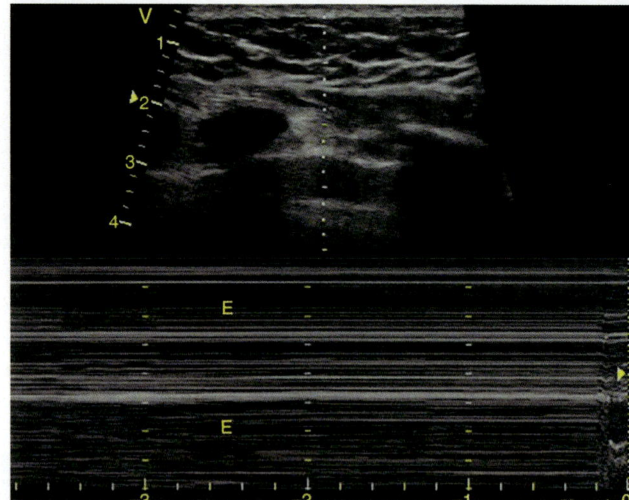

Image courtesy of Dr. Christine Butts and Dr. Matthew Bernard, Louisiana State University Health Sciences Center.

PEARL

Peak pressures and plateau pressures can be obtained only in volume-targeted modes.

Step 5. Observe ventilator waveforms.

The two most helpful ventilator waveforms are the flow-time and the pressure-time curves. The flow-time curve can be used to detect air trapping. The pressure-time curve can be used to determine plateau pressures with an inspiratory hold *(Figure 3-5)*.

A notching in the pressure-time curve during inspiration can signify air hunger. In this situation, the patient desires a higher flow rate than the ventilator is delivering *(Figure 3-6)*. It is commonly seen in volume-targeted modes. Increasing the flow rate will often alleviate this phenomenon. Another solution is changing to a pressure-targeted mode.

Double triggering can also be seen on ventilator waveforms, a complication that occurs when the patient desires a higher tidal volume than the ventilator is set to deliver. The patient is still inspiring when the first breath has finished cycling, and the ventilator immediately gives a second mechanical breath *(Figure 3-7)*. This is frequently seen in low-tidal-volume ventilation, as used for patients with ARDS and status asthmaticus. Double triggering is important to recognize because the actual tidal volume being provided is essentially twice the set tidal volume. This is especially critical in patients with ARDS and obstructive processes such as asthma and chronic obstructive pulmonary disease, who have lower tidal volume goals. Improved sedation — with an emphasis on blunting the respiratory drive using opiates — often alleviates double triggering. Other adjustments that may help include

FIGURE 3-5. Pressure-Time Curve Indicating Inspiratory Hold and Plateau Pressure

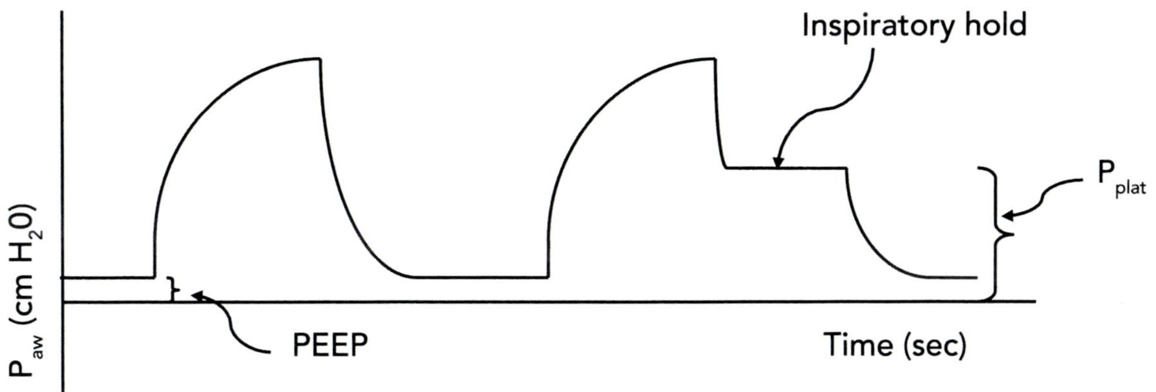

FIGURE 3-6. Air Hunger on Ventilator Waveform

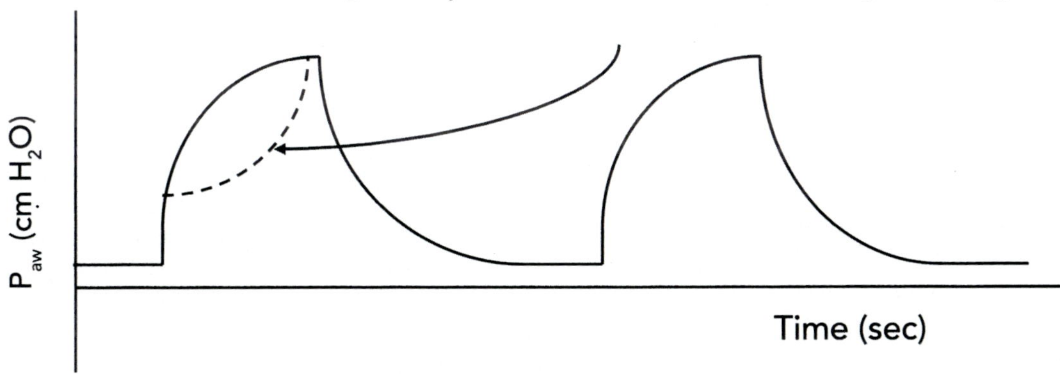

FIGURE 3-7. Double-Triggering Ventilator Waveform

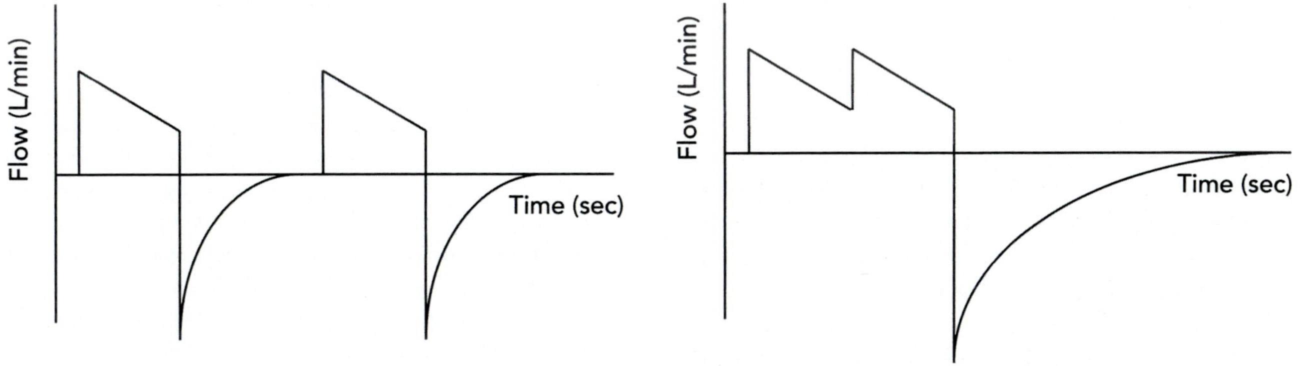

increasing the flow rate, increasing the tidal volume (1 mL/kg predicted body weight up to 8 mL/kg), or changing from a volume-targeted mode to a pressure-targeted mode.

Step 6. Order imaging studies.

Evaluate the chest radiograph for ET tube positioning, mainstem intubation, lung atelectasis, pneumothorax, and worsening parenchymal processes. Bedside ultrasonography is typically quicker in evaluating for pneumothorax, and it might provide information on the location of the ET tube, lung atelectasis, or parenchymal processes *(Figures 3-3* and *3-4).*

Step 7. Evaluate sedation.

Some patients, including those with drug overdoses or traumatic head injuries, might not require sedation. Others tolerate intubation quite well while almost fully awake. However, most patients require some form of sedation or analgesia to make the ET tube and ventilation tolerable.

Agents should be chosen based on the desired effect. If a patient appears agitated, a sedative-hypnotic such as propofol or dexmedetomidine, should be selected.[19] It is important to note that these agents do not provide an analgesic component.

Table 3-4. Special Scenarios

Children
ET tubes commonly migrate in and out of position with small manipulations of head position.
Place a cervical collar to help stabilize the patient's head position.
Document that the purpose is not for cervical spine protection.
Small ET tubes are uncuffed.
Most readily available intubating stylets and fiberoptic scopes are too large for pediatric ET tubes.
The Tracheostomy Patient — Unintentional Extubation
Determine if the patient had a laryngectomy.
Oral intubation is an option if the patient did not undergo a laryngectomy.
Determine the reason for tracheostomy.
Anatomical reason, difficult or failed airway — oral intubation might not be an option.
Traumatic brain injury, chronic respiratory failure — oral intubation might be an option.
Determine the age of the tracheostomy. If it is less than 1 week old, the site might not be mature enough for manipulation; high risk of creating a false tract.
Gently place a 6.0 ET tube in the stoma.
Placement can be confirmed with fiberoptic visualization. Stop if any resistance is encountered.
The Tracheostomy Patient — Obstruction
Remove the inner cannula and replace it with a same-sized cannula.

If a patient is being given adequate sedative doses and still appears agitated, consider pain as a cause. For example, an agitated patient with a femur fracture who is receiving high-dose benzodiazepines might simply need an opiate for pain control. Commonly prescribed opiates include fentanyl, hydromorphone, and morphine. The goal of sedation and anesthesia in ventilated patients is to achieve a state in which the patient will arouse to gentle stimulation but return to a sedated state when left alone. Patients who respond only to deep stimulation are oversedated. Current guidelines recommend titrating sedative and analgesic medications to achieve lighter levels of sedation.[19] Pain and agitation protocols have been shown to reduce the duration of mechanical ventilation and length of hospital stay. These scoring systems should be implemented to titrate sedative and analgesic medications in the intubated emergency department patient.[19]

Patients who display air hunger and a high respiratory rate can be given a trial of opiates to relieve symptoms. Proper sedation and analgesia are paramount in patients being treated with a strategy that allows or induces hypercapnia such as those with status asthmaticus and ARDS. Hypercapnia is a powerful stimulus to the respiratory drive, and opioids are often required to control respiratory rates. Patients who tend to be difficult to control (besides those with status asthmaticus and ARDS) include those with hepatic encephalopathy or intracranial processes, such as mass effect and hemorrhage. Patients who remain tachypneic despite a trial of sedation, analgesia, and ventilator changes may require chemical weakening with intermittently dosed paralytics. Careful consideration should be given prior to this step, as prolonged paralysis has been implicated in critical illness polyneuropathy.[20,21] An expert consultation should be obtained prior to initiating prolonged paralysis of neurosurgical patients. The goal of chemical paralysis in these patients is to weaken them enough to control their interactions with the ventilator. Usually, this does not require a full dose of the paralytic.

Hemodynamic instability in mechanically ventilated and sedated patients can be a result of medication; sedatives and analgesics can precipitate or worsen hypotension. As a general rule, continuous infusions should be held in these cases. Patients who are hypoxic and agitated but not hypotensive can benefit from improved sedation. It is possible that their pulmonary status is so tenuous that they are agitated from the hypoxia, and their condition is being worsened by the oxygen consumption caused by agitation. Patients who are agitated and hypotensive might respond well to a low-dose benzodiazepine and opiate if the agitation is a precipitant of hypotension. In all these cases, it is imperative to determine if sedation is a factor in the decompensation. Chemical paralysis should be reserved as a final option.

PEARL

Hemodynamic instability in mechanically ventilated and sedated patients can be a result of medication.

Special Scenarios

Two special scenarios should be mentioned. One is the crashing intubated child, and the second is the patient with a tracheostomy *(Table 3-4)*. The previously described approach, which can be used in pediatric patients, can be improved, with several caveats. The first is to recognize that ET tube migration is common with small movements of the head and neck. A simple solution is to use a cervical collar for immobilization. Second, small ET tubes are often uncuffed and do not have a pilot balloon. Air leaks in this scenario should prompt the clinician to consider whether the tube is dislodged or too small. Finally, specialized equipment such as intubating stylets and fiberoptic scopes, are typically not available in pediatric sizes.

There are several important questions that have ramifications for the care of the crashing ventilated patient with a tracheostomy:

- Does the patient have a laryngectomy?
- Why does the patient have a tracheostomy?
- How old is the tracheostomy?

The answers are significant because a patient with a laryngectomy cannot be intubated orally; a patient with a tracheostomy secondary to anatomical considerations or a difficult/failed airway can be hard to intubate orally; and the track in a patient with a recent tracheostomy (<1 week) may not have matured enough to allow the reintroduction of a tracheostomy tube.

Novel Ventilation Modes

Although specialized ventilation modes have not been shown to improve outcomes, their use has increased. These newer methods are designed to automatically adjust components such as tidal volume or pressure support, either within a breath (such as volume-assured pressure support) or from breath to breath (such as pressure-regulated volume control). The approach to the stable/near stable ventilated patient, described above, is not easily translatable; specifically, evaluating respiratory mechanics and waveforms in these modes is difficult. The format for the arrest/near arrest scenario is the same. Perhaps the most common pitfall associated with these approaches is the ventilator's ability to misinterpret patient effort as an improvement in respiratory dynamics. In these cases, the patient works harder and gets less support, resulting in discomfort.

Another mode used with increasing frequency is airway pressure release ventilation (APRV), which enables the patient to breathe spontaneously while the ventilator cycles between a pressure high and a pressure low. The difference between this mode and pressure-controlled ventilation is that the patient spends the majority of time at the high setting. Typically, 4 to 6 seconds is spent in pressure-high and 0.2

KEY POINTS

1. The initial step in managing the crashing ventilated patient is to determine the patient's hemodynamic stability. Important questions to ask:
   - How stable is the patient?
   - How rapidly is the patient deteriorating?
   - What is the patient's underlying pathophysiology?
   - How much time is available to determine the cause of the instability and address the problems?
2. The following patients are at risk for auto-PEEP (breath stacking): patients on volume-targeted modes with obstructive or reactive airway disease, those on volume-targeted modes receiving a high minute ventilation, and those receiving inverse-ratio ventilation.
3. If it is difficult or impossible to pass the suction catheter, the ET tube is dislodged, obstructed, or kinked or the patient is biting the tube.
4. Needle decompression:
   - Determine which side to decompress first.
   - Identify the fifth or sixth intercostal space in the anterior axillary line.
   - Prepare the area with chlorhexidine if time permits.
   - Anesthetize the area if the patient is conscious and time permits.
   - Insert an over-the-needle catheter over the rib.
   - A 14-gauge catheter, at least 5 cm, is preferred.
   - A different needle size might be needed, depending on the size of the patient.
   - Puncture the parietal pleura while listening for a sudden escape of air.
   - Remove the needle while leaving the catheter in place.
   - Secure the catheter with a bandage or small dressing.
   - Prepare for chest tube thoracostomy.
5. Is the ET tube in proper position?
   - Did it migrate out of the trachea?
   - Did it migrate down into the main bronchus?
   - Is it functioning properly?
6. Methods to manage whole-lung atelectasis:
   - Use recruitment maneuvers.
   - Disconnect from ventilator and provide hand ventilation at higher tidal volumes.
   - Provide frequent suctioning.
   - Rotate patient.
   - Perform chest percussion.
   - Administer bronchodilators.
   - Perform bronchoscopy.
7. The goal of sedation is a patient who arouses to gentle stimulation and returns to a sedated state when left alone. If deep stimulation is required to get a response, the patient is oversedated. Use validated scoring systems for pain and agitation to titrate analgesic and sedative medications.

to 1.5 seconds in pressure-low. Ventilation occurs with the "release" from pressure-high to pressure-low. Oxygenation is optimized by the alveolar recruitment obtained while at the pressure-high setting. APRV should not be used in patients with severe obstructive airway disease or those with a high ventilatory requirement due to the risk of hyperinflation, elevated alveolar pressure, and barotrauma. Auto-PEEP is an important consideration and the approach to the arrest/near arrest scenario with APRV is the same: disconnect the patient from the ventilator. The approach outlined in this chapter for the stable/near stable patient is not translatable to APRV, except for the evaluation of respiratory mechanics and waveforms. Finally, it should be noted that patients on APRV with pressure-high settings greater than 20 cm H_2O should remain on a ventilator during transport. Switching to hand ventilation could lead to hypoxia and hemodynamic compromise.

Conclusion

Mechanically ventilated patients are among the sickest that emergency clinicians must face. The underlying disease process that required intubation often is life-threatening. When patients become unstable, the physician should take a stepwise approach toward determining if the deterioration is prompted by the underlying disease process or interaction with the ventilator.

REFERENCES

1. Chen KY, Jerng JS, Liao WY, et al. Pneumothorax in the ICU: patient outcomes and prognostic factors. *Chest.* 2002;122:678-683.
2. Pepe PE, Marini JJ. Occult positive end-expiratory pressure in mechanically ventilated patients with airflow obstruction: the auto-PEEP effect. *Am Rev Respir Dis.* 1982;126:166-170.
3. O'Neill JF, Deakin CD. Do we hyperventilate cardiac arrest patients? *Resuscitation.* 2007;73:82-85.
4. Abella BS, Alvarado JP, Myklebust H, et al. Quality of cardiopulmonary resuscitation during in-hospital cardiac arrest. *JAMA.* 2005;293:305-310.
5. Aufderheide TP, Sigurdsson G, Pirrallo RG, et al. Hyperventilation-induced hypotension during cardiopulmonary resuscitation. *Circulation.* 2004;109:1960-1965.
6. Christie JM, Dethlefsen M, Cane RD. Unplanned endotracheal extubation in the intensive care unit. *J Clin Anesth.* 1996;8:289-293.
7. Bair AE, Laurin EG, Schmitt BJ. An assessment of a tracheal tube introducer as an endotracheal tube placement confirmation device. *Am J Emerg Med.* 2005;23:754-758.
8. Lichtenstein DA, Meziere G, Lascols N, et al. Ultrasound diagnosis of occult pneumothorax. *Crit Care Med.* 2005;33:1231-1238.
9. Blaivas M, Lyon M, Duggal S. A prospective comparison of supine chest radiography and bedside ultrasound for the diagnosis of traumatic pneumothorax. *Acad Emerg Med.* 2005;12:844-849.
10. Wilkerson RG, Stone MB. Sensitivity of bedside ultrasound and supine anteroposterior chest radiographs for the identification of pneumothorax after blunt trauma. *Acad Emerg Med.* 2010;17:11-17.
11. Harcke HT, Pearse LA, Levy AD, et al. Chest wall thickness in military personnel: implications for needle thoracentesis in tension pneumothorax. *Mil Med.* 2007;172:1260-1263.
12. Givens ML, Ayotte K, Manifold C. Needle thoracostomy: implications of computed tomography chest wall thickness. *Acad Emerg Med.* 2004;11:211-213.
13. Zengerink I, Brink PR, Laupland KB, et al. Needle thoracostomy in the treatment of a tension pneumothorax in trauma patients: what size needle? *J Trauma.* 2008;64:111-114.
14. Lee WW, Mayberry K, Crapo R, Jensen RL. The accuracy of pulse oximetry in the emergency department. *Am J Emerg Med.* 2000;18:427-431.
15. Bernard GR, Artigas A, Brigham KL, et al. The American-European Consensus Conference on ARDS. Definitions, mechanisms, relevant outcomes, and clinical trial coordination. *Am J Respir Crit Care Med.* 1994;149(3 Pt 1):818-824.
16. Ventilation with lower tidal volumes as compared with traditional tidal volumes for acute lung injury and the acute respiratory distress syndrome. The Acute Respiratory Distress Syndrome Network. *N Engl J Med.* 2000;342:1301-1308.
17. Tobin MJ. Advances in mechanical ventilation. *N Engl J Med.* 2001;344:1986-1996.
18. Tobin MJ. Respiratory monitoring. *JAMA.* 1990;264:244-251.
19. Barr J, Fraser GL, Puntillo K, et al. Clinical practice guidelines for the management of pain, agitation, and delirium in adult patients in the intensive care unit. *Crit Care Med.* 2013;41:263-306.
20. Douglass JA, Tuxen DV, Horne M, et al. Myopathy in severe asthma. *Am Rev Respir Dis.* 1992;146:517-519.
21. Kupfer Y, Namba T, Kaldawi E, Tessler S. Prolonged weakness after long-term infusion of vecuronium bromide. *Ann Intern Med.* 1992;117:484-486.

Fluid Management

4

IN THIS CHAPTER

- Fluid physiology
- Signs of hypovolemia
- Volume responsiveness
- Fluid selection
- Special circumstances
- Hemorrhagic shock
- Burn resuscitation
- Maintenance therapy

Alan C. Heffner

Fluid therapy is a cornerstone in the management of acute critical illness, which can be further complicated by relative and absolute hypovolemia. In practice, the clinician is routinely challenged with the tasks of assessing volume status, determining the need for fluid therapy, and choosing the best fluid and dose for each individual patient. Timely and appropriate fluid administration maintains macro- and microcirculation and reduces mortality.[1] In contrast, both the under- and overadministration of fluids adversely affect outcome. Inadequate fluid resuscitation can result in persistent organ malperfusion. Conversely, overaggressive fluid administration induces volume overload without improving oxygen delivery and is associated with diminished tissue oxygenation, impaired organ function, and adverse clinical outcomes. A thorough understanding of the appropriate selection, timing, and goals of fluid therapy is vital to optimize patient care.

General Principles

Fluid Distribution and Movement

Water is the most abundant constituent of the body, accounting for 50% to 70% of total body weight. Variations in total body water depend primarily on lean body mass since fat contains very little water *(Table 4-1)*. Water is distributed within intracellular and extracellular fluid compartments *(Table 4-2)*. Two-thirds of total body water resides in the intracellular space. The remainder is distributed to the extracellular space, which is further divided into interstitial and intravascular compartments in a 4:1 ratio. These two fluid compartments are not contiguous, but they can be treated as such because of their similar composition and behavior.

Water freely crosses cell membranes, and osmotic forces within fluid compartments determine its distribution within the body. Intracellular and extracellular fluid environments are iso-osmolar but are physiochemically distinct because of the tight regulation of dissolved solutes and proteins. Membrane-bound sodium-potassium ATPase pumps compartmentalize sodium and potassium to the extracellular and intracellular spaces, respectively. Active restriction of sodium to the extracellular space is the foundation for sodium-based resuscitation solutions.

Intravascular fluid, or plasma, differs from all other fluid compartments because it exists as a single continuous fluid collection and contains trapped protein moieties in a higher concentration than the surrounding interstitium. These trapped proteins and the endothelial glycocalyx layer produce the colloid oncotic pressure (COP) that favors fluid retention in the vascular space. Fluid flux across endothelial membranes is governed by Starling forces. In health, transcapillary hydrostatic force is nearly opposed by COP. Small net losses from the vascular space are returned to the systemic circulation via lymphatics. Supranormal hydrostatic pressure, hypoalbuminemia, and pathological endothelial permeability are common clinical conditions that enhance fluid extravasation. Alteration of COP with enhanced retention of intravascular volume is one

TABLE 4-1. Total Body Water Estimates

Adult male	60%
Adult female[a]	50%
Elderly[a]	50%
Obese[a]	50%
Infant	70%
Total body water represents 50% to 60% of lean body weight in adults.	

[a]Lower total body water proportional to skeletal muscle mass.

theoretic advantage of colloid-based fluids. Albumin typically accounts for 80% of COP, while large cellular moieties such as red cells and platelets, contribute less to oncotic effect. Therefore, blood products should be used for cellular replacement only when indicated and not for primary volume expansion when asanguineous solutions suffice.

Effective Circulating Volume

Effective circulating volume (ECV) is the portion of intravascular volume contributing to organ perfusion. ECV falls with hypovolemia but does not necessarily correlate with volume status, as organ perfusion is also dependent on cardiac output, arterial tone, and circulatory distribution. For example, ECV may be compromised by limited cardiac output (eg, heart failure) despite optimized volume status.

Pathophysiology

The immediate consequence of acute hypovolemia is impaired oxygen delivery, which triggers a swift compensatory response. Cardiac output is the most important determinant of oxygen delivery, with the normal flexibility to compensate for reduced oxygen-carrying capacity and/or increased metabolic demand *(Figure 4-1)*. In the setting of hypovolemia, the body defends itself through compensatory adjustments to maintain perfusion pressure and oxygen delivery.

At the macrocirculatory level, volume loss leads to decreased venous return and stroke volume. Reduced stretch sensed by aortic and carotid baroreceptors leads to swift sympathetic catecholamine release, resulting in vasoconstriction, tachycardia, and enhanced cardiac contractility in an attempt to maintain cardiac output. Venoconstriction shunts blood from capacitance vessels to maintain cardiac preload. Organ blood flow is proportional to perfusion pressure in most vascular beds, and peripheral arterial vasoconstriction maintains critical blood pressure (BP) to support the autoregulation of organ blood flow. Preferential perfusion simultaneously shunts limited cardiac output to vital organs by reducing blood flow to noncritical (hepatosplanchnic, renal, cutaneous) circulations. In this way, mean arterial pressure (MAP) can be maintained despite hypovolemia and organ hypoperfusion.

Volume depletion and hypovolemia describe the state of contracted extracellular fluid with clinical implications of compromised ECV and perfusion. It is distinguished from dehydration, which implies an intracellular water deficit characterized by plasma hypernatremia and hyperosmolarity. Hypovolemia can occur as a consequence of blood loss, water and electrolyte loss, or primary water loss.

Clinical Signs of Hypovolemia

Hypovolemia primarily manifests as circulatory insufficiency. Signs and symptoms reflect organ dysfunction and the counter-regulatory response to offset the hypovolemic state. Classically, hypovolemia is portrayed as a stepwise progression of signs and symptoms based on volume deficit *(Table 4-3)*. The clinical reality is that signs are highly variable, depending on the culprit disease, the speed of its evolution, and the individual's physiological reserve for compensation. Children and healthy adults with vigorous compensatory mechanisms can tolerate large volume loss in the absence of severe clinical symptoms. In contrast, patients with limited cardiac reserve may poorly tolerate even minimal fluid loss. Compared with primary volume loss or hemorrhage, sepsis presents a complicated state in which absolute fluid deficits are compounded by pathological vasodilation and accelerated end-organ dysfunction.

Shock

Shock is defined as the state of inadequate tissue perfusion in which oxygen delivery is unable to meet metabolic needs. Contrary to popular use, the term does not reflect perfusion pressure. In fact, blood pressure is an unreliable indicator of systemic oxygen delivery and perfusion. Malperfusion in the setting of normal blood pressure is termed *compensated shock*, reflecting the body's ability to maintain critical perfusion pressure. Most critically ill patients initially present in this state. Normotension should not be interpreted as a reliable indicator of normal perfusion. Difficulty in identifying these patients spawned the terms *occult hypoperfusion* and *cryptic shock* to describe normotensive patients with clinical or laboratory evidence of cardiovascular insufficiency.

PEARL

Blood pressure is an unreliable indicator of oxygen delivery and organ perfusion.

TABLE 4-2. Size and Composition of Body Fluid Compartments[a]

Compartment	% Body Weight	Volume (L)	H_2O (L)	Na (mmol/L)	K (mmol/L)	Cl (mmol/L)	HCO_3^- (mmol/L)
Total body	60	45	42				
Intracellular fluid	40	30	28 (60%)	16	160		10
Extracellular fluid	20	15	14 (40%)	140	4	103	26
Interstitial	16	12					
Plasma	4	3					
Blood	7	5					

[a]Values based on a 70-kg man.

TABLE 4-3. Classes of Acute Hemorrhagic Shock (estimated blood loss* based on patient's initial presentation)

	Class I	Class II	Class III	Class IV
Blood loss (mL)	Up to 750	750–1,500	1,500–2,000	>2,000
Blood loss (% blood volume)	Up to 15%	15%–30%	30%–40%	>40%
Pulse rate	<100	100–120	120–140	>140
Blood pressure	Normal	Normal	Decreased	Decreased
Pulse pressure	Normal or increased	Decreased	Decreased	Decreased
Respiratory rate	14–20	20–30	30–40	>35
Urine output (mL/hr)	>30	20–30	5–15	Negligible
CNS/mental status	Slightly anxious	Mildly anxious	Anxious, confused	Confused, lethargic
Fluid replacement	Crystalloid	Crystalloid	Crystalloid and blood	Crystalloid and blood

*Estimates based on a 70-kg man.

From: American College of Surgeons Committee on Trauma. *Advanced Trauma Life Support for Doctors.* 8th ed. Chicago, IL: American College of Surgeons; 2008. Used with permission.

Brief self-limited hypotension is a common clinical marker of progressive exhaustion of cardiovascular compensation and is the first sign of uncompensated shock.[4] Sustained hypotension defines uncompensated shock and is a late sign of developing illness when physiological attempts to maintain blood pressure are overwhelmed. Hypotension should always be considered pathological until proven otherwise even in the absence of immediately recognizable malperfusion. A mean arterial blood pressure (MAP) less than 65 mm Hg or a systolic blood pressure (SBP) less than 90 mm Hg classically defines absolute hypotension in adults. The degree and duration of hypotension correlate with adverse outcomes.[5]

The danger of defining a single threshold of critical hypotension rests in underrecognizing shock in some patients. Baseline BP is higher in the elderly, in whom hypotension portends a higher mortality rate. In addition to representing the threshold below which end-organ perfusion suffers, BP flags the need for intervention. Age-adjusted thresholds are most powerful; patients older than 65 are better identified using an SBP below 110 mm Hg to define uncompensated shock and risk of death.[6,7] Similarly, in patients with chronic hypertension, an SBP above 40 mm Hg and MAP more than 20 mm Hg below historic baseline constitute relative hypotension that warrants clinical concern.

FIGURE 4-1. Determinants of Systemic Oxygen Delivery

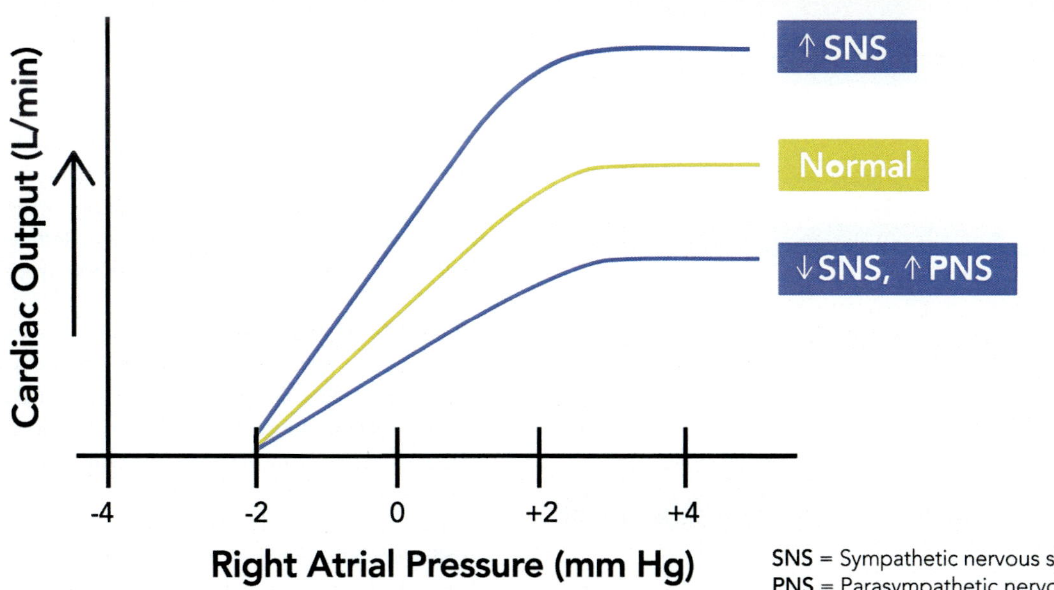

SNS = Sympathetic nervous system
PNS = Parasympathetic nervous system

Postural Vital Signs

The discriminative power of postural vital signs depends on appropriate testing and integration with additional clinical findings. Supine resting blood pressure and pulse rate should be reassessed at least 2 minutes after standing (standing triggers a brief orthostatic response in all patients). A postural pulse rise that is greater than 30 beats per minute is unusual in normovolemic patients.[8] Severe postural dizziness with intolerance of upright positioning confirms hypovolemia, in contrast to subjective symptoms that do not limit standing. Orthostatic hypotension, defined as SBP decline of more than 20 mm Hg, is observed in 10% to 30% of normovolemic patients. The postural hemodynamic response may also be altered by aging and medications. As many as 30% of elderly patients demonstrate an orthostatic response in the absence of volume depletion.[9]

Heart Rate and Shock Index

Sinus tachycardia is a nonspecific response, but its presence should prompt clinical suspicion for volume depletion. Heart rate normally increases in the early stages of hypovolemia to maintain cardiac output in the face of falling stroke volume. However, this response to acute volume loss is highly variable. In normal patients, volume loss of up to 20% fails to induce a tachycardic response.[8] This compensatory response may be further blunted by comorbid disease and medications, especially beta-blockers. Paradoxic and relative bradycardia occur in up to 30% of patients with traumatic and atraumatic hemoperitoneum.[10,11]

Shock index (SI) is the quotient of heart rate to systolic blood pressure. The normal range is 0.5 to 0.7. A rising SI signals declining cardiac performance. SI, which is a better marker of acute blood loss than either heart rate or SBP alone, assists in identifying early critical illness in patients with deceptively normal blood pressure.[12,13]

PEARL

- ✓ Shock index = Heart rate/systolic blood pressure.
- ✓ SI >0.9 is associated with adverse outcome and the need for therapeutic intervention in a number of critical conditions.

TABLE 4-4. Anatomical Sites of Nonhemorrhagic Fluid Loss

Gastrointestinal
Vomiting
Diarrhea
Drainage (ostomy, fistula, nasogastric)
Renal
Diuresis (medication, osmotic)
Salt wasting
Diabetes insipidus
Skin
Burn
Wound
Exfoliative rash
Sweat
Third-Space Sequestration
Intestinal obstruction
Peritonitis
Crush injury
Pancreatitis
Ascites
Pleural effusion
Capillary leak
Insensible Loss
Respiratory
Fever

Clinical Signs and Symptoms of Perfusion

Fatigue, dyspnea, postural dizziness, and near syncope are common symptoms of reduced cardiac output, including that stemming from hypovolemia. Organ dysfunction can be the heralding sign of hypovolemia and commonly occurs in the absence of gross hemodynamic instability (eg, compensated shock). Nonfocal confusion, agitation, and lassitude representing neurological dysfunction should prompt medical attention, especially in elderly patients. Oliguria, concentrated urine, and increased serum creatinine are exemplary signs of early renal dysfunction. Electrolyte and acid-base derangements associated with hypovolemia can also produce a constellation of associated symptoms.

Cutaneous malperfusion often represents sympathetic activation in response to shock. Subjective assessment of perfusion, including distal extremity temperature and mottling, is a practical noninvasive window into cardiovascular status.[14,15] In contrast, dry mucous membranes, abnormal skin turgor, and sunken eyes are classic — but imperfect — hallmarks of hypovolemia.

Fluid Resuscitation

Circulatory failure is the final common pathway of many diseases and carries a wide differential diagnosis. While hypovolemia is the most common primary cause of shock, inadequate circulating volume can complicate many shock states, including severe cardiac dysfunction. Restoration of the underlying fluid deficit is necessary to reverse hypoperfusion.

Intravenous Access

Appropriate intravenous access is vital to resuscitation. The determinants of flow through a rigid tube are listed in Table 4-5. The rate of volume infusion is determined by the size of the vascular catheter, not by the size of the cannulated vein. Flow is directly proportional to the fourth power of the catheter radius and inversely proportional to the catheter length. Therefore, doubling the catheter size results in a 16-fold increase in flow, whereas doubling the cannula length decreases flow by half.

Central venous catheters allow hemodynamic monitoring and provide a reliable portal for volume therapy, vasoactive drug infusion, and serial blood sampling. Because of differences in length, infusion rates through adult central venous catheters are up to 75% lower than through peripheral catheters of equal diameter. Many patients can be resuscitated adequately with peripheral venous access. In some circumstances, massive volume infusion may require the use of large-bore introducer catheters (8.5F to 9.5F) that support flow rates approaching those of intravenous tubing at almost 1 L/min *(Table 4-6)*.[16] Manual compression of the bag is an inefficient method of improving flow compared with use of an external pressure bag.[17]

PEARL

Infusion rates through central venous catheters can be up to 75% lower than through peripheral venous catheters.

Endpoints of Resuscitation

The immediate goal of cardiovascular support is to restore and maintain systemic oxygen delivery and organ perfusion. Structured resuscitation includes endpoints or targets to gauge the adequacy of management.[1,18] A rapid restoration of perfusion pressure is a priority to support the autoregulation of vital organ blood flow.[19] However, normalization of traditional markers of blood pressure and heart rate does not guarantee adequate organ perfusion and risks leaving the patient in persistent compensated shock.[20,21]

No single resuscitation endpoint is perfect for all patients or circumstances. Given the limitations of vital signs as indicators of cardiovascular wellness, it is most prudent to take a multimodal approach to normalizing global and regional perfusion markers *(Table 4-7)*.

Blood lactate concentration and base deficit are associated with illness severity and predict morbidity and mortality independent of hemodynamics.[22,23] They are similarly useful to corroborate an appropriate response to therapy. Rapid lactate clearance is associated with improved mortality rates across a number of critical conditions, while persistent hyperlactatemia is linked to higher rates of organ failure and death.[24] Therefore, serial lactate levels provide an important gauge of resuscitation. Lactate clearance greater than 10% per hour is a common goal, although lactate normalization (<2 mmol/L) is most strongly associated with survival.[25] Initial base deficit correlates with serum lactate but is confounded by resuscitation fluid and other therapies, limiting its utility as a serial maker of resuscitation.

Central venous oxygen saturation ($ScvO_2$) reflects the systemic balance of oxygen delivery and utilization. Limited oxygen delivery is compensated by enhanced tissue extraction, resulting in a fall in $ScvO_2$ below the normal 70%. Although subnormal $ScvO_2$ is associated with adverse outcomes, trials targeting this endpoint show mixed results.[18,26-28] Systematic central venous cannulation to measure this endpoint in the absence of another indication is not endorsed; however, it represents a pragmatic measure when access is available. In contrast to lactate kinetics, $ScvO_2$ response is rapid and dynamic, such that monitoring provides immediate feedback on resuscitation efforts (or clinical deterioration).

PEARL

Endpoint achievement signals the completion of immediate resuscitation; continued fluid resuscitation is not warranted unless the patient manifests recurrent malperfusion. Overresuscitation is associated with increases in morbidity and mortality.

The Empiric Fluid Challenge

The restoration of oxygen delivery via fluid resuscitation relies on the ability to optimize preload to maximize stroke volume. The empiric volume challenge remains the standard means of initial fluid resuscitation for overt clinical hypovolemia or acute undifferentiated shock. Volume expansion is achieved by infusing serial aliquots of isotonic fluid under direct observation at the bedside. Crystalloid (5–20 mL/kg) or colloid (5–10 mL/kg) boluses should be infused quickly (over 15–20 minutes). For adults, straight IV tubing and use of pressure bags are recommended, in contrast to rate-limiting IV pumps. Serial rapid boluses are titrated to clinical endpoint objectives while

TABLE 4-5. Determinants of Flow Through Rigid Tubing

Hagen-Poiseuille equation: $Q = (P_{in} - P_{out}) \times (\pi r^4/8\mu L)$

Q = Flow
$P_{in} - P_{out}$ = Pressure gradient
r = Radius
μ = Viscosity
L = Tube length

TABLE 4-6. Intravenous Fluid Flow Rate (through peripheral and central venous catheters)

Size of Cannula	Length (mm)	Internal Diameter (mm)	Flow Rate (mL/min)
20-gauge IV	32	0.7	54
18-gauge IV	32	0.9	104
18-gauge IV	45	0.9	90
16-gauge IV	32	1.2	220
16-gauge IV	45	1.2	186
14-gauge IV	32	1.6	302
14-gauge IV	45	1.6	288
9F sheath	100	2.5	838
IV tubing	3	3	1,030

the patient is monitored for adverse effects such as pulmonary edema. A positive clinical response to volume loading confirms volume responsiveness but does not predict further response to therapy. This can contribute to overly aggressive volume expansion and fluid excess, especially in the absence of clear resuscitation endpoints and monitoring.

PEARL

A positive clinical response to volume loading confirms volume responsiveness but does not predict further response to therapy.

Total volume requirements are difficult to predict at the onset of resuscitation and are often underestimated. Classic hypovolemia, as occurs with acute hemorrhage or fluid loss, may stabilize rapidly with appropriate volume expansion. The 3:1 rule of hemorrhage resuscitation suggests that three volumetric units of crystalloid are required to replete the extracellular fluid deficit of 1 unit of blood loss. However, experimental models demonstrate that fluid requirements in severely traumatized patients exceed the 3:1 suggestion. Pathologic vasodilation and transcapillary leak contribute to the need for ongoing volume replacement. Crystalloid requirements average 40 to 60 mL/kg in the first hours of septic shock but can be as high as 200 mL/kg to normalize perfusion parameters.[27,29]

Volume Responsiveness

The effectiveness of fluid administration in improving stroke volume depends on a number of variables, including venous tone and ventricular function. Following initial resuscitation, empiric fluid administration fails to improve macrocirculatory flow in 50% of critically ill patients.[30] Volume or preload responsiveness refers to the potential for fluid administration to augment stroke volume. Unlike an empiric volume challenge, volume responsiveness is gauged prior to fluid administration and can help determine whether fluid administration will contribute to reversing clinical hypoperfusion. Fluid loading in volume-unresponsive patients should be avoided, as it delays appropriate therapy and contributes to fluid excess with organ dysfunction, including hypoxemic respiratory failure and abdominal compartment syndrome.[2,31] Some patients remain hypoperfused despite the administration of crystalloid with an initial empiric volume greater than 40 mL/kg. In the absence of clinical hypovolemia, a more rational approach incorporates selecting and titrating subsequent therapy under the guidance of objective cardiovascular monitoring.

TABLE 4-7. Prioritized Clinical Questions and Endpoints of Goal-Directed Hemodynamic Support
1. Is volume resuscitation adequate?
Intravenous access
Evidence of volume responsiveness
2. Is systemic pressure sufficient to support major organ autoregulation?
Minimum MAP >65
Consider higher MAP goal in patients with persistent malperfusion.
3. Is oxygen delivery adequate to support organ function?
Systemic markers
Serum lactate clearance and normalization (<2 mmol/L)
$ScvO_2$ >70%
Regional markers
Cutaneous perfusion
Urine output >0.5 mL/kg/hr
Mental status

PEARL

Predicting volume responsiveness before fluid administration can identify patients likely to respond to fluid and avoids delays in appropriate therapy and fluid excess stemming from continued fluid administration in those unlikely to respond.

Predicting Volume Responsiveness

Invasive hemodynamic measurements are frequently used as surrogates of preload and predictors of volume responsiveness. Central venous pressure (CVP) monitoring is widely advocated. In the absence of conflicting data, a target CVP of 8 to 12 mm Hg is recommended to optimize preload prior to the institution of pressor and inotropic support.

Unfortunately, cardiac pressure surrogates of preload (CVP and pulmonary artery occlusion pressure) reflect the net influences of intravascular volume, venous tone, cardiac function, and intrathoracic pressure. These myriad influences confound their ability to reflect intravascular volume status or preload responsiveness in an individual patient. There is no consistent CVP threshold that reliably estimates response to fluid administration. Values considered low, normal, or high can be found in patients who respond positively to fluid.[30,32] Obstructive lung disease, positive-pressure ventilation, myocardial dysfunction, reflex venoconstriction, and erroneous measurements are examples of conditions that can elevate CVP despite hypovolemia. An increase in CVP coupled with clinical improvement following volume infusion corroborates fluid responsiveness but does not anticipate further effect.

PEARL

CVP is an unreliable surrogate for predicting volume status, preload, and response to fluid therapy.

Volumetric measures of preload, including stroke volume, right and global end-diastolic volume, and left ventricular end-diastolic area, can be obtained via several monitoring techniques. These volumetric surrogates of preload are intuitively more desirable, but they too have limited predictive value because discriminatory thresholds are imprecise and infrequent in clinical practice. Serial volumetric data in response to therapy can assist in individual patient management, but the dynamic nature of cardiovascular function during critical illness confounds their ability to predict fluid responsiveness.

Fluid responsiveness is best predicted by dynamic indices of preload reserve. Although respirophasic variation in stroke volume during positive-pressure mechanical ventilation is among the most reliable signs of preload responsiveness, it is limited by specific patient requirements. Positive-pressure ventilation induces cyclic alteration in preload. The resulting variation in left ventricular stroke volume is measured as variation in systolic pressure, pulse pressure, or ejected stroke volume using a number of devices. A variation greater than 13% identifies patients who are operating on the ascending limb of the ventricular function curve and are capable of augmenting stroke volume in response to fluid administration.[32]

Focused cardiac ultrasonography integrating biventricular function and vena cava size and collapsibility can also assist in a respiratory of volume responsiveness. In patients with shock, a respiratory variation of the inferior vena cava (IVC) greater than 50% during spontaneous breathing is generally recognized as an indicator for a safe and effective volume challenge. In contrast, minimal IVC variations are associated with supranormal CVP and a low probability of fluid responsiveness. See Chapter 22 (Bedside Ultrasound in the Critically Ill Patient) for additional information about IVC variation.

The Passive Leg Raise Test

The passive leg raise is a provocative maneuver to test whether a reversible volume challenge is capable of improving stroke volume. This is an attractive option because it provides immediate information to guide therapy without the administration of potentially unnecessary fluid. Passively raising both legs translocates blood from the lower extremities to the thorax to transiently augment preload *(Figure 4-2)*. The test is highly sensitive and specific in predicting volume responsiveness in a wide variety of situations, including ventilated and spontaneously breathing patients as well as those with irregular cardiac rhythms.[33] Volume-responsive patients show a temporary improvement in stroke volume (>15% within 3 minutes). A sensitive bedside stroke volume monitor is required to gauge the response to this maneuver.

PEARL

Respirophasic stroke volume variation is one of the most reliable tests of volume responsiveness but has specific requirements for interpretation:

- ✓ Positive-pressure ventilation (with the patient passive on the ventilator)
- ✓ Tidal volume >8 mL/kg
- ✓ Regular cardiac rhythm
- ✓ Stroke volume measurement device

Fluid Selection

The immediate goal of fluid resuscitation is vascular expansion to optimize stroke volume. Various fluid prescriptions are used for early resuscitation and the correction of fluid and electrolyte deficits. Each possesses specific benefits and disadvantages in given clinical scenarios. The composition of common resuscitation solutions is presented in Table 4-8. Randomized clinical trials of crystalloid versus colloid have not proved the clinical superiority of either; instead, they have shown comparable rates of mortality and organ function.[34,35]

Crystalloid

Isotonic sodium-based crystalloids preferentially distribute to the extracellular compartment, which includes the vascular volume. One liter of isotonic fluid distributes approximately 250 mL to the vascular compartment. This is the basis for the 3:1 rule often cited for resuscitation in acute hemorrhage. That ratio could more closely approximate 7:1 or 10:1 in patients with severe

FIGURE 4-2. Passive Leg Raise Maneuver

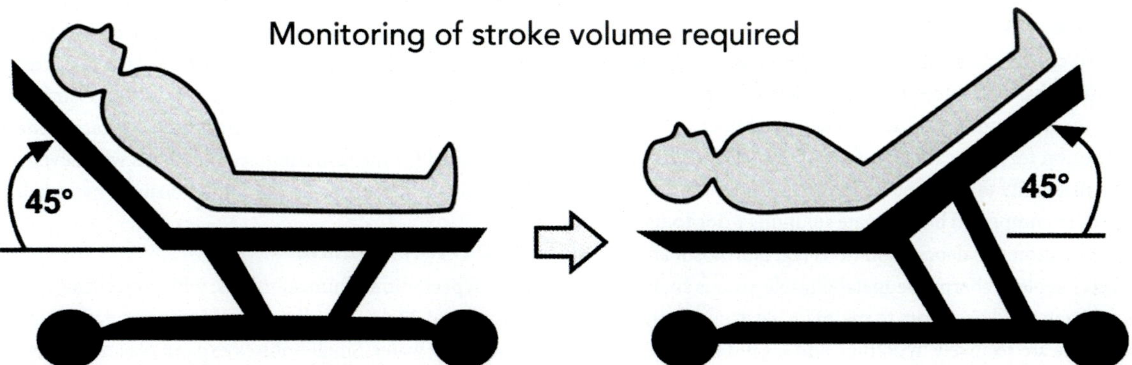

Stroke volume (SV) improvement greater than 15% is considered a positive challenge.

TABLE 4-8. Intravenous Fluid Composition

	Electrolytes (mEq/L)								
Solution	Na	Cl	HCO_3	K	Ca	Mg	Lactate	Osmolality mOsm/L	pH
Plasma	140	103	26	4	5	2		300	7.4
Crystalloid									
0.9% NaCl	154	154						308	5
Lactated Ringer's	130	109		4	2.7		28	273	6.5
Normosol R Plasma-Lyte	140	98		5		3		294	7.4
Isotonic bicarb (150 mEq NaHCO3 in 1 L water)	150		150					300	
3% NaCl	513	513						1,027	5
0.45% NaCl	77	77						154	5
0.20% NaCl	34	34						77	5
D_5W								278	4
Colloid									
6% Hetastarch (HESpan)	154	154						310	5.5
Human albumin, 5%	145	95						300	

hemorrhage, owing to decreased COP, transcapillary leak, and pathologic vasodilation. One unintended clinical consequence of ongoing fluid administration for cardiovascular support is the simultaneous evolution of tissue and pulmonary edema.

Isotonic fluid selection previously appeared less important than volume dosage titrated to an appropriate therapeutic endpoint. Although normal saline (0.9%) is the most widely used resuscitation solution, it provides a supraphysiological chloride load that induces metabolic acidosis in a dose-dependent manner.[36] This is likely more than a laboratory novelty, as growing evidence shows detrimental effects of induced hyperchloremia, including acute kidney dysfunction.[37]

Balanced Electrolyte Solutions

Balanced crystalloid solutions have a chemical composition approximating that of extracellular fluid. Lactated Ringer's and Hartmann solutions introduced lactate as a buffer to Ringer's solution for the treatment of metabolic acidosis in the 1930s. The instability of bicarbonate in plastic underlies the requirement to compound bicarbonate solutions prior to use. The new generation of balanced solutions (eg, Normosol and Plasma-Lyte) deploys alternative metabolizable anions such as lactate, acetate, and gluconate to maintain electroneutrality. Some solutions are relatively hypotonic and should be avoided if maintaining plasma osmolarity is a priority (eg, for patients with acute brain insult). Clinical concerns about inducing or exacerbating hyperkalemia as a result of potassium inclusion in these solutions are unsupported. In contrast, normal saline exacerbates hyperkalemia owing to its acidifying effect.[38] Calcium in these solutions can bind to medications and the citrated anticoagulant in blood, making them incompatible for co-administration with these agents.

The source of hypovolemia, associated electrolyte derangements, and volume requirements should influence fluid selection. The composition of balanced solutions supports their first-line use for most patients, especially those requiring large-volume resuscitation. Observational trials demonstrate fewer acid-base derangements and a lower incidence of major complications, including acute kidney injury, with the use of balanced crystalloids.[37,39] Normal saline is favored to correct the volume and electrolyte (chloride) disturbances seen in metabolic alkalosis, including those caused by a loss of gastric secretions (eg, vomiting, gastric outlet obstruction, or nasogastric suctioning). In contrast, isotonic bicarbonate is often formulated for the resuscitation of patients with severe coexisting bicarbonate-responsive metabolic acidosis or hyperkalemia.

Hypertonic Saline

Hypertonic sodium solutions, with concentrations ranging from 3% to 23.4%, rapidly expand intravascular volume by mobilizing water. Small boluses expand plasma by several times the infused volume at the expense of interstitial and intracellular fluid. The improved cardiovascular, vasoregulatory, and immunomodulating effects demonstrated in preclinical studies are not confirmed by outcomes during cardiovascular resuscitation. However, the improved and more prolonged clinical effect of hypertonic saline compared with mannitol for intracranial hypertension management favors its use in this setting.[40] Therefore, bolus dosing of 3% saline is often preferred for simultaneous intravascular expansion and cerebral osmotherapy in patients requiring attention to both issues. Multitraumatized patients are a common example, although outcome data are limited. Neurological complications such as pontine and extrapontine myelinolysis have not been reported following therapeutic use of hypertonic saline for these indications. Its use for management of hyponatremia requires vigilant monitoring to avoid overly rapid correction, a topic beyond the scope of this chapter.

Colloid

Colloid solutions are composed of electrolyte preparations fortified with large molecular-weight molecules. The presence of these large molecules contributes to COP, which favors retention of fluid in the vascular space. A vascular persistence of 12 to 24 hours makes colloids efficient volume expanders. The potency of colloid solutions on plasma volume differs with individual agents and concentrations: the higher the COP, the greater the expansion of plasma volume. Although equally effective when titrated to the same clinical endpoints, crystalloid solutions require 2 to 4 times more volume for equivalent resuscitation compared with iso-oncotic colloid. This volume-sparing effect theoretically limits interstitial and pulmonary edema. However, if endothelial integrity is disrupted following injury or illness, macromolecules might not be restricted to the vascular compartment.

Human Albumin

Human albumin is the reference colloid solution. Fractionated 4% or 5% human albumin is iso-oncotic to plasma, with more than 70% of infused volume retained within the vascular space. Use is often recommended as an adjunct for resuscitation based on the advantages outlined above, but outcome data are too limited to support the routine use of albumin over crystalloid.[34,35] Contemporary data on albumin use in specific patient populations have important implications. Albumin use in sepsis resuscitation has been associated with decreased mortality rates; however, this risk increases notably in patients with traumatic brain injuries.[41,42]

Hyperoncotic albumin solutions (20% to 25% albumin) were developed in the 1940s for the resuscitation of combat victims. Infusion of hyperoncotic albumin results in vascular expansion more than double the administered volume. In addition to the potential benefits of small-volume resuscitation, hyperoncotic albumin could offer other advantages. Antioxidant effects and synergistic interaction with administered drugs are hypothesized explanations for the reduction in morbidity and mortality linked to use in complicated hypoalbuminemic states. Examples include decompensated end-stage liver disease patients with spontaneous bacterial peritonitis, patients with hepatorenal syndrome, and those undergoing large-volume paracentesis.[44] The mobilization of interstitial edema supports hyperoncotic albumin matching with loop diuretic therapy to achieve negative fluid balance in hypoxemic respiratory failure.[45]

Semisynthetic Colloids

Semisynthetic colloids are polymerized starch solutions (eg, hydroxyethyl starch [HES], gelatin, and dextran) that were developed in response to the cost and limited supply of human albumin. The most widely used semisynthetic colloid is low molecular-weight HES. Several recent trials cast doubt on the safety of these agents because of the observed rates of nephrotoxicity and adverse outcomes.[46,47] The routine use of semisynthetic colloids is currently not recommended.

Special Circumstances

Hemorrhagic Shock

Hemorrhagic shock poses a unique clinical challenge: the timing and type of resuscitation must be balanced with the achievement of homeostasis. On one hand, hypotensive patients should be stabilized with rapid fluid infusion to maintain perfusion to essential organs. However, fluid resuscitation increases blood pressure, decreases blood viscosity, and dilutes clotting factors, which adversely impact natural hemostasis. Aggressive fluid resuscitation prior to surgical hemorrhage control can exacerbate blood loss.

Strategic limited-volume resuscitation reemerged in the 1980s when the value of early prehospital fluid resuscitation in penetrating trauma was questioned. Delayed fluid resuscitation in hypotensive patients with penetrating torso injuries reduced the rates of death and complications.[48] The detrimental effects of aggressive volume resuscitation to normalize BP in laboratory and human trials corroborate this concept.[49] Limited resuscitation with judicious use of fluids offers the optimal approach, with a conventional resuscitation ensuing after surgical hemostasis is achieved *(Table 4-9)*. The optimal degree and duration of permissive hypotension remain unclear, although current recommendations suggest a target MAP of 50 or SBP of 70 mm Hg. Patients with concomitant brain injury are not candidates for this strategy.

TABLE 4-9. Sources of Life-Threatening Hemorrhage (consider for limited volume resuscitation pending surgical control of bleeding)
Ectopic pregnancy
Gastrointestinal bleeding
Major hemoperitoneum
Major hemothorax
Penetrating torso trauma
Postpartum hemorrhage
Ruptured arterial aneurysm
Severe pelvic fracture
Traumatic aortic injury

Burn Resuscitation

Patients with second- and third-degree burns exhibit marked fluid shifts related to denuded skin, injured tissue, and a systemic inflammatory response. Aggressive fluid resuscitation is necessary to restore intravascular volume and maintain end-organ perfusion. Early anticipation of these large fluid requirements prevents underresuscitation. Initial fluid requirements are most commonly calculated according to the Parkland formula *(Table 4-10)*.

Formula calculations are based from the time of injury rather than from the time to medical attention and should incorporate prehospital fluid administration. Balanced resuscitation fluids are preferred to avoid iatrogenic metabolic acidemia from (ab)normal saline. Several formulas exist, but no single method is clearly superior. *All formulas are intended to provide an initial guide for resuscitation requirements.* The actual amount of fluid administered will vary, depending on the individual patient's status. Strict adherence to a calculated number can result in over- or underresuscitation. The over-administration of fluids is common and contributes to increased pulmonary complications and morbidity. Maintenance fluid requirements should be allocated in addition to burn formula replacement. Urine output greater than 1 mL/kg/hr is a traditional endpoint for acute burn resuscitation and may be augmented by the endpoints previously outlined *(Table 4-7)*.

TABLE 4-10. Parkland Burn Resuscitation Formula to Guide Acute Fluid Therapy

24-hour fluid requirement = 4 mL × weight (kg) × % body surface area burn.
Half of the fluid calculation is administered over the first 8 hours after injury.
The second half of the fluid calculation is administered over the subsequent 16 hours.
Maintenance fluid calculations should be added to burn resuscitation estimates.
Burn formulas estimate fluid requirements over the initial 24 hours of burn therapy.
Volume requirements may substantially exceed formula approximation.

Maintenance Fluid Therapy

In contrast to fluid resuscitation therapy, the goal of maintenance fluid is to sustain normal body fluid composition and volume. Fluid orders anticipate daily fluid requirements, ongoing losses, and coexisting electrolyte abnormalities. Although the two therapies are often ordered concurrently, daily physiological fluid requirements (true maintenance) should be consciously distinguished from therapy intended to slowly replace existing water and salt deficits.

Routine water and electrolyte maintenance needs are based on normal energy expenditure, sensible loss from urine and stool, and insensible loss from the respiratory tract and skin. Calculations assume euvolemia and are adjusted for body mass *(Table 4-11)*. In children, higher fluid requirements per kilogram are proportionate to total body water and metabolism. All maintenance prescriptions should be individualized. Energy expenditure, fluid losses, and electrolyte status vary with disease

KEY POINTS

1. Isotonic solutions maximize extracellular, including vascular, fluid retention and are indicated for volume resuscitation, regardless of accompanying electrolyte and water deficits.
2. Although hypotension should always be considered pathological, normotension does not guarantee normal perfusion.
3. Transient hypotension is an important clue to recognize, as it is associated with adverse outcomes and often heralds further hemodynamic deterioration in the absence of intervention.
4. Shock is defined by inadequate tissue perfusion, not systemic blood pressure.
5. Most patients requiring resuscitation initially present in compensated shock with normotension.
6. Normalization of vital signs does not ensure cardiovascular wellness or the completion of resuscitation.
7. A combination of global and regional targets should be used to guide the adequacy of therapy during resuscitation.
8. The solution to persistent malperfusion following initial fluid resuscitation is complex; hemodynamic monitoring is warranted to guide therapy.
9. In the absence of overt clinical hypovolemia, volume responsiveness should not be assumed and is best gauged by dynamic hemodynamic indices.
10. The targeted endpoint used to guide the dose of fluid resuscitation is more important than the individual fluid product (eg, crystalloid versus colloid) selection.
11. Isotonic crystalloids remain the standard initial resuscitation fluid and offer a significant cost advantage over colloid.
12. The choice of fluid should be individualized to normalize accompanying acid-base and electrolyte disturbances.
13. Despite its name, 0.9% normal saline is not a physiological fluid.
14. Balanced crystalloid solutions are recommended for fluid resuscitation in acute critical illness.

TABLE 4-11. Maintenance Fluid Estimate

Body Weight (kg)	Daily Maintenance	Hourly Maintenance
1–10	100 mL/kg	5 mL/kg/hour
10–20	1,000 mL plus 50 mL/kg	2 mL/kg/hour plus 40 mL
20–80	1,500 mL plus 20 mL/kg*	1 mL/kg/hour plus 60 mL

*To a maximum of 2,400 mL/day or 100 mL/hour
Sodium and chloride: 2 to 3 mEq/100 mL water
Potassium: 1 to 2 mEq/100 mL water
D5 ¼ normal saline with 20 mEq KCl is a common maintenance solution for most euvolemic pediatric patients and provides 20% of daily calories at routine maintenance rates. Comorbid conditions and/or electrolyte abnormalities may necessitate modification.

and dictate rate and electrolyte modifications. For example, exfoliative skin disease, increased work of breathing, and fever enhance insensible loss. Measurable nasogastric, fistula, ostomy, and urinary drainage can be estimated or replaced by drainage volume. The limitation of fluid and potassium is an important disease-specific modification for patients with renal insufficiency.

Hypotonic solutions with or without dextrose and potassium are popular fixed-combination maintenance solutions. Hospitalized patients often suffer from impaired free-water excretion due to a release of nonosmotic antidiuretic hormone, making them vulnerable to hyponatremia. The serum sodium concentration provides a simple and accurate marker of hydration status. Isotonic maintenance solutions should be considered in patients, including children, with a serum sodium concentration less than 138 mEq/L. Glucose infusions are best formulated by adding dextrose to an electrolyte solution (eg, Ringer's lactate, Normosol, normal saline, 0.45 normal saline, or 0.2 normal saline) rather than using 5% dextrose.

Conclusion

Fluid therapy is provided to virtually all acutely critically ill patients. Isotonic crystalloids remain the standard initial resuscitation fluid. Growing evidence of the advantages of balanced electrolyte solutions supports their use over normal saline, especially for patients requiring large-volume resuscitation. Normalization of vital signs does not guarantee adequate resuscitation. Rather, targeted endpoints, including clinical perfusion and lactate clearance, are useful to gauge the adequacy of resuscitation. For patients who remain in shock following initial empiric fluid resuscitation, dynamic markers of volume responsiveness should be deployed to guide further therapy.

REFERENCES

1. Jones AE, Brown MD, Trzeciak S, et al. The effect of a quantitative resuscitation strategy on mortality in patients with sepsis: a meta-analysis. *Crit Care Med.* 2008;36(10):2734-2739.
2. Wiedemann HP, Wheeler AP, Bernard GR, et al. Comparison of two fluid-management strategies in acute lung injury. *N Engl J Med.* 2006;354(24):2564-2575.
3. Murphy CV, Schramm GE, Doherty JA, et al. The importance of fluid management in acute lung injury secondary to septic shock. *Chest.* 2009;136(1):102-109.
4. Jones AE, Yiannibas V, Johnson C, Kline JA. Emergency department hypotension predicts sudden unexpected in-hospital mortality: a prospective cohort study. *Chest.* 2006;130(4):941-946.
5. Jones AE, Aborn LS, Kline JA. Severity of emergency department hypotension predicts adverse hospital outcome. *Shock.* 2004;22(5):410-414.
6. Edwards M, Ley E, Mirocha J, et al. Defining hypotension in moderate to severely injured trauma patients: raising the bar for the elderly. *Am Surg.* 2010;76(10):1035-1038.
7. Oyetunji TA, Chang DC, Crompton JG, et al. Redefining hypotension in the elderly: normotension is not reassuring. *Arch Surg.* 2011;146(7):865-869.
8. McGee S, Abernethy WB III, Simel DL. The rational clinical examination. Is this patient hypovolemic? *JAMA.* 1999;281(11):1022-1029.
9. Carlson JE. Assessment of orthostatic blood pressure: measurement technique and clinical applications. *South Med J.* 1999;92(2):167-173.
10. Demetriades D, Chan LS, Bhasin P, et al. Relative bradycardia in patients with traumatic hypotension. *J Trauma.* 1998;45(3):534-539.
11. Hick JL, Rodgerson JD, Heegaard WG, Sterner S. Vital signs fail to correlate with hemoperitoneum from ruptured ectopic pregnancy. *Am J Emerg Med.* 2001;19(6):488-491.
12. Rady MY, Rivers EP, Nowak RM. Resuscitation of the critically ill in the ED: responses of blood pressure, heart rate, shock index, central venous oxygen saturation, and lactate. *Am J Emerg Med.* 1996;14(2):218-225.
13. Birkhahn RH, Gaeta TJ, Terry D, et al. Shock index in diagnosing early acute hypovolemia. *Am J Emerg Med.* 2005;23(3):323-326.
14. Kaplan LJ, McPartland K, Santora TA, Trooskin SZ. Start with a subjective assessment of skin temperature to identify hypoperfusion in intensive care unit patients. *J Trauma.* 2001;50(4):620-627.
15. Schey BM, Williams DY, Bucknall T. Skin temperature and core-peripheral temperature gradient as markers of hemodynamic status in critically ill patients: a review. Heart Lung. 2010;39(1):27-40.
16. Jayanthi NV, Dabke HV. The effect of IV cannula length on the rate of infusion. *Injury.* 2006;37(1):41-45.
17. Stoneham MD. An evaluation of methods of increasing the flow rate of i.v. fluid administration. *Br J Anaesth.* 1995;75(3):361-365.
18. Jansen TC, van BJ, Schoonderbeek FJ, et al. Early lactate-guided therapy in intensive care unit patients: a multicenter, open-label, randomized controlled trial. *Am J Respir Crit Care Med.* 2010;182(6):752-761.
19. LeDoux D, Astiz ME, Carpati CM, Rackow EC. Effects of perfusion pressure on tissue perfusion in septic shock. *Crit Care Med.* 2000;28(8):2729-2732.
20. Wo CC, Shoemaker WC, Appel PL, et al. Unreliability of blood pressure and heart rate to evaluate cardiac output in emergency resuscitation and critical illness. *Crit Care Med.* 1993;21(2):218-223.
21. Rivers E, Nguyen B, Havstad S, et al. Early goal-directed therapy in the treatment of severe sepsis and septic shock. *N Engl J Med.* 2001;345(19):1368-1377.
22. Nichol AD, Egi M, Pettila V, et al. Relative hyperlactatemia and hospital mortality in critically ill patients: a retrospective multi-centre study. *Crit Care.* 2010;14(1):R25.
23. Howell MD, Donnino M, Clardy P, et al. Occult hypoperfusion and mortality in patients with suspected infection. *Intensive Care Med.* 2007;33(11):1892-1899.
24. Nguyen HB, Rivers EP, Knoblich BP, et al. Early lactate clearance is associated with improved outcome in severe sepsis and septic shock. *Crit Care Med.* 2004;32(8):1637-1642.
25. Puskarich MA, Trzeciak S, Shapiro NI, et al. Whole blood lactate kinetics in patients undergoing quantitative resuscitation for severe sepsis and septic shock. *Chest.* 2013;143(6):1548-1553.
26. Pope JV, Jones AE, Gaieski DF, et al. Multicenter study of central venous oxygen saturation (ScvO(2)) as a predictor of mortality in patients with sepsis. *Ann Emerg Med.* 2010;55(1):40-46.
27. Peake SL, Delaney A, Bailey M, et al. Goal-directed resuscitation for patients with early septic shock. *N Engl J Med.* 2014;371(16):1496-1506.
28. Yealy DM, Kellum JA, Huang DT, et al. A randomized trial of protocol-based care for early septic shock. *N Engl J Med.* 2014;370(18):1683-1693.
29. Carcillo JA, Davis AL, Zaritsky A. Role of early fluid resuscitation in pediatric septic shock. *JAMA.* 1991;266(9):1242-1245.
30. Michard F, Teboul JL. Predicting fluid responsiveness in ICU patients: a critical analysis of the evidence. *Chest.* 2002;121(6):2000-2008.
31. Balogh Z, McKinley BA, Cocanour CS, et al. Supranormal trauma resuscitation causes more cases of abdominal compartment syndrome. *Arch Surg.* 2003;138(6):637-642.
32. Marik PE, Baram M, Vahid B. Does central venous pressure predict fluid responsiveness? A systematic review of the literature and the tale of seven mares. *Chest.* 2008;134(1):172-178.
33. Monnet X, Rienzo M, Osman D, et al. Passive leg raising predicts fluid responsiveness in the critically ill. *Crit Care Med.* 2006;34(5):1402-1407.
34. Finfer S, Bellomo R, Boyce N, et al. A comparison of albumin and saline for fluid resuscitation in the intensive care unit. *N Engl J Med.* 2004;350(22):2247-2256.
35. Perel P, Roberts I, Ker K. Colloids versus crystalloids for fluid resuscitation in critically ill patients. *Cochrane Database Syst Rev.* 2013;2:CD000567.
36. Yunos NM, Kim IB, Bellomo R, et al. The biochemical effects of restricting chloride-rich fluids in intensive care. *Crit Care Med.* 2011;39(11):2419-2424.
37. Yunos NM, Bellomo R, Hegarty C, et al. Association between a chloride-liberal vs chloride-restrictive intravenous fluid administration strategy and kidney injury in critically ill adults. *JAMA.* 2012;308(15):1566-1572.
38. O'Malley CM, Frumento RJ, Hardy MA, et al. A randomized, double-blind comparison of lactated Ringer's solution and 0.9% NaCl during renal transplantation. *Anesth Analg.* 2005;100(5):1518-24, table.
39. Shaw AD, Bagshaw SM, Goldstein SL, et al. Major complications, mortality, and resource utilization after open abdominal surgery: 0.9% saline compared to Plasma-Lyte. *Ann Surg.* 2012;255(5):821-829.

40. Marko NF. Hypertonic saline, not mannitol, should be considered gold-standard medical therapy for intracranial hypertension. *Crit Care.* 2012;16(1):113.
41. Delaney AP, Dan A, McCaffrey J, Finfer S. The role of albumin as a resuscitation fluid for patients with sepsis: a systematic review and meta-analysis. *Crit Care Med.* 2011;39(2):386-391.
42. Rochwerg B, Alhazzani W, Sindi A, et al. Fluid resuscitation in sepsis: a systematic review and network meta-analysis. *Ann Intern Med.* 2014;161(5):347-355.
43. Myburgh J, Cooper DJ, Finfer S, et al. Saline or albumin for fluid resuscitation in patients with traumatic brain injury. *N Engl J Med.* 2007;357(9):874-884.
44. Sort P, Navasa M, Arroyo V, et al. Effect of intravenous albumin on renal impairment and mortality in patients with cirrhosis and spontaneous bacterial peritonitis. *N Engl J Med.* 1999;341(6):403-409.
45. Martin GS, Moss M, Wheeler AP, et al. A randomized, controlled trial of furosemide with or without albumin in hypoproteinemic patients with acute lung injury. *Crit Care Med.* 2005;33(8):1681-1687.
46. Perner A, Haase N, Guttormsen AB, et al. Hydroxyethyl starch 130/0.42 versus Ringer's acetate in severe sepsis. *N Engl J Med.* 2012;367(2):124-134.
47. Myburgh JA, Finfer S, Bellomo R, et al. Hydroxyethyl starch or saline for fluid resuscitation in intensive care. *N Engl J Med.* 2012;367(20):1901-1911.
48. Bickell WH, Wall MJ Jr, Pepe PE, et al. Immediate versus delayed fluid resuscitation for hypotensive patients with penetrating torso injuries. *N Engl J Med.* 1994;331(17):1105-1109.
49. Morrison CA, Carrick MM, Norman MA, et al. Hypotensive resuscitation strategy reduces transfusion requirements and severe postoperative coagulopathy in trauma patients with hemorrhagic shock: preliminary results of a randomized controlled trial. *J Trauma.* 2011;70(3):652-663.

Cardiac Arrest Updates

5

IN THIS CHAPTER

- General Management Considerations
- Circulatory Support
- Defibrillation
- Airway and Oxygenation
- Pharmacotherapy
- Systems Issues
- Future Directions

Joshua C. Reynolds and Benjamin J. Lawner

Out-of-hospital cardiac arrest (OHCA) represents a profound clinical and public health challenge, both in the United States and across the globe. Cardiovascular disease, which accounts for one-third of all US deaths, is the most common cause of OHCA.[1]

The overall occurrence of OHCA is highest in Australia (113:100,000), but its incidence from presumed cardiac cause is highest in North America (55:100,000).[2] These events are more likely to stem from cardiac disease in patients older than 35 years, and are more commonly attributable to "noncardiac" causes in patients younger than 35 years.[3] In fact, 83% of cardiac arrests occurring in patients younger than 19 years are noncardiac in origin.[4] Health care providers are notoriously inaccurate in predicting the cause of OHCA, often underestimating noncardiac etiologies.[5,6]

Epidemiological data from a large 10-site North American resuscitation research consortium has demonstrated marked regional variations in OHCA-related outcomes.[7] The median rate of survival to hospital discharge of cardiac arrest victims treated by emergency medical services (EMS) personnel is 8.4% (IQR: 5.4%, 10.4%), with rates ranging from 3.0% to 16.3%. This percentage is significantly higher in patients with ventricular fibrillation (VF) as the initial rhythm. The median rate of survival to hospital discharge in this subpopulation is 22.0% (IQR: 15.0%, 24.4%), with rates ranging from 7.7% to 39.9% across the same geographical locales.

Resuscitation science has evolved greatly since the inception of cardiopulmonary resuscitation (CPR). Guidelines for cardiac arrest resuscitation are updated every 5 years by the International Liaison Committee on Resuscitation (ILCOR), which provides treatment recommendations based on available evidence and expert opinion. ILCOR guidelines then are funneled through national and regional associations (eg, the American Heart Association [AHA]) and packaged as educational curricula (eg, basic life support [BLS] or advanced cardiac life support [ACLS]).

Emergency care providers and others tasked with leading resuscitation efforts must be aware of the source material for these curricula and understand the controversies, paradigms, and accumulated evidence behind the latest recommendations.

> **PEARL**
>
> A cardiac cause of cardiac arrest is more likely in patients over 35 years of age.

General Considerations

Cardiac arrest is a dynamic disease. Few other clinical presentations strain the leadership abilities of the emergency care provider to the same degree. Astute clinicians must realize, however, that they are orchestrating only one portion of a larger series of events, each of which directly affects patient outcomes. The achievement of return of spontaneous circulation (ROSC) is only one piece of this resuscitation puzzle.

Layperson recognition of cardiac arrest, activation of the EMS system, and provision of bystander CPR are equally important. In addition, the critical care, inpatient, and rehabilitation phases of treatment play crucial roles in patient survival. This overarching view of cardiac arrest care is embodied in the success of bundled postresuscitation care packages that improve outcomes among patients attaining ROSC.[8]

Circulatory Support

Pit Crew CPR

Prompt and effective cardiac arrest management can be difficult in the hectic and potentially austere environments in which it is required. To orchestrate efficient and effective resuscitation, regimented training and good working relationships between care providers are vitally important. "Pit crew" CPR (*Figure 5-1*) is an effective strategy for controlling the chaos of resuscitation, which — when bundled into a larger cardiac arrest management plan — can improve patient outcomes.[9]

Just as in motor sports, this technique is centered on a core group of providers with preassigned roles. The responsibility of each caregiver is determined by his or her location and proximity to the patient. For example, the provider at the head is always in charge of the airway, and the provider near the patient's left shoulder is always tasked with chest compressions. This concept is similar to strategies employed by trauma resuscitation teams.

Mechanical Devices

The management of human factors is one of the most challenging aspects of cardiac arrest resuscitation. With the proliferation of mechanical resuscitation devices, it is tempting to offload certain repetitive tasks to free up additional resources. Chest compressions and ventilations, for example, require a sizable investment of personnel and are prone to a great degree of interoperator variability in quality and effectiveness.

When working together, a mechanical chest compression device and ventilator can deliver sustained, uninterrupted, quality compressions and ventilations without deviating from specified parameters. This essentially eliminates the cognitive burden of constantly verifying the quality of procedure "performance," allowing the resuscitation leader to focus on detecting and addressing reversible causes. The feasibility of using mechanical CPR as a bridge to computed tomography (CT), cardiac catheterization, and percutaneous cannulation for extracorporeal membranous oxygenation (ECMO) is well demonstrated.[10-13]

PEARLS

- ✓ Consider offloading repetitive tasks to machines.
- ✓ When considering advanced diagnostic or interventional maneuvers, use a piston-driven or load-distributing band device when performing chest compressions.

The most common devices use either a piston or compression band system to decrease the volume of the thoracic cavity, pushing blood throughout the body. Designed to deliver efficient mechanized compressions comparable to those performed in manual CPR, these tools are timed to work in a 30:2 ratio or at rates suggested by the AHA. In select patients, mechanical CPR devices afford the opportunity for truly astounding resuscitations; however, the same benefits have not been observed in the general cardiac arrest population.[14]

A number of studies have been performed to evaluate these devices, but it should be noted that many were sponsored by manufacturers. Studies evaluating CPR metrics, including end-tidal carbon dioxide measurements, cerebral blood flow, and coronary perfusion pressure, demonstrate better results with mechanical CPR devices than with manual methods.[15-17] Randomized trials and a meta-analysis found a slight trend toward higher rates of ROSC but failed to show an outcome benefit for either technique.[18-21]

Application time appears to be the biggest issue with mechanical methods.[22,23] In most cases, a hands-off period is needed when applying the device; for an untrained rescuer, this could lead to significant time without compressions. Virtually every manufactured device has some posterior component that demands halting compressions to allow proper placement.

FIGURE 5-1. Pit Crew Model Positional Assignments

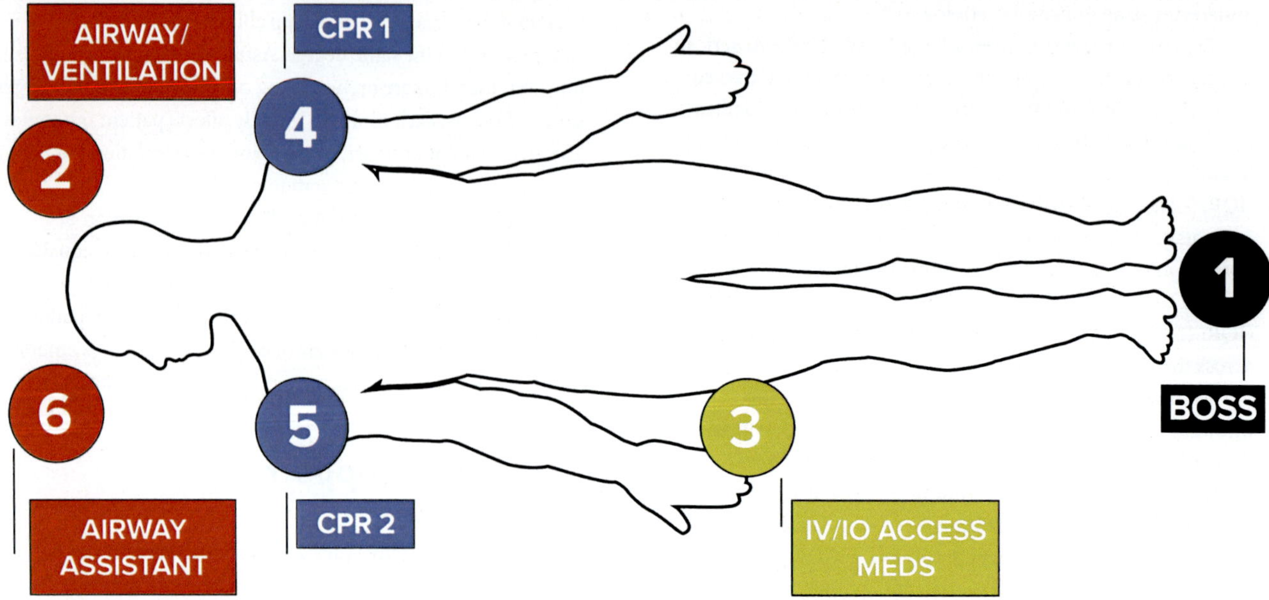

Although a number of device-related injuries have been reported, they have not been associated with untoward results.[24] Not surprisingly, most of these injuries are similar to those seen with manual CPR (eg, rib fractures, sternal fractures, liver lacerations, and pulmonary contusions). However, these tools typically are applied after some duration of manual CPR, so it is difficult to attribute specific injuries to the equipment alone.

Mechanical devices appear to provide benefit in prolonged resuscitations, during which providers tire; in situations where manual CPR is dangerous or not feasible; and as a bridge to percutaneous coronary intervention (PCI) or mechanical support.[21,25-27] There is no evidence for their routine use in the undifferentiated cardiac arrest patient.

Compression-Only CPR

Compression-only or hands-only CPR solely employs the chest compression portion of traditional CPR. The AHA suggests this method for lay rescuers, since it is simpler and better received by most people.[28] Reports are mixed regarding the efficacy of compression-only CPR performed by professional rescuers and hospital personnel. Some observational studies have suggested that patients whose cardiac arrest stems from a noncardiac cause might fare better with traditional CPR, whereas others report no difference in outcomes between the two techniques.[29-32] Although data regarding the need for rescue breaths are inconsistent, there is consensus on the need for prompt, effective chest compressions with limited interruptions — a point emphasized by current CPR guidelines.

Continuous CPR

The primary arguments for continuous chest compressions are similar to those for compression-only CPR. The term *continuous chest compressions* usually refers to the initial period of resuscitation, most notably the first 4 to 6 minutes following the loss of pulses. During this initial phase, myocardial and cerebral tissue is most sensitive to decreased blood flow; hypoperfusion during this fragile window will lead to worse outcomes.

It has been well demonstrated that any interruption in chest compressions — even a brief pause for ventilation — decreases coronary perfusion pressure and forward blood flow, which are vital to the heart and brain.[33] Quality, uninterrupted compressions not only perfuse vital organs, but also improve the probability of successful defibrillation. The combination of uninterrupted compressions and a minimal "preshock pause" may improve defibrillation success and neurological outcomes.[34]

When engaged in continuous compressions, care providers are prevented from employing advanced airway maneuvers or other interventions. The necessary distraction can dilute the focus on quality, minimally interrupted compressions and — at worst — can put patients at risk. A number of studies have questioned the use of advanced airways in cardiac arrest patients during the prehospital phase of care, a strategy that has been linked to poor outcomes.[36-38] Preclinical studies have found that even the two breaths given during a conventional 30:2 compression cycle increase intrathoracic pressures, decrease venous return, and reduce blood flow to the heart and brain.[39] While controversy continues about the best compression-to-breath ratio with a BLS or native airway, continuous compressions (>100 per minute) should be administered after placement of an advanced airway.

Defibrillation

Energy Selection

The original defibrillator was little more than a simple pair of electrodes that conducted 110 volts of alternating current through the exposed heart. Modern external defibrillators are available in a variety of designs with proprietary waveforms (eg, biphasic truncated exponential, pulsed biphasic, rectilinear biphasic, damped sinusoid monophasic, and monophasic truncated exponential) specific to the manufacturer. Most current models employ biphasic waveforms, which require less energy to terminate VF and improve first shock success.[40,41]

Clinicians should be familiar with the defibrillators available to them and the manufacturers' recommendations for use. The suggested energy for biphasic defibrillation depends on the manufacturer, varying between 150 and 360 joules.[43,44] However, concerns have arisen regarding the effectiveness of the recommended first shock energies, prompting some prehospital agencies to implement a "highest dose first" strategy.

Timing of Shock Delivery

Early defibrillation historically has been considered a key link in the "chain of survival" for its vitally important role in minimizing the interval until ROSC.[45] However, research suggests that defibrillating a myocardium depleted of high-energy phosphates may increase the incidence of post-defibrillation asystole — an observation that begs the question: should chest compressions be performed prior to defibrillation to restore high-energy phosphates and "prime" the myocardium?[46-48] Three studies designed to address this question have produced conflicting results. Two failed to demonstrate any benefit of CPR prior to defibrillation, but a third showed a survival benefit in a subgroup of patients for whom EMS response exceeded 4 minutes.[49-51] A 2011 international randomized trial involving nearly 10,000 patients failed to show a difference in the ability of the two strategies to improve survival rates with good neurological outcomes.[52]

Minimizing Peri-Shock Pauses

The peri-shock pause begins when compressions are stopped to allow defibrillation and ends when compressions are resumed *(Figure 5-2)*. Logistically, this period often includes a rhythm assessment, charging the defibrillator, delivering the defibrillation, and waiting for instructions to resume chest compressions.

The duration of the peri-shock pause is inversely associated with both ROSC and survival; it should be minimized as much as possible.[53] Reductions in the use of this strategy, particularly the preshock component (ie, for rhythm analysis and defibrillator charging), increase the likelihood of survival.[54]

The pit crew-style CPR techniques endorsed by the American Heart Association, including the "Seattle Switch" protocol *(Table 5-1)*, directly address the peri-shock pause. Care providers should communicate with each other to ensure that the device is charging while a compression cycle is finishing. Additionally, using a monitor defibrillator in "manual" mode (as opposed to "AED" mode) may help reduce the preshock pause and improve ROSC.

The primary activities during the postshock pause are rhythm and pulse checks after defibrillation. Notably, myocardial stunning is very common in the period after ROSC.[55] Even if successfully defibrillated, patients might be hypotensive initially, with weak or absent peripheral pulses. Furthermore, interrupting compressions to perform pulse checks may decrease a patient's odds of survival.[56] It is prudent to immediately follow a defibrillation attempt with an additional cycle (2 minutes) of chest compressions to minimize the postshock pause.[57] The pit-crew techniques discussed above can help facilitate coordination between the care providers.

Hands-on defibrillation — essentially continuing compressions while a shock is administered — is an alternative technique for eliminating the peri-shock pause altogether. A compelling study of patients undergoing elective cardioversion with a biphasic defibrillator demonstrated that rescuers, protected only by standard polyethylene gloves, could be in contact with the chest without exposure to dangerous levels of current.[58] Subsequent preclinical investigations have yielded conflicting results about the level of current to which caregivers are exposed; further study is necessary to determine the safety of this technique over the range of conditions encountered during resuscitation.[59,60]

Double-Sequence Defibrillation

In some cases of refractory fibrillation, successful restoration of a perfusing rhythm has been achieved through double-sequential defibrillation (ie, the discharge of two defibrillators nearly simultaneously [*Figure 5-3*]). The technique first was described in the electrophysiology lab as a strategy for terminating persistent atrial fibrillation. Since then, it has been used with some success in correcting out-of-hospital VF.[61,62]

PEARL

- ✓ Increased lengths of peri-shock pause are negatively associated with patient survival rates.
- ✓ Be careful and creative in choosing logistic maneuvers so as to minimize hands-off time.

Airway

Adjuncts

The two airway adjuncts most commonly available are oropharyngeal and nasopharyngeal devices — both of which have a long history of use, despite the lack of research supporting their utility in human CPR. In typical cases, the insertion of these noninvasive airway adjuncts will maximize the seal during positive-pressure ventilation and mitigate any obstruction caused by the patient's tongue and oropharyngeal structures. However, inadvertent intracranial insertion of a nasopharyngeal airway has been reported in patients with basal skull fractures.[63,64]

Cricoid Pressure

Cricoid pressure originally was proposed to reduce gastric inflation during ventilation with a bag-valve-mask (BVM); however, the studies that demonstrated its benefits used much higher tidal volumes than those currently recommended.[65,66] More recent research shows that cricoid pressure hampers

FIGURE 5-2. Schematic of Peri-Shock Pause

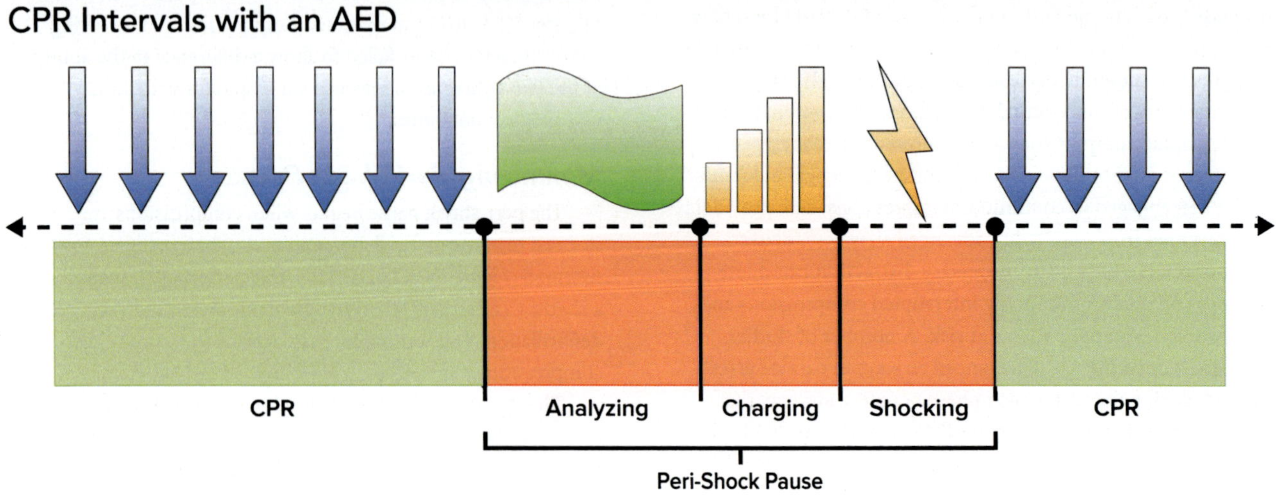

TABLE 5-1. The Seattle Switch Procedure

1. At the 1:45 mark, begin thinking about the next defibrillation. Tip: if doing 30:2, the heart rhythm can be seen during ventilations.
2. Ask aloud, "Who is next on chest compressions?" That individual should line up behind the rescuer doing CPR.
3. Precharge the defibrillator without interrupting chest compressions.
4. As soon as the defibrillator begins charging, the BVM should be removed from the patient's face.
5. Once the defibrillator has charged, announce "Stop CPR."
6. The provider doing chest compressions should clear out of the way (this is the start of the peri-shock pause).
7. The provider on the monitor should quickly verify that the rhythm is shockable and press "shock."
8. Once the shock has been delivered (or if the rhythm is nonshockable), announce, "Continue CPR."
9. A new rescuer should start compressions (this is the end of the peri-shock pause and the start of a new 2-minute cycle).
10. IVs, drugs, and advanced airway procedures are acceptable, provided they do not interfere with expertly performed BLS!
11. Once an advanced airway is in place, deliver asynchronous ventilations every 6 seconds (that's slow).
12. If the patient fails to respond to pit crew CPR (>5 cycles and still no ROSC), consider switching to another resuscitation system.

the placement of both supraglottic and endotracheal airways, and hinders laryngeal mask airway placement and subsequent ventilation.[67-74] The method also increases the time to intubation and reduces laryngoscopic views.[67-82] Cricoid pressure should not be applied routinely during airway management in cardiac arrest.

Advanced Airways

Prehospital advanced airway management is a controversial topic beyond the scope of this chapter. There is no clear evidence of its benefit, and the incidence of adverse events during intubation attempts becomes unacceptably high when prehospital personnel do not receive active, ongoing skill training.[35, 83-88] Whether in the prehospital setting or in the emergency department, prolonged attempts at advanced airway management unnecessarily interrupt chest compressions, especially when acceptable alternatives are available. Evidence is mixed regarding the optimal timing of advanced airway management during cardiac arrest resuscitation; however, earlier airway management (<5 minutes) has been associated with an improved rate of 24-hour survival.[89]

Intubations performed less than 12 minutes into the resuscitation have been associated with better survival rates than those initiated after 13 minutes.[90] However, a bundled protocol that includes delayed intubation, passive oxygen delivery via nonrebreather mask during CPR, and minimally interrupted chest compressions appears to improve neurological survival to hospital discharge in adults with witnessed OHCA who present with a shockable rhythm.[91]

Supraglottic airways are acceptable alternatives to endotracheal intubation during cardiac arrest resuscitation. Ventilation through a variety of these devices results in similar arterial blood gas values compared with traditional BVM ventilation.[92,93] Additionally, ventilation through a laryngeal mask airway results in less regurgitation (3.5%) than ventilation with a bag-valve-mask (12.4%).[94]

Supraglottic airways perform as well as, or better than, endotracheal intubation in terms of insertion success, time to insertion, and ventilation parameters.[95-103] They also can serve as rescue devices for difficult/failed intubations in cardiac arrest; however, their routine use, especially in cases of prehospital cardiac arrest, is discouraged.[96,97,101,104-109] One retrospective study comparing endotracheal intubation with an esophageal-tracheal Combitube found no difference in the rates of ROSC or survival.[102] A 2013 Japanese study of more than 600,000 OHCA events independently linked advanced airway management via endotracheal tube or supraglottic device to worsened neurological outcomes.[37]

Another retrospective study of more than 10,000 cardiac arrest cases found survival was highest among patients receiving airway management via bag-valve-mask. The worst neurological outcomes were found in those who were ventilated with a supraglottic device.[36] Given the mixed evidence related to optimal airway management in cardiac arrest, a randomized pragmatic trial of airway management in OHCA (supraglottic airway vs. endotracheal intubation) recently was initiated (NIH: 8793277).

Regardless of the airway management strategy employed, confirmation of advanced airway placement is crucial. The best available standard is continuous waveform capnography, which has 100% sensitivity and 100% specificity in cardiac arrest.[112,113] If this modality is unavailable, the combination of a colorimetric end-tidal carbon dioxide (CO_2) detector and clinical assessment is an acceptable alternative. When arrest occurs secondary to a suspected cardiac cause, advanced airway management does not appear to confer a distinct advantage over less invasive techniques such as bag-valve-mask ventilation. Indeed, important considerations with respect to initial airway management include avoiding interruptions in compressions and achieving airway patency.

Oxygenation

Current convention dictates oxygenating with 100% fraction of inspired oxygen (FiO_2) during CPR, although preclinical animal research suggests that the higher percentage results in worse neurological outcomes than 21% FiO_2.

Passive oxygenation is one technique that can help

minimize interruptions in chest compressions. It is predicated on cycles of successive chest wall compressions and recoil that generate passive airflow while applying high-flow oxygen via a nonrebreather mask. If the tidal volumes generated are greater than the dead space, oxygenated air is moved into the lungs. If these volumes are insufficient, however, the turbulent mixing of air can result in molecular diffusion and subsequent gas exchange (much like the effects seen in high-frequency oscillatory ventilation).

FIGURE 5-3. Pad Placement for Double-Sequence Defibrillation

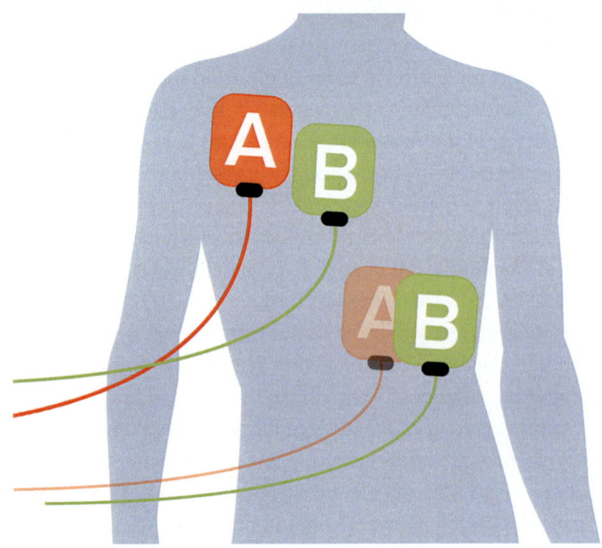

A simplified cardiac arrest protocol consisting of passive oxygenation via a nonrebreather mask and continuous chest compressions has been shown to improve rates of neurologically intact survival to hospital discharge in adults with witnessed cardiac arrest and a shockable initial rhythm.[114,115]

Ventilation

The human data on ventilation parameters during CPR focus solely on respiratory rate and do not address minute ventilation or peak inspiratory pressure. The ventilatory rate frequently is too high during cardiac arrest resuscitation, and the use of real-time CPR feedback devices results in ventilation rates closer to those recommended in the guidelines.[50] Preliminary animal studies have associated hyperventilation with diminished hemodynamics and survival, but there are no human studies to support the avoidance of hyperventilation.[39]

End-tidal carbon dioxide monitoring is a noninvasive method of obtaining physiological feedback during resuscitation; increases in CO_2 values typically herald ROSC.[116,117] Additionally, values greater than 10 mm Hg during CPR are associated with ROSC, whereas those below 10 mm Hg may predict nonsurvival.[118-124] End-tidal CO_2 has not been evaluated specifically as a tool to guide resuscitation interventions in real time.

Pharmacotherapy

General Principles

There is a shifting deemphasis on pharmacological interventions based on a growing body of literature that acknowledges short-term improvements in ROSC but has yet to demonstrate long-term benefits. This lack of treatment effect in clinical studies is in contrast to the benefits observed in preclinical animal trials.[125] Pharmacotherapy in cardiac arrest originated from a canine model of VF in the 1960s, in which animals receiving epinephrine demonstrated an improved survival rate. The use of epinephrine primarily was intended to boost systemic vascular resistance, leading to increased cardiac preload, thus augmenting the ability of CPR to produce coronary perfusion pressure and end-organ perfusion.[126] Human investigations have found the same improvements in ROSC or short-term survival, but no resuscitation medication ever has been linked to improvements in survival to hospital discharge or favorable neurological outcomes.

Epinephrine

Despite nearly 50 years of continuous clinical use, there is equipoise regarding epinephrine for cardiac arrest. In recent years, the medication has been associated with lower survival rates and poor neurological outcomes.[127-130] Speculation about the cause of these unfavorable long-term effects centers on compromised microvascular perfusion, beta-adrenergic-mediated toxicity, and the futility of transient survival in otherwise nonviable patients.[131]

The first study to directly investigate the use of epinephrine was a 2009 randomized controlled trial of IV line placement during resuscitation. Patients who received an infusion of the drug experienced a higher rate of ROSC (40%) compared with those who did not (25%); however, the rates of survival to discharge at 1 year did not differ between the groups.[132] A post-hoc analysis of epinephrine administration yielded a negative association between the drug and good neurological outcomes.[133] A more recent propensity-matched, population-based study of more than 400,000 Japanese patients also linked the prehospital administration of epinephrine to an improved rate of ROSC but a decreased rate of survival to hospital discharge with favorable neurological outcomes.[134]

Critics of this work point out variability in the dosing of epinephrine, the timing of its administration, and the post-arrest care of resuscitated patients. The standard dose of epinephrine used in resuscitation (1 mg or 0.05–0.1 mg/kg) was originally derived from a study of 20- to 30-kg dogs. This dose is tremendously supraphysiological and roughly 1,000 times the maximum dose used as a vasopressor in the resuscitation of patients in shock. Several studies in the 1990s explored even higher doses of epinephrine (3–5 mg).[136-139] Not surprisingly, most found no improvement in long-term survival. A lower dose (<1 mg) might mitigate concerns regarding toxicity and microvascular compromise.[131]

Two recent retrospective studies addressed the timing of

epinephrine administration. In one cohort of more than 3,000 patients who were stratified by the first documented cardiac rhythm, those who received epinephrine within 10 minutes after the emergency call had a higher survival rate and better neurological outcomes than those who received the drug after 10 minutes.[140] Similarly, another study reported improved rates of ROSC and survival if epinephrine was administered within 10 minutes after the onset of cardiac arrest.[141] Although the original observational studies of epinephrine were conducted before the era of therapeutic hypothermia and protocolized postarrest care, follow-up studies have addressed these concerns, yielding similar results.[133,134] A robust, randomized, placebo-controlled trial of epinephrine in cardiac arrest is urgently warranted.

Vasopressin

A potent vasoconstrictor, vasopressin is associated with improved end-organ and cerebral blood flow and lacks the beta toxicity associated with epinephrine. Nonetheless, in head-to-head comparisons, vasopressin alone offers no survival advantage over epinephrine.[142-144] Furthermore, the combination of the two drugs offers no survival advantage over epinephrine alone.[145,146] In contrast, a recent trial of vasopressin, epinephrine, and methylprednisolone demonstrated improved survival rates and neurological outcomes.[147,148] Several confounders (postarrest care protocols that include stress-dose steroids) make it difficult to assess the isolated effects of vasopressin.

Atropine

At best, atropine offers no survival benefit; at worst, it may diminish survival.[149-154] The agent confers no mechanistic advantage during resuscitation from asystole and pulseless electrical activity, so its routine use cannot be recommended.

Antiarrhythmics

Current guidelines recommend the administration of an antiarrhythmic medication if VF or ventricular tachycardia (VT) persists after one defibrillation attempt and 2 minutes of CPR. Amiodarone is the preferred agent, but lidocaine can be given if amiodarone is unavailable. Several studies point to an improved rate of survival to hospital admission in patients receiving amiodarone versus lidocaine for refractory or recurrent VF/VT; however, neither drug has been shown to improve long-term survival or neurological function.[133,155-157] A three-arm, randomized, blinded, multicenter study of 3,000 OHCA patients with shock-resistant ventricular dysrhythmias found no difference in survival or favorable neurological outcome between patients taking amiodarone, lidocaine, or placebo. A subgroup analysis of patients with witnessed cardiac arrest found that those receiving active drugs (amiodarone or lidocaine) were more likely to survive than those receiving placebo.[158]

Systems Issues

Termination of Resuscitation

Advances in resuscitation science continue to shed light on which patient populations are most likely to survive a cardiac arrest event. Factors consistently linked to survival include prompt bystander CPR, quality uninterrupted chest compressions, and early defibrillation.

In an attempt to develop universally applicable guidelines for the prehospital termination of resuscitation (TOR), a team of researchers prospectively validated a previously established set of rules for BLS providers in a cohort of 2,145 OHCA patients (*Table 5-2*).[159] These rules demonstrated 100% specificity for recommending transport of potential survivors and a positive predictive value of 100% for death. The predicted transport rate was 46%.

A set of universal TOR rules could minimize practice variations among physicians providing online medical control. Established protocols also could improve resource utilization and EMS safety by reducing the number of patients transported to hospitals; however, this reduction could impede the development of new strategies and techniques for managing those currently deemed unresuscitatable. Universal TOR rules also open the possibility for occasional — albeit rare — premature terminations of resuscitation.

Regionalization of Care

Patients in cardiac arrest and those who have been resuscitated should be managed at a regionalized cardiac arrest center. This is not a new model of care for time-sensitive interventions. Trauma, ST-elevation myocardial infarction (STEMI), and acute stroke all take advantage of established, regionalized systems of care that coordinate prehospital units with receiving centers. Several case-control studies have highlighted the effectiveness of bundled postresuscitation care, demonstrating improved results compared with historical controls.[8,160-165] Typical hospital-based physicians treat postcardiac arrest patients infrequently, given the low rates of resuscitation in communities. Regionalized cardiac arrest centers increase referral volumes and thereby the experience of clinicians.[166] The positive correlation between care providers' experience (or procedural volume) with complex diagnoses (or procedures) and better patient outcomes is well documented.[167]

An accumulating body of evidence points to improved outcomes when cardiac arrest patients are treated at regionalized centers.[168] Several studies have described the great influence these transportation decisions can have on outcomes.[169] In one German study, the patients treated in a PCI center were more than 3 times as likely to survive with a favorable neurological outcome. Another study investigated 27,000 Korean patients who were transported to hospitals with CPR in progress.[170] Even with longer transport intervals, those

TABLE 5-2. Validated Universal Rules for Prehospital Termination of Resuscitation
No return of spontaneous circulation prior to transport
No shock administered
Arrest not witnessed by EMS personnel

TABLE 5-3. Proposed Clinical Services for Regionalized Cardiac Arrest Centers

Neurological Services
Induced hypothermia
Continuous EEG monitoring
Seizure management
Neurology consultation
Neurosurgical consultation
Cerebral imaging (CT, MRI, perfusion studies)
Neurophysiological testing (evoked potentials)
Prognostication services
Critical care Services
Ventilator management
Glucose control
Goal-directed hemodynamic management
Cardiovascular Services
Cardiac catheterization/percutaneous coronary intervention
Coronary artery bypass grafting
Intraaortic balloon pump
Cardiovascular mechanical support devices
Extracorporeal membranous oxygenation (ECMO)
Transplant surgery consultation
Electrophysiology consultation
ICD placement
Other Services
Physical medicine and rehabilitation consultation
Physical and occupational therapy
Social work
Organ donation
Outpatient physical and occupational therapy
Outpatient neurological rehabilitation
Outpatient psychological services

transferred to high-volume centers were more likely to survive to hospital discharge than those treated in low-volume centers.

One of the common barriers to the implementation of regionalized cardiac arrest care is patient transport. The decision to bypass a local hospital to transport a patient to a more distant resuscitation center is controversial. However, two recent studies indicate that prehospital transfer time does not independently affect patient outcomes after cardiac arrest, suggesting the feasibility of a modest increase in transport intervals.[172,173] Likewise, patients who achieve ROSC at a local hospital should be strongly considered for interfacility transfer to a regional cardiac arrest center, which also is far likelier to offer organ donation and procurement services for those who do not survive *(Table 5-2)*.[171]

A study of 248 resuscitated patients transferred to tertiary care facilities with a median transport time of 63 minutes found that rearrest was uncommon (6%) and critical events (eg, hypotension and/or hypoxia) affected 23% of patients during transport.[174] Most critical events took place within the first hour of transport, and 27% occurred at the referring facility prior to departure. Patients taking vasopressors were most likely to suffer critical events. When weighing the risk of transport against the overall survival rate (53%) and survival rate of patients suffering a critical event (29%), the researchers found that those referred to a cardiac arrest center from an outlying facility derived benefit, with an acceptable risk of decompensation en route.

Special Populations

Traumatic Cardiac Arrest

Most causes of traumatic cardiac arrest, which historically has carried a dismal prognosis, are related to airway maintenance, thoracic trauma that impedes adequate oxygenation/ventilation, hemorrhage, or intracranial injury. Diagnostic and therapeutic interventions should be tailored to these underlying factors.

KEY POINTS

1. Achieving return of spontaneous circulation is one component of an effective cardiac arrest strategy. Comprehensive resuscitation care requires the engagement of both emergency health care practitioners and the lay public.
2. There is no evidence to support the routine use of mechanical chest compression devices in the prehospital setting for undifferentiated cardiac arrest.
3. In select patients, mechanical chest compression devices provide a bridge to invasive therapies.
4. Although data regarding the need for rescue breaths during CPR are inconsistent, there is consensus on the need for prompt, effective chest compressions with limited interruptions.
5. Know the defibrillator model used in your institution as well as the manufacturer's recommended energy selection.
6. For witnessed arrests with a shockable rhythm, it is reasonable to defibrillate before starting CPR. For unwitnessed arrests with a shockable rhythm, it is reasonable to perform CPR before defibrillating.
7. Increasing lengths of the peri-shock pause are negatively associated with the survival rate.
8. Be careful and creative in choosing logistic maneuvers so as to minimize hands-off time.
9. Cricoid pressure impairs laryngoscopy and the placement of advanced airways; it should not be performed routinely.
10. Evidence for advanced airway management in the setting of out-of-hospital cardiac arrest is lacking. Supraglottic devices and endotracheal intubation have been associated with an increase in mortality rate.

In the setting of traumatic cardiac arrest, the clinician should focus on prompt airway management, empiric chest tube placement, hemorrhage control, the transfusion of blood products, and consideration of resuscitative thoracotomy. Conventional ACLS measures are unlikely to add value in cases of traumatic cardiac arrest. In advanced centers, extracorporeal membranous oxygenation (ECMO) or resuscitative endovascular balloon occlusion of the aorta (REBOA) may be considered for select patients.

Poisoned Patients

Since resuscitation of the critically ill patient often is undertaken without the benefit of a complete medical history, consideration of underlying causes is of prime importance. Certain toxidromes are associated with myocardial depression, lethal arrhythmias, and high fatality rates. In specific cases, the administration of a particular ACLS drug can counteract a poison's deleterious effects. Consider consulting with a regional poison control center when appropriate. (*Also see Chapter 16.*)

Pediatric Patients

All providers who perform resuscitation must maintain proficiency in pediatric emergency skills. In children, cardiac arrest typically results from hypoxic insult (as opposed to lethal arrhythmia), so special attention to airway management is of extreme importance when managing these vulnerable patients. In general, pediatric resuscitation emphasizes airway management and the correction of underlying pathology. More detailed information is provided in Chapter 25.

The value of quality compressions and BLS cannot be overstated. Lengthy attempts to establish intravenous access are discouraged in favor of quicker modalities such as intraosseous needle insertion. Devices such as the E-Z IO drill (Vidacare, Shavano Park, TX) minimize the technical difficulty of placing a catheter into the bone marrow.

Some tertiary care centers report favorable results with extracorporeal membrane oxygenation in victims of refractory arrest.[175] This technology can enhance the resuscitation armamentarium in hospitals with specialized personnel and equipment. Finally, adequate preparation and training are essential. Pediatric supplies must be readily accessible and familiar to all clinicians charged with leading resuscitation. Weight-based drug regimens and color-coded kits containing appropriately sized equipment can minimize stress during an arrest scenario.

Future Directions

Extracorporeal Life Support

Extracorporeal life support (ECLS) — the incorporation of ECMO into cardiac arrest resuscitation — is a resource-intensive therapy that has been deployed successfully to boost neurological survival in select patients suffering OHCA. Japan, which boasts one of the most sophisticated ECLS systems in the world, determines patient eligibility using the following criteria:

- Age 18 to 74 years
- Bystander-witnessed cardiac arrest
- Presumed cardiac etiology
- Less than 15 minutes from collapse until EMS arrival
- Shockable rhythm
- Persistent cardiac arrest on arrival[176]

Eligible patients are cannulated percutaneously for ECMO in the emergency department while CPR is in progress. Once life support is initiated, patients are cooled rapidly with the ECMO circuit while receiving urgent coronary angiography, PCI (if indicated), and insertion of an intraaortic balloon pump.

There is a clear stepwise relationship between outcomes and quartiles of the intervals. The optimal cutoffs in the Japanese ECLS system are 55.5 minutes for the collapse-to-ECMO interval and 21.5 minutes for the ECMO-to-34°C (93.2°F) interval. The odds of survival with a positive neurological outcome is 50% or higher when the ECMO-to-34°C (93.2°F) interval is less than 21.5 minutes, regardless of the collapse-to-ECMO interval. A cumulative review of the Japanese ECLS literature through 2011

KEY POINTS

11. Prehospital airway management should not take precedence over the performance of high-quality uninterrupted chest compressions.
12. Endotracheal tube placement should be confirmed with continuous waveform capnography.
13. After return of spontaneous circulation, oxygenation and ventilation strategies should aim for minimally necessary FiO_2 and normocarbia. There is little evidence to guide these strategies during resuscitation.
14. Indications for resuscitation drugs need to be reevaluated in the context of modern postresuscitation care.
15. Although the routine use of vasopressors can improve the rate of ROSC, there is no evidence that the practice improves survival rates or neurological outcomes. These agents might, in fact, worsen long-term outcomes.
16. Antiarrhythmic medications might offer short-term benefits, but they never have been associated with survival or favorable neurological outcomes.
17. Sodium bicarbonate does not improve outcomes and could be harmful.
18. Calcium, magnesium, and fibrinolytic agents should be reserved for the treatment of an underlying pathology in special cases of cardiac arrest.
19. When geographically feasible, patients with OHCA should be transported to a cardiac arrest center.
20. Patients resuscitated at a local hospital should be evaluated for transfer to a facility capable of the providing the full spectrum of postcardiac arrest care.

found 1,282 patients who experienced OHCA between 1983 and 2008 and received ECLS.[177] Among the 516 patients with available data, 27% survived to hospital discharge. Approximately 50% of the cases resulted in mild or no neurological disabilities. Another propensity-adjusted analysis of ECLS in patients with witnessed OHCA of cardiac origin found a 3-fold improvement in the 90-day neurologically intact survival rate (29% vs. 8%).[178] A randomized comparison of ECLS and traditional resuscitation is being planned by investigators in Prague, Czech Republic.[179]

The success of any ECLS program hinges on patient selection and collaboration among prehospital, emergency department, and critical care personnel. ECLS is a resource-intensive endeavor in which successful outcomes are extremely time dependent.

Goal-Directed Intraarrest Resuscitation

Preclinical research and small human studies have explored the possibility of hemodynamic-directed CPR as a model for individually tailored resuscitation.[126,180-184] In contrast to the "one-size-fits-all" prescription for advanced cardiac life support, hemodynamic-directed CPR attempts to account for an individual patient's response to resuscitative efforts. This approach requires invasive hemodynamic monitoring and will be best tested in patients who experience an in-hospital cardiac arrest. In theory, CPR metrics and vasopressors can be used to target specific hemodynamic goals such as diastolic blood pressure or coronary perfusion pressure. Targeting these endpoints might reduce vasopressor use, thereby increasing cerebral perfusion pressure and brain tissue oxygenation.

Waveform-Guided Defibrillation

Preclinical data suggest that the VF waveform can be used to guide the timing of defibrillation — the success of which can be predicted using a quantitative analysis of the waveform. Certain waveform characteristics (eg, amplitude, frequency, periodicity) are associated with coronary perfusion pressure and myocardial ATP concentration.[185-187] Many clinicians are familiar with the practice of delaying shock delivery for "fine" VF to provide CPR, improve perfusion of the myocardium, and increase the "coarseness" of the waveform.[50,188,189] Real-time, automated waveform analysis currently is not available, and the ability of providers to interpret the information has not been studied.

Conclusion

Cardiac arrest is a complex disease. As resuscitation professionals, emergency care providers should move beyond the rote memorization of protocols and understand the science and evidence behind the latest treatment guidelines. In addition, they must be diligent in hunting for treatable causes of cardiac arrest during the brief window afforded by resuscitative measures. Despite technological advances and the maturity of resuscitation science, the priorities of resuscitation remain unchanged.

Careful attention to high-quality minimally interrupted compressions affords patients the best chance for surviving neurologically intact. Intraarrest advanced airway management must not interrupt the delivery of compressions. High-performing prehospital EMS systems have implemented interventions such as "pit crew" CPR to improve survival and preserve a patient's functional neurological status through the initiation of compressions, defibrillation, and goal-directed postarrest care.

PEARL

Extracorporeal life support is an option for a subset of patients whose cardiac arrest was witnessed and who receive quality CPR, but are refractory to initial resuscitative measures. ECLS requires a significant investment of time and resources and is feasible only at select centers.

REFERENCES

1. Sayre MR, Koster RW, Botha M, et al. Part 5: Adult basic life support: 2010 International Consensus on Cardiopulmonary Resuscitation and Emergency Cardiovascular Care Science With Treatment Recommendations. *Circulation.* 2010;122(16 suppl 2):S298-S324.
2. Writing Group Members, Roger VL, Go AS, Lloyd-Jones DM, et al. Heart disease and stroke statistics — 2012 update: a report from the American Heart Association. *Circulation.* 2012;125:e2-220.
3. Herlitz J, Svensson L, Engdahl J, et al. Characteristics of cardiac arrest and resuscitation by age group: an analysis from the Swedish cardiac arrest registry. *Am J Emerg Med.* 2007;25:1025-1031.
4. Ong ME, Stiell I, Osmond MH, et al. Etiology of pediatric out-of-hospital cardiac arrest by coroner's diagnosis. *Resuscitation.* 2006;68:335-342.
5. Kuisma M, Alaspaa A. Out-of-hospital cardiac arrests of non-cardiac origin: epidemiology and outcome. *Eur Heart J.* 1997;18:1122-1128.
6. Kurkciyan I, Meron G, Behringer W, et al. Accuracy and impact of presumed cause in patients with cardiac arrest. *Circulation.* 1998;98:766-771.
7. Nichol G, Thomas E, Callaway CW, et al. Regional variation in out-of-hospital cardiac arrest incidence and outcome. *JAMA.* 2008;300:1423-1431.
8. Sunde K, Pytte M, Jacobsen D, et al. Implementation of a standardised treatment protocol for post resuscitation care after out-of-hospital cardiac arrest. *Resuscitation.* 2007;73:29-39.
9. Bobrow BJ, Vadeboncoeur TF, Stolz U, et al. The influence of scenario-based training and real-time audiovisual feedback on out-of-hospital cardiopulmonary resuscitation quality and survival from out-of-hospital cardiac arrest. *Ann Emerg Med.* 2013;62:47-56.
10. Perkins GD, Brace S, Gates S. Mechanical chest-compression devices: current and future roles. *Curr Opin Crit Care.* 2010;16:203-210.
11. Wagner H, Terkelsen CJ, Friberg H, et al. Cardiac arrest in the catheterisation laboratory: a 5-year experience of using mechanical chest compressions to facilitate PCI during prolonged resuscitation efforts. *Resuscitation.* 2010;81:383-387.
12. Larsen AI, Hjørnevik AS, Ellingsen CL, Nilsen DW. Cardiac arrest with continuous mechanical chest compression during percutaneous coronary intervention: a report on the use of the LUCAS device. *Resuscitation.* 2007;75:454-459.
13. Stub D, Bernard S, Pellegrino V, et al. Refractory cardiac arrest treated with mechanical CPR, hypothermia, ECMO and early reperfusion (the CHEER trial). *Resuscitation.* 2014 Oct 2. pii: S0300-9572(14)00751-5. doi: 10.1016/j.resuscitation.2014.09.010. [Epub ahead of print]
14. Zimmermann S, Rohde D, Marwan M, et al. Complete recovery after out-of-hospital cardiac arrest with prolonged (59 min) mechanical cardiopulmonary resuscitation, mild therapeutic hypothermia and complex percutaneous coronary intervention for ST-elevation myocardial infarction. *Heart Lung.* 2014;43:62-65. doi:10.1016/j.hrtlng.2013.10.011.
15. McDonald JL. Systolic and mean arterial pressures during manual and mechanical CPR in humans. *Ann Emerg Med.* 1982;11:292-295.
16. Ward KR, Menegazzi JJ, Zelenak RR, et al. Comparison of chest compressions between mechanical and manual CPR by monitoring end-tidal PCO2 during human cardiac arrest. *Ann Emerg Med.* 1993;22:669-674.
17. Rubertsson S, Karlsten R. Increased cortical cerebral blood flow with LUCAS; a new device for mechanical chest compressions compared to standard external compressions during experimental cardiopulmonary resuscitation. *Resuscitation.* 2005;65:357-363.
18. Rubertsson S, Lindgren E, Smekal D, et al. Mechanical chest compressions and simultaneous defibrillation vs conventional cardiopulmonary resuscitation in out-of-hospital cardiac arrest: the LINC randomized trial. *JAMA.* 2014;311:53-61.
19. Axelsson C, Nestin J, Svensson L, et al. Clinical consequences of the introduction of mechanical chest compression in the EMS system for treatment of out-of-hospital cardiac arrest — a pilot study. *Resuscitation.* 2006;71:47-55.
20. Smekal D, Johansson J, Huzevka T, Rubertsson S. A pilot study of mechanical chest compressions with the LUCAS device in cardiopulmonary resuscitation. *Resuscitation.* 2011;82:702-706.
21. Westfall M, Krantz S, Mullin C, Kaufman C. Mechanical versus manual chest compressions in out-of-hospital cardiac arrest: a meta-analysis. *Crit Care Med.* 2013;41:1782-1789. doi: 10.1097/CCM.0b013e31828a24e3.

22. Yost D, Phillips RH, Gonzales L, et al. Assessment of CPR interruptions from transthoracic impedance during use of the LUCAS mechanical chest compression system. *Resuscitation.* 2012;83:961-965.
23. Ong ME, Annathurai A, Shahidah A, et al. Cardiopulmonary resuscitation interruptions with the use of a load-distrib*uting band device during emergency department cardiac arrest. Ann Emerg Med.* 2010;56:233-241.
24. Krischer JP, Fine EG, Davis JH, Nagel EL Complications of cardiac resuscitation. *Chest.* 1987;92:287-291.
25. Bonnemeier H, Simonis G, Olivecrona G, et al. Continuous mechanical chest compression during in-hosptial cardiopulmonary resuscitation of patients with pulseless electrical activity. *Resuscitation.* 2011;82:155-159.
26. Wyss CA, Fox J, Franzeck F, et al. Mechanical versus manual chest compression during CPR in a cardiac catherisation setting. *Cardiovascular Med.* 2010;12:92-96.
27. Grogaard HK, Wik L, Eriksen M, et al. Continuous chest compressions during cardiac arrest to facilitate restoration of coronary circulation with percutaneous coronary intervention. *J Am Coll Cardiol.* 2007;50:1093-1094.
28. Sayre MR, Berg RA, Cave DM, et al. Hands-only (compression only) cardiopulmonary resuscitation: a call to action for bystander response to adults who experience out-of-hospital sudden cardiac arrest: a science advisory for the public from the American Heart Association Emergency Cardiovascular Care Committee. *Circulation.* 2008;117:2162-2167.
29. Rea T, Fahrenbruch C, Culley L, et al. CPR with chest compression alone or with rescue breathing. *N Engl J Med.* 2010;363:423-433.
30. Kitamura T, Iwami T, Kawamura T, e al. Bystander-initiated rescue breathing for out-of-hospital cardiac arrests of noncardiac origin. *Circulation.* 2010;122:293-299.
31. Japanese Circulation Society Resuscitation Science Study Group. Chest-compression-only bystander cardiopulmonary resuscitation in the 30:2 compression-to-ventilation ratio era. *Circ J.* 2013;77:2742-2750.
32. Yao L, Wang P, Zhou L, Chen M, et al. Compression-only cardiopulmonary resuscitation vs standard cardiopulmonary resuscitation: an updated meta-analysis of observational studies. *Am J Emerg Med.* 2014;32:517-523.
33. Mader TJ, Paquette AT, Salcido DD, et al. The effect of the preshock pause on coronary perfusion pressure decay and rescue shock outcome in porcine ventricular fibrillation. *Prehosp Emerg Care.* 2009;13:487-494.
34. Kern KB, Ewy GA, Voorhees WD, et al. Myocardial perfusion pressure: a predictor of 24-hour survival during prolonged cardiac arrest in dogs. *Resuscitation.* 1998;16:241-250.
35. Carlson JN, Reynolds JC. Does advanced airway management improve outcomes in adult out-of-hospital cardiac arrest? *Ann Emerg Med.* 2014;64:163-164.
36. McMullan J, Gerecht R, Bonomo J, et al; CARES Surveillance Group. Airway management and out-of-hospital cardiac arrest outcome in the CARES registry. *Resuscitation.* 2014;85:617-622.
37. Hasegawa K, Hiraide A,Chang Y, Brown DF. Association of prehospital advanced airway management with neurologic outcome and survival in patients with out-of-hospital cardiac arrest. *JAMA.* 2013;309:257-266.
38. Shin SD, Ahn KO, Song KJ, et al. Out-of-hospital airway management and cardiac arrest outcomes: a propensity score matched analysis. *Resuscitation.* 2012;83:313-319.
39. Aufderheide TP, Sigurdsson G, Pirrallo RG, et al. Hyperventilation-induced hypotension during cardiopulmonary resuscitation. *Circulation.* 2004;109:1960-1965.
40. Schneider T, Martens PR, Paschen H, et al. Multicenter, randomized, controlled trial of 150-J biphasic shocks compared with 200- to 360-J monophasic shocks in the resuscitation of out-of-hospital cardiac arrest victims. Optimized Response to Cardiac Arrest (ORCA) Investigators. *Circulation.* 2000;102:1780-1787.
41. van Alem AP, Chapman FW, Lank P, et al. A prospective, randomised and blinded comparison of first shock success of monophasic and biphasic waveforms in out-of-hospital cardiac arrest. *Resuscitation.* 2003;58:17-24.
42. Kudenchuk PJ, Cobb LA, Copass MK, et al. Transthoracic incremental monophasic versus biphasic defibrillation by emergency responders (TIMBER): a randomized comparison of monophasic with biphasic waveform ascending energy defibrillation for the resuscitation of out-of-hospital cardiac arrest due to ventricular fibrillation. *Circulation.* 2006;114:2010-2018.
43. Stiell IG, Walker RG, Nesbitt LP, et al. BIPHASIC Trial: a randomized comparison of fixed lower versus escalating higher energy levels for defibrillation in out-of-hospital cardiac arrest. *Circulation.* 2007;115:1511-1517.
44. Walsh SJ, McClelland AJ, Owens CG, et al. Efficacy of distinct energy delivery protocols comparing two biphasic defibrillators for cardiac arrest. *Am J Cardiol.* 2004;94:378-380.
45. Cummins RO, Ornato JP, Thies WH, Pepe PE. Improving survival from sudden cardiac arrest: the "chain of survival" concept. A statement for health professionals from the Advanced Cardiac Life Support Subcommittee and the Emergency Cardiac Care Committee, American Heart Association. *Circulation.* 1991;83:1832-1847.
46. Weaver WD, Cobb LA, Dennis D, et al. Amplitude of ventricular fibrillation waveform and outcome after cardiac arrest. *Ann Intern Med.* 1985;102:53-55.
47. Reynolds JC, Salcido DD, Menegazzi JJ. Conceptual models of coronary perfusion pressure and their relationship to defibrillation success in a porcine model of prolonged out-of-hospital cardiac arrest. *Resuscitation.* 2012;83:900-906.
48. Reynolds JC, Salcido DD, Menegazzi JJ. Coronary perfusion pressure and return of spontaneous circulation after prolonged cardiac arrest. *Prehosp Emerg Care.* 2010;14:78-84.
49. Cobb LA, Fahrenbruch CE, Walsh TR, et al. Influence of cardiopulmonary resuscitation prior to defibrillation in patients with out-of-hospital ventricular fibrillation. *JAMA.* 1999;281:1182-1188.
50. Wik L, Hansen TB, Fylling F, et al. Delaying defibrillation to give basic cardiopulmonary resuscitation to patients with out-of-hospital ventricular fibrillation: a randomized trial. *JAMA.* 2003;289:1389-1395.
51. Jacobs IG, Finn JC, Oxer HF, et al.CPR before defibrillation in out-of-hospital cardiac arrest: a randomized trial. *Emerg Med Australas.* 2005;17:39-45. Erratum in *Emerg Med Australas.* 2009;21:430.
52. Stiell IG, Nichol G, Leroux BG, et al; ROC Investigators. Early versus later rhythm analysis in patients with out-of-hospital cardiac arrest. *N Engl J Med.* 2011;365:787-797.
53. Cheskes S, Schmicker RH, Christenson J, et al; Resuscitation Outcomes Consortium (ROC) Investigators. Perishock pause: an independent predictor of survival from out-of-hospital shockable cardiac arrest. *Circulation.* 2011;124:58-66.
54. Cheskes S, Schmicker RH, Verbeek PR, et al; Resuscitation Outcomes Consortium (ROC) Investigators. The impact of peri-shock pause on survival from out-of-hospital shockable cardiac arrest during the Resuscitation Outcomes Consortium PRIMED trial. *Resuscitation.* 2014;85:336-342.
55. Zia A, Kern KB. *Management of postcardiac arrest myocardial dysfunction. Curr Opin Crit Care.* 2011;17:241-246.
56. Eftestøl T, Sunde K, Steen PA. Effects of interrupting precordial compressions on the calculated probability of defibrillation success during out-of-hospital cardiac arrest. *Circulation.* 2002;105:2270-2273.
57. Rea TD, Helbock M, Perry S, et al. Increasing use of cardiopulmonary resuscitation during out-of-hospital ventricular fibrillation arrest: survival implications of guideline changes. *Circulation.* 2006;114:2760-2765.
58. Lloyd MS, Heeke B, Walter PF, Langberg JJ. Hands-on defibrillation: an analysis of electrical current flow through rescuers in direct contact with patients during biphasic external defibrillation. *Circulation.* 2008;117:2510-2514.
59. NeumannT, Gruenewald M, Lauenstein C, et al. Hands-on defibrillation has the potential to improve the quality of cardiopulmonary resuscitation and is safe for rescuers — a preclinical study. *J Am Heart Assoc.* 2012;1:e001313.
60. Deakin CD, Lee-Shrewsbury V, Hogg K, Petley GW. Do clinical examination gloves provide adequate electrical insulation for safe hands-on defibrillation? I: Resistive properties of nitrile gloves. *Resuscitation.* 2013;84:895-899.
61. Alaeddini J, Feng Z, Feghali G, et al. Repeated dual external direct cardioversions using two simultaneous 360-J shocks for refractory atrial fibrillation are safe and effective. *Pacing Clin Electrophysiol.* 2005;28:3-7.
62. Leacock BW. Double simultaneous defibrillators for refractory ventricular fibrillation. *J Emerg Med.* 2014;46:472-474.
63. Schade K, Borzotta A, Michaels A. Intracranial malposition of nasopharyngeal airway. *J Trauma.* 2000;49:967-968.
64. Muzzi DA, Losasso TJ, Cucchiara RF. Complication from a nasopharyngeal airway in a patient with a basilar skull fracture. *Anesthesiology.* 1991;74:366-368.
65. Petito SP, Russell WJ. The prevention of gastric inflation: a neglected benefit of cricoid pressure. *Anaesth Intensive Care.* 1988;16:139-143.
66. Lawes EG, Campbell I, Mercer D. Inflation pressure, gastric insufflation and rapid sequence induction. *Br J Anaesth.* 1987;59:315-318.
67. Asai T, Barclay K, Power I, Vaughan RS. Cricoid pressure impedes placement of the laryngeal mask airway and subsequent tracheal intubation through the mask. *Br J Anaesth.* 1994;72:47-51.
68. Asai T, Barclay K, Power I, Vaughan RS. Cricoid pressure impedes placement of the laryngeal mask airway. *Br J Anaesth.* 1995;74: 521-525.
69. Ansermino JM, Blogg CE. Cricoid pressure may prevent insertion of the laryngeal mask airway. *Br J Anaesth.* 1992;69:465–467.
70. Aoyama K, Takenaka I, Sata T, Shigematsu A. Cricoid pressure impedes positioning and ventilation through the laryngeal mask airway. *Can J Anaesth.* 1996;43:1035-1040.
71. Brimacombe J, White A, Berry A. Effect of cricoid pressure on ease of insertion of the laryngeal mask airway. *Br J Anaesth.* 1993;71: 800-802.
72. Gabbott DA, Sasada MP. Laryngeal mask airway insertion using cricoid pressure and manual in-line neck stabilisation. *Anaesthesia.* 1995;50:674-676.
73. Xue FS, Mao P, Li CW, et al. Influence of pressure on cricoid on insertion ProSeal laryngeal mask airway and ventilation function [in Chinese]. *Zhongguo Wei Zhong Bing Ji Jiu Yi Xue.* 2007;19:532-535.
74. Li CW, Xue FS, Xu YC, et al.Cricoid pressure impedes insertion of, and ventilation through, the ProSeal laryngeal mask airway in anesthetized, paralyzed patients. *Anesth Analg.* 2007;104:1195-1198.
75. McNelis U, Syndercombe A, Harper I, Duggan J. The effect of cricoid pressure on intubation facilitated by the gum elastic bougie. *Anaesthesia.* 2007;62:456-459.
76. Harry RM, Nolan JP. The use of cricoid pressure with the intubating laryngeal mask. *Anaesthesia.* 1999;54:656-659.
77. Noguchi T, Koga K, Shiga Y, Shigematsu A. The gum elastic bougie eases tracheal intubation while applying cricoid pressure compared to a stylet. *Can J Anaesth.* 2003;50:712-717.
78. Asai T, Murao K, Shingu K. Cricoid pressure applied after placement of laryngeal mask impedes subsequent fibreoptic tracheal intubation through mask. *Br J Anaesth.* 2000;85:256-261.
79. Snider DD, Clarke D, Finucane BT. The "BURP" maneuver worsens the glottic view when applied in combination with cricoid pressure. *Can J Anaesth.* 2005;52:100-104.
80. Smith CE, Boyer D. Cricoid pressure decreases ease of tracheal intubation using fibreoptic laryngoscopy (WuScope System). *Can J Anaesth.* 2002;49:614-619.
81. Heath ML, Allagain J. Intubation through the laryngeal mask: a technique for unexpected difficult intubation. *Anaesthesia.* 1991;46: 545-548.
82. Levitan RM, Kinkle WC, Levin WJ, Everett WW. Laryngeal view during laryngoscopy: a randomized trial comparing cricoid pressure, backward-upward-rightward pressure, and bimanual laryngoscopy. *Ann Emerg Med.* 2006;47:548-555.
83. Bradley JS, Billows GL, Olinger ML, et al. Prehospital oral endotracheal intubation by rural basic emergency medical technicians. *Ann Emerg Med.* 1998;32:26-32.
84. Sayre MR, Sakles JC, Mistler AF, et al. Field trial of endotracheal intubation by basic EMTs. *Ann Emerg Med.* 1998;31:228-233.
85. Katz SH, Falk JL. Misplaced endotracheal tubes by paramedics in an urban emergency medical services system. *Ann Emerg Med.* 2001;37: 32–37.

86. Jones JH, Murphy MP, Dickson RL, et al. Emergency physician-verified out-of-hospital intubation: miss rates by paramedics. *Acad Emerg Med.* 2004;11:707-709.
87. Wirtz DD, Ortiz C, Newman DH, Zhitomirsky I. Unrecognized misplacement of endotracheal tubes by ground prehospital providers. *Prehosp Emerg Care.* 2007;11:213-218.
88. Timmermann A, Russo SG, Eich C, et al. The out-of-hospital esophageal and endobronchial intubations performed by emergency physicians. *Anesth Analg.* 2007;104:619-623.
89. Wong ML, Carey S, Mader TJ, Wang HE. Time to invasive airway placement and resuscitation outcomes after inhospital cardiopulmonary arrest. *Resuscitation.* 2010;81:182-186.
90. Shy BD, Rea TD, Becker LJ, Eisenberg MS. Time to intubation and survival in prehospital cardiac arrest. *Prehosp Emerg Care.* 2004;8:394-399.
91. Bobrow BJ, Ewy GA, Clark L, et al. Passive oxygen insufflation is superior to bag-valve-mask ventilation for witnessed ventricular fibrillation out-of-hospital cardiac arrest. *Ann Emerg Med.* 2009;54:656-662.e651.
92. Rumball CJ, MacDonald D. The PTL, Combitube, laryngeal mask, and oral airway: a randomized prehospital comparative study of ventilatory device effectiveness and cost-effectiveness in 470 cases of cardiorespiratory arrest. *Prehosp Emerg Care.* 1997;1:1-10.
93. SOS-KANTO Study Group. Comparison of arterial blood gases of laryngeal mask airway and bag-valve-mask ventilation in out-of- hospital cardiac arrests. *Circ J.* 2009;73:490-496.
94. Stone BJ, Chantler PJ, Baskett PJ. The incidence of regurgitation during cardiopulmonary resuscitation: a comparison between the bag valve mask and laryngeal mask airway. *Resuscitation.* 1998;38:3-6.
95. Frass M, Frenzer R, Rauscha F, et al. Ventilation with the esophageal tracheal Combitube in cardiopulmonary resuscitation: promptness and effectiveness. *Chest.* 1988;93:781-784.
96. Atherton GL, Johnson JC. Ability of paramedics to use the Combitube in prehospital cardiac arrest. *Ann Emerg Med.* 1993;22:1263-1268.
97. Rabitsch W, Schellongowski P, Staudinger T, et al. Comparison of a conventional tracheal airway with the Combitube in an urban emergency medical services system run by physicians. *Resuscitation.* 2003;57:27-32.
98. Rumball C, Macdonald D, Barber P, et al. Endotracheal intubation and esophageal tracheal Combitube insertion by regular ambulance attendants: a comparative trial. *Prehosp Emerg Care.* 2004;8:15-22.
99. Samarkandi AH, Seraj MA, el Dawlatly A, et al. The role of laryngeal mask airway in cardiopulmonary resuscitation. *Resuscitation.* 1994;28:103-106.
100. Staudinger T, Brugger S, Watschinger B, et al. Emergency intubation with the Combitube: comparison with the endotracheal airway. *Ann Emerg Med.* 1993;22:1573-1575.
101. Staudinger T, Brugger S, Roggla M, et al. Comparison of the Combitube with the endotracheal tube in cardiopulmonary resuscitation in the prehospital phase [in German]. *Wien Klin Wochenschr.* 1994;106:412-415.
102. Cady CE, Weaver MD, Pirrallo RG, Wang HE. Effect of emergency medical technician-placed Combitubes on outcomes after out-of- hospital cardiopulmonary arrest. *Prehosp Emerg Care.* 2009;13:495-499.
103. Verghese C, Prior-Willeard PF, Baskett PJ. Immediate management of the airway during cardiopulmonary resuscitation in a hospital without a resident anaesthesiologist. *Eur J Emerg Med.* 1994;1:123-125.
104. Deakin CD, Peters R, Tomlinson P, Cassidy M. Securing the prehospital airway: a comparison of laryngeal mask insertion and endotracheal intubation by UK paramedics. *Emerg Med J.* 2005;22:64-67.
105. Calkins TR, Miller K, Langdorf MI. Success and complication rates with prehospital placement of an esophageal-tracheal combitube as a rescue airway. *Prehosp Disaster Med.* 2006;21:97-100.
106. Guyette FX, Wang H, Cole JS. King airway use by air medical providers. *Prehosp Emerg Care.* 2007;11:473-476.
107. Tentillier E, Heydenreich C, Cros AM, et al. Use of the intubating laryngeal mask airway in emergency pre-hospital difficult intubation. *Resuscitation.* 2008;77:30-34.
108. Timmermann A, Russo SG, Rosenblatt WH, et al. Intubating laryngeal mask airway for difficult out-of-hospital airway management: a prospective evaluation. *Br J Anaesth.* 2007;99:286-291.
109. Martin SE, Ochsner MG, Jarman RH, et al. Use of the laryngeal mask airway in air transport when intubation fails. *J Trauma.* 1999;47:352-357.
110. Hasegawa K, Hiraide A, Chang Y, Brown DF. Association of prehospital advanced airway management with neurologic outcome and survival in patients with out-of-hospital cardiac arrest. *JAMA.* 2013;309:257–266.
111. McMullan J, Gerecht R, Bonomo J, et al. Airway management and out-of-hospital cardiac arrest outcome in the CARES registry. *Resuscitation.* 2014;85:617-622.
112. Grmec S. Comparison of three different methods to confirm tracheal tube placement in emergency intubation. *Intensive Care Med.* 2002;28:701-704.
113. Silvestri S, Ralls GA, Krauss B, et al. The effectiveness of out-of-hospital use of continuous end-tidal carbon dioxide monitoring on the rate of unrecognized misplaced intubation within a regional emergency medical services system. *Ann Emerg Med.* 2005;45:497-503.
114. Kellum MJ, Kennedy KW, Barney R, et al. Cardiocerebral resuscitation improves neurologically intact survival of patients with out-of-hospital cardiac arrest. *Ann Emerg Med.* 2008;52:244-252.
115. Kellum MJ, Kennedy KW, Ewy GA. Cardiocerebral resuscitation improves survival of patients with out-of-hospital cardiac arrest. *Am J Med.* 2006;119:335-340.
116. Bhende MS, Thompson AE. Evaluation of an end-tidal CO2 detector during pediatric cardiopulmonary resuscitation. *Pediatrics.* 1995;95:395-399.
117. Sehra R, Underwood K, Checchia P. End tidal CO2 is a quantitative measure of cardiac arrest. *Pacing Clin Electrophysiol.* 2003;26(part 2):515-517.
118. Grmec S, Kupnik D. Does the Mainz Emergency Evaluation Scoring (MEES) in combination with capnometry (MEESc) help in the prognosis of outcome from cardiopulmonary resuscitation in a pre-hospital setting? *Resuscitation.* 2003;58:89-96.
119. Grmec S, Klemen P. Does the end-tidal carbon dioxide (ETCO2) concentration have prognostic value during out-of-hospital cardiac arrest? *Eur J Emerg Med.* 2001;8:263-269.
120. Kolar M, Krizmaric M, Klemen P, Grmec S. Partial pressure of end-tidal carbon dioxide successful predicts cardiopulmonary resuscitation in the field: a prospective observational study. *Crit Care.* 2008;12:R115.
121. Levine RL, Wayne MA, Miller CC. End-tidal carbon dioxide and outcome of out-of-hospital cardiac arrest. *N Engl J Med.* 1997;337:301-306.
122. Wayne MA, Levine RL, Miller CC. Use of end-tidal carbon dioxide to predict outcome in prehospital cardiac arrest. *Ann Emerg Med.* 1995;25:762-767.
123. Ahrens T, Schallom L, Bettorf K, et al. End-tidal carbon dioxide measurements as a prognostic indicator of outcome in cardiac arrest. *Am J Crit Care.* 2001;10:391-398.
124. Sanders AB, Kern KB, Otto CW, et al. End-tidal carbon dioxide monitoring during cardiopulmonary resuscitation: a prognostic indicator for survival. *JAMA.* 1989;262:1347-1351.
125. Reynolds JC, Rittenberger JC, Menegazzi JJ. Drug administration in animal studies of cardiac arrest does not reflect human clinical experience. *Resuscitation.* 2007;74:13-26.
126. Paradis NA, Martin GB, Rivers EP, et al. Coronary perfusion pressure and the return of spontaneous circulation in human cardiopulmonary resuscitation. *JAMA.* 1990;263:1106-1113.
127. Herlitz J, Ekström L, Wennerblom B, et al. Adrenaline in out-of-hospital ventricular fibrillation. Does it make any difference? *Resuscitation.* 1995;29:195-201.
128. Behringer W, Kittler H, Sterz F, et al. Cumulative epinephrine dose during cardiopulmonary resuscitation and neurologic outcome. *Ann Intern Med.* 1998;129:450-456.
129. Holmberg M, Holmberg S, Herlitz J. Low chance of survival among patients requiring adrenaline (epinephrine) or intubation after out-of-hospital cardiac arrest in Sweden. *Resuscitation.* 2002;54:37-45.
130. Ong ME, Tan EH, Ng FS, et al; Cardiac Arrest and Resuscitation Epidemiology Study Group. Survival outcomes with the introduction of intravenous epinephrine in the management of out-of-hospital cardiac arrest. *Ann Emerg Med.* 2007;50:635-642.
131. Callaway CW. Epinephrine for cardiac arrest. *Curr Opin Cardiol.* 2013;28:36-42.
132. Olasveengen TM, Sunde K, Brunborg C, et al. Intravenous drug administration during out-of-hospital cardiac arrest: a randomized trial. *JAMA.* 2009;302:2222-2229.
133. Olasveengen TM, Wik L, Sunde K, Steen PA. Outcome when adrenaline (epinephrine) was actually given vs. not given - post hoc analysis of a randomized clinical trial. *Resuscitation.* 2012;83:327-332.
134. Jacobs IG, Finn JC, Jelinek GA, et al. Effect of adrenaline on survival in out-of-hospital cardiac arrest: a randomised double-blind placebo-controlled trial. *Resuscitation.* 2011;82:1138-1143.
135. Hagihara A, Hasegawa M, Abe T, et al. Prehospital epinephrine use and survival among patients with out-of-hospital cardiac arrest. *JAMA.* 2012;307:1161-1168.
136. Brown CG, Martin DR, Pepe PE, et al. A comparison of standard-dose and high-dose epinephrine in cardiac arrest outside the hospital. The Multicenter High-Dose Epinephrine Study Group. *N Engl J Med.* 1992;327:1051-1055.
137. Gueugniaud PY, Mols P, Goldstein P, et al. A comparison of repeated high doses and repeated standard doses of epinephrine for cardiac arrest outside the hospital. European Epinephrine Study Group. *N Engl J Med.* 1998;339:1595-1601.
138. Callaham M, Madsen CD, Barton CW, et al. A randomized clinical trial of high-dose epinephrine and norepinephrine vs standard-dose epinephrine in prehospital cardiac arrest. *JAMA.* 1992;268:2667-2672.
139. Stiell IG, Hebert PC, Weitzman BN, et al. High-dose epinephrine in adult cardiac arrest. *N Engl J Med.* 1992;327:1045-1050.
140. Hayashi Y, Iwami T, Kitamura T, et al. Impact of early intravenous epinephrine administration on outcomes following out-of-hospital cardiac arrest. *Circ J.* 2012;76:1639-1645.
141. Koscik C, Pinawin A, McGovern H, et al. Rapid epinephrine administration improves early outcomes in out-of-hospital cardiac arrest. *Resuscitation.* 2013;84:915-920.
142. Wenzel V, Krismer AC, Arntz HR, et al; European Resuscitation Council Vasopressor during Cardiopulmonary Resuscitation Study Group. A comparison of vasopressin and epinephrine for out-of-hospital cardiopulmonary resuscitation. *N Engl J Med.* 2004;350:105-113.
143. Stiell IG, Hébert PC, Wells GA, et al. Vasopressin versus epinephrine for inhospital cardiac arrest: a randomised controlled trial. *Lancet.* 2001;358:105-109.
144. Aung K, Htay T. Vasopressin for cardiac arrest: a systematic review and meta-analysis. *Arch Intern Med.* 2005;165:17-24.
145. Callaway CW, Hostler D, Doshi AA, et al. Usefulness of vasopressin administered with epinephrine during out-of-hospital cardiac arrest. *Am J Cardiol.* 2006;98:1316-1321.
146. Gueugniaud PY, David JS, Chanzy E, et al. Vasopressin and epinephrine vs. epinephrine alone in cardiopulmonary resuscitation. *N Engl J Med.* 2008;359:21-30.
147. Mentzelopoulos SD, Zakynthinos SG, Tzoufi M, et al. Vasopressin, epinephrine, and corticosteroids for in-hospital cardiac arrest. *Arch Intern Med.* 2009;169:15-24.
148. Mentzelopoulos SD, Malachias S, Chamos C, et al. Vasopressin, steroids, and epinephrine and neurologically favorable survival after in-hospital cardiac arrest: a randomized clinical trial. *JAMA.* 2013;310:270-279.
149. Coon GA, Clinton JE, Ruiz E. Use of atropine for brady-asystolic prehospital cardiac arrest. *Ann Emerg Med.* 1981;10:462-467.
150. Tortolani AJ, Risucci DA, Powell SR, Dixon R. In-hospital cardiopulmonary resuscitation during asystole: therapeutic factors associated with 24-hour survival. *Chest.* 1989;96:622-626.
151. Stiell IG, Wells GA, Hebert PC, et al. Association of drug therapy with survival in cardiac arrest: limited role of advanced cardiac life support drugs. *Acad Emerg Med.* 1995;2:264-273.

152. Engdahl J, Bang A, Lindqvist J, Herlitz J. Can we define patients with no and those with some chance of survival when found in asystole out of hospital? *Am J Cardiol.* 2000;86:610-614.
153. Engdahl J, Bang A, Lindqvist J, Herlitz J. Factors affecting short- and long-term prognosis among 1069 patients with out-of-hospital cardiac arrest and pulseless electrical activity. *Resuscitation.* 2001;51:17-25.
154. van Walraven C, Stiell IG, Wells GA, et al. Do advanced cardiac life support drugs increase resuscitation rates from in-hospital cardiac arrest? The OTAC Study Group. *Ann Emerg Med.* 1998;32:544-553.
155. Kudenchuk PJ, Cobb LA, Copass MK, et al . Amiodarone for resuscitation after out-of-hospital cardiac arrest due to ventricular fibrillation. *N Engl J Med.* 1999;341:871-878.
156. Dorian P, Cass D, Schwartz B, et al. Amiodarone as compared with lidocaine for shock-resistant ventricular fibrillation. *N Engl J Med.* 2002;346:884-890. Erratum in: *N Engl J Med.* 2002;347:955.
157. Glover BM, Brown SP, Morrison L, et alDorian P; Resuscitation Outcomes Consortium Investigators. Wide variability in drug use in out-of-hospital cardiac arrest: a report from the resuscitation outcomes consortium. Resuscitation. 2012;83:1324-1330.
158. Kudenchuk PJ, Brown SP, Daya M, et al. Amiodarone, lidocaine, or placebo in out-of-hospital cardiac arrest. *N Engl J Med* 2016;374:1711-1722.
159. Morrison LJ, Verbeek PR, Zhan C, et al. Validation of a universal prehospital termination of resuscitation clinical prediction rule for advanced and basic life support providers. *Resuscitation.* 2009;80:324-328.
160. Gaieski DF, Band RA, Abella BS, et al. Early goal-directed hemodynamic optimization combined with therapeutic hypothermia in comatose survivors of out-of-hospital cardiac arrest. *Resuscitation.* 2009;80:418-424.
161. Rittenberger JC, Kelly E, Jang D, et al. Successful outcome utilizing hypothermia after cardiac arrest in pregnancy: a case report. *Crit Care Med.* 2008;36:1354-1356.
162. Knafelj R, Radsel P, Ploj T, Noc M. Primary percutaneous coronary intervention and mild induced hypothermia in comatose survivors of ventricular fibrillation with ST-elevation acute myocardial infarction. *Resuscitation.* 2007;74:227-234.
163. Wolfum S, Pierau C, Radke PW, et al. Mild therapeutic hypothermia in patients after out-of-hospital cardiac arrest due to ST-segment elevation myocardial infarction undergoing immediate percutaneous coronary intervention. *Crit Care Med.* 2008;36:1780-1786.
164. Oddo M, Schaller MD, Feihl F, et al. From evidence to clinical practice: effective implementation of therapeutic hypothermia to improve patient outcome after cardiac arrest. *Crit Care Med.* 2006;34:1865-1873.
165. Reynolds JC, Rittenberger JC, Callaway CW. Methylphenidate and amantadine to stimulate reawakening in comatose patients resuscitated from cardiac arrest. *Resuscitation.* 2013;84:818-824.
166. Donnino MW, Rittenberger JC, Gaieski D, et al. The development and implementation of cardiac arrest centers. *Resuscitation.* 2011;82:974-978.
167. Birkmeyer JD, Stukel TA, Siewers AE, et al. Surgeon volume and operative mortality in the United States. *N Engl J Med.* 2003;349:2117-2127.
168. Callaway CW, Schmicker RH, Brown SP, et al. Early coronary angiography and induced hypothermia are associated with survival and functional recovery after out-of-hospital cardiac arrest. *Resuscitation.* 2014;85:657-663.
169. Wnent J, Seewald S, Heringlake M, et al. Choice of hospital after out-of-hospital cardiac arrest - a decision with far-reaching consequences: a study in a large German city. *Crit Care.* 2012;16(5):R164.
170. Cha WC, Lee SC, Shin SD, et al. Regionalisation of out-of-hospital cardiac arrest care for patients without prehospital return of spontaneous circulation. *Resuscitation.* 2012;83:1338-1342.
171. Reynolds JC, Rittenberger JC, Callaway CW; Post Cardiac Arrest Service. Patterns of organ donation among resuscitated patients at a regional cardiac arrest center. *Resuscitation.* 2014;85:248-252.
172. Spaite DW, Bobrow BJ, Vadeboncoeur TF, et al The impact of prehospital transport interval on survival in out-of-hospital cardiac arrest: implications for regionalization of post-resuscitation care. *Resuscitation.* 2008;79:61-66.
173. Spaite DW, Stiell IG, Bobrow BJ, et al. Effect of transport interval on out-of-hospital cardiac arrest survival in the OPALS study: implications for triaging patients to specialized cardiac arrest centers. *Ann Emerg Med.* 2009;54:256-257.
174. Hartke A, Mumma BE, Rittenberger JC, et al. Incidence of re-arrest and critical events during prolonged transport of post-cardiac arrest patients. *Resuscitation.* 2010;81:938-942.
175. Huang SC, Wu ET, Chen YS, et al. Extracorporeal membrane oxygenation rescue for cardiopulmonary resuscitation in pediatric patients. *Crit Care Med.* 2008;36:1607-1613.
176. Nagao K, Kikushima K, Watanabe K, et al. Early induction of hypothermia during cardiac arrest improves neurological outcomes in patients with out-of-hospital cardiac arrest who undergo emergency cardiopulmonary bypass and percutaneous coronary intervention. *Circ J.* 2010;74:77-85.
177. Morimura N, Sakamoto T, Nagao K, et al. Extracorporeal cardiopulmonary resuscitation for out-of-hospital cardiac arrest: a review of the Japanese literature. *Resuscitation.* 2011;82:10-14.
178. Maekawa K, Tanno K, Hase M, et al. Extracorporeal cardiopulmonary resuscitation for patients with out-of-hospital cardiac arrest of cardiac origin: a propensity-matched study and predictor analysis. *Crit Care Med.* 2013;41:1186-1196.
179. Belohlavek J, Kucera K, Jarkovsky J, et al. Hyperinvasive approach to out-of hospital cardiac arrest using mechanical chest compression device, prehospital intraarrest cooling, extracorporeal life support and early invasive assessment compared to standard of care. A randomized parallel groups comparative study proposal. "Prague OHCA study." *J Transl Med.* 2012;10:163.
180. Martin GB, Carden DL, Nowak RM, et al. Aortic and right atrial pressures during standard and simultaneous compression and ventilation CPR in human beings. *Ann Emerg Me.* 1986;15:125-130.
181. Sanders AB, Ogle M, Ewy BA. Coronary perfusion pressure during cardiopulmonary resuscitation. *Am J Emerg Med* 1985;3:11-14.
182. Sutton RM, Friess SH, Maltese MR, et al. Hemodynamic-directed cardiopulmonary resuscitation during in-hospital cardiac arrest. *Resuscitation.* 2014;85:983-986.
183. Friess SH, Sutton RM, French B, et al. Hemodynamic directed CPR improves cerebral perfusion pressure and brain tissue oxygenation. *Resuscitation.* 2014;85:1298-1303.
184. Salcido DD, Menegazzi JJ, Suffoletto BP, et al. Association of intramyocardial high energy phosphate concentrations with quantitative measures of the ventricular fibrillation electrocardiogram waveform. *Resuscitation.* 2009;80:946-950.
185. Reynolds JC, Salcido DD, Menegazzi JJ. Correlation between coronary perfusion pressure and quantitative ECG waveform measures during resuscitation of prolonged ventricular fibrillation. *Resuscitation.* 2012;83:1497-1502.
186. Callaway CW, Sherman LD, Mosesso VN Jr, et al. Scaling exponent predicts defibrillation success for out-of-hospital ventricular fibrillation cardiac arrest. *Circulation.* 2001;103:1656-1661.
187. Eftestøl T, Losert H, Kramer-Johansen J, et al. Independent evaluation of a defibrillation outcome predictor for out-of-hospital cardiac arrested patients. *Resuscitation.* 2005;67:55-61.
188. Snyder DE, White RD, Jorgenson DB. Outcome prediction for guidance of initial resuscitation protocol: shock first or CPR first. *Resuscitation.* 2007;72:45-51.

Postcardiac Arrest Management

6

IN THIS CHAPTER

- Oxygenation and ventilation
- Circulatory support
- Targeted temperature management
- Cardiac catheterization
- Ventilator-associated pneumonia
- Stress-related mucosal injury
- Blood transfusions
- Deep venous thrombosis prophylaxis

Evie G. Marcolini and Michael C. Bond

Successful resuscitation of a patient from sudden cardiac death is one of the most gratifying experiences of the emergency physician. Although this achievement is exciting, the initial enthusiasm at the return of spontaneous circulation (ROSC) quickly is tempered by the challenges clinicians face during the immediate postcardiac arrest period. With the persistent epidemic of hospital crowding, an expeditious transfer to the intensive care unit (ICU) following a successful resuscitation is no longer an option for most patients, many of whom are forced to remain in the emergency department for exceedingly long periods.

As a result, provision of postcardiac arrest treatment largely falls to the emergency physician, who must be adept at managing these critically ill patients. Essential elements in this care include mechanical ventilation, circulatory support, invasive and noninvasive hemodynamic monitoring, neuroprotective strategies, cardiac catheterization, and appropriate supportive care.

Definition

The term *postresuscitation disease* was coined in the 1970s when Dr. Vladimir Negovsky attempted to describe the unique pathophysiology of a patient resuscitated from cardiopulmonary arrest.[1,2] In 2008, the International Liaison Committee on Resuscitation (ILCOR) used the term *postcardiac arrest syndrome* (PCAS) to differentiate the disorder from the resuscitation of patients with sepsis or shock caused by other critical illnesses. PCAS consists of three general processes: postcardiac arrest brain injury, postcardiac arrest myocardial dysfunction, and systemic ischemia and reperfusion syndrome.[3]

Cardiopulmonary arrest essentially is the ultimate shock state, resulting in markedly impaired oxygen delivery and extraction, endothelial activation, systemic inflammation, multiorgan failure, and death. Once ROSC is achieved, patient management is directed at reversing these detrimental pathophysiological processes.

Acute Management

Oxygenation and Ventilation

Once successfully resuscitated, the patient should be intubated, and mechanical ventilation (of primary importance for the prevention of hypoxia and maintenance of normocapnia) should be initiated. Like any medical therapy, mechanical ventilation can directly injure patients if it is not applied and managed correctly. *Ventilator-induced lung injury* is the term used to describe a series of pathophysiological mechanisms such as alveolar overdistension (volutrauma), sheer stress from repeated opening and closing of alveolar units (atelectrauma), barotrauma, and the systemic release of inflammatory mediators (biotrauma) that result in lung injury. Initially, the ventilator should be set to limit ventilator-induced lung injury by achieving lower and safer distending pressures. These initial settings (*Figure 6-1*) are a starting point for ventilatory support. The ventilator can be adjusted based on serial measurements of pH, partial pressure of carbon dioxide ($PaCO_2$), oxygen saturation (SpO_2), and plateau pressure.

A natural consequence of using these initial recommended settings is the accumulation of carbon dioxide. Hypercapnia can increase intracranial pressure (ICP), diminish cerebral perfusion pressure, and exacerbate an existing acidosis. Similarly, hypocapnia can propagate cerebral injury by causing cerebral vasoconstriction, leading to ischemia. Given the emphasis on neuroprotective strategies in the PCAS patient, the ventilator should be adjusted to achieve a $PaCO_2$ between 40 and 45 mm Hg.

Capnography can be a useful tool to maintain the neuroprotective goal for $PaCO_2$.[4] End-tidal carbon dioxide values

FIGURE 6-1. Flow Diagram for Postarrest Management

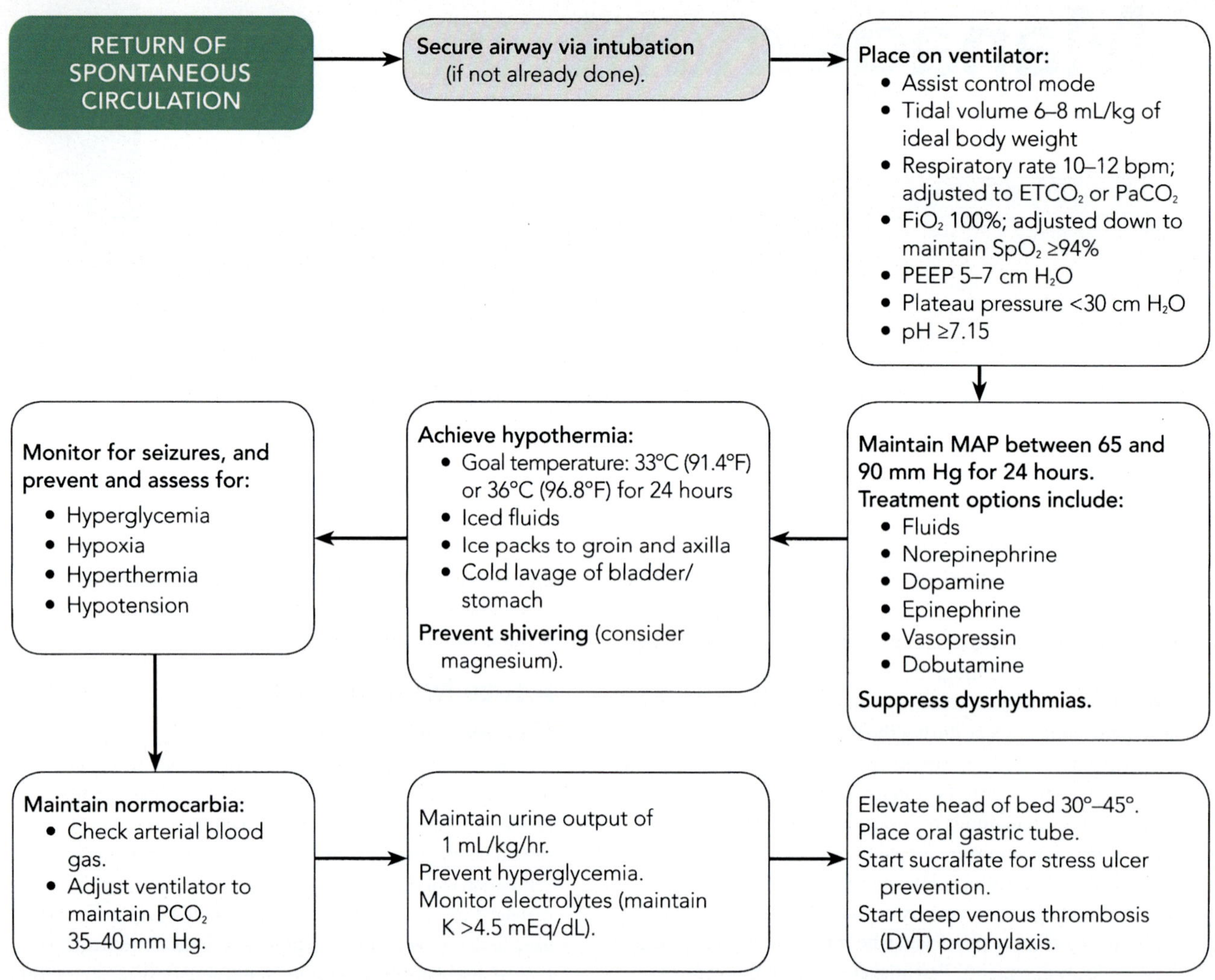

should be maintained between 35 and 40 mm Hg.[4] To prevent oxygen toxicity, the initial fraction of inspired oxygen (FiO_2) setting of 100% should be titrated down as tolerated to a goal oxygen saturation of 94% or more.[4] Evidence suggests that severe hyperoxia (partial pressure of oxygen [PaO_2] >300 mm Hg) may increase the inpatient mortality rates of post-ROSC patients, and moderate or probable hyperoxia (PaO_2 101-299 mm Hg) may improve organ function without negatively affecting survival rates.[5,6]

Circulatory Support

All PCAS patients should receive continuous cardiac and pulse oximetry monitoring, a Foley catheter for measuring urine output, and serial laboratory diagnostic testing that includes cardiac enzymes, lactate, and arterial blood gases. Most patients with PCAS have a tenuous cardiovascular status at best. Hemodynamic instability can be caused by hypovolemia, impaired vasoregulation, myocardial dysfunction, dysrhythmias, and even iatrogenic complications such as the initiation of therapeutic hypothermia.

Achieving an adequate circulating volume should be the first priority when managing such cases. The administration of intravenous fluids is the initial strategy for correcting intravascular volume depletion. Although the debate over crystalloid versus colloid therapy seems endless, isotonic crystalloids currently are the recommended fluid of choice in these patients.[3]

The decision to administer fluid therapy should be based on a multifactorial assessment of tissue perfusion, including parameters such as hypotension, oliguria, elevated lactate levels, and prolonged capillary refill. Dynamic tools for measuring changes in cardiac output or stroke volume, including pulse contour analysis, ultrasound techniques, or the passive leg raise maneuver, can be used to assess fluid responsiveness. It is important to recognize the limitations of central venous pressure (CVP) and static measurements, which can be altered by tricuspid valve disease, arrhythmias, pericardial effusion, right ventricular dysfunction, or simply the reference level of the transducer.

A more detailed discussion of these methods can be found in the chapters on fluid management (*Chapter 4*) and bedside ultrasound (*Chapter 22*). A urine output of at least 0.5 mL/kg/hr should be achieved and maintained when titrating fluid therapy in these patients.

PEARL

CVP should not be used routinely to guide fluid therapy in postcardiac arrest patients.

It is essential to maintain adequate oxygen delivery to vital organs when treating patients following cardiac arrest. Oxygen delivery to the tissues directly depends on organ perfusion pressure. The best physiological estimate of organ perfusion pressure is the mean arterial pressure (MAP), which must be monitored continuously. An elevated MAP significantly correlates with improved neurological outcomes in PCAS patients.[8]

After cardiac arrest, cerebral blood flow appears to depend on elevated MAP to maintain adequate cerebral perfusion. Current recommendations suggest maintaining pressures between 65 and 90 mm Hg in the first 24 hours following ROSC; however, better neurological outcomes have been associated with pressures targeted to 70 mm Hg.[8] If the goal MAP cannot be achieved with intravenous fluids alone, vasopressors should be initiated and blood pressure should be monitored continuously with the use of an arterial line.[3]

PEARL

Although the optimal MAP for the postarrest patient has not been defined, research suggests that MAP should be maintained between 70 and 90 mm Hg in the initial period following ROSC.

The efficacy of vasopressors in the management of PCAS has not been formally studied. Based on the authors' experience, norepinephrine is a reasonable first-line agent, given that it increases MAP through vasoconstriction and has minimal effects on the heart rate and cardiac index. In addition, norepinephrine has been shown to improve renal perfusion and lactate clearance.[9]

Dopamine also is a reasonable first-line vasopressor medication; however, its effects of increased heart rate and contractility can increase myocardial workload in an already compromised heart. Phenylephrine is at best a second-line agent, given its increase in MAP without elevating the heart rate or cardiac index.

A continuous infusion of epinephrine can increase MAP through an elevated heart rate and systemic resistance. Compared with other vasopressor medications, however, epinephrine also results in a greater degree of impaired splanchnic perfusion and an increase in lactate levels.

Vasopressin is a hormone that acts synergistically with other catecholamines to raise MAP by increasing systemic vascular resistance. Much like epinephrine, it has the potential to decrease splanchnic perfusion, thereby increasing lactate levels. This medication should be used as a last resort only after other agents have proven unsuccessful, and care must be taken to ensure adequate intravascular volumes.

If fluid therapy and vasopressor medications fail, inotropic agents can be used to achieve hemodynamic goals. Inotrope-responsive myocardial stunning can be present for up to 72 hours in survivors of cardiac arrest.[10] The duration of myocardial stunning correlates to the length of cardiac arrest; echocardiography can help determine cardiac function.[10]

Dobutamine, the longtime inotrope of choice, can be used to support hemodynamics (either by itself or in conjunction with norepinephrine). The drug can increase the cardiac index by as much as 50% and escalate cardiac consumption with a concomitant decrease in pulmonary artery occlusion pressure. However, dobutamine can exacerbate tachycardia in hypovolemic patients; adequate fluid resuscitation should be ensured.

The success of resuscitation should be monitored via serial laboratory assessments while intravenous fluids, vasopressor medications, and inotropic therapy are provided. Lactate values have been studied extensively and can be used to gauge the success of therapeutic efforts. The time to lactate clearance directly correlates to PCAS patient outcomes.[11,12] In addition to lactate, which should be measured every 3 to 4 hours, central venous oxygen saturation also has been proposed as an endpoint for resuscitation of the critically ill. However, new evidence indicates no survival benefit to central venous oxygen saturation ($ScvO_2$) monitoring in patients with severe sepsis or septic shock; its routine use is no longer recommended.[13-15]

For patients who remain hemodynamically unstable despite fluid, vasopressor medications, and inotropic therapy, the placement of an intraaortic balloon pump, initiation of extracorporeal membrane oxygenation, or placement of a transthoracic ventricular assist device should be considered. These potential lifesaving therapies, which require appropriate consultation and resources, might not be possible in many emergency departments.

PEARL

Up to 70% of postarrest patients will demonstrate myocardial dysfunction in the first few hours after ROSC. Initiate inotropic therapy if intravenous fluids and vasopressors fail to achieve the target MAP.

Neuroprotective Strategies

Brain injury is the most common cause of death in those who survive a cardiac arrest.[16] Targeted temperature management — the only therapy shown to increase survival in this patient population — improves short-term neurological recovery and survival in cases of PCAS of presumed cardiac origin.[17-22] The number needed to treat for one survivor to leave the hospital with good neurological function is between 4 and 13.

Animal studies show that earlier implementation leads to better outcomes.[23]

Targeted temperature management consists of induction, maintenance, and rewarming phases. Methods for achieving goal temperatures include administering ice-cold intravenous fluids, applying ice packs to the groin and axilla, and using surface or internal cooling devices. There is no evidence to support the superiority of one method of induction over another.[17-19,22]

While the "ideal" temperature remains up for debate, elevated temperatures have been linked to more severe brain injury in PCAS patients. Sedation and neuromuscular blockade can be used to prevent shivering, and warming the skin will reduce the core temperature threshold for this side effect.[24] During the induction and rewarming phases, fluid and electrolyte shifts occur and must be monitored. Decreased core temperatures cause vasoconstriction with increased central venous pressure and subsequent diuresis, which will reverse upon rewarming.

The maintenance phase of treatment requires continuous feedback of temperature to avoid significant fluctuations. Rewarming can be regulated by most cooling devices. Current recommendations suggest rewarming at 0.25°C (77°F) to 0.5°C (33°F) per hour to minimize the rapid changes in electrolyte concentrations, metabolic rate, and hemodynamic stability.[25]

PEARL

Monitor electrolytes (especially potassium, magnesium, and calcium) during the induction and rewarming phases of targeted temperature management.

Patients in whom targeted temperature management is induced must be monitored and treated for shivering. Adequate sedation can be achieved with benzodiazepines or propofol. Other therapies used for shivering include dexmedetomidine, buspirone, meperidine, and skin counterwarming.[26] If this side effect continues despite the titration of sedative medications, neuromuscular blockers should be used. However, these agents have a longer duration of action in the setting of hypothermia, and continuous electroencephalographic monitoring might be necessary to watch for seizure activity.

Both sedation and hypothermia are neuroprotective in that they decrease oxygen consumption. Magnesium sulfate has been shown to increase the shivering threshold. Magnesium increases the cooling rate via vasodilation and — in animal studies — demonstrates neuroprotection during therapeutic hypothermia.[27,28]

Contraindications to targeted temperature management include severe systemic infection, preexisting coagulopathy, and established multiorgan failure.[29] Complications include infection, hemodynamic instability, decreased cardiac output, arrhythmia (most commonly bradycardia), coagulopathy, hyperglycemia, increased amylase, hypophosphatemia, hypocalcemia, hypokalemia, and hypomagnesemia.

In addition to targeted temperature management, other neuroprotective strategies should be used in the PCAS patient. Seizures should be treated aggressively with standard medications such as benzodiazepines, phenytoin, valproate, propofol, or barbiturates. Hypotension, the most common adverse effect of these medications, must be avoided. Myoclonus is best treated with clonazepam. Electroencephalography should be used frequently or continuously to monitor the patient for subclinical seizure activity. Hyperthermia, hypoxemia, and hyperglycemia should be avoided because they worsen neurological outcomes. With every degree the temperature rises, so does the risk of a poor outcome (with an odds ratio of 2.26).[12]

Thrombolytic Therapy

Massive pulmonary embolus has been reported as the second leading cause of nontraumatic out-of-hospital deaths.[30] Smaller pulmonary emboli can lead to a hypoxemic cardiac arrest, manifesting an electromechanical dissociation rhythm that is responsive to adequate oxygenation. Although thrombolysis after cardiac arrest appears to be safe, prospective studies of thrombolytics show no improvement in patient outcomes.[31,32]

Cardiac arrest results in endothelial dysfunction, which causes an increase in fibrin generation and impaired anticoagulation.[33] Although clear prospective data are lacking, thrombolytic agents may aid neurological recovery in PCAS patients who survive ventricular fibrillation arrest and reasonably can be considered for the treatment of suspected pulmonary embolus.[34]

Acute Coronary Syndrome/Cardiac Catheterization

Acute myocardial infarction is the most common cause of sudden cardiopulmonary arrest.[35] Standard therapy with antiplatelet medication and anticoagulation should be started in patients who have suspected acute coronary syndrome. Ideally, emergency department care should be coordinated with the patient's cardiologist. It is reasonable to withhold anticoagulation until all central venous access or arterial lines are placed to prevent bleeding complications.

According to the 2013 American College of Cardiology Foundation (ACCF)/American Heart Association (AHA) guidelines, immediate angiography and, when indicated, percutaneous coronary intervention (PCI) should be performed in resuscitated out-of-hospital cardiac arrest patients whose initial ECG indicates STEMI.[36] Furthermore, the 2014 ACCF/AHA guidelines for the management of NSTEMI recommend early revascularization in patients with cardiogenic shock. (Both are Class I recommendations.)[37]

Use caution when starting beta-blockers in patients who already have a labile blood pressure or who might require vasopressor support. It is imperative to maintain an adequate MAP to ensure sufficient cerebral perfusion pressure. Although beta-blockers can be protective and decrease the long-term mortality rate in patients with acute coronary syndrome, hypotension can have detrimental effects on the patient's neurological recovery.

Research supports early angiography along with targeted

temperature management for any PCAS patient whose arrest likely is secondary to sequelae from coronary artery disease.[21] Establishing inclusion and exclusion criteria in such a protocol can be challenging, as there are no reliable indicators of acute myocardial infarction in PCAS patients. Taking all other physiological factors into consideration, it is reasonable to begin targeted temperature management and consider early angiography.

If percutaneous coronary interventions are unavailable, thrombolytic therapy may be a viable option for the treatment of PCAS, although it has not been studied in patients receiving targeted temperature management. Possible risks include ineffective thrombolysis and hemorrhage. As in cases of ST-segment elevation myocardial infarction, coronary artery bypass grafting is recommended in patients with left main coronary artery thrombosis or three-vessel disease.

Supportive Care

Prevent Ventilator-Associated Pneumonia

Ventilator-associated pneumonia, a leading cause of morbidity and mortality in the ICU population, is defined as pneumonia occurring more than 48 hours after intubation. The mortality rate for this complication ranges from 20% to 50%. Although all intubated PCAS patients are vulnerable to this infection, several low- to no-cost interventions markedly decrease the risk. These include semirecumbent positioning (head of bed elevated 30°-40°), frequent suctioning of the oropharynx, maintaining adequate endotracheal cuff pressures to prevent aspiration (between 20 and 30 cm H_2O), oral care with chlorhexidine rinses, and gastric decompression with an orogastric tube.[38,39]

Prevent Stress-Related Mucosal Injury

Stress-related mucosal injury is present in up to 75% of intubated patients who arrive in the ICU. Clinically significant bleeding occurs in up to 25% of this population (2%-5% require transfusion). As a result, the initiation of stress ulcer prophylaxis is indicated for intubated PCAS patients at high risk for gastrointestinal hemorrhage (eg, those with coagulopathy, mechanical ventilation >48 hours, or a history of peptic ulcer disease, gastritis, or gastrointestinal hemorrhage). Other patients at risk include those with sepsis, severe head injury, renal failure, hepatic failure, hypotension, and multisystem trauma.

Maintain Adequate Hemoglobin Levels

Goals for hemoglobin concentration have not been well studied in PCAS patients. In septic patients, early goal-directed therapy guidelines recommend maintaining Hgb above 10 g/dL during the initial 6 hours of resuscitation. However, several recent studies show no advantage to using a restrictive transfusion strategy (transfusion trigger of Hgb <7 g/dL) over a liberal transfusion strategy (transfusion trigger of Hgb <10 g/dL).[40-45] At present, there is no specific target hemoglobin level for the postarrest patient.[3] However, liberal transfusion strategies have been associated with fewer major cardiac events and deaths; therefore, it is reasonable to maintain Hgb above 8 g/dL in patients with active myocardial ischemia.

Prevent Deep Venous Thrombosis

Early prophylaxis against deep venous thrombosis is recommended in all ICU patients. In PCAS patients who do not have a high risk of bleeding, low-dose heparin, low-molecular-weight heparin, or mechanical compression devices are recommended, depending on the individual's comorbidities, medication allergies, presence of bleeding, and clinical stability.[47]

Monitor Glucose Concentrations

Blood glucose levels are independently associated with survival in cases of PCAS.[48] Tight glucose control has improved outcomes in surgical and medical ICU patients, whereas moderate control reduces the incidence of hypoglycemia in those resuscitated from ventricular fibrillation.[49-51] Observational research has shown a direct correlation between hyperglycemia and poor neurological outcomes in patients with PCAS, but the optimal glucose concentration has not been defined.[52] Hyperglycemia and hypoglycemia should be avoided, and until a standard protocol for managing hyperglycemia has been validated, ICU physicians and institutional protocols should be consulted.[4]

KEY POINTS

1. Use capnography to monitor ventilation in the postarrest patient. Adjust the ventilator respiratory rate to achieve an end-tidal carbon dioxide measurement of 35 to 40 mm Hg.
2. Decrease the FiO_2 to the lowest fraction of inspired oxygen that maintains SpO_2 ≥94%.
3. Maintain the patient's PaO_2 between 100 and 300 mm Hg, as severe hyperoxia is associated with increased mortality.
4. Consider thrombolytic therapy in patients with suspected massive pulmonary embolism.
5. Postarrest patients with evidence of an ST-elevation myocardial infarction (MI) on either the prearrest or postarrest ECG should be sent for emergent cardiac catheterization.
6. Postarrest patients with evidence of a non-ST-elevation MI with hemodynamic or electrical instability should be considered for emergent cardiac catheterization.
7. Administer deep venous thrombosis prophylaxis.
8. Avoid hypoglycemia and hyperglycemia.

Conclusion

Although ROSC remains the hallmark of successful resuscitation, emergency physicians are developing a heightened appreciation for the significant role they play in governing the outcome of patients with PCAS.[21] Clinicians from a variety of health care disciplines also should be involved in the care of these patients, including emergency medicine and critical care, and subspecialties such as cardiology, neurology, and nephrology. By implementing a standardized approach, providers can build upon the work that already has been done to achieve ROSC and further improve long-term survival.

REFERENCES

1. Negovsky VA. The second step in resuscitation — the treatment of the 'post-resuscitation disease.' *Resuscitation.* 1972;1:1-7.
2. Negovsky VA, Gurvitch AM. Post-resuscitation disease — a new nosological entity. Its reality and significance. *Resuscitation.* 1995; 30:23-27.
3. Neumar RW, Nolan JP, Adrie C, et al. Post-cardiac arrest syndrome: epidemiology, pathophysiology, treatment, and prognostication. A consensus statement from the International Liaison Committee on Resuscitation (American Heart Association, Australian and New Zealand Council on Resuscitation, European Resuscitation Council, Heart and Stroke Foundation of Canada, InterAmerican Heart Foundation, Resuscitation Council of Asia, and the Resuscitation Council of Southern Africa); the American Heart Association Emergency Cardiovascular Care Committee; the Council on Cardiovascular Surgery and Anesthesia; the Council on Cardiopulmonary, Perioperative, and Critical Care; the Council on Clinical Cardiology; and the Stroke Council. *Circulation.* 2008;118:2452-2483.
4. Callaway CW, Donnino MW, Fink EL, et al. Part 8: Post-Cardiac Arrest Care: 2015 American Heart Association Guidelines Update for Cardiopulmonary Resuscitation and Emergency Cardiovascular Care. *Circulation.* 2015;132(18 suppl 2): S465–482.
5. Wang CH, Chang WT, Huang CH, et al. The effect of hyperoxia on survival following adult cardiac arrest: a systematic review and meta-analysis of observational studies, *Resuscitation.* 2014;85:1142-1148.
6. Elmer J, Scutella M, Pullalarevu R, et al. The association between hyperoxia and patient outcomes after cardiac arrest: analysis of a high-resolution database. *Intensive Care Med.* 2015;41:49-57.
7. McIntyre LA, Fergusson DA, Hutchison JS, et al. Effect of a liberal versus restrictive transfusion strategy on mortality in patients with moderate to severe head injury. *Neurocrit Care.* 2006;5:4-9.
8. Kilgannon JH, Roberts BW, Jones AE, et al. Arterial blood pressure and neurologic outcome after resuscitation from cardiac arrest. *Crit Care Med.* 2014;42:2083-2091.
9. Balk R, Casey L. Sepsis and septic shock. Philadelphia, PA: W.B. Saunders; 2000.
10. Laurent I, Monchi M, Chiche JD, et al. Reversible myocardial dysfunction in survivors of out-of-hospital cardiac arrest. *J Am Coll Cardiol.* 2002;40:2110-2116.
11. Donnino MW, Andersen LW, Giberson T, et al. Initial lactate and lactate change in post-cardiac arrest: a multicenter validation study. *Crit Care Med.* 2014;42:1804-1811.
12. Donnino MW, Miller J, Goyal N, et al. Effective lactate clearance is associated with improved outcome in post-cardiac arrest patients. *Resuscitation.* 2007;75:229-234.
13. ARISE Investigators; ANZICS Clinical Trials Group, Peake SL, et al. Goal-directed resuscitation for patients with early septic shock. *N Engl J Med.* 2014;371:1496-1506.
14. Mouncey PR, Osborn TM, Power GS. et al. Trial of early, goal-directed resuscitation for septic shock. *N Engl J Med.* 2015;372:1301-1311.
15. Pro CI, Yealy DM, Kellum JA, et al. A randomized trial of protocol-based care for early septic shock. *N Engl J Med.* 2014;370:1683-1693.
16. Fink M. Textbook of critical care. Philadelphia, PA: Elsevier Saunders; 2005.
17. Bernard SA, Gray TW, Buist MD, et al. Treatment of comatose survivors of out-of-hospital cardiac arrest with induced hypothermia. *N Engl J Med.* 2002;346:557-563.
18. Holzer M, Bernard SA, Hachimi-Idrissi S, et al. Hypothermia for neuroprotection after cardiac arrest: systematic review and individual patient data meta-analysis. *Crit Care Med.* 2005;33:414-418.
19. Hypothermia After Cardiac Arrest Study Group. Mild therapeutic hypothermia to improve the neurologic outcome after cardiac arrest. *N Engl J Med.* 2002;346:549-556.
20. Nolan JP, Morley PT, Hoek TL, et al. Therapeutic hypothermia after cardiac arrest. An advisory statement by the Advancement Life Support Task Force of the International Liaison Committee on Resuscitation. *Resuscitation.* 2003;57:231-235.
21. Sunde K, Pytte M, Jacobsen D, et al. Implementation of a standardised treatment protocol for post resuscitation care after out-of-hospital cardiac arrest. *Resuscitation.* 2007;73:29-39.
22. Nielsen N, Wetterslev J, Cronberg T, et al. Targeted temperature management at 33 degrees C versus 36 degrees C after cardiac arrest. *N Engl J Med.* 2013;369:2197-2206.
23. Kuboyama K, Safar P, Radovsky A, et al. Delay in cooling negates the beneficial effect of mild resuscitative cerebral hypothermia after cardiac arrest in dogs: a prospective, randomized study. *Crit Care Med.* 1993;21:1348-1358.
24. Cheng C, Matsukawa T, Sessler DI, et al. Increasing mean skin temperature linearly reduces the core-temperature thresholds for vasoconstriction and shivering in humans. *Anesthesiology.* 1995;82:1160-1168.
25. Arrich J; European Resuscitation Council Hypothermia After Cardiac Arrest Registry Study Group. Clinical application of mild therapeutic hypothermia after cardiac arrest. *Crit Care Med.* 2007;35:1041-1047.
26. Choi HA, Ko SB, Presciutti M, et al. Prevention of shivering during therapeutic temperature modulation: the Columbia anti-shivering protocol. *Neurocrit Care.* 2011;14:389-394.
27. Wadhwa A, Sengupta P, Durrani J, et al. Magnesium sulphate only slightly reduces the shivering threshold in humans. *Br J Anaesth.* 2005;94:756-762.
28. Zhu H, Meloni BP, Moore SR, et al. Intravenous administration of magnesium is only neuroprotective following transient global ischemia when present with post-ischemic mild hypothermia. *Brain Res.* 2004;1014:53-60.
29. Soar J, Nolan JP. Mild hypothermia for post cardiac arrest syndrome. *BMJ.* 2007;335:459-460.
30. Courtney DM, Kline JA. Identification of prearrest clinical factors associated with outpatient fatal pulmonary embolism. *Acad Emerg Med.* 2001;8:1136-1142.
31. Abu-Laban RB, Christenson JM, Innes GD, et al. Tissue plasminogen activator in cardiac arrest with pulseless electrical activity. *N Engl J Med.* 2002;346:1522-1528.
32. Bottiger BW, Bode C, Kern S, et al. Efficacy and safety of thrombolytic therapy after initially unsuccessful cardiopulmonary resuscitation: a prospective clinical trial. *Lancet.* 2001;357:1583-1585.
33. Gando S, Kameue T, Nanzaki, S, et al. Massive fibrin formation with consecutive impairment of fibrinolysis in patients with out-of-hospital cardiac arrest. *Thromb Haemost.* 1997;77:278-282.
34. Schreiber W, Gabriel D, Sterz F, et al. Thrombolytic therapy after cardiac arrest and its effect on neurological outcome. *Resuscitation.* 2002;52:63-69.
35. Huikuri HV, Castellanos A, Myerburg RJ. Sudden death due to cardiac arrhythmias. *N Engl J Med.* 2001;345:1473-1482.
36. American College of Emergency Physicians; Society for Cardiovascular Angiography and Interventions, O'Gara PT, et al. 2013 ACCF/AHA guideline for the management of ST-elevation myocardial infarction: a report of the American College of Cardiology Foundation/American Heart Association Task Force on Practice Guidelines. *J Am Coll Cardiol.* 2013;61:e78-e140.
37. Amsterdam EA, Wenger NK, Brindis RG, et al. 2014 AHA/ACC guideline for the management of patients with non-ST-elevation acute coronary syndromes: a report of the American College of Cardiology/American Heart Association Task Force on Practice Guidelines. *J Am Coll Cardiol.* 2014;64:e139-e228.
38. Gaussorgues P, Gueugniaud PY, Vedrinne JM, et al. Bacteremia following cardiac arrest and cardiopulmonary resuscitation. *Intensive Care Med.* 1988;14:575-577.
39. Rello J, Diaz E, Roque M, et al. Risk factors for developing pneumonia within 48 hours of intubation. *Am J Respir Crit Care Med.* 1999;159:1742-1746.
40. Restrictive approach to transfusion best in upper gastrointestinal bleeding. *BMJ.* 2013;346:f71.
41. Carson JL, Grossman BJ, Kleinman S, et al. Red blood cell transfusion: a clinical practice guideline from the AABB. *Ann Intern Med.* 2012;157:49-58.
42. Carson JL, Terrin ML, Noveck H, et al. Liberal or restrictive transfusion in high-risk patients after hip surgery. *N Engl J Med.* 2011;365:2453-2462.
43. Goodnough LT, Maggio P, Hadhazy E, et al. Restrictive blood transfusion practices are associated with improved patient outcomes. *Transfusion.* 2014;54(10 Pt 2):2753-2759.
44. Hebert PC, Wells G, Blajchman MA, et al. A multicenter, randomized, controlled clinical trial of transfusion requirements in critical care. Transfusion Requirements in Critical Care Investigators, Canadian Critical Care Trials Group. *N Engl J Med.* 1999;340:409-417.
45. McIntyre L, Hebert PC, Wells G, et al. Is a restrictive transfusion strategy safe for resuscitated and critically ill trauma patients? *J Trauma.* 2004;57:563-568.
46. Carson JL, Brooks MM, Abbott JD, et al. Liberal versus restrictive transfusion thresholds for patients with symptomatic coronary artery disease. *Am Heart J.* 2013;165:964-971 e961.
47. Geerts W, Selby R. Prevention of venous thromboembolism in the ICU. *Chest.* 2003;124(6 suppl):357S-363S.
48. Skrifvars MB, Pettila V, Rosenberg PH, et al. A multiple logistic regression analysis of in-hospital factors related to survival at six months in patients resuscitated from out-of-hospital ventricular fibrillation. *Resuscitation.* 2003;59:319-328.
49. Oksanen T, Skrifvars MB, Varpula T, et al. Strict versus moderate glucose control after resuscitation from ventricular fibrillation. *Intensive Care Med.* 2007;33:2093-2100.
50. Van den Berghe G, Schoonheydt K, Becx P, et al. Insulin therapy protects the central and peripheral nervous system of intensive care patients. *Neurology.* 2005;64:1348-1353.
51. Van den Berghe G, Wilmer A, Hermans G, et al. Intensive insulin therapy in the medical ICU. *N Engl J Med.* 2006;354:449-461.
52. Mullner M, Sterz F, Binder M, et al. Blood glucose concentration after cardiopulmonary resuscitation influences functional neurological recovery in human cardiac arrest survivors. *J Cereb Blood Flow Metab.* 1997;17:430-436.

Deadly Arrhythmias

7

IN THIS CHAPTER

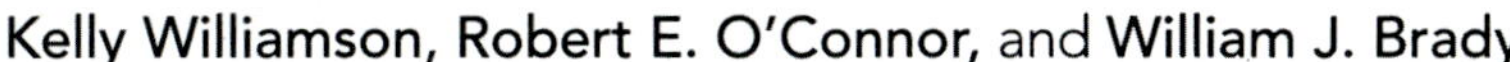

- Bradycardia
- Atrioventricular block
- Narrow complex tachycardia
- Wide complex tachycardia
- Sudden death syndromes

Kelly Williamson, Robert E. O'Connor, and William J. Brady

Abnormal heart rhythms are encountered frequently in the emergency department, and it is incumbent upon the clinician to differentiate between unstable arrhythmias that require an urgent evaluation and management plan, and stable presentations that allow more time for a comprehensive workup. The patient with chronic rate-controlled atrial fibrillation who presents with an unrelated complaint, for example, might not require additional cardiovascular care. However, the patient with an ST-segment elevation myocardial infarction (STEMI) associated with ventricular tachycardia (VT) requires emergent intervention. Advanced cardiovascular life support (ACLS) guidelines point to the following indicators of instability: hypotension or systemic hypoperfusion, altered mentation, ischemic chest pain, and respiratory distress (*Table 7-1*).[1]

Electrocardiography, the interpretation of the electrical activity of the heart using rhythm-monitoring techniques, is essential to the timely diagnosis and treatment of arrhythmias. Any rhythm must be evaluated in the context of the presentation, with particular consideration given to specific patient characteristics such as age and medical history. For instance, an elderly man with a previous myocardial infarction (MI) who presents with a wide complex tachycardia is likely to be experiencing ventricular tachycardia, as both age and preexisting MI place him at risk for this malignant arrhythmia.

Bradyarrhythmias

Bradyarrhythmia is a general descriptive term for rhythms with a ventricular rate slower than 60 beats/min in the adult. Age-related norms define pediatric bradyarrhythmias, which are the result of sinus node dysfunction or atrioventricular (AV) conduction disorders that lead to such pathologies as sinus bradycardia, junctional rhythm, idioventricular rhythm, and atrial fibrillation with a slow ventricular response. Atrioventricular blocks, or impaired conduction of the electrical signal between the atria and the ventricles, also can lead to bradyarrhythmia. These rhythms are caused by decreased automaticity with increased refractoriness of cardiac cells and abnormal conduction of impulses within the system, and are affected in disease processes such as myocardial ischemia, hypothermia, drug toxicity, and electrolyte abnormalities.

In a review of patients with unstable bradycardia or AV block, 80% of the rhythm abnormalities could be attributed to a secondary cause.[3,4] The most frequently identified underlying causes were acute coronary syndrome (ACS) and toxicological exposures; multifactorial events (eg, hypoxia with hypoperfusion) also were frequently encountered.[3,4] In this same series, bradycardias were encountered significantly more often than AV block. In fact, 66% of patients demonstrated sinus, junctional, or idioventricular bradycardia. The vast majority of AV blocks seen in this population were third-degree heart blocks (82% of AV blocks); first- and second-degree AV blocks were seen much less commonly.[3,4] Among patients with ACS, sinus bradycardia and third-degree AV block were the most common bradyarrhythmias encountered.

TABLE 7-1. Instability Considerations in the Arrhythmic Patient
Hypotension and/or hypoperfusion
Altered mental status
Ischemic chest discomfort
Dyspnea resulting from pulmonary edema
Extremely rapid rate (approaching 300 beats/min)

Pharmacological Management

Management issues in the bradyarrhythmic patient are multifactorial and can range from the initiation of general supportive measures (eg, oxygen delivery, intravenous fluids) to the administration of various medications (eg, atropine, adrenergic agonists), or electrical therapy in the form of cardiac pacing to specific therapeutic maneuvers (eg, treatment of hyperkalemia).[1] Atropine often is the first-line agent for the treatment of bradyarrhythmias in patients not in cardiac arrest (eg, cases of symptomatic sinus bradycardia or AV block). Its administration increases the heart rate by enhancing the automaticity of the sinoatrial (SA) node and AV nodal conduction by means of a direct vagolytic mechanism.

Atropine administration has inherent limitations, as patients are more likely to respond appropriately to the first dose than to subsequent doses. In addition, bradyarrhythmias secondary to AV block may have a limited response to atropine.[2-4]

Although there are theoretic concerns about the medication, there is limited evidence to refute its cautious use in the appropriate clinical situation. Controversy exists surrounding its potential to worsen ischemia or lead to the development of malignant ventricular arrhythmias in patients with ACS. While the increase in heart rate theoretically might exacerbate ischemia if given during an acute coronary event, sustained systemic and coronary hypoperfusion from an unstable bradyarrhythmia also could lead to adverse outcomes.[2-4] In addition, the development of malignant ventricular arrhythmias after the administration of atropine for unstable bradyarrhythmia is infrequent in the prehospital setting (2%–4%).[3,4,7]

PEARL

Paradoxic slowing of the heart rate following atropine administration is rare in patients with infranodal AV block, particularly those with Mobitz type II second-degree AV block and third-degree AV block with a wide QRS complex. This adverse effect is uncommon, but the emergency care provider should be aware of its potential in patients with unstable bradyarrhythmias.

Glucagon, a naturally occurring hormone, has positive inotropic and chronotropic effects. Its use in patients experiencing bradyarrhythmias has been most extensively delineated in those with toxic exposure to cardioactive medications, including cases of calcium channel antagonist and beta-blocker overdose.[8,9] Recommended doses in the setting of toxicity from these drugs are variable; generally, an initial intravenous bolus of 2 to 10 mg is suggested, with continuous infusion at 2 to 5 mg/hr if necessary. In infants and small children, the bolus dose is 50 mcg/kg. Adverse effects include nausea, emesis, hypokalemia, and inconsequential hyperglycemia.

The use of adrenergic agents such as dopamine, epinephrine, and isoproterenol also has been explored in the pharmacologic management of unstable bradyarrhythmias. These agents are potent chronotropes that can increase the heart rate in certain situations, and can elevate conduction velocity within the AV node and the intraventricular conduction system. Unfortunately, these drugs also can markedly increase myocardial work and oxygen demand in patients with conditions such as ACS. As a result, they should be used only temporarily to provide a bridge to more definitive management with transcutaneous or transvenous cardiac pacing.

Cardiac Pacing

Cardiac pacing can be accomplished either transcutaneously or transvenously. Transcutaneous pacing is markedly easier to perform and frequently effective, but it is quite uncomfortable for the patient unless ample pain medication or continuous sedation is administered. Because sedative-hypnotic agents might worsen perfusion in the already unstable patient, this technique typically is reserved as a temporizing measure in emergent situations.

Transcutaneous pacemakers generally have two connections to the patient: a set of pads for delivering the pacing current and leads for monitoring. If feasible, the pads should be placed in an anteroposterior position, with the anterior pad as close as possible to the point of maximum cardiac impulse, and the posterior pad directly opposite the anterior in the left perithoracic region. Two variables require adjustment: the energy output required to pace the patient and the rate at which pacing occurs. "Electrical capture" is manifested by the rhythm produced by the pacing unit, and "mechanical pacing" is determined if a pulse is felt corresponding to the paced electrical rhythm. Complications include pain, local tissue injury, and failure to detect underlying ventricular arrhythmias.

The more definitive transvenous pacing is highly effective yet quite invasive. Central venous access is required and best established via the right internal jugular or left subclavian vein. The pacing electrode is then advanced through the vein under electrocardiographic guidance. The balloon-tipped catheter is inserted into the central line and advanced approximately 10 cm. At this point, the pulse generator is activated in the "sense" mode, and the pacing wire is further advanced into the ventricle until cardiac electrical activity is detected.

At this time, the balloon is deflated, the generator is switched to the "pace" mode, and the current is increased from the minimal setting used during the first phase (eg, <0.2 mA) to a setting that is likely to electrically capture the ventricle (eg, 4–5 mA). This electrical capture should be apparent on the rhythm monitor as the wire is advanced up to 10 cm and placement in the right ventricle can be confirmed by recognition of a left-bundle branch block pattern. If capture does not occur, the wire should be withdrawn back to the initial 10-cm mark and the process should be repeated.

PEARL

The right internal jugular route is preferred for transvenous cardiac pacing so that the left central veins remain "device free" in the event that permanent cardiac pacing is needed.

Specific Bradyarrhythmias

Sinus Bradycardia

Sinus bradycardia (SB) is a very common arrhythmia, defined by the presence of a ventricular rate of less than 60 beats/min in the adult patient; age-adjusted rates are used in infants and children. In sinus bradycardia, the SA node still functions normally, generating impulse formation with appropriate transmission through the atria and the AV node and into the ventricles.

SB is encountered in a number of scenarios and must be interpreted within the context of the presentation, as rates less than 60 beats/min are not always pathological. For instance, highly trained endurance athletes can have a resting heart rate in the range of 40 to 50 beats/min. However, the presence of SB also can be indicative of an evolving clinical situation that requires emergent action. It is frequently observed in early ACS presentations (an inferior wall STEMI can cause SB because of heightened parasympathetic tone).

In addition, adverse medication effects can trigger sinus bradycardia, either through unintentional exposure or purposeful ingestion. These situations require immediate diagnosis and emergent intervention to prevent cardiovascular collapse.[2-4] Prompt initiation of general supportive care, including appropriate volume resuscitation, vasopressor support for perfusion, and adequate oxygenation, is important in the early management of clinically significant SB, regardless of its underlying pathophysiology.

Electrocardiographical Diagnosis

As previously discussed, SB is defined as a sinus rhythm with a rate below 60 beats/min in an adult. All other electrocardiographical characteristics of this rhythm are normal: P wave, PR interval, and P-QRS relationship. The P wave is upright in the limb leads. The PR interval is fixed in length; it can be normal or abnormally prolonged in the presence of a first-degree AV block. It is important to note, however, that the P-wave-to-QRS-complex relationship is normal, with all sinus node-originated P waves conducted to the ventricles, creating a QRS complex (*Figure 7-1*).

Specific Management Considerations

SB is the most common arrhythmia encountered in early ACS presentations, particularly in patients with inferior-wall STEMI. In these situations, atropine has demonstrated significant efficacy via its direct vagolytic action on the SA node; its use should be considered early in patients with symptomatic SB related to ACS. An initial dose of 0.5 to 1 mg should be administered intravenously, followed by three additional doses at 3- to 5-minute intervals as needed for persistent pathology (for a total dose of 3 mg).[5] Higher

FIGURE 7-1. Sinus Bradycardia

Sinus bradycardia is defined as the presence of sinus rhythm with a rate slower than 60 beats/min. The P wave is upright in the limb leads and in leads I, II, and III. The PR interval is fixed in length; it can be normal or abnormally prolonged with a coexisting first-degree AV block. Importantly, however, the P-wave-to-QRS-complex relationship is normal, with all sinus node-originated P waves conducted to the ventricles, with a resultant QRS complex.

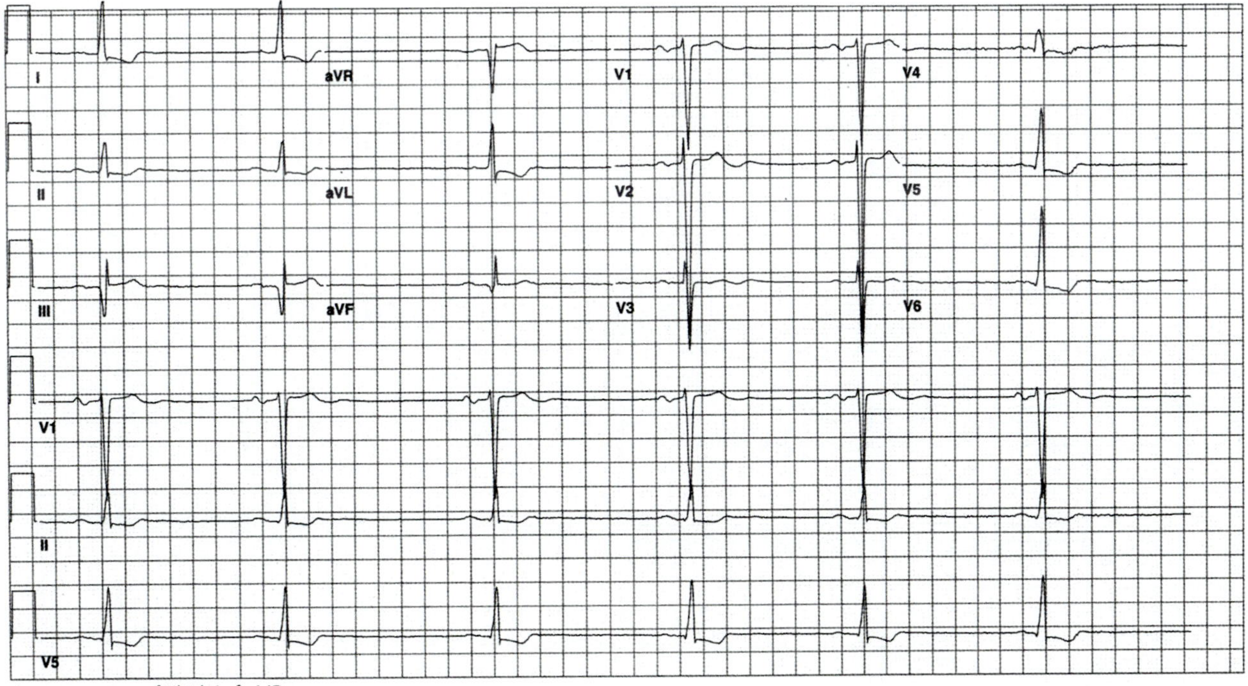

Image courtesy of Ulrich Luft, MD.

individual doses, larger cumulative amounts, and more frequent use of atropine have demonstrated prompt, beneficial responses in this clinical scenario.[3,4]

Junctional Bradycardia

The AV node can be considered as the first default pacemaker if the sinus node becomes dysfunctional. As a result, junctional bradycardia most often originates at the AV node; however, on occasion, the proximal bundle of His may be the focus. The resulting escape rhythm is a junctional rhythm with a narrow QRS complex. As with SB, the junctional rhythm commonly is seen in patients with ACS and toxicological exposures; it occasionally is encountered in trained athletes.[2-4]

ECG Diagnosis

A junctional rhythm demonstrates a regular, narrow QRS complex at a rate of roughly 40 to 60 beats/min (*Figure 7-2*). Junctional rhythms that originate from the AV node typically have a ventricular rate of 45 to 60 beats/min, while slower junctional rhythms (35–45 beats/min) have been found to originate in the proximal bundle of His.[3] P waves usually are absent; if present, they will be retrograde. "Retrograde" refers to conduction from — rather than to — the AV node; the AV nodal impulse moves in a retrograde fashion back into the atria, producing this type of P wave. The retrograde P wave can be found before, during, or after the QRS complex; frequently, it is inverted.

Specific Management Considerations

Junctional bradycardia, the second most common arrhythmia in patients with ACS, responds reasonably well to atropine via the drug's direct vagolytic action. Junctional bradycardic rhythms also are seen frequently in poisoned patients. Although they are less likely to respond to atropine than are ACS-mediated rhythms, such therapy is still recommended.[3,4] When managing a patient with a compromising junctional rhythm, the clinician should consider the administration of atropine while other targeted treatments are being prepared.

PEARL

Atropine is more likely to work at the AV-node level of the conduction system; it is less likely to be effective if the rhythm originates below the AV node.

Idioventricular Rhythm (Bradycardia)

An idioventricular rhythm results from a pacemaker site located in the distal intraventricular conduction system or within the ventricular myocardium. In either case, this type of rhythm should be considered a secondary default pacemaker after failure of both the SA and AV nodes. With rates of less than 40 beats/min, the idioventricular rhythm will support marginal perfusion at best. This rhythm is most common in cardiac arrest patients who demonstrate electrical activity on the cardiac monitor yet have no palpable pulse.

FIGURE 7-2. Junctional Rhythm

A junctional rhythm demonstrates a regular, narrow QRS complex at a rate of roughly 40 to 60 beats/min. Slower junctional rhythms (35–45 beats/min) have been found to originate in the bundle of His. The QRS complex remains narrow in these presentations. P waves are usually not present.

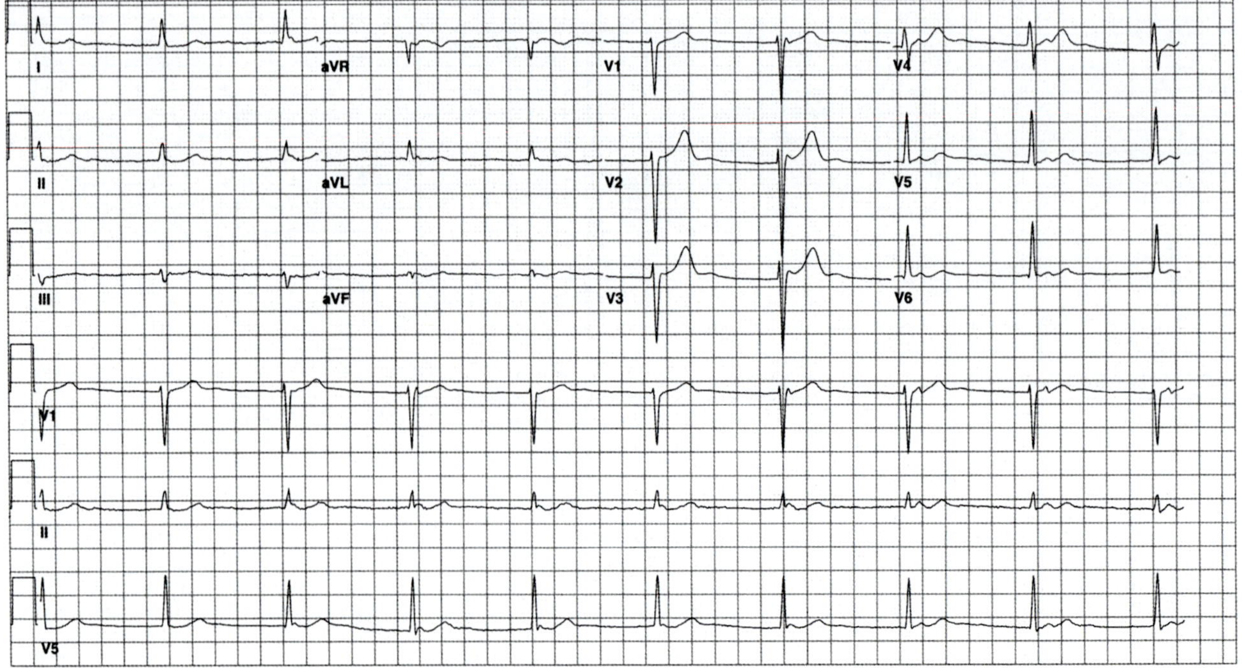

Image courtesy of Ulrich Luft, MD.

ECG Diagnosis

Idioventricular rhythms are very slow (usually between 30 and 40 beats/min). The QRS complexes are abnormally widened if the pacemaker site is found in the more distal portions of the ventricular conduction system or within the ventricular myocardium itself. However, if the pacemaker site is in the ventricular septum, the complexes may be only minimally widened. In either case, they occur at a regular frequency. Preexisting intraventricular conduction delay (ie, bundle-branch block) accompanied by a junctional escape rhythm is indistinguishable from a faster idioventricular rhythm.[10]

Specific Management Considerations

General resuscitative management is crucial in this particular rhythm scenario; adequate oxygenation, appropriate intravascular volume status, and sufficient perfusion are key considerations in patients with idioventricular rhythms. Atropine and other medications are unlikely to restore appropriate perfusion in patients with compromising idioventricular rhythms; cardiac pacing likely will become necessary in these presentations. Specific therapies (eg, attention to hyperkalemia or cardioactive medication poisonings) also should be considered.

PEARL

Atropine and other medications are unlikely to restore perfusion in patients with compromising idioventricular rhythms.

Atrioventricular Block

The *site* of an AV conduction block helps predict the likelihood that it will progress to *complete* AV block and potential hemodynamic collapse. More proximal locations (namely at or above the AV node) are associated with first- and second-degree type I block and typically pose low risk. First-degree AV block rarely — if ever — is symptomatic or worrisome; it is, in fact, considered a normal variant condition. A patient with first-degree AV block who lacks symptoms, signs, or a troubling clinical presentation needs no further attention or therapy for the conduction issue.

The same is true for second-degree type I AV block. Conversely, distal sites of dysfunction within or below the AV node are encountered in second-degree type II and third-degree AV block and should be considered pathologic. These abnormalities are most common in acutely ill patients with significant hemodynamic compromise. Patients with second-degree type II AV block are at high risk of progressing to complete heart block. These "high-grade" presentations frequently are seen in patients with STEMIs; the presence of third-degree AV block is predictive of STEMI in chest pain patients.[3,4]

ECG Diagnosis

From the electrocardiographical perspective, AV block is diagnosed based on the PR interval and the relationship of the P wave to the QRS complex. In **first-degree AV block** (*Figure 7-3*), the PR interval is prolonged from the normal 0.12 to 0.2 seconds. While minimal variability can be seen because of changes in heart rate and autonomic tone, this prolongation typically is fixed and unchanging. In addition, the rhythm is regular with uniform, consistent P-P and R-R intervals.

Second-degree AV block is usually, though not always, an irregular rhythm. There are two types of second-degree AV block: Mobitz type I and Mobitz type II. Both feature intermittent failure of atrial impulses to reach the ventricles (ie, some P waves are not followed by QRS complexes). **Second-degree type I AV block** is characterized by an initially normal PR interval that progressively lengthens (*Figure 7-4*). Initially, each P wave is associated with a QRS complex. The PR interval lengthens until a beat is not conducted to the ventricle during which time a P wave will be noted without an associated QRS complex. As this pattern progresses, the R-R interval shortens. This pattern then repeats itself at varying intervals. Grouped beating of Wenckebach is observed in this form of AV block when the QRS complexes occur in groups separated by a pause, yielding the apparent irregularity of the rhythm. The morphology of the P waves and the QRS complexes generally is normal.

Second-degree type II AV block (*Figure 7-5*) also features intermittently blocked P waves but with a different pattern. In this form, each P wave initially is associated with a QRS complex and a fixed PR interval. This pattern continues until, ultimately, a P wave occurs without conduction to the ventricle; thus no QRS complex is seen. As with type I block, the pattern then repeats at varying intervals. Most patients with type II AV block have an associated bundle-branch block, meaning the block is distal to the bundle of His, producing a widened QRS complex. Less often, the block is intra-Hisian or in the AV node, demonstrating a narrow QRS complex.

The magnitude of AV block is expressed as a ratio of P waves to QRS complexes (the conduction ratio). When the conduction ratio is 2:1, it is impossible to differentiate the two types of second-degree AV blocks since the conduction of every other P wave is obstructed, preventing a lengthening assessment of the PR interval. If the conduction ratio is other than 2:1, the rhythm can appear irregular with grouping of conducted beats separated by the nonconducted beat. The descriptor "highgrade" is applied when more than one P wave in a row is nonconducted.

Third-degree AV block is called complete atrioventricular dissociation or complete heart block (*Figure 7-6*). In this case, the atria and ventricles are working independently without any electrical communication. The SA node usually produces regularly occurring P waves; therefore, the P-P intervals are constant and unchanging. In complete heart block, the atrial pacemaker is faster than the escape pacemaker, which can be either junctional or ventricular; therefore, the atrial rate is faster

FIGURE 7-3. First-Degree AV Block

Showing fixed prolongation of the PR interval. Note that the normal PR interval is 0.12–0.2 seconds. The PR interval does not change appreciably from beat to beat. The P-wave-to-QRS-complex relationship is normal, with each P wave producing a QRS complex.

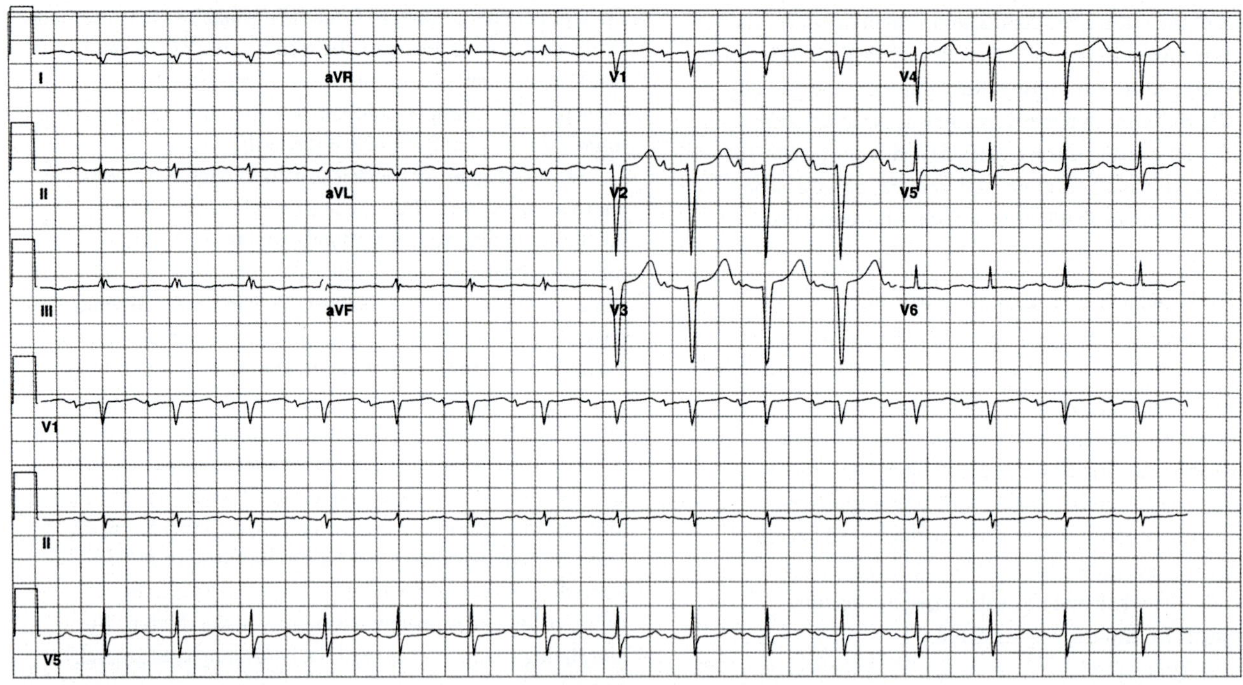

Image courtesy of Ulrich Luft, MD.

FIGURE 7-4. Second-Degree Type I AV Block

Progressive prolongation of PR interval until a beat is not conducted (ie, a QRS complex is dropped).

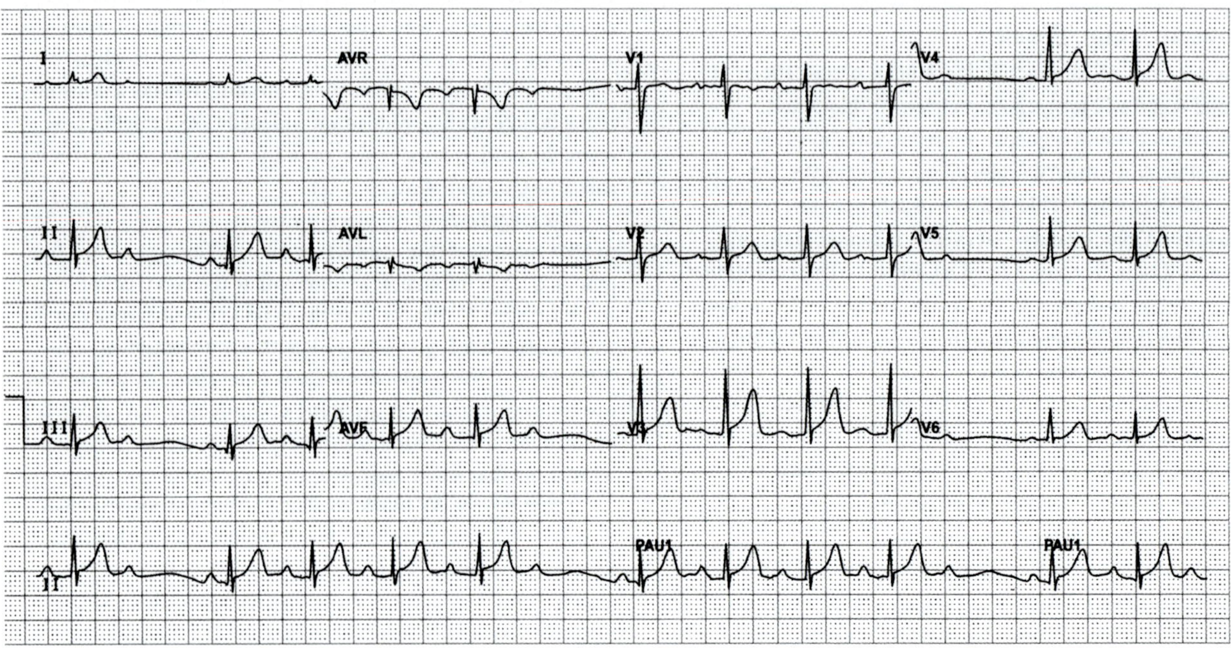

Image courtesy of lifeinthefastlane.com

FIGURE 7-5. Second-Degree Type II AV Block

Fixed PR interval with sudden dropped beat. The ventricular depolarization can be a narrow or wide QRS complex. In this particular example, the first four conducted beats demonstrate 2-1 conduction, meaning that a non-conducted P wave follows each conducted beat; in this sequence, we cannot conclusively determine the type of second-degree AV block, either type I or II. It is only at the fifth QRS complex that the clinician can determine the presence of second-degree type II AV block. In this sequence, we have two consecutive QRS complexes followed by the non-conducted beat.

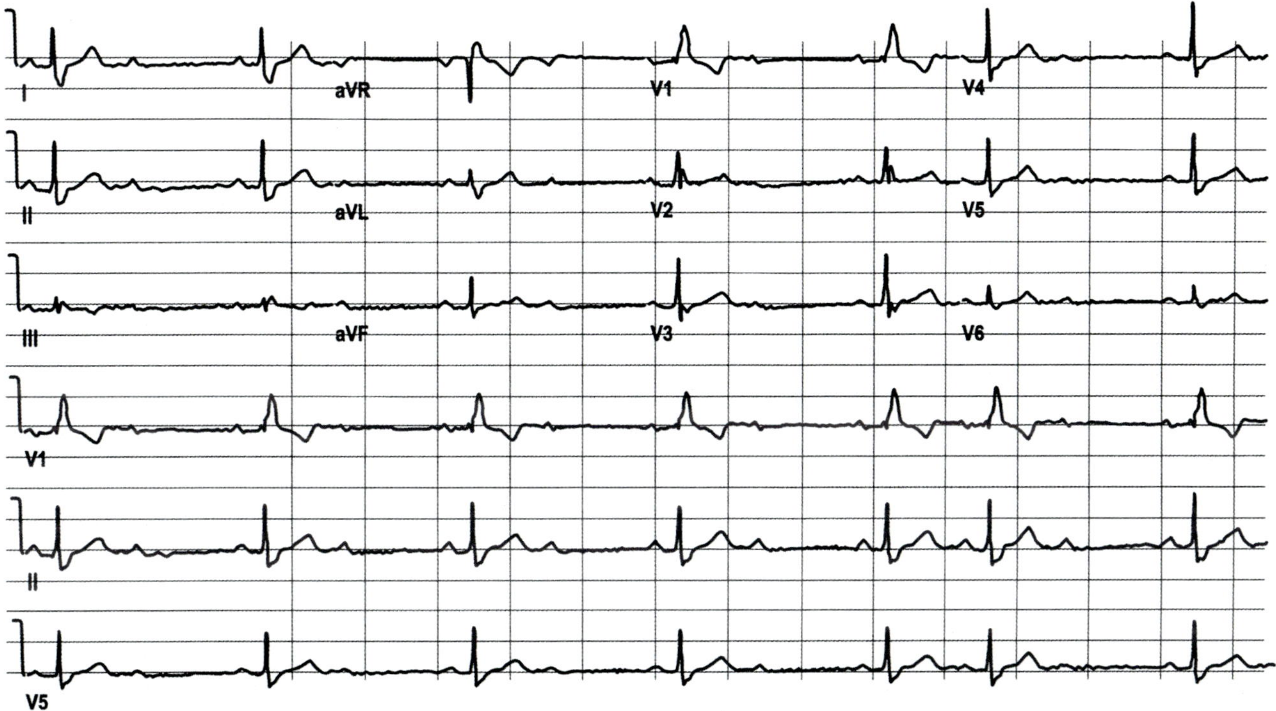

than the ventricular rate. The escape rhythm most often occurs in a regular manner as well, again with constant and unchanging R-R intervals. Depending on the site of the conduction block, the escape rhythm can be either junctional (narrow QRS complex) or idioventricular (wide QRS complex). The PR interval is variable, constantly changing without a consistent pattern due to the complete lack of electrical communication between the atria and the ventricles.

Specific Management Considerations

Isolated first- and second-degree type I AV blocks rarely require intervention unless the patient has an acute clinical condition that can affect cardiac conduction (eg, ACS or toxicologic overdose). Even in these cases, the block is not of concern in and of itself; rather, its presence can be predictive of a more significant conduction abnormality. In this situation, the clinician should consider increasing the level of patient surveillance and prepare for more aggressive resuscitative therapy.

The "high-grade" AV blocks (second-degree type II and third degree) can have significant negative effects on perfusion and often require emergent management. Medications such as atropine are less likely to be of benefit in these situations, and the clinician must consider prompt initiation of cardiac pacing if the patient's hemodynamic status is compromised. Transcutaneous pacing pads should be applied even on asymptomatic patients out of concern for deterioration while other causes of the abnormality (eg, hyperkalemia) are explored. Empiric therapy should be initiated at the discretion of the treating clinician.[2]

Tachyarrhythmias

Narrow Complex Tachycardia

Narrow complex tachycardia (NCT) refers to a cardiac rhythm with a ventricular rate above 100 beats/min and a QRS complex width less than or equal to 0.08 seconds in an adult patient; as with the bradyarrhythmias, age-appropriate rates and widths exist for pediatric patients with NCT.[11] NCTs are a diverse group of rhythm disturbances with varying acuity levels, natural histories, management strategies, and outcomes. Rhythms in this category include sinus tachycardia (ST), paroxysmal supraventricular tachycardia (PSVT), atrial fibrillation (AF), atrial flutter, and multifocal atrial tachycardia (MAT).

ECG Diagnosis

Each of these rhythm disturbances can present as cardiovascular collapse, either directly related to the arrhythmia or because of its causative syndrome. For instance, the patient with PSVT can present with significant hypotension, with the circulatory shock resulting from

FIGURE 7-6. Third-Degree AV Block

Also known as complete heart block. There is a complete lack of electrical communication between the atria and the ventricles. Note the regular rates of both the P waves and QRS complexes, with the atrial rate exceeding the ventricular rate. At times, the P wave is "lost" within the larger QRS complex.

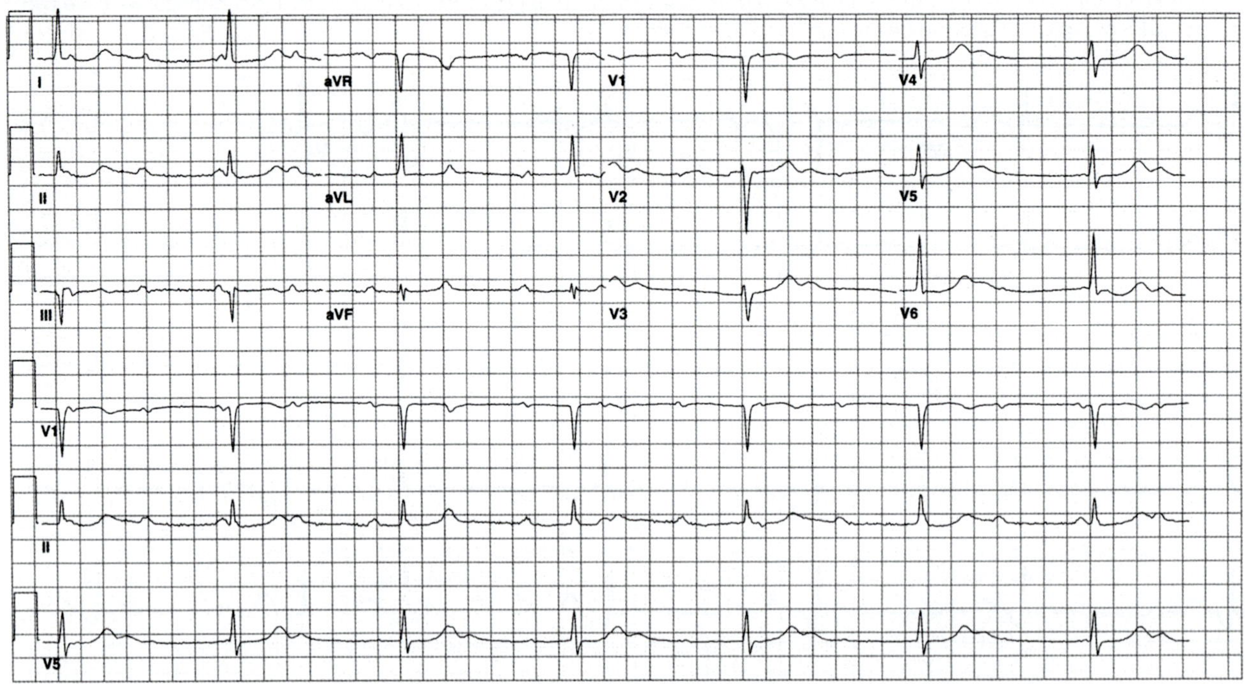

Image courtesy of Ulrich Luft, MD.

the rhythm itself. Conversely, a patient with significant hypotension secondary to gastrointestinal hemorrhage can present with ST — the circulatory shock in this case being a result of the hemorrhage, with the rhythm solely a manifestation of the hemodynamic compromise.

Specific Management Considerations

Certain tachyarrhythmias require urgent rhythm-specific therapy, whereas others need treatment aimed at correction of the underlying cause of the dysrhythmia. Determination of patient stability, or lack thereof, will guide early management decisions. A number of therapeutic maneuvers can be employed in the treatment of NCT, including intravenous fluids, supplemental oxygen, vagal maneuvers, adenosine, beta-blockers, calcium channel blockers, and electrical cardioversion. It must be emphasized, however, that the therapeutic approach varies, depending on the rhythm; this list of interventions does not apply to all NCTs.

In some cases, the first appropriate treatment is the vagal maneuver, including carotid massage or initiation of the diving reflex. This intervention can be considered in the patient with PSVT, AF, or NCT associated with the Wolff-Parkinson-White (WPW) syndrome. Vagal maneuvers can be curative; if performed correctly and early in the patient's clinical course, this intervention will convert the rhythm in approximately 20% of such presentations.

PEARL

Vagal maneuvers should be considered in the patient with PSVT, AF, or NCT related to WPW syndrome.

For PSVT and WPW-related NCT, adenosine is the next most appropriate therapeutic agent, although it is unlikely to be of benefit in other NCT presentations. Adenosine is a very short-acting agent that blocks the AV node and interrupts the reentrant circuit responsible for propagating the tachycardia. It generally is a safe choice with an excellent record of successful arrhythmia termination in this setting. It should be given initially as a rapid 6-mg IV bolus; if that is unsuccessful, a 12-mg rapid bolus can be given and repeated if no response occurs. Dosing for children is 0.1 mg/kg, with a maximum first dose of 6 mg; a second dose of 0.2 mg/kg, with a maximum of 12 mg, may be administered if the first fails to terminate the arrhythmia.[6]

A lower initial dose of 3 mg should be used in the following scenarios: 1) recent use of either dipyridamole or carbamazepine (these two medications potentiate the effects of adenosine), 2) administration of adenosine via central venous line, allowing a higher concentration of medication to arrive quickly at the heart, and 3) in patients with a transplanted heart (the graft heart is more sensitive to effects of the drug). In each of these presentations, prolonged pauses or short periods of asystole have been observed. In other clinical situations, the effects of

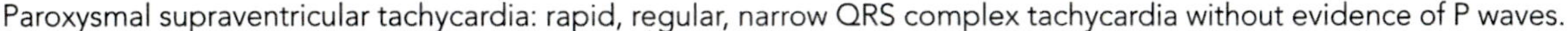

FIGURE 7-7. Paroxysmal Supraventricular Tachycardia

Paroxysmal supraventricular tachycardia: rapid, regular, narrow QRS complex tachycardia without evidence of P waves.

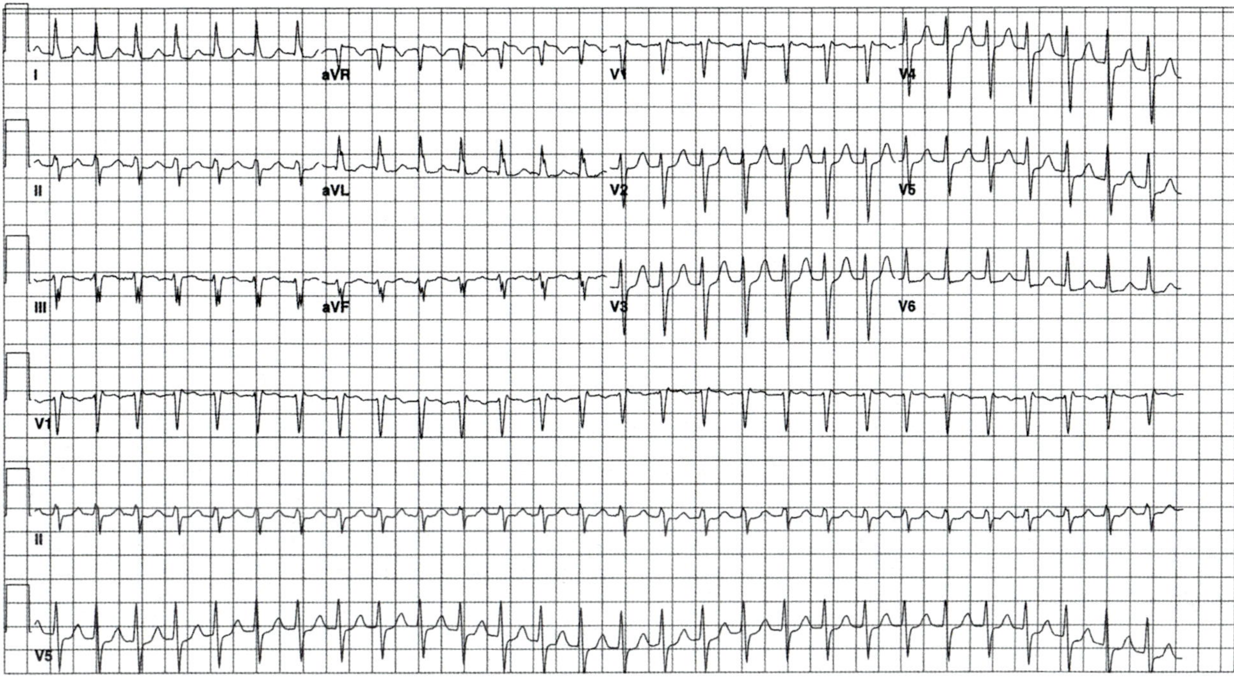

Image courtesy of Ulrich Luft, MD.

adenosine are antagonized by methylxanthines such as caffeine and theophylline. In the presence of these substances, larger doses of the drug might be required (ie, an 18-mg IV bolus); in extreme cases, adenosine might be ineffective.

It is important to correctly define a "failure" in the administration of adenosine. The serum half-life of the drug is very short, leading to a profound yet brief AV nodal blocking effect. Thus, a transient period of AV nodal blockade with near-immediate recurrence of the PSVT is not a treatment failure, but merely a consequence of the medication's brief duration of effect. In such situations, repeat dosing at the same level is unlikely to succeed; a higher dose should be given if possible.[12]

For refractory PSVT, AF, atrial flutter, and WPW-related NCT, longer-acting AV nodal blocking agents such as beta-blockers and calcium channel blockers can be given intravenously to achieve direct control of the ventricular rate. Metoprolol is a reasonable beta-blocker for managing such situations. It is given intravenously at a dose of 5 mg, and can be repeated two additional times at appropriate intervals if the desired effect is not observed. Esmolol, a parenteral beta-blocker with a relatively short duration of effect, also can be used in place of the longer-duration agents if hypotension is a concern. Diltiazem, administered at a dose of 0.25 mg/kg IV over several minutes, is an appropriate calcium channel blocker for such arrhythmias. If the desired clinical response does not occur, it can be repeated at a dose of 0.35 mg/kg IV.[5]

Finally, electrical cardioversion can be considered in patients with PSVT, AF, atrial flutter, and WPW-related NCT who are unstable or do not respond to initial pharmacological measures. Caution must be exercised regarding hemodynamic stability; not all patients who present with one of these arrhythmias require electrical cardioversion. AF, for example, can prompt hemodynamic instability; however, it is far more likely to be a manifestation of instability, rather than a cause.

Paroxysmal Supraventricular Tachycardia

PSVT is second only to AF as the most common pathological supraventricular tachycardia (SVT) encountered in the emergency department.[13] Although younger patients are more likely to experience PSVT in the absence of known cardiovascular disease, no definitive conclusions can be drawn regarding the influence of age or sex on the mechanism of the tachycardia. AV nodal reentrant tachycardia (AVNRT) appears to be the most common mechanism of SVT in patients of all ages; and age may not be a reliable predictor of tachycardia.[14]

The incidence of PSVT is evenly distributed between men and women for the most part; however, there appears to be a higher prevalence of AVNRT among women, with the proportion ranging from 68% to 76% in three studies. The reason for this unbalanced distribution is unclear. Regardless of

FIGURE 7-8. Sinus Tachycardia

Sinus tachycardia with a rate of 150 beats/min. This abnormality should be considered a "reactive rhythm," and treatment should be focused on the cause(s), including hypovolemia, hypoxia, fever, medication/toxin effect, and pain/ anxiety (a diagnosis of exclusion).

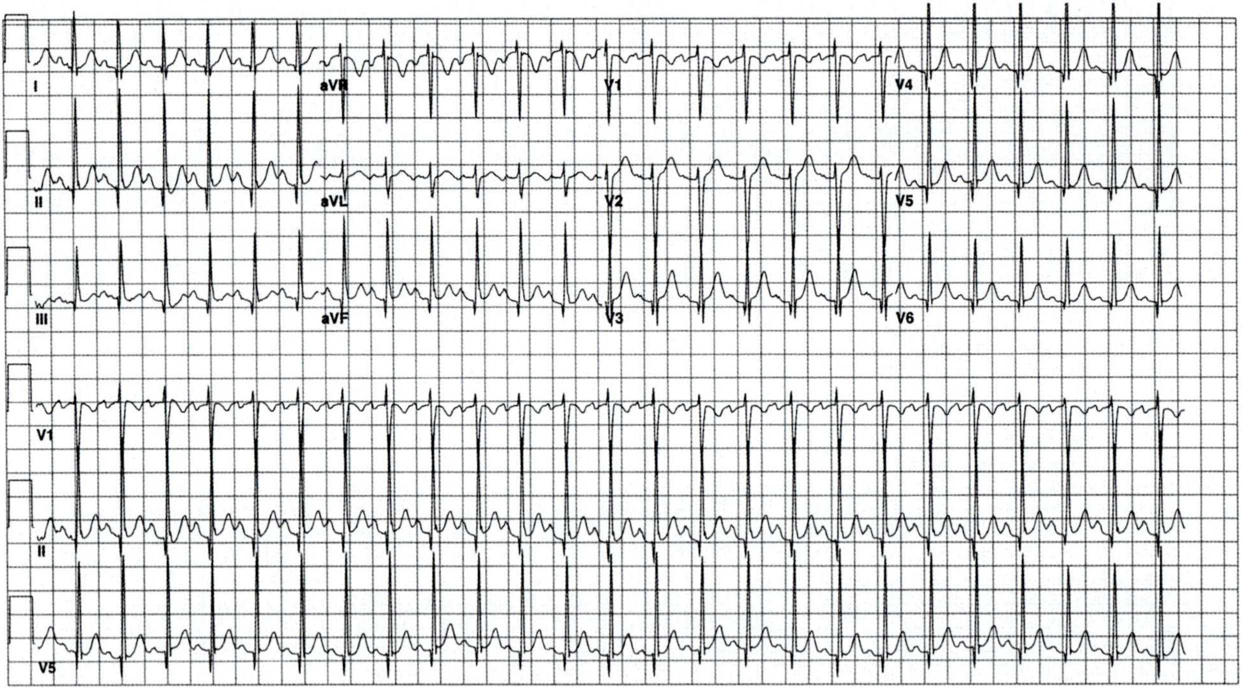

Image courtesy of Ulrich Luft, MD.

the mechanism, the rhythm is only a nuisance in most cases of PSVT and not a threat to life; management of the arrhythmia is all that is required. The rare patient who presents with PSVT as a manifestation of an underlying issue will require management of the arrhythmia and the causative pathology.[13]

Approximately 80% of patients with PSVT have an arrhythmia focus in the AV node; the remaining patients have PSVT with an atrial focus. It is estimated that 2% to 3% of PSVT-appearing arrhythmias are, in fact, WPW-related NCT. Because the vast majority of PSVT cases result from a problem in the AV node, it is not surprising that adenosine and other AV nodal-blocking agents are successful in rhythm management with chemical conversion.

ECG Diagnosis

PSVT is a narrow QRS complex tachycardia with a complex duration of less than 0.08 seconds. PSVT is rapid and regular; in the adult patient, the rate usually is 170 to 180 beats/min but can range from as low as 130 beats/min to as high as 300 beats/min. In children, the rate can approach 240 to 260 beats/min, particularly in infants.

P waves usually are not seen; because atrial and ventricular depolarizations occur almost simultaneously, the P waves frequently are buried in the QRS complex and totally obscured. In fact, the P wave is not observed on ECG in 70% of PSVT cases. In a minority of presentations, the so-called retrograde P wave is noted. As with junctional bradycardia, the term "retrograde P waves" refers to conduction from — rather than to — the AV node. The AV nodal impulse moves in a retrograde direction back into the atria. The retrograde P wave can be found before, during, or after the QRS complex; frequently, it is inverted in the limb leads. If the P wave occurs after the QRS complex, it can distort the terminal portion of the complex, producing a "pseudo" S wave in the inferior leads and a "pseudo" R wave in V_1. PSVT and rapid ST can be compared in Figures 7-7 and 7-8.

Specific Management Considerations

The management of PSVT usually results in favorable patient outcomes. In most cases, vagal maneuvers and intravenous adenosine are curative. It is the uncommon patient who requires a beta-blocker or calcium channel blocker. The use of an agent with a longer serum half-life can assist in the conversion to sinus rhythm; this therapy can be used in full or partial dose, combined with repeat adenosine administration. In the rare patient with recalcitrant PSVT or an unstable presentation, electrical cardioversion can be employed.[13]

Atrial Fibrillation and Atrial Flutter

AF remains the most prevalent form of NCT, affecting more than 2.3 million Americans.[15] Patients can present with worsening of their chronic AF as a result of poorly controlled ventricular rates; with paroxysmal AF associated with hyperthyroidism, hypokalemia, or hypomagnesemia; or

FIGURE 7-9. Atrial Fibrillation

ECG demonstrating an irregularly irregular rhythm with wide complexes secondary to left bundle-branch block.

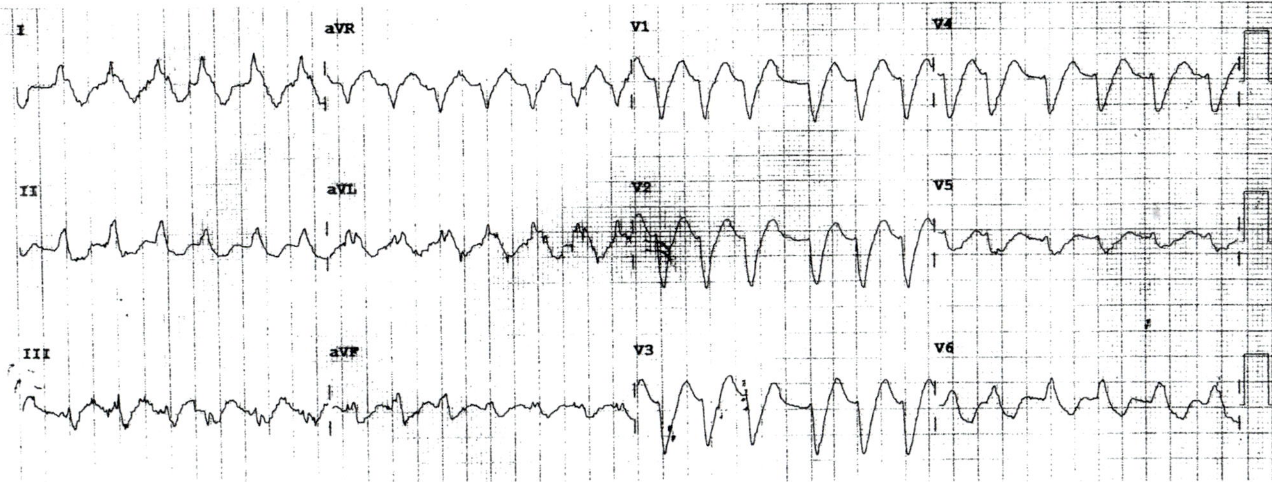

following excessive ethanol intoxication (the holiday heart syndrome).[16] The mechanism of AF appears to be multiple microreentrant wavelets in the atria. Paroxysms of AF can be triggered by preceding alterations in autonomic tone[17] or ectopic foci, which frequently are located in or around the pulmonary veins.[18]

AF is the second most common tachycardia in patients with WPW syndrome, occurring in 20% to 25% of these patients. Atrial flutter, another common NCT that shares many etiological features with AF, most commonly is caused by a macroreentrant circuit within the right atrium. An NCT that is regular (150 beats/min) strongly suggests atrial flutter with 2-to-1 conduction, as this is the "natural" rate for atrial flutter when unaffected by other disease states or medications.

ECG Diagnosis

AF usually can be diagnosed on an ECG. The rhythm is irregular with absent P waves. The baseline can be isoelectric or exhibit fibrillatory waves of varying morphologies at a rate of 400 to 700 beats/min. The amplitude of the fibrillatory waves is suggestive of the underlying pathology. Fine fibrillatory waves (defined as an amplitude <0.5 mm) are associated with ischemic heart disease, whereas coarse waves (>0.5 mm in amplitude) signify left atrial enlargement likely related to chronic hypertension. The rate varies, but a ventricular response of approximately 170 beats/min is common, representing the "natural" rate of atrial fibrillation (ie, not altered by another disease state or medications). The QRS complex is narrow in most presentations; however, preexisting bundle-branch block or rate-related bundle dysfunction can produce a widened QRS complex (*Figure 7-9*).

Atrial flutter can be regular or irregular. As with AF, the QRS complex is narrow unless affected by a preexisting bundle-branch block. P waves are present and of a single morphology. Typically, the P waves appear as downward deflections called flutter waves, which are marked by a characteristic "sawtooth" appearance. These waves are best seen in the inferior leads and lead V_1. Most commonly, the atrial rate is regular, usually 300 beats/min, with a range from 250 to 350 beats/min.

Although one-to-one conduction is possible, some form of fixed AV block usually is present, leading to a ventricular rate that corresponds with the degree of the block. Two-to-one AV block, which is most common, will produce a ventricular rate of about 150 beats/min, while a 3-to-1 AV block will result in a rate of 100 beats/min. Irregularity in the rhythm occurs when the degree of AV block is variable.

Specific Management Considerations

AF affects hemodynamic stability in two principal ways. The majority of symptoms, including weakness, dizziness, palpitations, chest discomfort, and dyspnea, are a result of the rapid rate. Therefore, the most important treatment consideration in these patients is control of the ventricular response. However, the continued presence of AF at a controlled rate still can produce unwanted clinical effects. An organized atrial contraction contributes to appropriate left ventricular filling; the loss of this "atrial kick" can continue to produce unpleasant manifestations despite adequate rate control.

In the setting of AF, hemodynamic stability must be considered along a spectrum ranging from the asymptomatic patient with an incidentally discovered arrhythmia to the individual with new-onset tachyarrhythmia in profound shock caused by a rapid ventricular response. In profoundly unstable patients with AF, urgent electrical cardioversion is the most appropriate therapy. In the mildly unstable patient, a trial of rate control can be attempted with calcium channel or beta-adrenergic blockade; additional agents include digoxin and amiodarone.

The final consideration for emergency care providers regarding AF focuses on the cardioversion of patients who are otherwise clinically stable. Numerous studies have suggested that a significant portion of patients with new-onset AF spontaneously convert to sinus rhythm within 24 hours after onset and evaluation.[19-22] This high rate of spontaneous conversion, coupled with the results of numerous AF trials, demonstrates the similarities between rate control and rhythm control in regard to several key endpoints.[21,22] In fact, there appear to be no significant differences between the two in terms of quality of life, control of symptoms, and the occurrence of adverse events.[21,22]

There are, however, several benefits to performing cardioversion in patients who present with AF, namely enabling discharge and follow up without the need for inpatient admission. The success rate for emergency department cardioversion is high (85.5%–97%, according to recent research),[23] and the risk of thromboembolic events and AF relapse following the intervention appears to be low.[24]

Wide Complex Tachycardia

Ventricular Tachycardia

In general, *wide complex tachycardia* (WCT) describes a rhythm scenario characterized by a broad QRS complex (>0.12 seconds) and a ventricular rate over 100 beats/min. In particular, VT is a malignant rhythm disturbance that originates from the myocardium or conduction system below the AV node. In most instances, VT presents with a wide QRS complex and a rate greater than 120 beats/min; in rare cases, VT presents as a "normal-appearing" QRS complex such as in children with an age-related "narrow" QRS complex width and adults with cardiac glycoside toxicity.[25,26]

VT frequently is encountered as a complication of coronary artery disease related to either active ischemia or the presence of scar tissue, which can create a substrate for ventricular arrhythmias. Patients with cardiomyopathy are the second most frequently encountered group presenting with VT. Electrolyte abnormalities, particularly those related to potassium, also can lead to VT. Medications, particularly type IA antiarrhythmic agents, digoxin, phenothiazines, and tricyclic antidepressants, also can produce ventricular arrhythmias.

This diagnosis has several classification systems. The first (sustained or nonsustained) refers to the persistence of the arrhythmia. The second (stable versus unstable) evaluates the hemodynamic impact of the arrhythmia. Finally, the appearance of the QRS complex is described by the designation *monomorphic* or *polymorphic*.

ECG Diagnosis

Monomorphic VT usually is regular, most often with rates ranging from 140 to 180 beats/min (*Figure 7-10a*). Polymorphic VT is characterized by an unstable (frequently varying) QRS complex morphology in any single ECG lead (*Figure 7-10b*). Variations in the R-R interval and electrical axis also are noted in this ventricular arrhythmia. Torsade de pointes, literally translated as "twisting of the points," is identified when polymorphic VT occurs in the setting of delayed myocardial repolarization manifested on the sinus rhythm ECG by a prolongation of the QT interval. Thus torsade de pointes is a subtype of polymorphic VT and not a synonym for the entire category of polymorphic VT (*Figure 7-10c*).

Specific Management Considerations

Patients with ventricular tachycardia should be managed much like those with any other NCT, and treatment should be based on the individual's presentation and related clinical issues. Attention should be paid to underlying inciting conditions, including electrolyte disorders (potassium and magnesium), medication toxicities, acute coronary ischemia, genetic issues (long QT syndrome), and other cardiac and noncardiac ailments. In the stable patient, pharmacological agents may be considered the first-line therapy. These drugs include procainamide, amiodarone, lidocaine, and magnesium.[5]

Procainamide is an effective agent for stable VT patients with preserved left ventricular function; it is preferred over amiodarone, sotalol, and lidocaine for the treatment of stable monomorphic VT.[5] Procainamide is given at 20 to 50 mg/min until the arrhythmia terminates or one of the following criteria is achieved: hypotension (systolic blood pressure <90 mm Hg), the QRS complex duration is prolonged by 50% from its original duration, the tachycardia accelerates, or a total of 17 mg/kg has been given.[5] An alternative dosing protocol requires 10 minutes for the maximum dose of 10 mg/kg; in this regimen, procainamide is administered at 100 mg/min until a maximum of 10 mg/kg or one of the above criteria is reached. Procainamide should not be used in patients with a prolonged QT interval.[5]

In patients with a tenuous hemodynamic status, amiodarone is the antiarrhythmic of choice, with lidocaine as the acceptable alternative. In such patients, amiodarone is given as a dose of 150 mg IV over 10 minutes, and lidocaine is given as a bolus of 1.5 mg/kg IV over 2 minutes. Magnesium also can be considered as a primary antiarrhythmic agent, but its use should be reserved for various "niche" applications (eg, in patients with known hypomagnesemia, QT interval prolongation, or polymorphic VT). Magnesium can be given at a dose of 1 to 2 grams (8–16 mEq) IV over 20 to 30 minutes to a stable patient and more rapidly to an unstable patient. Its main adverse effect is altered mentation with associated respiratory depression. Regardless of the agent used, careful cardiovascular monitoring is required.

In addition to these commonly accepted medications, adenosine can be used for undifferentiated, regular monomorphic WCT to aid in the detection of SVT with aberrancy (the agent is capable of slowing or converting this rhythm to sinus rhythm).[5] When used for this indication, the dosing is as described above for the treatment of PSVT.[5] Note that adenosine also can convert VT (adenosine-sensitive VT), so great caution should be used; the medication should not be given to patients with irregular or polymorphic VT.[5]

Synchronized cardioversion is the ultimate treatment of choice in the event of antiarrhythmic drug failure for significantly hemodynamically unstable patients and those with ongoing ACS.

FIGURE 7-10. Ventricular Tachycardia

A. Monomorphic ventricular tachycardia

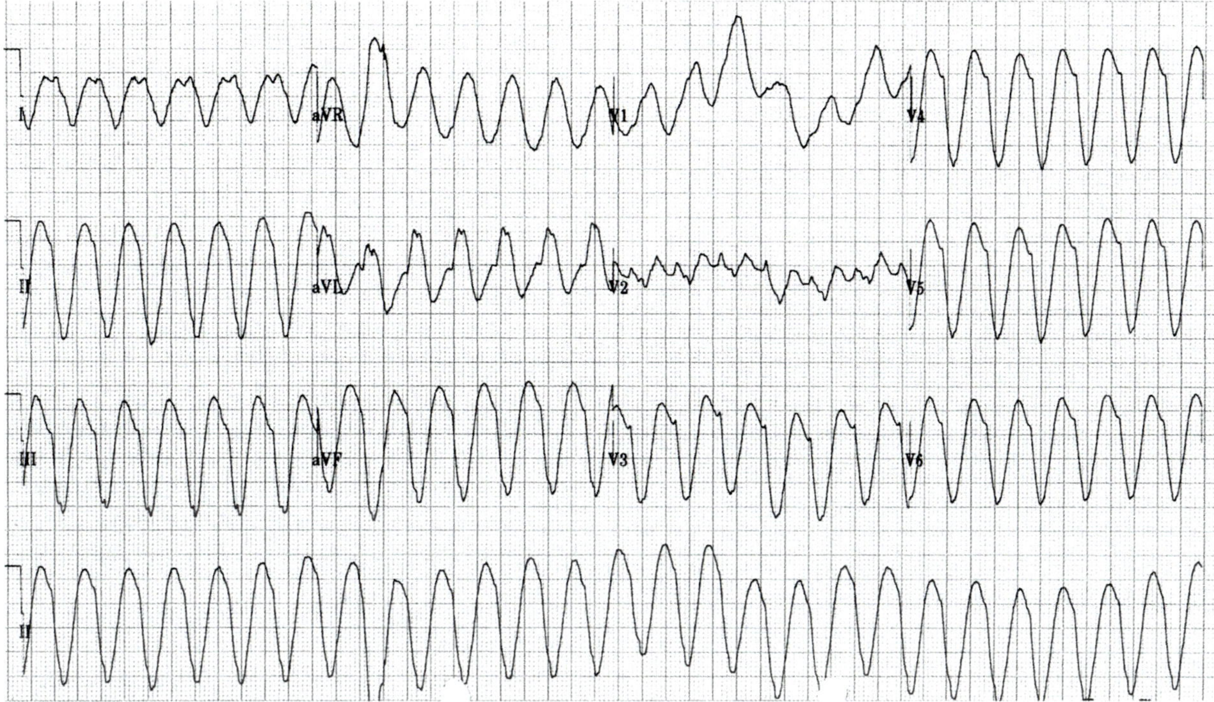

B. Polymorphic ventricular tachycardia

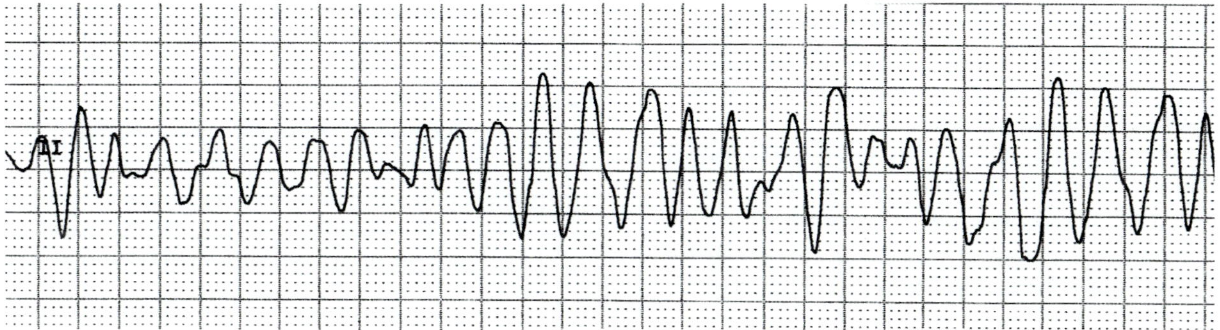

C. Polymorphic ventricular tachycardia, torsade de pointes subtype

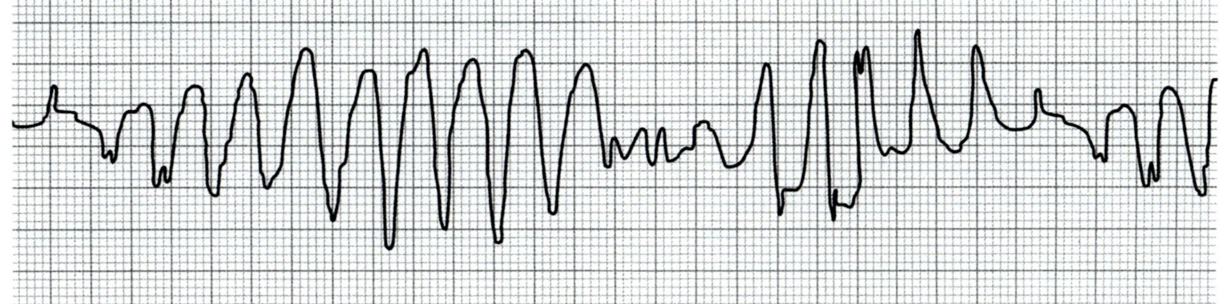

Ventricular versus Supraventricular Tachycardia with Aberrant Conduction

A wide QRS complex tachycardia (defined electrocardiographically in the adult patient as an arrhythmia with a QRS complex greater than 0.12 seconds and a ventricular rate above 120 beats/min) presents diagnostic challenges for the emergency physician. The electrocardiographical differential diagnosis of WCT includes VT versus SVT with aberrant ventricular conduction. The aberrant ventricular conduction of SVT can be caused by a preexisting bundle-branch block; a functional (rate-related) bundle malfunction, resulting in a widened QRS complex when the heart rate exceeds a characteristic maximum for that patient; or accessory atrioventricular conduction, as encountered in preexcitation syndromes such as those described by Wolff, Parkinson, and White.

Other clinical syndromes less frequently encountered in this WCT differential include rapid sinus tachycardia with preexisting bundle-branch block configuration, sodium-channel blockade (eg, tricyclic antidepressant ingestion), or hyperkalemia. If one considers all patients encountered with WCT from the perspective of the cardiologist, approximately 80% will receive a diagnosis of VT. This preponderance of VT probably reflects referral bias of difficult cases to electrophysiology centers.[27-31] Emergency clinicians are likely to encounter a much broader range of etiologies in undifferentiated WCT presentations. Numerous strategies aimed at assisting the clinician with the proper diagnosis have been proposed, emphasizing various data, including the patient's age and cardiovascular history,[31,32] physical examination findings, ECG,[32-38] and response to therapeutic interventions. Although these principles are useful, they largely have centered on criteria suggestive of VT.

Correctly diagnosing WCT is critical for appropriate patient management. For instance, an AV nodal blocking agent such as diltiazem could cause cardiovascular collapse and death in a VT patient incorrectly diagnosed with aberrant SVT. Examination of a variety of clinical features, including the patient's age, medical history, and ECG, is more useful in establishing a diagnosis of VT than aberrant SVT. VT is a more likely diagnosis in older individuals with WCT; age greater than 50 years is a reasonably strong predictor that the WCT is VT. Furthermore, a WCT patient with a prior myocardial infarction and significant left ventricular dysfunction is more likely to experience VT.[31,32] It must be emphasized that these two clinical features are not absolute criteria for this diagnosis — they only support its statistical likelihood.

In regard to electrocardiographical findings, AV dissociation (though uncommon) can be useful in ruling in a diagnosis of VT. In patients without retrograde conduction to the atria, the sinus node continues to initiate atrial depolarization. Since atrial depolarization is completely independent of ventricular activity, the resulting P waves will be dissociated from the QRS complexes. In the patient with VT, an independent atrial impulse occasionally can cause ventricular depolarization via the normal conducting system. Such a supraventricular impulse, if able to trigger depolarization within the ventricle, will result in wide QRS complex beats (a morphology that differs from other wide QRS complex beats).

If the resulting QRS complex occurs earlier than expected and is narrow, the complex is called a *capture beat*. The supraventricular impulse electrically captures the ventricle, producing a narrow complex. The presence of capture beats strongly supports a diagnosis of VT. Fusion beats occur when a sinus beat conducts to the ventricles via the AV node and joins, or fuses, with a ventricular beat originating from the abnormal ectopic focus. These two electrical beats combine, resulting in a QRS complex of intermediate width and a unique morphology that differs from the other beats of monomorphic VT. The presence of fusion beats also is strongly suggestive of VT. Fusion and capture beats occur infrequently (seen in <10% of patients with VT).

QRS concordance, which addresses the relationship of the polarity of the QRS complexes across the precordium, can assist with rhythm diagnosis. Concordance of the QRS complexes in the chest leads that are either predominantly positive or negative suggests a ventricular origin of the tachycardia.

Wolff-Parkinson-White Syndrome

WPW syndrome is a form of ventricular preexcitation that involves an accessory conduction pathway between the atria and the ventricles. In the patient with WPW syndrome, the accessory pathway bypasses the AV node to create a direct electrical connection between the atria and ventricles, thereby removing the protection against excessively rapid rates traditionally provided by the AV node. Furthermore, the accessory pathway will conduct any impulse that presents itself (ie, nondecremental conduction), again in marked contrast to the AV node. While many patients remain asymptomatic throughout their lives, they are prone to a variety of supraventricular tachyarrhythmias, including reentrant tachyarrhythmias (PSVT [narrow and wide QRS complex tachycardias], 70%), AF (25%), and ventricular fibrillation (rare).[41]

PEARL

AF occurs more frequently in patients with WPW syndrome than in the general population.

ECG Diagnosis

The diagnosis of WPW syndrome relies on the electrocardiographical features listed in Table 7-2. The PR interval is shortened because the impulse progressing down the accessory pathway is not subject to the physiological slowing that occurs in the AV node. Consequently, the ventricular myocardium is activated by two pathways, which results in a fused or widened QRS complex (*Figure 7-11*). The initial part of the complex, the delta wave, represents aberrant activation through the accessory pathway, while the terminal portion of the QRS represents normal activation through the His-Purkinje

FIGURE 7-11. Wolff-Parkinson-White Syndrome in Normal Sinus Rhythm

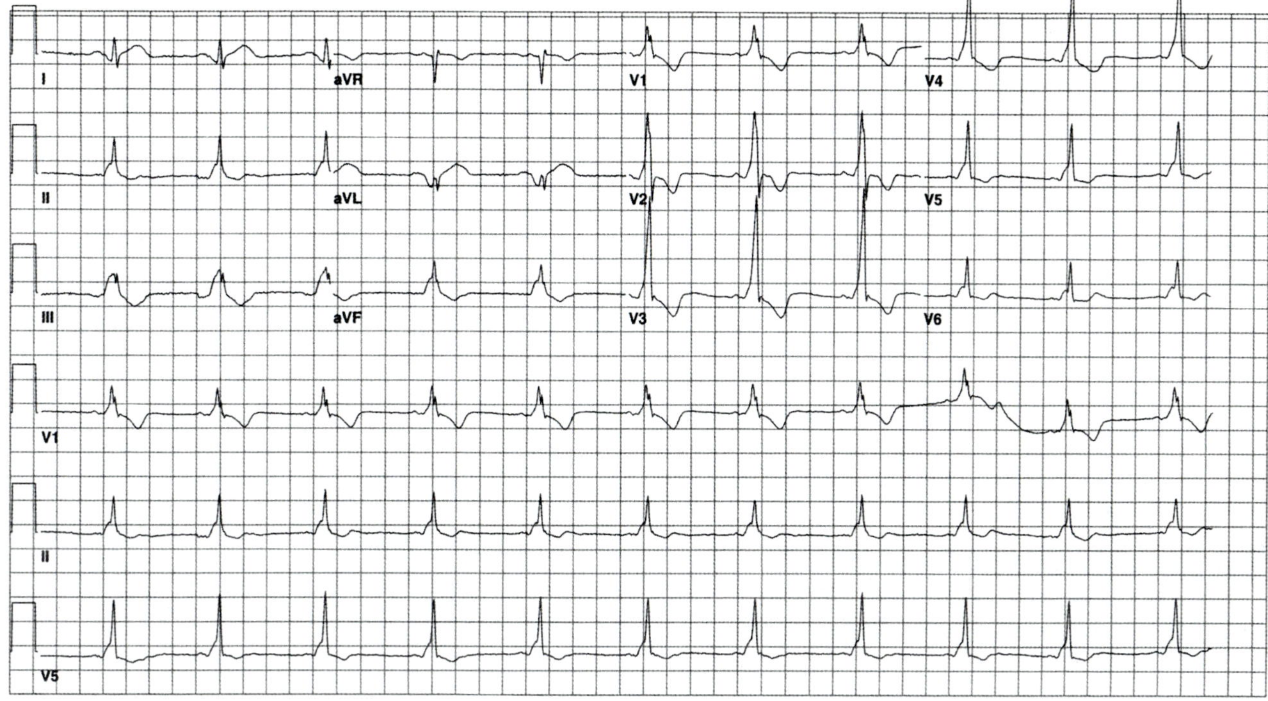

Image courtesy of Ulrich Luft, MD.

system — the result of impulses traveling through both the AV node and the accessory pathway.

The most frequently encountered rhythm disturbance seen in cases of WPW is AV reciprocating tachycardia (AVRT). In this setting, the ventricle is activated through either the normal conduction system or the accessory pathway, with return of the impulse to the atrium by the other pathway. Such AVRT is referred to as either orthodromic (anterograde conduction via the AV node) or antidromic (retrograde conduction via the AV node). Orthodromic conduction represents approximately 90% of AVRT seen in WPW patients. With antidromic conduction, the QRS complexes appear wide, and the 12-lead ECG displays a very rapid WCT that is nearly indistinguishable from VT.

AF is found in up to 20% of WPW patients presenting with a symptomatic arrhythmia.[42] As with the two forms of AVRT, the accessory pathway lacks the feature of slow, decremental conduction; therefore, the pathway can conduct atrial beats at a rate of 300 beats/min or more, subjecting the ventricle to very rapid rates. In addition to the rapid ventricular response, the electrocardiographical features of this rhythm include wide QRS complexes and the delta wave. Significant beat-to-beat variations are seen in the QRS complex morphologies — a result of the two impulses arriving at the ventricle and fusing to form a composite depolarization and, thus, potentially different QRS complex configurations.

Specific Management Considerations

The initial treatment of all three arrhythmias (narrow QRS complex AVRT, wide QRS complex AVRT, and AF) in the WPW patient depends on the patient's clinical stability and the electrocardiographical features of the arrhythmia.

In the hemodynamically stable patient, the next step must include consideration of the QRS complex width and regularity of the rhythm. In a stable patient with a regular narrow QRS complex tachycardia (ie, orthodromic AVRT), the performance of vagal maneuvers should be the first step in therapeutic intervention. If this therapy fails, the next step should be the administration of adenosine, a short-acting agent that blocks the AV node and interrupts the reentrant circuit. Adenosine generally is safe and has an excellent record of successful arrhythmia termination in this setting. The drug should be given initially as a rapid 6-mg IV bolus; if unsuccessful, a 12-mg rapid bolus can be administered and may be repeated if no response occurs.

TABLE 7-2. Electrocardiographical Features of WPW Syndrome
PR interval <0.12 seconds
Slurring and slow rising of the initial segment of the QRS complex (a delta wave)
Widened QRS complex with total duration >0.12 seconds
Secondary repolarization changes reflected in ST-segment/T-wave changes that are generally directed opposite (discordant) to the major delta wave and QRS complex

If adenosine fails, other longer-acting AV nodal blocking agents may be given intravenously. Procainamide can be considered as a drug of last resort. The medication, which blocks the accessory conduction pathway, acts more slowly than calcium channel antagonists and beta-adrenergic blocking agents. If all medications fail, the patient can be electrically cardioverted after appropriate sedation.

In summary, the first therapeutic maneuver in stable patients with a wide QRS complex tachycardia — either regular (ie, orthodromic AVRT) or irregular (AF) — should be administration of procainamide. If that is unsuccessful, electrical cardioversion after appropriate sedation should be considered. AV nodal blocking interventions and agents such as vagal maneuvers, adenosine, amiodarone, beta-blockers, and calcium channel blockers should be avoided. These therapies can potentiate conduction via the accessory pathway, leading to the development of extremely rapid ventricular rates and, ultimately, cardiovascular decompensation.

The Sudden Death Syndromes

A number of clinical syndromes predispose patients to sudden cardiac death, including both monomorphic and polymorphic ventricular tachycardia and ventricular fibrillation. In certain clinical settings, a subset of these syndromes can be suspected based on the patient's presentation and electrocardiographical abnormalities. These entities are not detectable or obvious all of the time, however, even when the ECG is interpreted within the context of the clinical presentation. Three such diagnoses worthy of discussion are Brugada syndrome, long QT syndrome, and hypertrophic cardiomyopathy.[43-45]

Brugada Syndrome

Brugada syndrome[43] is an inherited disorder that predisposes patients, most often young individuals, to sudden death. Its pathophysiology involves abnormal depolarization resulting from dysfunctional membrane-based ion channels; in fact, the disorder frequently is referred to as a channelopathy. The prevalence of Brugada syndrome varies dramatically among ethnic groups; it is highest in Asian populations and markedly lower in those originating from Western Europe. Fevers and medications with potent sodium-channel blocking effects can exacerbate the underlying defect, potentially increasing the chance of dysrhythmia.

The vast majority of Brugada patients are asymptomatic; the syndrome is discovered only incidentally via an ECG obtained for other clinical reasons. A minority of these patients is symptomatic, with signs ranging from episodic dizziness and palpitations to syncope, convulsions, and cardiac arrest. In each of these presentations, the clinical manifestations result from a malignant ventricular dysrhythmia. Characteristic electrocardiographical changes (*Figure 7-12a*) are necessary to confirm the diagnosis, but such manifestations are variable and not always evident, making the diagnosis difficult.

The ECG will demonstrate right bundle branch block, either incomplete or complete, and characteristic ST-segment elevation in leads V_1 and V_2. The ST-segment elevation is grouped into three subtypes: type 1 with coved-shaped elevation greater than 2 mm, followed by an inverted T wave; type 2 with elevation above 2 mm followed by a positive or biphasic T wave, producing a "saddle" configuration; and type 3, coved-shaped elevation of only 1 to 2 mm and a "saddle" configuration. Provocative testing with a sodium-channel blocker can accentuate the ST-segment elevation.

Patient management depends on each clinical presentation. The stable patient in whom the syndrome is suspected should be referred promptly to an appropriate cardiologist. In cases of aborted sudden cardiac death (ie, a self-limited episode or successfully treated dysrhythmia), the risk of recurrent ventricular fibrillation is more than 50% within 5 years. For cases of suspected or known Brugada syndrome who present in cardiac arrest, standard management for the presenting rhythm is suggested.

In those patients with a confirmed diagnosis via electrophysiological study, the only proven therapy to terminate malignant ventricular arrhythmias and prevent sudden death is placement of an implantable cardioverter defibrillator. Quinidine, a class Ia antiarrhythmic, sometimes is used as an adjunct with an implantable cardioverter defibrillator; antiarrhythmic agents alone do not reduce the occurrence of sudden death.

Long QT Syndrome

Long QT syndrome (LQTS) is characterized by prolongation of the QT interval and an increased risk of malignant ventricular dysrhythmias.[44] The abnormality is divided into congenital and acquired varieties. Congenital LQTS is an inherited disorder with an estimated prevalence of 1 in 2,000 live births; it can occur as 1 of 13 variants. Congenital LQTS results in abnormal ion movement across the cell membrane, producing another channelopathy, QT interval prolongation, and sudden cardiac death. Acquired LQTS can result from electrolyte abnormalities (eg, hypokalemia, hypomagnesemia), medication effects, and other disease states, including acute coronary syndrome and severe left ventricular dysfunction. In situations where the genetic trait is not fully penetrant, the inherited tendency toward QT interval prolongation can be unmasked or accentuated with electrolyte abnormalities, medication use, or acute illness, all of which can complicate the diagnosis.

As with Brugada syndrome, a diagnosis of LQTS can be considered based on clinical and electrocardiographical findings. The syndrome can manifest in many different ways — from palpitations and sudden dizziness to syncope, seizure, and sudden death; syncope is the most common symptom and torsade de pointes is the most common dysrhythmia. As its name implies, the syndrome is marked by an abnormally long QT interval (*Figure 7-12b*). The normal QT interval corrected for heart rate (QTc) is up to 440 milliseconds (ms) in men and 460 ms in women. In general, a QTc interval greater than 450 ms should be considered potentially abnormal, assuming the appropriate clinical presentation exists. In general, the risk of malignant ventricular dysrhythmia escalates as the QTc interval

FIGURE 7-12. The Sudden Death Syndromes

A. Brugada syndrome with characteristic electrocardiographical abnormalities. i. Incomplete RBBB with coved-type ST-segment elevation in lead V_1. ii. Incomplete RBBB with saddle-type ST segment elevation in lead V_1.

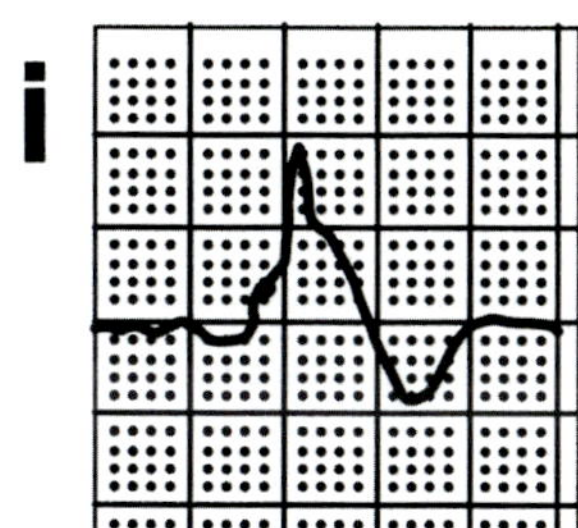

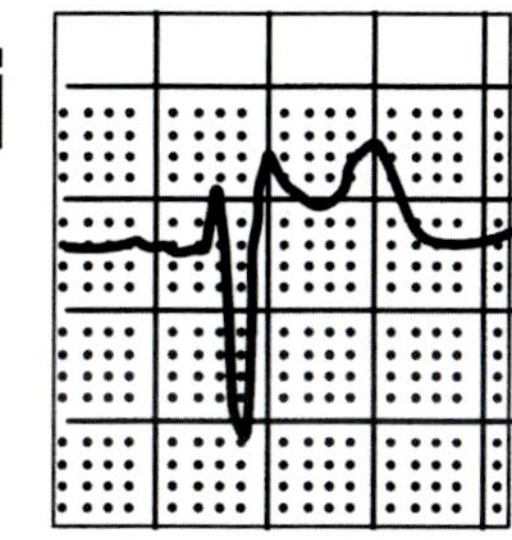

B. Normal sinus rhythm in the long QT syndrome.

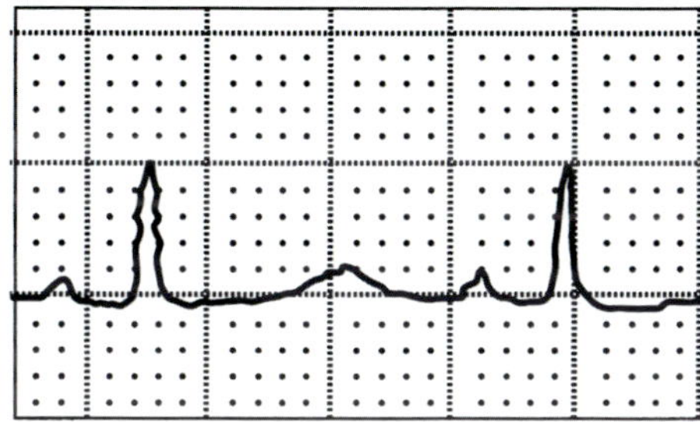

C. Electrocardiographical findings of hypertrophic cardiomyopathy. i. Prominent R wave with ST-segment elevation in leads V_1 and V_2. ii. Q waves in the lateral leads, leads I aVl, V_5, and V_6. In this example, only Q waves in lateral leads V_5 and V_6 are shown.

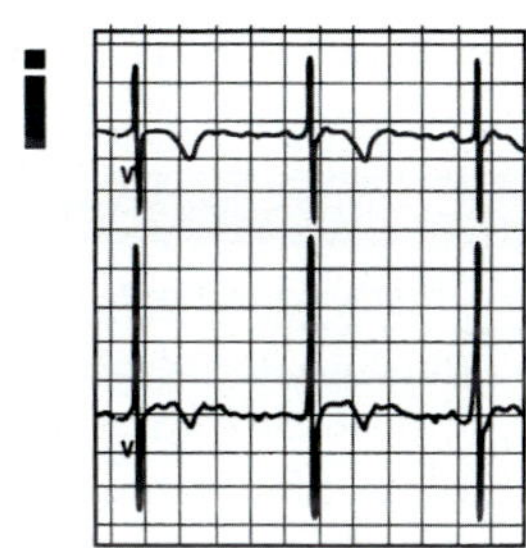

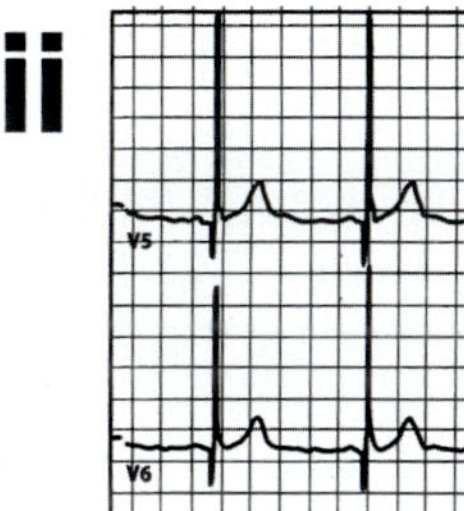

D. Concerning rhythm, also known as polymorphic ventricular tachycardia, which can occur in the situations depicted in figures A–C.

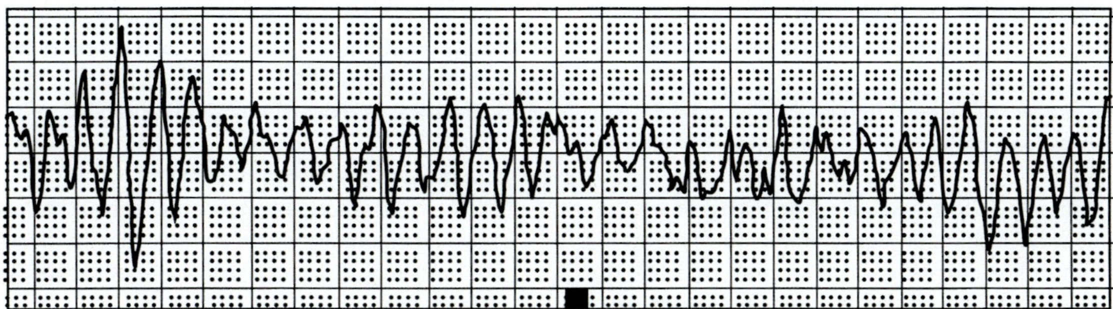

increases; a moderate risk is encountered when the QTc is between 480 and 499 ms and is significantly higher when the QTc interval is greater than 500 ms.[26]

Treatment priorities for LQTS mirror those for Brugada syndrome. Address exacerbating factors and avoid creating more of them, including electrolyte abnormalities and medications with pronounced QT-interval-prolonging properties. The management of malignant ventricular dysrhythmias should follow standard guidelines for the particular dysrhythmia, with additional attention paid to electrolyte abnormalities. Referral to a cardiologist for additional management is warranted.

Hypertrophic Cardiomyopathy

Hypertrophic cardiomyopathy (HCM)[45] is one of the most common inherited primary cardiac disorders and the most frequent cause of sudden cardiac death in young athletes. The specific risk of sudden cardiac death is related to an individual's risk profile, including historical, familial, and clinical features. Risk factors include recurrent syncope associated with events producing significant adrenergic stimulation; sustained ventricular tachycardia; prior cardiac arrest; a family history of sudden, explained death in a young person; and various cardiac findings (extreme anatomical left ventricular hypertrophy; the presence of a left ventricular outflow obstruction gradient greater than 30 mm Hg; and the presence of nonsustained ventricular tachycardia during cardiac monitoring). The annual rate of sudden cardiac death is very low (0.5%–1.0%) in patients with a minimal (0 or 1) risk factor; however, the rate is significantly higher in those with two or more.

The presenting symptoms associated with HCM are variable, owing in part to its significant genetic heterogeneity. Presentations can result from abnormal ventricular function caused by left ventricular outflow obstruction, diastolic dysfunction, or malignant ventricular dysrhythmia with sudden cardiac death. A family history of HCM or unexplained sudden death in a young person should raise suspicion for the disorder.

Various stimuli that heighten sympathetic nervous system activity can increase the risk of malignant dysrhythmia, including physical exertion and extreme emotion (eg, anger or fright). The concept of adrenergically mediated near syncope or syncope should prompt consideration of this diagnosis. The ECG will be abnormal in most patients with HCM, with a range of findings (*Figure 7-12c*), including ST-segment elevation in the right to midprecordial leads; right ventricular hypertrophy with prominent R waves in leads V_1 and V_2; left ventricular hypertrophy; and deep, narrow Q waves in the lateral leads (I, aVL, V_5, and V_6). The clinically suspected diagnosis should be confirmed by echocardiography.

For patients presenting in stable condition, referral to a cardiologist for further testing and risk assessment is warranted. Any patient with symptoms suggestive of HCM and an abnormal ECG can be considered for admission, further monitoring, and definitive evaluation. As with the other two sudden death syndromes, cardiac arrest should be managed based on standard protocols and the unique clinical presentation of each patient.

Conclusion

Critically ill emergency department patients often present with arrhythmias. For some, the arrhythmia is the primary reason for critical illness, but for others, it is a reflection of illness severity. Regardless, the emergency care provider must

KEY POINTS

1. The vast majority of bradyarrhythmias are secondary events, meaning that they are external to the cardiac pacemaker-conduction system.[2]
2. In adults, the initial dose of atropine is 0.5 mg to 1 mg intravenously, repeated every 3 to 5 minutes to a maximum total dose of 3 mg; the pediatric dose is 0.02 mg/kg.[5,6]
3. The administration of dopamine, epinephrine, and isoproterenol should be considered temporary therapy providing a medical bridge to more definitive management with transcutaneous or transvenous cardiac pacing.[5]
4. Sinus bradycardia is seen frequently in early ACS presentations, particularly in patients with inferior-wall STEMI.
5. Patients with ACS, a metabolic abnormality, or a cardioactive medication ingestion who demonstrate new-onset first-degree or second-degree type I AV block should be considered at risk of progression to complete heart block and managed accordingly.
6. The management of NCTs is based on the rhythm, the patient's presentation, and related clinical issues.
7. If electrical cardioversion is considered, its use should be coupled with the administration of a sedative with or without analgesic effect.
8. Adequate rate control is a primary concern in all patients with AF.
9. Aberrantly conducted SVT often is the default diagnosis in the event that none of the criteria for VT are met — a major flaw in medical decisionmaking that is fraught with the potential for serious adverse consequences.[29,30,39,40]
10. Electrical cardioversion should be applied to all patients with hemodynamic instability regardless of the features of the tachyarrhythmia.
11. In cases of syncope or new-onset convulsion, an ECG should be obtained with consideration of rhythm and morphological findings suggestive of the sudden death syndromes.

possess quintessential skills for diagnosing and managing potentially lethal rhythm disturbances, including accurate ECG interpretation and the rapid initiation of lifesaving therapy.

REFERENCES

1. Sinz E, Navarro K. *Advanced Cardiovascular Life Support Provider Manual.* Dallas, TX: American Heart Association; 2011.
2. Brady WJ, Harrigan RA. Diagnosis and management of bradycardia and atrioventricular block associated with acute coronary ischemia. *Emerg Med Clin North Am.* 2001;19:371-384.
3. Brady WJ, Swart G, DeBehnke DJ, et al. The efficacy of atropine in the treatment of hemodynamically unstable bradycardia and atrioventricular block: prehospital and emergency department considerations. *Resuscitation.* 1999;41:47-55.
4. Swart G, Brady WJ, DeBehnke DJ, Ma OJ, Aufderheide TP. Acute myocardial infarction complicated by hemodynamically unstable bradyarrhythmia: prehospital and emergency department treatment with atropine. *Am J Emerg Med.* 1999;17:647-652.
5. Neumar RW, Otto CW, Link MS, et al. Part 8: adult advanced cardiovascular life support: 2010 American Heart Association Guidelines for Cardiopulmonary Resuscitation and Emergency Cardiovascular Care. *Circulation.* 2010;122(suppl 3):S729-S767.
6. Kleinman ME, Chameides L, Schexnayder SM, et al. Part 14: pediatric advanced life support: 2010 American Heart Association Guidelines for Cardiopulmonary Resuscitation and Emergency Cardiovascular Care. *Circulation.* 2010;122(suppl 3):S876-S908.
7. Richman S. Adverse effect of atropine during myocardial infarction. *JAMA.* 1974;228:1414-1416.
8. Fernandes CM, Daya MR. Sotalol-induced bradycardia reversed by glucagon. *Can Fam Phys.* 1995;41:659-660.
9. Love JN, Howell JM. Glucagon therapy in the treatment of symptomatic bradycardia. *Ann Emerg Med.* 1997;29:181-183.
10. Chou T, Knilans TK. *Electrocardiography in Clinical Practice: Adult and Pediatric.* 4th ed. Philadelphia, PA: WB Saunders; 1996.
11. Borloz MP, Mark DG, Pines JM, Brady WJ. Electrocardiographic differential diagnosis of narrow QRS complex tachycardia: an ED-oriented algorithmic approach. *Am J Emerg Med.* 2010;28:378-381.
12. Brady WJ, DeBehnke DJ, Wickman LL, Lindbeck G. Treatment of out-of-hospital supraventricular tachycardia: adenosine vs. verapamil. *Acad Emerg Med.* 1996;3:574-585.
13. Luber S, Brady WJ, Joyce T, Perron AD. Paroxysmal supraventricular tachycardia: outcome after emergency department care. *Am J Emerg Med.* 2001;19:40-42.
14. Brembilla-Perrot B, Houriez P, Beurrier D, et al. Influence of age on the electrophysiological mechanism of paroxysmal supraventricular tachycardias. *Int J Cardiol.* 2001;78:293-298.
15. McDonald AJ, Pelletier AJ, Ellinor PT, Camargo CA. Increasing US emergency department visit rates and subsequent hospital admissions for atrial fibrillation from 1993 to 2004. *Ann Emerg Med.* 2008;51:58-65.
16. Crozier I, Melton I, Pearson S. Management of atrial fibrillation in the emergency department. *Int Med J.* 2003;33:182-185.
17. Bettoni M, Zimmerman M. Autonomic tone variations before the onset of paroxysmal atrial fibrillation. *Circulation.* 2002;105:2753-2759.
18. Haïssaguerre M, Jaïs P, Shah DC, et al. Spontaneous initiation of atrial fibrillation by ectopic beats originating in the pulmonary veins. *N Engl J Med.* 1998;339:659-666.
19. Ergene U, Ergene O, Fowler J, et al. Must antidysrhythmic agents be given to all patients with new-onset atrial fibrillation? *Am J Emerg Med.* 1999;17:659-662.
20. Digitalis in Acute Atrial Fibrillation (DAAF) Trial Group. Intravenous digoxin in acute atrial fibrillation: results of a randomized, placebo-controlled multicentre trial in 239 patients. *Eur Heart J.* 1997;18:649-654.
21. Olshansky B, Rosenfeld LE, Warner AL, et al. The atrial fibrillation follow-up investigation of rhythm management (AFFIRM) study. *J Am Coll Cardiol.* 2004;43:1209-1210.
22. Hagens VE, Van Gelder IC, Crijins HJ, et al. The RACE study in perspective of randomized studies on management of persistent atrial fibrillation. *Card Electrophysiol Rev.* 2003;7:118-121.
23. Cohn BJ, Keim SM, Yealy DM. Is emergency department cardioversion of recent-onset atrial fibrillation safe and effective? *J Emerg Med.* 2013;45:117-127.
24. von Besser K, Mills AM. Is discharge to home after emergency department cardioversion safe for the treatment of recent-onset atrial fibrillation? *Ann Emerg Med.* 2011;58:517-520.
25. Hudson KB, Brady WJ, Chan TC, et al. Electrocardiographic features of ventricular tachycardia. *J Emerg Med.* 2003;25:303-314.
26. Meldon SW, Brady WJ, Berger S, Mannenbach M. Pediatric ventricular tachycardia: a report of three cases with a review of the acute diagnosis and management. *Pediatr Emerg Care.* 1994;10:294-300.
27. Steinman RT, Herrera C, Schluger CD, et al. Wide QRS tachycardia in the conscious adult: ventricular tachycardia is the most frequent cause. *JAMA.* 1989;261:1013-1016.
28. Morady F, Baerman JM, DiCarlo LA, et al. A prevalent misconception regarding wide complex tachycardias. *JAMA.* 1985;254:2790-2792.
29. Stewart RB, Bardy GH, Greene HL. Wide complex tachycardia: misdiagnosis and outcome after emergent therapy. *Ann Intern Med.* 1986;104:766-771.
30. Akhtar M, Shenasa M, Jazayeri M, et al. Wide QRS complex tachycardia: reappraisal of a common clinical problem. *Ann Intern Med.* 1988;109:905-912.
31. Tchou P, Young P, Mahmud R, et al. Useful clinical criteria for the diagnosis of ventricular tachycardia. *Am J Med.* 1988;84:53-56.
32. Baerman JM, Morady F, DiCario LA, de Buitleir M. Differentiation of ventricular tachycardia from supraventricular tachycardia with aberration: value of the clinical history. *Ann Emerg Med.* 1987;16:40-43.
33. Falk RH, Knowlton AA, Bernard SA, et al. Digoxin for converting recent-onset atrial fibrillation to sinus rhythm. *Ann Intern Med.* 1987;106:503-506.
34. Levitt MA. Supraventricular tachycardia with aberrant conduction versus ventricular tachycardia: differentiation and diagnosis. *Am J Emerg Med.* 1988;6:273-277.
35. Antunes E, Brugada J, Steurer G, et al. The differential diagnosis of a regular tachycardia with a wide QRS complex on the 12-lead ECG: ventricular tachycardia, supraventricular tachycardia with aberrant intraventricular conduction, and supraventricular tachycardia with anterograde conduction over an accessory pathway. *Pacing Clin Electrophysiol.* 1994;17:1515-1524.
36. Wellens HJ, Bar FW, Lie KI. The value of the electrocardiogram in the differential diagnosis of a tachycardia with a widened QRS complex. *Am J Med.* 1978;64:27-33.
37. Steurer G, Gursoy S, Frey B, et al. The differential diagnosis on the electrocardiogram between ventricular tachycardia and preexcited tachycardia. *Clin Cardiol.* 1994;17:306-308.
38. Brugada P, Brugada J, Mont L, et al. A new approach to the differential diagnosis of a regular tachycardia with a wide QRS complex. *Circulation.* 1991;83:1649-1659.
39. Drew BJ, Scheinman MM. ECG criteria to distinguish between aberrantly conducted supraventricular tachycardia and ventricular tachycardia: practical aspects for the immediate care setting. *Pacing Clin Electrophysiol.* 1995;18:2194-2208.
40. Herbert ME, Votey SR, Mortan MT, et al. Failure to agree on the electrocardiographic diagnosis of ventricular tachycardia. *Ann Emerg Med.* 1996;27:35-38.
41. Mark DG, Brady WJ, Pines JM. Pre-excitation syndromes: diagnostic consideration in the emergency department. *Am J Emerg Med.* 2009;27:878-888.
42. Wellens HJ, Durrer D. Wolff-Parkinson-White syndrome and atrial fibrillation. Relation between refractory period of AP and ventricular rate during atrial fibrillation. *Am J Cardiol.* 1974;34:777-782.
43. Mattu A, Rogers RL, Kim H, et al. The Brugada syndrome. *Am J Emerg Med.* 2003;21:146-151.
44. Mancuso EM, Brady WJ, Harrigan RA, et al. Electrocardiographic manifestations: long QT syndrome. *J Emerg Med.* 2004;27:385-393.
45. Kelly BS, Mattu A, Brady WJ. Hypertrophic cardiomyopathy: electrocardiographic manifestations and other important considerations for the emergency physician. *Am J Emerg Med.* 2007;25:72-79.

Cardiogenic Shock

8

IN THIS CHAPTER

- Pathophysiology and etiologies
- Initial resuscitation and stabilization
- Reperfusion therapy
- Mechanical devices
- Experimental therapies
- Special causes and treatments

Jehangir Meer and Amal Mattu

Cardiogenic shock is an extreme cardiac disorder that results from left ventricular (LV) or right ventricular (RV) failure, which culminates in a state of end-organ hypoperfusion (*Table 8-1*).[1] In 97% of cases, the left ventricle is the site of compromise.[2] Patients presenting in cardiogenic shock can be extremely challenging to manage, as they often require multiple, time-dependent interventions. Historically, the mortality rate associated with cardiogenic shock was 80% to 90%.[3] Although the rate has decreased with recent advances in treatment, it remains as high as 50%, a statistic that has not improved in 15 years.[3,4]

The most common cause of cardiogenic shock is acute coronary syndrome (ACS), specifically ST-segment elevation myocardial infarction (STEMI). Cardiogenic shock complicates 7% to 10% of cases of acute STEMI and 2.5% of non-STEMI and is the most common cause of death in patients with acute myocardial infarction (AMI).[5,6] In select cases, aggressive treatment with reperfusion therapy and surgical treatment is life-saving. Patients who live long enough to be admitted have an excellent chance of long-term survival and good functional status.[7]

The pathogenesis of cardiogenic shock is thought to occur simultaneously at the macrocellular and microcellular levels. Patients who develop cardiogenic shock classically have had a large anterior myocardial infarction (MI) or a reinfarction, resulting in a substantial area of nonfunctioning myocardium. This causes a significant decrease in stroke volume and arterial pressure and a modest depression in ejection fraction. It is thought that a series of neurohormonal responses then becomes activated, with the sympathetic nervous system and renin-angiotensin systems signaling peripheral vasoconstriction as well as salt and water retention. In addition, a systemic inflammatory response state develops, with release of cytokines and excessive nitric oxide production, further depressing myocardial function. These pathways lead to a vicious cycle that exacerbates myocardial ischemia and necrosis, resulting in lower arterial pressure, anaerobic metabolism, lactic acidosis, multiorgan failure, and death.[8,9]

Between 10% and 15% of patients are in cardiogenic shock when they arrive in the emergency department. In most cases, shock develops within 48 hours after the onset of infarction; however, the complication can be delayed for as long as 2 weeks.[9,10] Patients who develop shock early tend to have a lower 30-day mortality rate.[9]

The most common cause of cardiogenic shock is myocardial depression from an AMI or ACS. Other causes are presented in Table 8-2. In most cases, the culprit can be established through the interpretation of 12-lead electrocardiogram (ECG) tracing and a point-of-care echocardiography examination.[11]

Initial Resuscitation and Stabilization

When assessing patients in cardiogenic shock, clinicians must rapidly determine if pump failure is to blame or if the disorder is of a hypovolemic, hemorrhagic, obstructive, distributive, or septic nature *(Figure 8-1)*. Because many patients present in extremis, the available history is often limited; however, descriptions of chest pain or its anginal equivalents (eg, dyspnea, diaphoresis, presyncope, arm pain) should

TABLE 8-1. Clinical Markers of Hypoperfusion
Cool extremities
Decreased urine output (<0.5 mL/kg/hr)
Change in mental status
Hypotension (SBP <90 mm Hg) for at least 30 minutes
Decreased cardiac index (<2.2 L/min/m²)

FIGURE 8-1. General Approach to Cardiogenic Shock

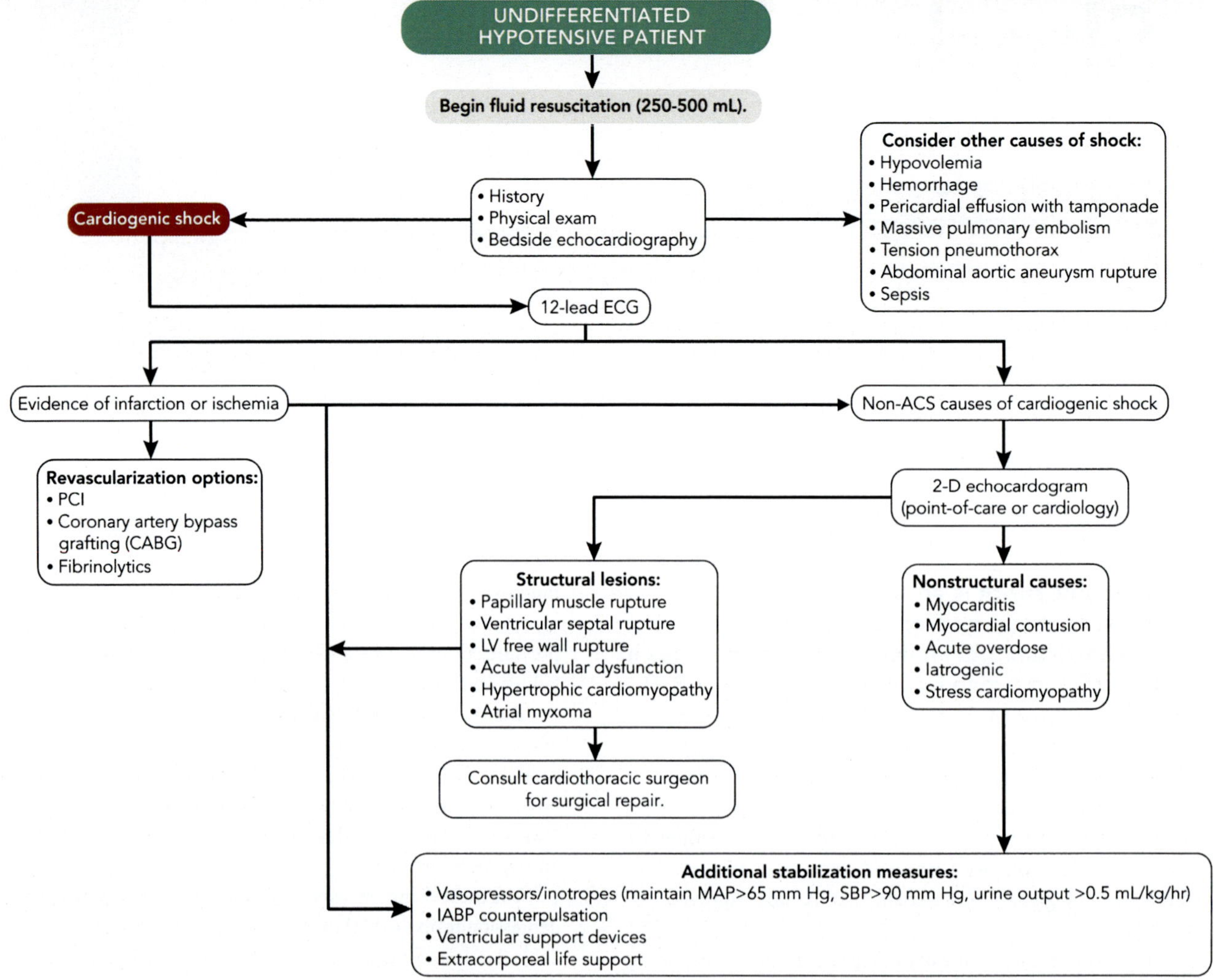

be elicited. Information from emergency medical services personnel or family members is often very helpful. On physical examination, these patients often have abnormal vital signs such as tachycardia, rapid and faint pulses, hypotension, and tachypnea (caused by congestive heart failure or respiratory compensation for metabolic acidosis). They can appear agitated or confused. The cardiovascular examination may reveal jugular venous distention and pulmonary rales (found in LV pump failure) or jugular venous distention and absent rales (found in RV failure). Third or fourth heart sounds might be heard. The presence of a systolic murmur suggests mechanical complications such as ventricular septal rupture or acute mitral regurgitation.[8]

A 12-lead ECG can provide evidence of ACS and should be obtained urgently after the patient's arrival *(Table 8-3)*. Patients should be placed on continuous cardiac monitoring to detect arrhythmias or atrioventricular blocks. Tachyarrhythmias should be managed with electrical cardioversion, as antiarrhythmic medications can worsen hypotension. Bradycardic rhythms should be treated with atropine and transcutaneous or transvenous pacing. In addition, blood samples should be drawn for a laboratory analysis of cardiac biomarkers, serum lactate level, coagulation studies, complete blood count (CBC), and chemistries. A portable chest radiograph should be ordered, and a point-of-care echocardiogram should be obtained and assessed for global contractility and other causes of shock (eg, pericardial effusion with tamponade, dilated aortic root or detection of intimal flap with thoracic aortic dissection, or signs of acute RV strain with pulmonary embolism).

Several studies have shown that emergency providers can, with little training, accurately identify depressed LV contractility

TABLE 8-3. Potential ECG Abnormalities in Cardiogenic Shock

STEMI	ST-segment elevation or new left bundle-branch block
ACS	Hyperacute or inverted T waves ± ST-segment depression, ST elevation in lead aVR in the presence of diffuse ST-segment depression

using bedside ultrasound.[12,13] Ideally, a formal echocardiogram (transthoracic or transesophageal) performed by a cardiologist should be obtained to help evaluate for structural etiologies requiring surgical intervention. The use of pulmonary artery catheters is a class I recommendation by the American College of Cardiology/American Heart Association (ACC/AHA) in patients with hypotension not responding to fluid administration. However, their use has declined in many centers and have largely been replaced with two-dimensional echocardiography.[14,15]

PEARL

To identify cardiogenic shock, look for evidence of pump failure and exclude other causes of shock. Point-of-care echocardiography performed by an emergency physician can confirm pump failure (by showing decreased global contractility) and exclude other etiologies (pericardial effusion with tamponade *[Figure 8-2]*, massive pulmonary embolism *[Figure 8-3]*, and valvular regurgitation *[Figure 8-4]*).

Initial resuscitation should focus on the patient's airway, breathing, and circulation. Those who are hypoxic or in significant respiratory distress require respiratory support using positive-pressure, noninvasive, or mechanical ventilation. Because of the nature of shock (pump failure), most resuscitation efforts will be directed at improving circulation, with the aim of keeping systolic arterial pressure above 90 mm Hg, the mean arterial pressure above 65 mm Hg, and a urine output greater than 0.5 mL/kg/hr. An initial fluid bolus should be given to optimize preload and improve ventricular filling. This is particularly true in patients with RV failure (eg, those with RV infarction who are preload dependent) in whom additional fluid might be required. Nitrates, beta-blockers, and morphine should be avoided. Unlike in the management of sepsis, the amount of intravenous fluid administered should be monitored cautiously. Most patients require treatment with some combination of inotropes and vasopressors *(Table 8-4)*; placement of a central line also is recommended.

The ACC/AHA recommends dobutamine as a first-line agent (an inotrope with selective beta-agonist and arterial dilator properties) if the systolic blood pressure (SBP) is above 90 mm Hg. If the systolic pressure is below 90 mm Hg, then dopamine — which has both inotropic and vasopressor properties — should be started and titrated to maintain

TABLE 8-2. Causes of Cardiogenic Shock

Myocardial Ischemia/Infarction (Mechanical Complications)
Acute mitral regurgitation secondary to papillary muscle rupture
Ventricular septal rupture
LV free wall rupture
Nonischemic Depression of Myocardial Contractility
Myocarditis
Takotsubo (stress-induced) cardiomyopathy
Sepsis
Myocardial contusion
Acute overdose of cardiotoxic drug (beta-blockers, calcium channel blocker, digoxin)
Iatrogenic
Postcardiotomy shock
Valvular Pathology
Acute aortic regurgitation
Aortic and mitral stenosis
LV Outflow Tract Obstruction
Hypertrophic obstructive cardiomyopathy
Left atrial myxoma

FIGURE 8-2. Pericardial Effusion with Tamponade

Echocardiogram using a parasternal long-axis window to show a large pericardial effusion with tamponade and RV collapse.

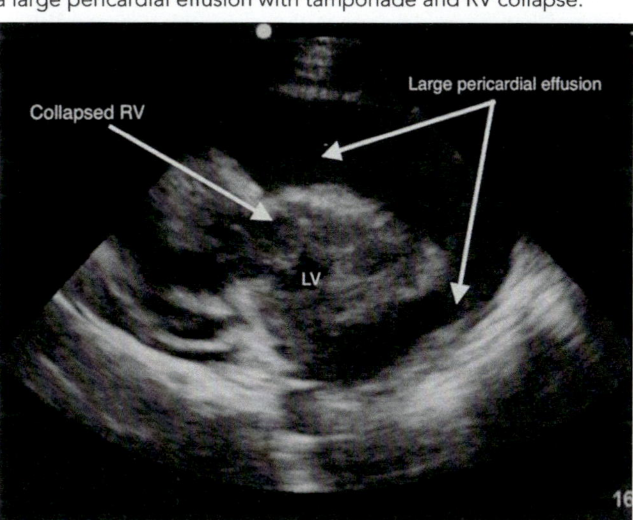

FIGURE 8-3. Massive Pulmonary Embolism

Echocardiogram using an apical four-chamber window showing dilated RV, with the RV:LV ratio approximately 1:1, suggesting RV strain.

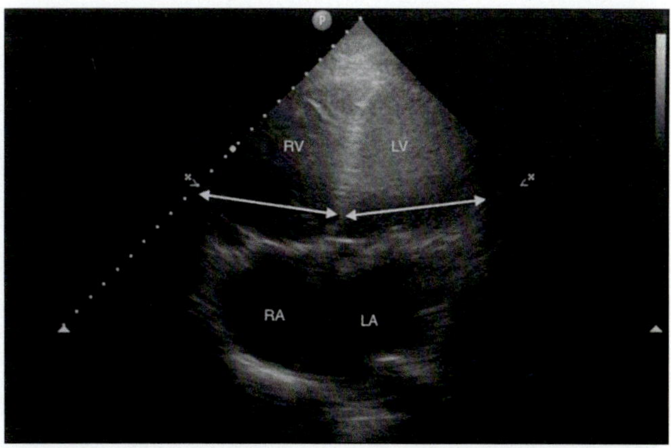

TABLE 8-4. Vasoactive Agents Used in Cardiogenic Shock

Drug	Dose	Use
Norepinephrine	Initial dose: 0.5–1 mcg/min Titrate by: 1–2 mcg/min Maximum dose: 30 mcg/min	First-line agent added to dopamine if SBP remains <90 mm Hg
Dobutamine	Initial dose: 2.5 mcg/kg/min Titrate by: 2.5 mcg/kg/min Maximum dose: 20 mcg/kg/min	First-line inotropic agent to use if SBP >90 mm Hg
Dopamine	Initial dose: 5 mcg/kg/min Titrate by: 5–10 mcg/kg/min Maximum dose: 20 mcg/kg/min	Second-line agent (vasopressor/inotrope) to use if SBP <90 mm Hg

adequate pressure. If the response to dopamine is insufficient, norepinephrine (which has stronger vasopressor action than dopamine) may be added. (The previous statement is based largely on consensus without substantial evidence to support it.) The smallest possible dose of these inotropes/vasopressors should be administered. Although these agents improve contractility and increase arterial pressure, they also increase myocardial oxygen demand and can worsen ischemia and arrhythmias. A subgroup analysis from one recent randomized trial suggests that norepinephrine is associated with a lower mortality rate than dopamine in patients with cardiogenic shock.[16] Pure vasopressors such as phenylephrine should be avoided because they increase myocardial oxygen demand without improving contractility. Phenylephrine can also induce bradycardia.

Calcium-sensitizing agents (eg, levosimendan) also have been studied. Their mechanism of action is thought to be the binding of cardiac troponin C, resulting in a vasodilatory effect on vascular smooth muscle. Although these agents appear to improve disease outcomes (eg, BNP and symptoms), they may worsen patient prognosis (eg, higher rates of death, hypotension, and cardiac dysrhythmias).[17]

Additional medications to consider include aspirin,

FIGURE 8-4. Valvular Regurgitation

Echocardiogram using an apical four-chamber window showing mitral regurgitation jet during systole, when the mitral valve is closed.

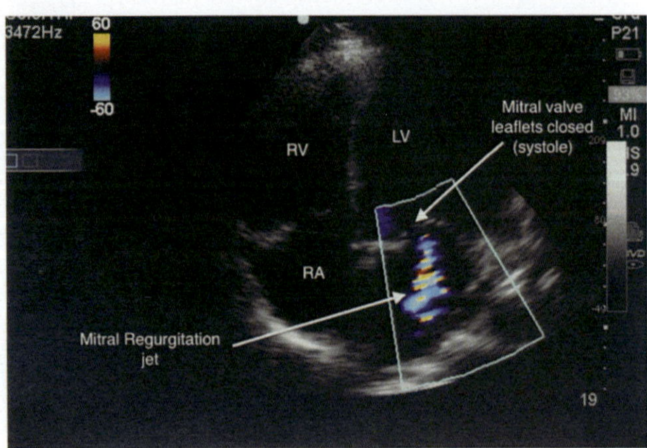

intravenous heparin, and glycoprotein IIb/IIIa (GpIIb-IIIa) inhibitors. No randomized trials have evaluated the use of GpIIb-IIIa inhibitors in the setting of cardiogenic shock, yet they are commonly used as adjunctive therapy.[8] Clopidogrel should be given only after consultation with an interventional cardiologist; its administration prior to percutaneous coronary intervention (PCI) is controversial.[8] About 25% of patients in cardiogenic shock have severe triple-vessel disease or left main coronary artery disease that requires urgent coronary artery bypass grafting (CABG). The administration of clopidogrel prior to the procedure has been associated with increased perioperative bleeding and morbidity.[8]

Medications to avoid in patients in cardiogenic shock include nitroglycerin, beta-blockers, calcium channel blockers, and diuretics because they are likely to worsen hypotension.

Reperfusion Therapy

Since ischemia is the most common cause of cardiogenic shock, reperfusion therapy logically is a cornerstone of its management. Several trials have examined whether PCI is superior to fibrinolytic therapy or CABG in improving outcomes among patients in cardiogenic shock.

The large-scale SHOCK trial showed that early revascularization decreased the mortality rate compared with medical management alone.[1] Although 30-day mortality was lower in patients who received early revascularization (PCI or CABG) compared to those who were treated with an intraaortic balloon pump (IABP), the difference did not reach statistical significance. However, in a 6-year follow up, overall survival was significantly higher in the early intervention group.[16] Of the survivors at 1 year, 83% met the characteristics of the heart failure functional class I or II of the New York Heart Association (NYHA).[17] Both PCI and CABG are class I recommendations for STEMI patients younger than 75 years who develop cardiogenic shock within 36 hours after infarction.[14,18] In patients older than 75, early revascularization did not yield any benefit and was associated with increased mortality. However, because early revascularization has been associated with improved outcomes for those older than 75 elsewhere, a selective approach of offering revascularization to previously high-functioning individuals with good physiological reserve is justified.[15,19]

The SHOCK registry also demonstrated a short-term survival benefit from revascularization with PCI/CABG compared to the use of fibrinolytics.[20-22] The reduced benefits are hypothesized to be due to several factors, including reduced penetration of the fibrinolytic to the occluded vessel in hypotensive patients and a higher rate of reocclusion of the infarcted vessel after thrombolysis administration.[23-25] The ACC/AHA issued a class I recommendation that thrombolytics be used in STEMI patients in cardiogenic shock if they do not qualify for revascularization or if transportation to a catheterization laboratory would cause significant delays.[14] PCI is preferred for thrombolysis if it is available.

PEARL

The mortality rate is lower in patients in cardiogenic shock who undergo revascularization (PCI/CAGB) than in those who receive fibrinolytics.

Patients are more likely to be referred for primary CABG versus PCI if they are found to have left main coronary artery disease or severe triple-vessel disease on cardiac catheterization. Cardiogenic shock patients with AMI are more likely to have left main coronary artery disease or severe triple-vessel disease than their hemodynamically stable counterparts and therefore have a higher need for CABG.[6] Unfortunately, there have been no randomized head-to-head trials comparing outcomes for PCI versus CABG. In patients with moderate triple-vessel disease, it is reasonable to perform PCI on the infarct-related artery and defer CABG of the other diseased vessels.[15]

In patients with severe triple-vessel or left main coronary artery disease, emergent CABG is recommended. The timing of reperfusion is simple: the faster a patient can get to PCI or CABG, the lower the mortality rate.[27,28] A survival benefit of revascularization was still noted up to 18 hours after the onset of shock.[28]

TABLE 8-5. Mechanical Support Devices
Intraaortic balloon pump counterpulsation
Ventricular assist devices
Extracorporeal life support

TABLE 8-6. Class I Indications for IABPs[12]
For cardiogenic shock not reversed with pressors prior to angiography and revascularization
For acute mitral regurgitation and ventricular septal rupture complicating AMI prior to angiography and surgical repair
For refractory post-MI angina as a bridge to angiography and revascularization

Mechanical Support Devices

Patients in cardiogenic shock who require mechanical support are at the most critically ill spectrum of disease severity. These patients remain hemodynamically unstable despite aggressive supportive care and vasopressor therapy. The initiation of mechanical support can be a key therapeutic step toward definitive therapy with revascularization or surgical repair *(Table 8-5).*

Intraaortic Balloon Pump Counterpulsation

Intraaortic balloon pump (IABP) counterpulsation can be life-saving in patients with hemodynamic instability requiring vasopressors to maintain perfusion *(Table 8-6).* The pump, which typically is placed by an interventional cardiologist, can improve diastolic coronary flow by as much as 30% by increasing diastolic blood pressure.[29] IABPs also decrease afterload (which lowers myocardial oxygen consumption) and improve subendocardial blood flow. The device should be placed as early as possible, ideally before definitive revascularization, especially if the patient requires transfer to another facility for PCI.[6] Not every patient shows hemodynamic improvement with IABP counterpulsation, but a response predicts a better outcome.[30]

Some evidence suggests that there is no benefit to IABPs prior to the initiation of early revascularization with PCI or CAGB.[31] One study found no difference in the 30-day mortality rate or in secondary outcomes and disease markers (such as lactate levels and length of stay in the ICU).[31] However, the study had several limitations, including an atypically small sample size, fewer sick patients (evidenced by a lower 30-day mortality rate), and asymmetry in the crossover intention-to-treat principles.[32]

IABP counterpulsation is beneficial in patients with structural causes of cardiogenic shock such as mitral regurgitation or ventricular septal rupture.[8] Although IABPs improve survival after thrombolytic therapy, their use without revascularization has not been shown to reduce the risk of death.[33-36] Complications of IABP counterpulsation occur in 10% to 30% of cases.[8,37,38] Contraindications and complications related to the placement of balloon pumps are listed in Table 8-7. IABP is listed as a Level IIa recommendation in the 2013 ACCF/AHA guidelines for the management of STEMI.[39]

Ventricular Assist Devices

Ventricular assist devices (VADs) are used in selected patients who remain unstable despite supportive care, IABP counterpulsation, and revascularization. These patients usually have very low cardiac outputs (<1.2 L/min/m^2).[25] The devices can be inserted percutaneously or implanted surgically. They can assist the left ventricle, the right ventricle, or both. Although there is no difference in 30-day mortality between IABP counterpulsation and percutaneous VADs in patients undergoing PCI for cardiogenic shock secondary to AMI, patients experienced higher complication rates after use of a VAD.[40]

Percutaneous VADs can be inserted rapidly but they cannot be left in place for a long time. The device can be an appropriate bridge to an implantable VAD or a more definitive therapy such as revascularization, CABG, or cardiac transplantation.[42] The implantation procedure should be performed in a catheterization lab by an interventional cardiologist. For example, when placing TandemHeart percutaneous VAD (Cardiac Assist, Inc., Pittsburgh, PA), a 21F femoral catheter is placed transseptally across the interatrial septum into the left atrium, which unloads the left atrium and ventricle.[41] Blood is then pumped back to the patient via a 15F to 17F catheter inserted into the femoral artery. Flows of 3.5 to 4 L/min have been reported.[41]

Implantable VADs are placed by a cardiothoracic surgeon in the operating room and can support patients for longer periods, including those waiting for cardiac transplantation.[43] Given the limited supply of donor hearts, the use of VADs as longterm, definitive therapy is appealing, but more research is needed.[44,45] Because the resources to place percutaneous and implantable VADs are not widely available, patients in whom IABP counterpulsation and revascularization fail must be transported to a tertiary care center that has the equipment and personnel needed to perform these specialized procedures.

Extracorporeal Life Support

Two types of extracorporeal life support (ECLS) are used in patients in cardiogenic shock: cardiopulmonary bypass and extracorporeal membrane oxygenation (ECMO). Percutaneous cardiopulmonary bypass can be instituted rapidly at the bedside using the femoral artery and vein to provide nonpulsatile flow of 3 to 5 L/min. This type of support can only be used short term (hours) because of red blood cell destruction.[46] Survival to discharge for ECLS patients has been documented at 33%.[47] Both types of ECLS require specialized teams and equipment, so many patients who require this type of intervention must be transported to tertiary care hospitals.

TABLE 8-7. Precautions for IABPs

Contraindications
Aortic regurgitation
Aortic dissection
Severe peripheral vascular disease
Complications
Hemorrhage
Limb ischemia
Femoral artery laceration
Aortic dissection
Infection
Hemolysis
Thrombocytopenia
Thrombosis
Embolism

PEARL

Consider ventricular assist devices and extracorporeal life support in patients who remain in shock despite aggressive supportive care, IABP counterpulsation, and revascularization.

Novel Therapies

L-N^G-monomethyl-arginine

L-N^G-monomethyl-arginine (L-NMMA) is a nitric oxide inhibitor that is thought to improve outcomes by competitively blocking the compound in patients with shock. High levels of nitric oxide have been associated with decreased contractility. In a small trial of patients with severe cardiogenic shock (on mechanical ventilator, IABP, and pressors) improvements in hemodynamic measurements (ie, raised mean arterial pressure and lowered wedge pressure) were observed after treatment with L-NMMA. All but 1 of the 11 patients were weaned off the ventilator, and 7 were alive at 1 month.[48] The subsequent TRIUMPH trial did not reveal any benefit of L-NMMA.[49] The SHOCK-2 trial showed improvement in hemodynamic markers but no improvement in survival rate.[50]

Hypothermia

Although therapeutic hypothermia exerts cerebral protection and improves mortality after resuscitation from circulatory arrest, its application in patients in cardiogenic shock has been discouraged due to concerns it could worsen hemodynamics. Improvements in hemodynamic and cardiac function parameters have been observed in ICU patients with cardiogenic shock who were cooled to 33°C (91.4°F) for either 1 or 24 hours.[51] However, the small body of evidence makes it difficult to draw definitive conclusions. Controlled studies are required to show differences in mortality and patient outcomes before the treatment can be considered in clinical practice.

Structural Abnormalities

Although LV failure from MI is the most common cause of cardiogenic shock, structural etiologies also must be ruled out. These include papillary muscle rupture, LV free wall rupture, and ventricular septal rupture *(Table 8-8)*.[7] Together, these three conditions are responsible for 12% of cardiogenic shock cases and warrant cardiac surgical repair.[52] These complications should be suspected in any patient presenting in shock after a nonanterior MI, especially if it is the individual's first event. Echocardiography should be used to detect these complications.[7]

Papillary Muscle Rupture

Rupture occurs when an MI produces ischemia at the head of the papillary muscle and usually is preceded by severe mitral regurgitation. It is a relatively uncommon condition, associated with 7% of patients in cardiogenic shock in the SHOCK trial registry.[52,53] It is more likely to occur in patients with acute inferior or posterior MIs and within the first 24 hours after the onset of AMI. Risk factors include female gender and age greater than

65 years.[54] Patients present with acute pulmonary edema and often have a loud pansystolic cardiac murmur. Urgent formal echocardiography should be ordered when the diagnosis is suspected. Surgical repair is listed as a class I recommendation by the ACC/AHA. Without surgical repair, these patients have a very high mortality rate (71% in the SHOCK trial registry). Even with surgery, the mortality rate remains approximately 40%.[54] Temporary afterload reduction can improve cardiac output while the patient awaits surgery.[55] Because this is difficult to accomplish when patients are already hypotensive, a combination of vasopressors (for blood pressure support) and afterload reducers is needed.

TABLE 8-8. Structural Causes of Cardiogenic Shock[7]

Three structural causes account for 12% of cases of cardiogenic shock:
Papillary muscle rupture
Left ventricular free wall rupture
Ventricular septal rupture
All are associated with very high mortality rates if they are not surgically repaired; therefore, early diagnosis is imperative.
Echocardiography has a vital role in diagnosing/excluding structural causes:
Severe mitral regurgitation and/or papillary muscle abnormalities suggest papillary muscle rupture.
A large pericardial effusion in a patient with an acute anterior wall MI suggests left ventricular free wall rupture.
A left-to-right shunt across the ventricular septum with acute right ventricular dilatation suggests acute ventricular septal rupture.

Left Ventricular Free Wall Rupture

LV free wall rupture is a rare but lethal complication of acute anterior MI. A substantial majority of patients die immediately from pulseless electrical activity arrest, but a small subset develop a contained hemorrhagic cardiac tamponade and might be salvageable. This diagnosis has decreased in incidence from 6% to 1% in the revascularization era.[52] Rupture occurs in the first 24 hours after AMI in about 50% of cases and within 1 week in the remainder.[56] Patients develop nonspecific symptoms such as refractory or recurrent chest pain, nausea, vomiting, syncope, and paradoxic bradycardia.[57] Echocardiography is required for diagnosis and will show a significant pericardial effusion.

Ventricular Septal Rupture

Rupture of the intraventricular septum is a very rare complication of AMI and cardiogenic shock and usually develops within 24 hours after infarction. [14,15] Patients typically present with acute pulmonary edema and a loud pansystolic murmur. An urgent echocardiogram is required to make the diagnosis; right ventricular overload is seen, with left-to-right shunting of blood though the rupture.[35] Urgent surgical repair is a class I recommendation by the ACC/AHA; however, even with surgery, the mortality rate exceeds 80%.[15]

Conclusion

Cardiogenic shock, most frequently a complication of AMI, requires timely diagnosis and resuscitation. A sound knowledge of the various options for aggressive supportive treatment can make the difference between life and death. Early referral for revascularization or cardiac surgical repair in selected cases is often necessary for survival.

KEY POINTS

1. Point-of-care echocardiography performed by an emergency physician can confirm pump failure (by showing decreased global contractility) and exclude other causes of shock (pericardial effusion with tamponade, massive pulmonary embolism, and valvular regurgitation).
2. Place all patients in whom cardiogenic shock is suspected on cardiac monitors for the evaluation of arrhythmias.
3. Treat tachyarrhythmias with electrical cardioversion; antiarrhythmic medications can worsen hypotension.
4. Treat symptomatic bradycardia with atropine and transcutaneous or transvenous pacing.
5. Pure vasopressors such as phenylephrine should be avoided because they increase myocardial oxygen demand without improving contractility.
6. The initial treatment of cardiogenic shock includes:
   - Correct hypotension with a fluid bolus (250–500 mL, or more if RV infarction is suspected).
   - Add vasopressors/inotropes early to keep mean arterial pressure >65 mm Hg, SBP >90 mm Hg, and urine output >0.5 mL/kg/hr.
7. Reperfusion therapy is the mainstay treatment in most cardiogenic shock patients.
   - PCI is preferred over fibrinolytic therapy.
   - Fibrinolytics are indicated in patients who are not candidates for revascularization and in those who would experience significant delays in getting to the catheterization lab.
   - CABG is the preferred method of revascularization if coronary angiography reveals left main coronary artery disease or severe triple-vessel disease.
   - "Time is muscle" — the faster the revascularization, the lower the mortality risk.

REFERENCES

1. Nieminen MS, Bohm C, Cowie MR, et al. Executive summary of the guidelines on the diagnosis and treatment of acute heart failure: the Task Force on Acute Heart Failure of the European Society of Cardiology. *Eur Heart J.* 2005;26:384-416.
2. Hochman JS, Sleeper LA, Webb JG, et al. Early revascularization in acute myocardial infarction complicated by cardiogenic shock. SHOCK Investigators. Should we emergently revascularize occluded coronaries for cardiogenic shock? *N Engl J Med.* 1999;341:625-634.
3. Goldberg RJ, Samad NA, Yarzdbska J, et al. Temporal trends in cardiogenic shock complicating acute myocardial infarction. *N Engl J Med.* 1999;340:1162-1168.
4. Aissaoui N, Puymirat E, Simon T et al. Long-term outcome in early survivors of cardiogenic shock at the acute stage of myocardial infarction: a landmark analysis from the French registry of Acute ST-elevation and non-ST-elevation Myocardial Infarction (FAST-MI) Registry. *Crit Care.* 2014;18:516-525.
5. Holmes DR Jr, Berger PB, Hochman JS, et al. Cardiogenic shock in patients with acute ischemic syndromes with and without ST-segment elevation. *Circulation.* 1999;100:2067-2073.
6. Jacobs AK, French JK, Col J, et al. Cardiogenic shock with non-ST-segment elevation myocardial infarction: a report from the SHOCK Trial Registry. Should we emergently revascularize occluded coronaries for cardiogenic shock? *J Am Coll Cardiol.* 2000;36:1091-1096.
7. Reynolds HR, Hochman JS. Cardiogenic shock: current concepts and improving outcomes. *Circulation.* 2008;117:686-697.
8. Gurm HS, Bates ER. Cardiogenic shock complicating myocardial infarction. *Crit Care Clin.* 2007;23:759-777.
9. Lindholm MG, Kober L, Boesgaard S, et al. Cardiogenic shock complicating acute myocardial infarction. *Eur Heart J.* 2003;24:258-265.
10. Sanborn TA, Sleeper LA, Bates ER, et al. Impact of thrombolysis, intra-aortic balloon pump counterpulsation, and their combination in cardiogenic shock complicating acute myocardial infarction: a report from the SHOCK trial registry. *J Am Coll Cardiol.* 2000;36:1123-1129.
11. Labovitz A, Noble V, Bierig M, et al. Focused cardiac ultrasound in the emergent setting: A consensus statement of the American Society of Echocardiography and American College of Emergency Physicians. *J Am Soc Echocardiogr.* 2010;23:1225-1230.
12. Niendorff DF, Rassias AJ, Palac R, et al. Rapid cardiac ultrasound of inpatients suffering PEA arrest performed by nonexpert sonographers. *Resuscitation.* 2005;67:81-87.
13. Randazzo MR, Snoey ER, Levitt MA, et al. Accuracy of emergency physician assessment of left ventricular ejection fraction and central venous pressure using echocardiography. *Acad Emerg Med.* 2003;10:973-977.
14. Antman EM, Anbe DT, Armstrong PW, et al. ACC/AHA guidelines for the management of patients with ST-elevation myocardial infarction: a report of the American College of Cardiology/American Heart Association Task Force on Practice Guidelines (Committee to Revise the 1999 Guidelines for the Management of Patients with Acute Myocardial Infarction). *J Am Coll Cardiol.* 2004;44:E1-E211.
15. Menon V, Hochman JS. Management of cardiogenic shock complicating acute myocardial infarction. *Heart.* 2003;88:531-537.
16. Ohman EM, Chang PP. Improving the quality of life after cardiogenic shock: do more revascularization. *J Am Coll Cardiol.* 2005;46:274-276.
17. Menon V, Webb JC, Hillis LD, et al. Outcome and profile of ventricular septal rupture with cardiogenic shock after myocardial infarction: a report from the SHOCK registry trial. *J Am Coll Cardiol.* 2000;36:1110-1116.
16. De Backer D, Biston P, Devriendt J, et al. Comparison of dopamine and norepinephrine in the treatment of shock. *N Engl J Med.* 2010;362:779-789.
17. Nativi-Nicolau J, Selzman C, Fang J, et al. Pharmacologic therapies for acute cardiogenic shock. *Curr Opin Cardiol.* 2014;29:250-257.
18. Eagle KA, Guyton RA, Davidoff R, et al. ACC/AHA 2004 guideline update for coronary artery bypass graft surgery. A report of the American College of Cardiology/American Heart Association Task Force on Practice Guidelines (Committee to Revise the 1999 Guidelines for Coronary Artery Bypass Surgery). *Circulation.* 2004;100:e340-e437.
19. Dzavik V, Sleeper LA, Cocke TP, et al. Early revascularization is associated with improved survival in elderly patients with acute myocardial infarction complicated by cardiogenic shock: a report from the SHOCK trial registry. *Eur Heart J.* 2003;24:828-837.
20. Sanborn TA, Feldman T. Management strategies for cardiogenic shock. *Curr Opin Cardiol.* 2004;19:608-612.
21. Naples RM, Harris JW, Ghaemmahami CA. Critical care aspects in the management of patients with acute coronary syndromes. *Emerg Med Clin North Am.* 2008;26:685-702.
22. Holmes DR Jr, Bates ER, Kleiman NS, et al. Contemporary reperfusion therapy for cardiogenic shock: the GUSTO-I Investigators Global Utilization of Streptokinase and Tissue Plasminogen Activator for Occluded Coronary Arteries. *J Am Coll Cardiol.* 1995;26:668-674.
23. Hollenberg SM, Kavinsky CJ, Parillo JE. Cardiogenic shock. *Ann Intern Med.* 1999;131:47-59.
24. Ellis TC, Lev E, Yasbek NF, et al. Therapeutic strategies for cardiogenic shock, 2006. *Current Treat Options Cardiovasc Med.* 2006;8:79-94.
25. Duvernoy CS, Bates ER. Management of cardiogenic shock attributable to acute myocardial infarction in the reperfusion era. *J Intensive Care Med.* 2005;4:188-198.
26. Bates ER, Moscussi M. Postmyocardial infarction cardiogenic shock. In: Brown DL, ed. *Cardiac Intensive Care.* Philadelphia, PA: WB Saunders; 1998:215-227.
27. Zeymer U, Neuhaus KL. Predictors of in-hospital mortality in 1333 patients with acute myocardial infarction complicated by cardiogenic shock treated with primary percutaneous coronary intervention (PCI): results of the primary PCI registry of the Arbeitsgemeinschaft Leitende Kardiologische Krankenhausarzte (ALKK). *Eur Heart J.* 2004;25:322-328.
28. Hochman JS, Sleeper LA, Webb JG, et al. Early revascularization and long-term survival in cardiogenic shock complicating acute myocardial infarction. *JAMA.* 2006;295:2511-2515.
29. Scheidt S, Wilner G, Mueller H, et al. Intra-aortic balloon counterpulsation in cardiogenic shock: report of a co-operative clinical trial. *N Engl J Med.* 1973;288:979-984.
30. Ramanathan K, Cosmi J, Harkness SM, et al. Reversal of systemic hypoperfusion following intra aortic balloon pumping is associated with improved 30-day survival independent of early revascularization in cardiogenic shock complicating an acute myocardial infarction. *Circulation.* 2003;108(suppl 1):I-672.
31. Thiele H, Zeymer U, Neurmann F, et al. Intraaortic balloon support for myocardial infarction with cardiogenic shock. *N Engl J Med.* 2012;367:1287-1296.
32. O'Connor C, Rogers G. Editorial: evidence for overturning the guidelines in cardiogenic shock. *N Engl J Med.* 2012;367:1349-1350.
33. Anderson RD, Ohman EM, Holmes DR, et al. Use of intra-aortic balloon counterpulsation in patients presenting with cardiogenic shock: observations from the GUSTO-I study. *J Am Coll Cardiol.* 1997;30:708-715.
34. Webb JG. Interventional management of cardiogenic shock. *Can J Cardiol.* 1998;14:233-244.
35. Hochman JS, Sleeper LA, White HD, et al. One-year survival following early revascularization for cardiogenic shock. *JAMA.* 2001;285:190-192.
36. Hudson MP, Ohman EM. Intra-aortic balloon counterpulsation for cardiogenic shock complicating acute myocardial infarction. In: Hollenberg SM, Bates ER, eds. *Cardiogenic Shock.* Armonk, NY: Futura; 2002:81-102.
37. Trost JC, Hillis LD. Intra-aortic balloon counterpulsation. *Am J Cardiol.* 2006;97:J391-J398.
38. Stone GW, Ohman EM, Miller MF, et al. Contemporary utilization and outcomes of intra aortic balloon counterpulsation in acute myocardial infarction: the benchmark registry. *J Am Coll Cardiol.* 2003;41:1940-1945.
39. O'Gara P, Kushner F, Ascheim D, et al. 2013 ACCF/AHA Guideline for Management of ST-Elevation Myocardial Infarction: Executive Summary: A report of the American College of Cardiology Foundation/American Heart Association Task Force on Practice Guidelines. *Circulation.* 2013;127:529-555.
40. Thiele H, Sick P, Boudriot E, et al. Randomized comparison of intra-aortic balloon support with a percutaneous left ventricular assist device in patients with revascularized acute myocardial infarction complicated by cardiogenic shock. *Eur Heart J.* 2005;26:1276-1283.
41. Topalian S, Ginsberg F, Parrilo J. Cardiogenic shock. *Crit Care Med.* 2008;36(suppl):S66-S74.
42. Kar B, Adkins LE, Civitello AB, et al. Clinical experience with the TandemHeart percutaneous ventricular assist device. *Tex Heart Inst J.* 2006;33:111-115.
43. Tayara W, Starling RC, Yamani MH, et al. Improved survival after acute myocardial infarction complicated by cardiogenic shock with circulatory support and transplantation: comparing aggressive intervention with conservative treatment. *J Heart Lung Transplant.* 2006;25:504-509.
44. Burkoff D, O'Neill W, Brunckhorst C, et al. Feasbility study of the use of the TandemHeart percutaneous ventricular assist device for the treatment of cardiogenic shock. *Catheter Cardiovasc Interv.* 2006;68:211-217.
45. Meyns B, Dens J, Sergeant P, et al. Initial experience with the Impella device in patients with cardiogenic shock: Impella support for cardiogenic shock. *Thorac Cardiovasc Surg.* 2003;51:312-317.
46. Nichol G, Karmy-Jones R, Salerno C, et al. Systematic review of percutaneous cardiopulmonary bypass for cardiac arrest or cardiogenic shock states. *Resuscitation.* 2006;70:381-394.
47. Bartlett RH, Roloff DW, Custer JR, et al. Extracorporeal life support: the University of Michigan experience. *JAMA.* 2000;283:904-908.
48. Cotter G, Kaluski E, Blatt A, et al. L-NMMA (a nitric oxide synthase inhibitor) is effective in the treatment of cardiogenic shock. *Circulation.* 2000;101:1358-1361.
49. TRIUMPH investigators, Alexander JH, Reynolds HR, et al. Effect of tilarginine acetate in patients with acute myocardial infarction and cardiogenic shock: the TRIUMPH randomized controlled trial. *JAMA.* 2007;297:1657-1666.
50. Dzavik V, Cotter G, Reynolds HR, et al. Effect of nitric oxide synthase inhibition on hemodynamics and outcome of patients with persistent cardiogenic shock complicating acute myocardial infarction: a phase II dose-ranging study. *Eur Heart J.* 2007;28:1009-1016.
51. Schmidt-Schweda S, Ohler A, Post H, et al. Moderate hypothermia for severe cardiogenic shock (COOL Shock Study I & II). *Resuscitation.* 2013;85:319-325.
52. Hochman JS, Buller CE, Sleeper LA, et al. Cardiogenic shock complicating acute myocardial infarction–etiologies, management and outcome: a report from the SHOCK registry trial. *J Am Coll Cardiol.* 2000;36:1063-1070.
53. Thompson CR, Buller CE, Sleeper LA, et al. Cardiogenic shock due to acute severe mitral regurgitation complicating acute myocardial infarction: a report from the SHOCK trial registry. *J Am Coll Cardiol.* 2000;36:1104-1109.
54. Bates ER, Topol EJ. Limitations of thrombolytic therapy for acute myocardial infarction complicated by congestive heart failure and cardiogenic shock. *J Am Coll Cardiol.* 1991;18:1077-1084.
55. Aronson D, Goldsher N, Zukermann R, et al. Ischemic mitral regurgitation and risk of heart failure after myocardial infarction. *Arch Intern Med.* 2006;166:2362-2368.
56. Wehrens XH, Doevendans PA. Cardiac rupture complicating myocardial infarction. *Int J Cardiol.* 2004;95:285-292.
57. Birnbaum Y, Wagner GS, Gates KB, et al. Clinical and electrocardiographic variables associated with increased risk of ventricular septal defect in acute anterior myocardial infarction. *Am J Cardiol.* 2000;86:830-834.
58. Slater J, Brown RJ, Antonelli TA, et al. Cardiogenic shock due to cardiac free wall rupture or tamponade after acute myocardial infarction: a report from the SHOCK trial registry. *J Am Coll Cardiol.* 2000;36:1117-1122.

Extracorporeal Membrane Oxygenation

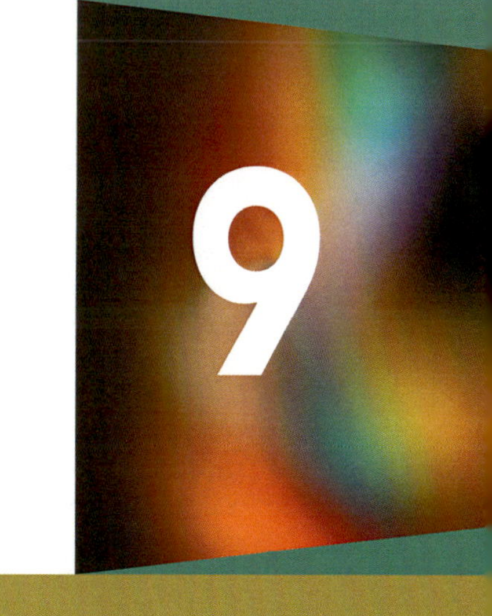

IN THIS CHAPTER

- Extracorporeal cardiopulmonary resuscitation
- ECMO for respiratory failure
- ECMO for cardiogenic shock
- ECMO in trauma

Zack Shinar and Joe Bellezzo

Extracorporeal membrane oxygenation (ECMO) involves the use of an artificial membrane oxygenator to oxygenate and remove carbon dioxide (CO_2) from the blood. The method is performed in two distinct configurations: venoarterial (VA-ECMO) and venovenous (VV-ECMO). VA-ECMO also can be referred to as cardiopulmonary support (CPS), extracorporeal life support (ECLS), and cardiopulmonary bypass (CPB).

Extracorporeal cardiopulmonary resuscitation (ECPR) describes the initiation of VA-ECMO during cardiac arrest. Observational studies support the effectiveness of ECPR.[1-5] VA-ECMO requires both arterial and venous cannulation and is used to treat cardiac failure. VV-ECMO, on the other hand, is used to manage respiratory failure when conventional ventilator strategies are unsuccessful; it requires only venous cannulation. Common conditions for the use of VV-ECMO include adult respiratory distress syndrome (ARDS), influenza, and status asthmaticus.[6,7]

Patients with refractory shock are an emerging population that might benefit from ECMO; however, the benefits of the procedure must be coupled with an analysis of its potential risks and complications.[9] Additional information can be found at the authors' website, www.edecmo.org.

Extracorporeal Cardiopulmonary Resuscitation

ECPR involves the initiation of ECMO during cardiac arrest, and functionally is performed in parallel with traditional resuscitative efforts. The application of ECMO in the arresting patient is inherently more challenging than in more elective applications (eg, refractory respiratory failure).

Indications

ECPR provides the patient in cardiac arrest with a temporary bridge until definitive therapy can be provided. When cardiac arrest occurs because of an intrinsic problem within the heart (eg, an occluded coronary artery), an extrinsic problem with the heart (eg, metabolic disturbances), or a problem with the lung (eg, pulmonary embolism), ECPR allows bypass of those organs. The procedure also maintains perfusion to the brain, heart, and other organs. However, it is important to note that ECPR is not inherently therapeutic.

A scarcity of time and resources necessitates the rapid and correct identification of patients who might benefit from ECMO. Patients in cardiac arrest often arrive with very little information, except what can be provided by emergency medical services personnel and witnesses. Essential to the decision to initiate ECPR is delineation of the goals of therapy. If the patient is believed to be potentially curable, aggressive therapy should be initiated. If the patient's condition is deemed irreversible, then palliative therapy should be chosen.

Ideal candidates for ECPR are often younger patients who were neurologically intact prior to the onset of cardiac arrest. Other key determinants include immediate bystander CPR, witnessed arrest, and short downtime. It can be problematic to eliminate patients algorithmically; it is best to make the decision to initiate ECMO based on an overall understanding of each particular case. Major ECMO centers in Japan and Australia, as well as the authors' center in San Diego, have published inclusion and exclusion criteria *(Table 9-1)*. Though there are minor variations between centers, common inclusion criteria include a short transport time (<10 minutes), a total cardiac arrest time from start of procedure of less than 60 minutes, bystander CPR within 10 minutes of a witnessed arrest, and reasonable prearrest neurological function. In the future, the ability to neuroprognosticate a patient rapidly upon presentation could greatly increase the utility of ECPR.

Procedure

Starting ECPR involves obtaining percutaneous vascular access, transitioning to ECMO cannulae, priming the machine, and initiating the pump. The cannulae are inserted in three stages:

- **Stage 1** involves placement of commercially available vascular access catheters via the Seldinger technique. Ultrasound should be used for proper identification and cannulation of the vessels. Successful cannulation of both the femoral artery and femoral vein marks the completion of this stage. While the resuscitationist is contemplating ECMO, the femoral venous central line is used for delivery of fluids and drugs. The arterial line is transduced to guide vasoactive therapy, determine the validity of the arrest state, and manage pressures after arrest.
- **Stage 2** involves the exchange of traditional central venous catheters with larger ECMO cannulae. A series of progressive dilators is used until the vessel will accept the ECMO cannula chosen (15F–19F arterial; 17F–23F venous [*Figures 9-1* and 9-2]). Stage 2 is complete when an ECMO cannula is properly positioned and secured into each respective femoral vessel.
- **Stage 3** involves connecting the ECMO cannulae to the primed ECMO machine. Air is removed from the circuit, and the pump is started *(Figure 9-3)*. Successful initiation of total cardiopulmonary bypass marks the completion of this stage.

Cannulating the femoral vessels in a patient receiving active chest compressions is difficult. After circulatory arrest, the pressures in the venous and arterial systems begin to equalize, rendering a larger-than-normal femoral vein and a smaller-than-normal femoral artery. During chest compressions, both femoral vessels can appear pulsatile when visualized with ultrasound, making identification of the artery and vein problematic. The femoral artery should be given priority because it is more difficult to cannulate. Every effort should be made to secure each vessel on the "first stick." Each failed attempt increases the risk of hematoma formation, a complication that makes further cannulation attempts more challenging. Some practitioners advocate a brief pause in chest compressions during arterial cannulation *(Figure 9-3)*.

Once cardiopulmonary bypass has been established, the next step is to optimize flow through the circuit. Circuit flow is accomplished by increasing the revolutions per minute (RPM) of the centrifugal pump. Increasing the RPM beyond the capacity of the circuit causes hemolysis of red blood cells and creates "chatter" as increased negative pressure on the venous line pulls the inferior vena cava (IVC) edges onto the cannula, resulting in substantial trauma. When this occurs, the RPM should be decreased enough to eliminate chatter. If the lower RPM does not generate sufficient blood flow, other factors should be addressed such as kinked lines or clamps, venous line placement, and circulating volume. Continued chatter with reduction of the pump's RPM suggests hypovolemia or a poorly placed venous cannula.

TABLE 9-1. ECMO Criteria

Inclusion Criteria
Persistent cardiopulmonary arrest despite traditional resuscitative efforts
Shock (SBP <70 mm Hg) refractory to standard therapies
Exclusion Criteria
Initial rhythm asystole
Chest compressions not initiated within 10 min after arrest (either bystanders or EMS personnel)
Estimated EMS transport time >10 min
Total arrest time >60 min
Suspicion of shock due to sepsis or hemorrhage
Preexisting severe neurological disease prior to arrest (including traumatic brain injury, stroke, or severe dementia)

PEARL

Arterial cannulation during active chest compressions is difficult to achieve. Care should be taken to make the first attempt successful.

Physiology

Once placed on VA-ECMO, the physiology of a patient's circulatory system changes dramatically. The venous cannula draws blood from the right atrium. Ideally, all blood is removed with this cannula, but limitations of its size and placement make complete blood removal unlikely. The venous blood is then pumped through a gas exchanger, which adds oxygen and removes carbon dioxide. Two types of pumps are used for ECMO: pressure limited and volume limited. Roller pumps are an example of volume-limited pumps and are more commonly used in the operating room. These pumps push the same volume each cycle and can produce excess pressure in the arterial portion of the extracorporeal perfusion system if obstructions occur. This liability does not, however, exist with current generation ECPR pressure-limited pumps. Pressure-limited pumps must have accurate flow determinations since the rotary speed can fail to generate flow if an obstruction is present. These pumps use rotational spin to create a centrifugal vortex, which causes flow to decrease or cease if downward obstruction occurs in the circuitry. One of the resulting complications of this scenario is hemolysis secondary to heat generation within the pump, especially under low-flow, high-RPM conditions.

After blood flows through the oxygenator and pump, it

FIGURE 9-1. Dilation

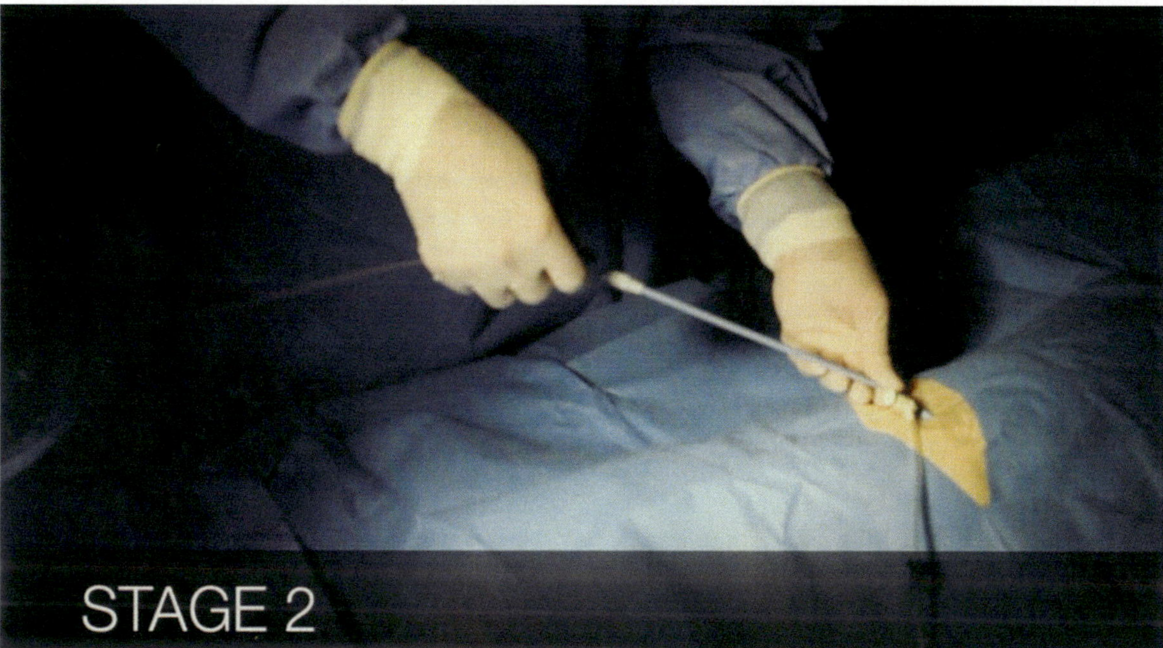

FIGURE 9-2. Cannula Insertion

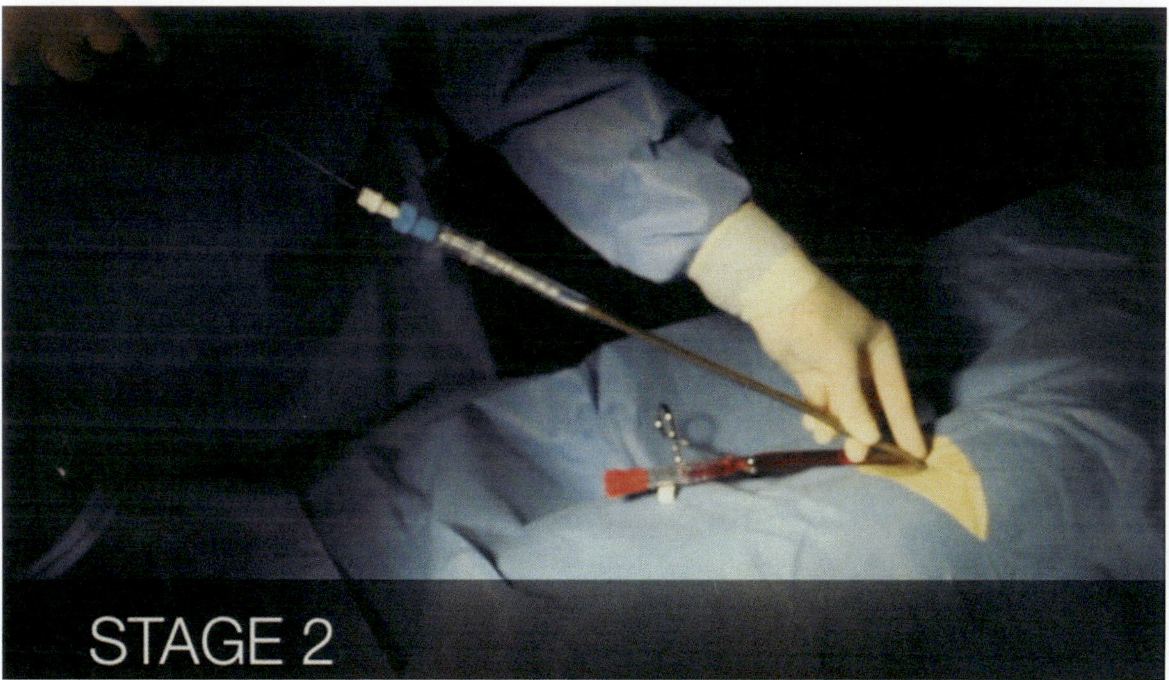

returns to the body through the femoral arterial cannula. This cannula ends at or near the level of the iliac bifurcation, enabling oxygenated blood to flow through the renal and splanchnic arteries. Blood then returns to the upper body retrograde through the aorta. It can also travel via the iliac artery to the lower extremity, where the arterial cannula has been placed. Flow to the ipsilateral lower extremity can be decreased significantly due to mechanical obstruction from the arterial cannula diameter. This problem can be addressed by placing an additional catheter distal to the arterial ECMO cannula. The second catheter is then fed by a side port on the arterial ECMO cannula, allowing perfusion of the leg distal to the cannula. Even with this additional catheter, the extremity must be assessed frequently for adequate perfusion. Perfusion deficits to the leg can significantly increase the risk of morbidity and mortality.

The blood traveling retrograde up the aorta perfuses the kidneys and brain. Importantly, perfusion to the area around the ascending aorta can be variable. Depending on the patient's native heart function, flow could be antegrade from the contracting left ventricle or completely reliant on the retrograde flow from the ECMO pump. The latter scenario occurs with cardiac standstill and results in a closed aortic valve due to the pressure gradient. A persistently closed aortic valve causes the left ventricle to become a cul-de-sac, where venous blood accumulates after entering the lungs from the systemic arterial system. Bronchial flow averages 2% to 5% of the systemic flow. Both can distend the ventricle and cause pulmonary volume sequestration. Some patients will have varying degrees of aortic insufficiency, which can exacerbate the problem even further. Failure to decompress the pulmonary vascular system often results in iatrogenic pulmonary edema or hemorrhage, which can be fatal.

PEARLS

- ✓ Flow on VA-ECMO is retrograde through the aorta.
- ✓ On VA-ECMO, severe pulmonary edema can occur from incomplete venous withdrawal, unejected bronchial blood flow, and/or aortic insufficiency. Urgent decompression of the left ventricle might be necessary.

Coronary perfusion depends on the diastolic pressure gradient within the left ventricle, and therefore should be improved by initiation of bypass. The pump provides nonpulsatile flow retrograde up the aorta. One question that has not been fully answered is whether pulsatile flow is important to the coronary circulation and other vascular beds. Depending on the patient's native heart function, coronary perfusion might be fed predominantly by the native circulation rather than ECMO blood flow. For this reason, adequate ventilation of the lungs is important.

Complications

Several factors can contribute to blood loss, a major complication of ECPR. Patients are systemically heparinized prior to the initiation of bypass. In addition, the ECMO circuits commonly are treated with a heparin-bonding system to prevent thrombosis of the oxygenator and pump. A heparinized patient combined with trauma from femoral cannulae placement make monitoring of hemoglobin essential.

Blood transfusions are expected in the patient undergoing ECPR; minimizing blood loss is important. One helpful tip is to avoid "hubbing" the cannulae during placement. ECMO cannulae are tapered for the portions that lay outside the patient. Overly aggressive insertion will cause a larger diameter vessel injury. During normal patient care, these cannulae can move, creating a vessel hole larger in diameter than the cannula. This can lead to substantial blood loss in a heparinized patient receiving high-pressure blood flow.

Another significant complication of ECMO is pulmonary edema. The physiology of a patient undergoing the procedure involves retrograde flow of blood to the aorta from the femoral arterial cannula. The retrograde flow will close the aortic valve if the native heart has insufficient contractility. If the aortic valve is even slightly incompetent, retrograde flow can enter the left ventricle and lead to pulmonary edema. Significant pulmonary

FIGURE 9-3. Connecting Cannulae to ECMO Circuit

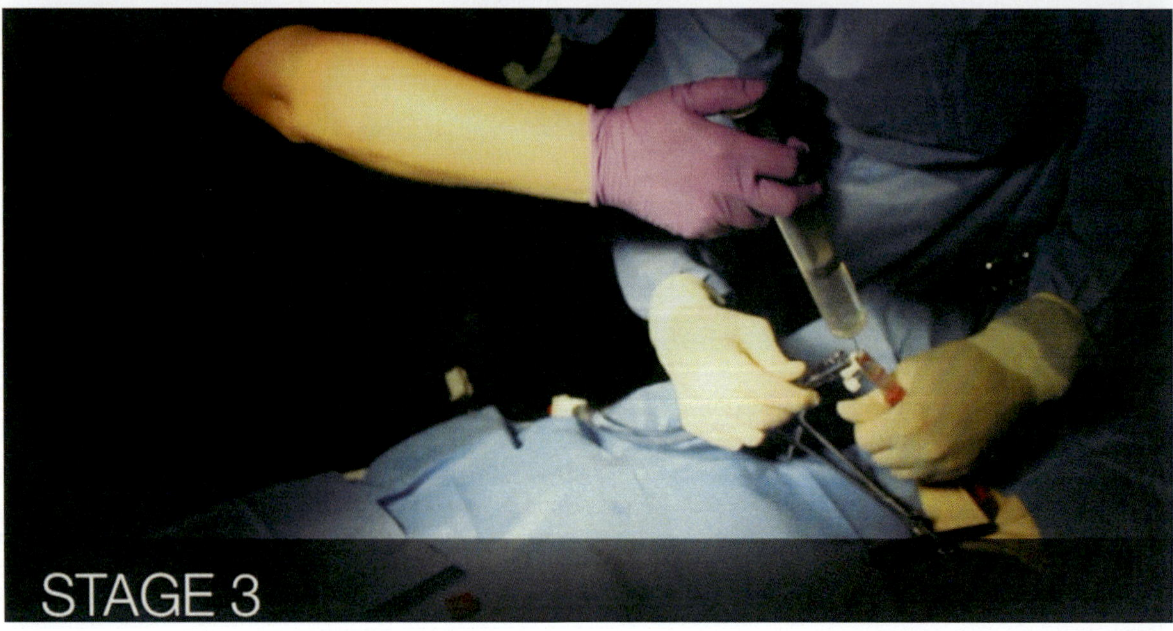

vascular congestion can cause life-threatening pulmonary hemorrhage. Occasionally, the left ventricle may need to be decompressed.

Additionally, right ventricular pressures can increase if insufficient blood is removed from the venous ECMO cannula. This is another cause of pulmonary edema — a risk that underscores the importance of the adequate removal of blood from the right atrium by the venous cannula in patients with poor native heart function. Maximizing the RPM and ensuring proper placement of the venous cannula within the right atrium can help achieve sufficient blood removal. In practice, pulmonary edema becomes a bigger problem each day a patient remains on bypass. Procedures such as septoplasty or the placement of pulmonary artery drains should be considered when edema cannot be controlled.

Postbypass Care

In addition to monitoring for complications, several factors should be considered when managing a patient on ECMO. First, additional central venous lines should be placed only if absolutely necessary and then with extreme caution. The negative pressure in the venous system created by the ECMO circuit can cause significant air emboli. Second, flow and gas exchange should be monitored diligently. A common ECMO error is the accidental placement of two venous cannulae, resulting in ineffective venovenous bypass. Adequate flows follow, as indicated by the bright red color in both the arterial and venous cannulae, but there is no effect on the patient's blood pressure or arterial oxygenation.

Another common error is the inadvertent obstruction of the ECMO circuit — a complication that should prompt the clinician to suspect a clamped section of the ECMO circuit. Failure to unclamp circuit sections or the presence of spontaneous kinks in the tubing will result in poor flows with high arterial pressures on the ECMO machine. The final common miscalculation is inadequate oxygenation. In this scenario, good flows are evident, but no color change is discernible between the arterial and venous systems. Forgetting to connect the oxygenator to oxygen or neglecting to turn the oxygen on will result in this failure. Insertion of a right radial arterial line is especially helpful to measure the nonpulsatile pressures created by ECMO support.

PEARL

Troubleshooting a malfunctioning circuit includes monitoring blood flow and observing blood color within the circuit.

The Evidence

Many institutions use ECPR to resuscitate patients from cardiac arrest, but is this method better than conventional resuscitative measures? Comparison of interventions for cardiac arrest is problematic over large populations. The difficulty in obtaining conclusive evidence is compounded by the fact that only a small fraction of the world uses ECPR. To date, several case series, observational studies, and retrospective reviews have suggested a benefit, yet no randomized control trial has been conducted into the role of ECPR in the resuscitation of dying patients. The large Extracorporeal Life Support Organization (ELSO) registry has shown a 27% survival rate with ECPR; this rate is similar to survival data on ECMO used for in-hospital cardiac arrest.[3,4] More recently, we demonstrated that emergency physicians can perform ECPR without assistance from specialists.[2,10]

Remarkably, one Japanese study found that 52% of patients who undergo combination treatment with ECPR and therapeutic hypothermia survive with intact neurological function.[4] Another study found that 30-day survival for out-of-hospital cardiac arrest (OHCA) patients in facilities using ECPR was 8 times greater than that of patients who did not receive ECPR.[5] Finally, one study used case matching to minimize the differences in decisions to initiate ECPR. Researchers found a highly significant hazard ratio of 0.51 for survival to discharge for in-patient cardiac arrests.[1]

PEARL

Case studies and prospective observational studies have supported the efficacy of ECPR in cardiac arrest patients; however, a randomized control trial remains necessary to prove its efficacy.

The Future of ECPR

Although extracorporeal circulation has been used to treat cardiac arrest for more than two decades, initial trials failed to demonstrate its effectiveness in such cases.[14] Only in the past decade has ECMO been shown to be effective for improving postarrest outcomes. Explanations for this increase in ECPR success include advancements in ECMO technology, improved postarrest care, targeted temperature management, and improved bystander CPR. Also, the introduction of implantable mechanical devices has called into question the importance of postresuscitative cardiac function and increased the emphasis on preserved neurological function. ECMO has been used successfully as a bridge to left ventricular assist device implantation in patients who do not regain sufficient cardiac function.[2,17]

The ability to produce neurologically intact survivors is multifactorial. In OHCA patients, providing rapid and adequate perfusion to the brain is paramount. Prehospital ECPR has shown promise using a trained on-call resuscitationist for certain OHCA patients.[21,23] In this scenario, a physician arrives at the scene of the initially dispatched ambulance to determine if ECMO is needed. If summoned, the ECMO team (a physician and trained nurse) brings a bypass machine and thawed blood products to the scene.

The time to bypass also can be reduced by decreasing prehospital scene times. This strategy entails transferring patients — following 15 minutes of on-scene resuscitation — to a center capable of performing ECPR.[22] The decision to transport

TABLE 9-2. CESAR Trial Inclusion Criteria for VV-ECMO

Murray score >3
Ventilation <7 days
Age <65 years
Reversibility

a patient in cardiac arrest must be made by weighing the benefits of ECPR performed at the receiving hospital against the disadvantages of potentially suboptimal CPR during transport.

Despite great technological advancements, it remains a struggle to accurately identify patients who will benefit from ECPR. There is much more to learn as researchers worldwide continue to expand the boundaries of resuscitation. Induced profound hypothermia (10°C, 50°F) combined with extracorporeal resuscitation is being studied in a traumatic arrest model.[15] Such advances will force a paradigm shift in resuscitation methods in arresting medical patients.

PEARL

Prehospital ECMO and ECMO-induced profound hypothermia are exciting possibilities for the future of resuscitation.

Respiratory Failure

VV-ECMO provides oxygenation and CO_2 removal via venous cannulae. Cannulation can be achieved with femoral-jugular, femoral-femoral, or dual-lumen single jugular catheters. Increasing oxygenation and removing CO_2 is analogous to the role of the body's native lungs. Because blood can be completely saturated with the ECMO oxygenator, oxygenation is elevated by increasing the blood flow over the membranes of the oxygenator. CO_2 is removed by escalating the countercurrent sweep gas. Conceptually, this is similar to increasing minute ventilation in a patient on mechanical ventilation.

VV-ECMO for the treatment of patients in refractory, recoverable respiratory failure has been used extensively worldwide. Indications include insufficient oxygenation despite maximal ventilatory management and refractory respiratory acidosis. Recent use in acute respiratory distress syndrome (ARDS) and the H1N1 pandemic yielded supported — yet controversial — data.[7,8] The CESAR trial was a randomized control trial in which patients with severe ARDS were either managed traditionally or transferred to an ECMO center *(Table 9-2)*. Of the patients who were transferred, 63% had neurologically intact survivorship at 6 months compared with 47% of the traditional therapy group.[7] The ANZ-ECMO trial, an observational study performed during the peak of the 2009 H1N1 influenza outbreak in Australia and New Zealand, demonstrated a mortality rate lower than expected for patients treated for severe respiratory failure from presumptive influenza.[8]

VV-ECMO is less cumbersome than ECPR for several reasons. First, VV-ECMO patients usually undergo a trial of mechanical ventilation before bypass is initiated, which yields time to set up the proper equipment in the proper location. Second, these patients are not undergoing chest compressions, making insertion of the cannula far easier. Third, the difficult task of cannulating and dilating a central artery is not necessary in VV-ECMO. Either one large dual-lumen or two smaller single-lumen venous catheters are used in cases of isolated respiratory failure. Finally, the complication of pulmonary edema should not be seen with VV-ECMO. Weaning a patient off the procedure involves decreasing the sweep gas until no further augmentation of the native lung is underway. During this phase, flows are maintained to prevent clot formation within the circuit.

PEARL

Consider VV-ECMO in patients with reversible respiratory disease in whom traditional respiratory support measures are failing.

Cardiogenic Shock

Research demonstrates that ECMO may benefit patients with cardiogenic shock.[11,12] As with VV-ECMO, initiating VA-ECMO is far easier and safer in the absence of active chest compressions. If VA-ECMO can be started before perfusion is lost, neurological function can be salvaged, thereby avoiding the risk of anoxic encephalopathy seen with ECPR. Disadvantages to using bypass in this patient population are related to the risks of ECMO, which include perforation of central vessels resulting in exsanguination and refractory pulmonary edema. The decision to initiate bypass should be based on a risk-benefit assessment comparing the dangers of ECMO to those of vasopressors. While no randomized control trial has compared these two treatments, data suggest that patients in cardiogenic shock may be appropriate candidates for ECMO.[9,11]

PEARL

Consider ECMO in cases of cardiogenic shock, which carries a high risk of death.

Trauma

Although the use of ECMO in trauma patients remains controversial, benefits have been described in those with isolated lung injuries and lung injuries following multisystem trauma.[2] ARDS and transfusion-related acute lung injury (TRALI) are two indications for VV-ECMO in the postresuscitation phase of trauma. Long-term (10-year) data demonstrate increased survival compared to predicted survival in patients with significant lung injuries.[16] In the acutely bleeding patient, anticoagulation is a major barrier to ECMO implementation. Several institutions have shown success without systemic anticoagulation.[18,19] Trauma patients are subject to many of the same pathologies (eg, hypothermia, pulmonary embolism, and refractory ventricular fibrillation) seen in nontrauma patients. When considering ECMO in this population, the benefits should be weighed against the risk of bleeding. Novel techniques for ECMO in trauma are being pioneered in Stockholm and Baltimore.

PEARL

ECMO can be considered in trauma patients with acute lung injury.

Pediatric Cardiac Arrest

ECMO has been used extensively in pediatric patients, especially in those with newborn respiratory disease and congenital heart disease. The use of ECPR in the arresting pediatric patient is more limited; however, studies from major children's hospitals and registry data have reported survival to discharge rates greater than 40% with good neurological outcomes. Children with preexisting cardiac abnormalities or newborn respiratory disease tend to do better than those with other disorders.[24] Many children require a cannula size typically not stocked by adult ECMO centers. In addition, the location of cannulation may be different in younger patients, in whom the carotid and jugular vessels frequently are used.

Conclusion

Worldwide experience with ECMO is growing for both respiratory and circulatory distress. For each patient, a thoughtful assessment of the risk versus benefit of ECMO initiation needs to be made. Observational and case matching studies have shown benefit and the future of ECMO will continue to be refined with device enhancements, better cannulation techniques, and increased knowledge in pump management.

PEARL

Pediatric ECPR might require equipment not stocked by adult ECMO hospitals.

Special thanks to Dr. Walter Dembitsky, Ms. Suzanne Chillcott, Dr. David Willms, Dr. Maryam Naim, and Dr. Cyrus Olsen, who helped prepare this chapter.

REFERENCES

1. Chen YS, Lin JW, Yu HY, et al. Cardiopulmonary resuscitation with assisted extracorporeal life-support versus conventional cardiopulmonary resuscitation in adults with in-hospital cardiac arrest: an observational study and propensity analysis. *Lancet.* 2008;372:554-561.
2. Bellezzo J, Shinar Z, Davis D, et al. Emergency physician-initiated extracorporeal cardiopulmonary resuscitation. *Resuscitation.* 2012;83:966-970.
3. Jaski BE, Ortiz B, Alla KR, et al. A 20-year experience with urgent percutaneous cardiopulmonary bypass for salvage of potential survivors of refractory cardiovascular collapse. *J Thorac Cardiovasc Surg.* 2010;139:753-757.
4. Nagao K, Hayashi N, Kanmatsuse K, et al. Cardiopulmonary cerebral resuscitation using emergency cardiopulmonary bypass, coronary reperfusion therapy and mild hypothermia in patients with cardiac arrest outside the hospital. *J Am Coll Cardiol.* 2000;36:776-783.
5. Sakamoto T, Morimura N, Nagao K, et al. Extracorporeal cardiopulmonary resuscitation versus conventional cardiopulmonary resuscitation in adults with out-of-hospital cardiac arrest: a prospective observational study. *Resuscitation.* 2014;85:762-768.
6. Stub D, Bernard S, Pellegrino V, et al. Refractory cardiac arrest treated with mechanical CPR, hypothermia, ECMO and early reperfusion (the CHEER trial). *Resuscitation.* 2015;86:88-94.
7. Peek GJ, Mugford M, Tiruvoipati R, et al. Efficacy and economic assessment of conventional ventilatory support versus extracorporeal membrane oxygenation for severe adult respiratory failure (CESAR): a multicentre randomised controlled trial. *Lancet.* 2009;374:1351-1363.
8. Noah MA, Peek GJ, Finney SJ, et al. Referral to an extracorporeal membrane oxygenation center and mortality among patients with severe 2009 influenza A (H1N1). *JAMA.* 2011;306:1659-1668.
9. Min HK, Lee YT. Role of percutaneous cardiopulmonary support (PCPS) in patients with unstable hemodynamics during the peri-coronary-intervention period. In Baškot B, ed. *Coronary Angiography — The Need for Improvement in Medical and Interventional Therapy.* Rijeka: InTech; 2011:135.
10. Shinar Z, Bellezzo J, Paradis N, et al. Emergency department initiation of cardiopulmonary bypass: case report and review of literature. *J Emerg Med.* 43 2012;43:83-86.
11. Combes A, Leprince P, Luyt CE, et al. Outcomes and long-term quality-of-life of patients supported by extracorporeal membrane oxygenation for refractory cardiogenic shock. *Crit Care Med.* 2008;36:1404-1411.
12. Schwarz B, Mair P, Margreiter J, et al. Experience with percutaneous venoarterial cardiopulmonary bypass for emergency circulatory support. *Crit Care Med.* 2003;31:758-764.
13. Thiagarajan RR, Brogan TV, Scheurer MA, et al. Extra-corporeal membrane oxygenation to support cardiopulmonary resuscitation in adults. *Ann Thorac Surg* 2009;87:778-785.
14. Pretto E, Safar P, Saito R, et al. Cardiopulmonary bypass after prolonged cardiac arrest in dogs. *Ann Emerg Med.* 1987;16:611-619.

KEY POINTS

1. ECMO is effective in cardiac arrest (ECPR), respiratory failure (VV-ECMO), and refractory cardiogenic shock (VA-ECMO).
2. Pulmonary bypass (VV-ECMO) involves only venous access, whereas cardiopulmonary bypass (VA-ECMO) requires both venous and arterial cannulation.
3. The three steps of initiating ECMO are 1) femoral arterial and venous cannulation using standard central line kits, 2) dilation and insertion of ECMO cannulae, and 3) connecting ECMO cannulae to the primed machine and starting the circuit.
4. Increasing the RPM of the pump increases flow. Generally, higher flow rates are preferred.
5. Chatter can be eliminated by decreasing the RPM of the machine. Volume assessment and position of cannulae should be reevaluated if the chatter continues.
6. ECPR pumps are pressure limited. They are safer than volume-limited pumps but require close monitoring for distal circuit obstruction.
7. Monitoring perfusion to the cannulated lower extremity is extremely important and usually requires an additional perfusion catheter distal to the primary arterial ECMO cannula.
8. Blood loss and pulmonary edema are the two major complications of ECMO.
9. Avoid "hubbing" the cannula during insertion to minimize blood loss at the cannulation site and limit bleeding complications during hospitalization.
10. VV-ECMO is pure pulmonary support, whereas VA-ECMO is total cardiopulmonary bypass.
11. VV-ECMO may benefit patients with refractory respiratory failure due to severe influenza and ARDS.

15. Wu X, Drabek T, Kochanek PM, et al. Induction of profound hypothermia for emergency preservation and resuscitation allows intact survival after cardiac arrest resulting from prolonged lethal hemorrhage and trauma in dogs. *Circulation.* 2006;113:1974-1982.
16. Ried M, Bein T, Philipp A, et al. Extracorporeal lung support in trauma patients with severe chest injury and acute lung failure: a 10-year institutional experience. *Crit Care.* 2103;17:R110.
17. Chen YS, Ko WJ, Lin FY, et al. Preliminary result of an algorithm to select proper ventricular assist devices for high-risk patients with extracorporeal membrane oxygenation support. *J Heart Lung Transplant.* 2001;20:850-857.
18. Mullenbach RM, Kredel M, Kunze E, et al. Prolonged heparin-free extracorporeal membrane oxygenation in multiple injured acute respiratory distress syndrome patients with traumatic brain injury. *J Trauma Acute Care Surg.* 2012;72:1444-1447.
19. Arlt M, Philipp A, Voelkel S, et al. Extracorporeal membrane oxygenation in severe trauma patients with bleeding shock. *Resuscitation.* 2012;81:804-809.
20. Guirand DM, Okoye OT, Schmidt BS, et al. Venovenous extracorporeal life support improves survival in adult trauma patients with acute hypoxemic respiratory failure: a multicenter retrospective cohort study. *J Trauma Acute Care Surg.* 2014;76:1275-1281.
21. Lamhaut L, Jouffroy R, Kalpodjian A, et al. Successful treatment of refractory cardiac arrest by emergency physicians using pre-hospital ECLS. *Resuscitation.* 2012;83:e177-e178.
22. Poppe M, Schober A, Weiser C, et al. "Load & Go" Criteria in out-of-hospital cardiac arrest patients for the use of emergency-extracorporeal life support at the emergency department [abstract]. Resuscitation Science Symposium, American Heart Association; November 2014.
23. Lamhout L, Jouffroy R, Soldan M, et al. Safety and feasibility of prehospital extra corporeal life support implementation by non-surgeons for out-of-hospital refractory cardiac arrest. *Resuscitation.* 2013;84:1525-1529.
24. Naim MY, Topjian AA, Nadkami VM. CPR and E-CPR: What is new? *World J Pediatr Congenit Heart Surg.* 2012;3:48-53.

Cardiac Tamponade

10

IN THIS CHAPTER

- Evaluating the signs and etiologies of tamponade
- Managing hemodynamically stable and unstable patients
- Treating traumatic tamponade
- Pericardiocentesis
- Diagnostic imaging

Semhar Z. Tewelde

For patients with cardiac tamponade, survival hinges on the emergency clinician's ability to promptly diagnosis and manage the disorder, identify its cause, and prevent the recurrence of pericardial effusion. Without appropriate treatment, the disorder commonly leads to obstructive and cardiogenic forms of shock, pulseless electrical activity, and ultimately death. The diagnosis and evaluation of tamponade is challenging given its numerous etiologies, nonspecific symptoms, and variable clinical progression. Management is further complicated by a lack of validated indicators that signal whether patients require immediate, urgent, or delayed treatment.

Critical Considerations

Cardiac tamponade is a complex clinical syndrome that results from a variety of causes that trigger the accumulation of fluid in the finite pericardial space *(Table 10-1)*.[1-3] Analogous to the syndrome itself, symptoms fall along a continuum ranging from incipient to ominous.[2,4,5] An accurate diagnosis depends on the manifestation of symptoms as well as the results of diagnostic imaging. It is critical to confirm the presence or absence of cardiac tamponade when evaluating a patient with a new pericardial effusion. The following questions can guide diagnosis and serve as an outline for the remainder of this chapter:

- How rapidly has the effusion developed and what is its most likely cause?
- What are the echocardiographic findings?
- Are there clinical manifestations that suggest tamponade?
- Does the patient have unique clinical confounders that make the diagnosis of tamponade problematic?

Hemodynamic Stability

The circulatory status of any patient with tamponade is best defined as fragile. Paramount in determining a patient's future hemodynamic stability is the rate of pericardial fluid accumulation *(Figure 10-1)*.[6-8] The pericardium affixes the heart to surrounding structures within the thoracic cavity. It consists of two layers: an inner visceral and an outer parietal cover. The space within the two-layer envelope normally contains a small amount of fluid.

PEARL

The rate of volume expansion, not the total volume accrued, is crucial to hemodynamic stability.

Tamponade occurs when the intrapericardial fluid accumulation exceeds ventricular diastolic pressures, resulting in reduced compliance of the myocardium and intracardiac chambers.[10] The pericardial pressure ultimately limits cardiac filling and reduces cardiac output.[11] The heart's response during respiratory variation becomes exaggerated, and extreme ventricular interdependence develops.[1,9,11,12] The definitive indicator of tamponade physiology is the equalization of the diastolic pressures seen on right heart catheterization. Certain populations with altered baseline physiologies do not exhibit the classic manifestations of tamponade *(Table 10-2)*.[3,9] This absence is most typical in cases of hypovolemia (caused by hemorrhage, dehydration, or aggressive dialysis/diuresis) because the ventricular filling pressure necessary to exhibit tamponade physiology is decreased in response to the patient's reduced blood volume.[3,13] This condition is called *low-pressure tamponade.*

FIGURE 10-1. Pericardial Pressure/Volume Curve

A. illustrates a smaller volume of quickly accumulating pericardial fluid, leading to cardiac tamponade. This can be compared to the slow accumulation depicted in **B.**, where cardiac tamponade is reached only with larger volumes.

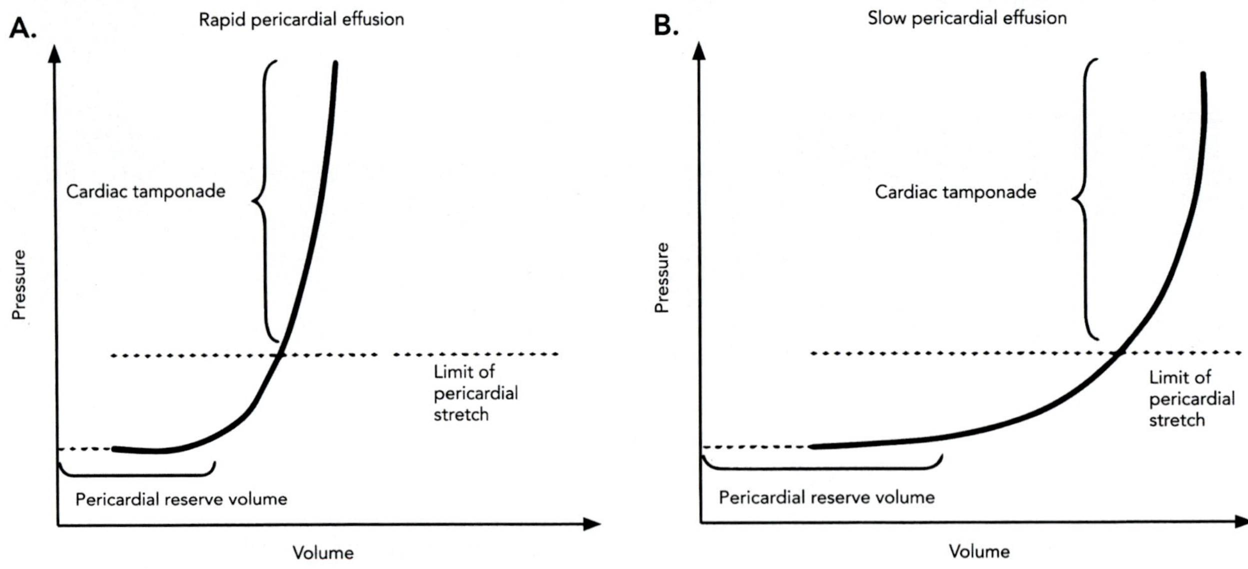

Reproduced from Imazio M, Adler Y. Management of pericardial effusion. *Eur Heart J.* 2013;34:1186-1197.

> **PEARL**
> Certain populations will not exhibit the characteristic signs of tamponade because of variations in their physiologies secondary to comorbidities.

Etiology

A wide array of conditions can cause pericardial effusion and ensuing cardiac tamponade. The most obvious are traumatic in nature since these cases often progress rapidly and can be linked to a clear mechanism of injury. A reported 10% of blunt and 2% of penetrating cardiac injuries result in tamponade.[9] Unlike traumatic etiologies, medical causes are numerous and have a latent course, making them more challenging to diagnose. The most common culprits include malignancy, renal dysfunction, infection, rheumatologic/connective tissue disease, radiation/chemotherapeutic therapy, and idiopathic sources.[4,8]

TABLE 10-1. Causes of Tamponade

Causes of Tamponade
Collagen-vascular disease: systemic lupus erythematosus, scleroderma
Hypothyroidism
Idiopathic
Infection: viral, bacterial, fungal, parasitic
Malignancy (most common in developed countries)
Medication
Metabolic imbalances: uremia
Post-myocardial infarction: Dressler syndrome, free wall rupture
Postoperative phase: postpericardiotomy, device implantation (pacemaker lead, central venous catheter)
Radiation
Traumatic events: blunt or penetrating injuries, aortic dissection

> **PEARL**
> In developed countries, metastatic malignancy involving the pericardium is the most common cause of tamponade.

Uremia, a once common and ubiquitously fatal cause of tamponade, has become rare in recent years. The declining incidence of the disease is thought to be secondary to the earlier identification of renal disease and improved hemodialysis; however, the exact etiology of uremic pericarditis remains unclear. Despite regular compliance with medical therapy and dialysis, a number of these patients still go on to develop uremic pericarditis without the classic signs and symptoms (eg, chest pain, fever, and electrocardiographic changes). Therefore, a high degree of suspicion is necessary.

Signs and Symptoms

Other than traumatic pericardial effusions, the presentation of tamponade can be subtle; symptoms are neither specific nor sensitive and are easily mistaken for other clinical entities. If overt signs and symptoms are readily

FIGURE 10-2. Pulsus Paradoxus

Pulsus paradoxus can be detected using fingertip pulse oximeter plethysmography. Inspiration decreases the magnitude of the waveform with each QRS, and expiration increases its magnitude.

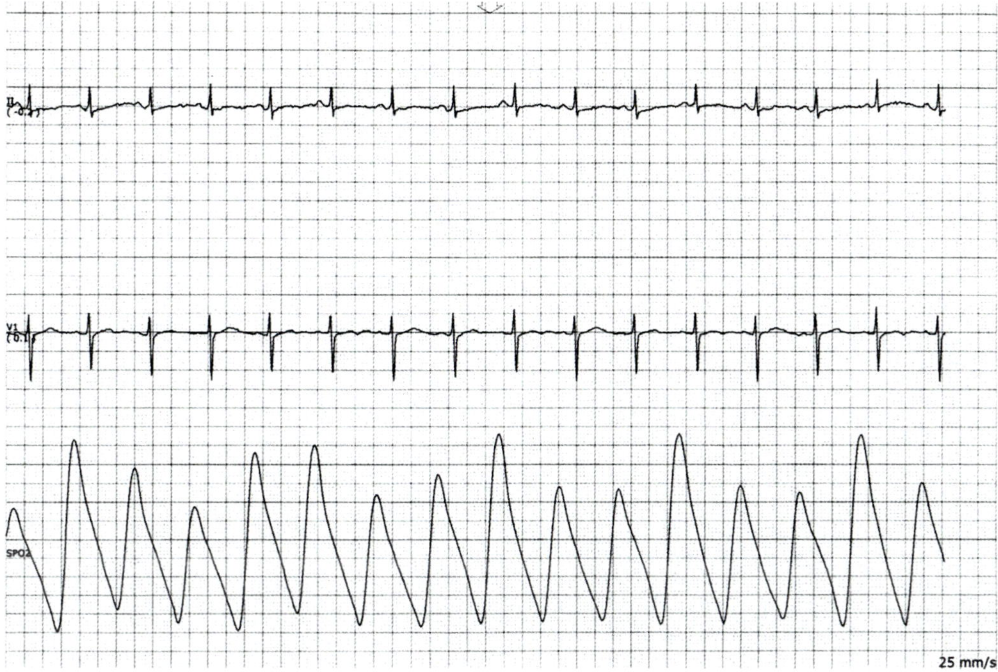

observed, the clinician should anticipate deterioration and circulatory collapse. The detection of the Beck triad (muffled heart sounds, jugular venous distension, and hypotension) is considered pathognomonic for cardiac tamponade. However, this description is based on traumatic pericardial hemorrhage and is typically not evident in other forms of the disease.[11] Dyspnea is the most common symptom, followed by chest pain, palpitation, weakness, and early satiety.[2,5,9] The most common physical finding is tachycardia. Tachypnea, jugular venous distension, and pulsus paradoxus are also notable findings in many patients.[2,4,5,9]

TABLE 10-2. Nonclassic Manifestations of Cardiac Tamponade
Effusive-constrictive tamponade
Pressures do not improve after pericardiocentesis
Low-pressure tamponade
Hemorrhage
Dehydration
Aggressive dialysis
Aggressive diuresis
Regional tamponade
Postoperative
Focal thrombus
Taut pericardium
Right-heart tamponade (right atrial pressure > left atrial pressure)

Most patients with tamponade experience an exaggerated decrease in blood pressure with inspiration. This complication, known as pulsus paradoxus, can be detected using a stethoscope and manual sphygmomanometer.[14] The difference in blood pressure between the first expiratory Korotkoff sound and the first Korotkoff sound that no longer disappears with inspiration is the pulsus. If the difference is more than 10 mm Hg, pulsus paradoxus is present. A novel use of pulse oximetry can aid in identifying the disorder *(Figure 10-2)*.[14] The difference between the inspiratory decrease in magnitude of the waveform and the expiratory increase has been shown to correlate with intraarterially measured pulsus paradoxus.[15] Unfortunately, the finding is not pathognomonic for cardiac tamponade; it is linked to a number of clinical conditions and may be absent in some patients who actually have tamponade.

PEARL

The novel use of pulse-oximetry waveforms can more easily and rapidly identify a pulsus paradoxus.

Clinical examination findings that should raise concern for imminent deterioration include a decline in mental status or agitation, worsening tachypnea (reflecting acidosis), decline in tachycardia (circulatory fatigue), decreased urine output, and pallor with poor extremity perfusion. The absence of hypotension should not be comforting, however. This sign is a late finding and often not seen until arrest is imminent due to natural compensatory mechanisms such as sympathetic tone and catecholamine response.

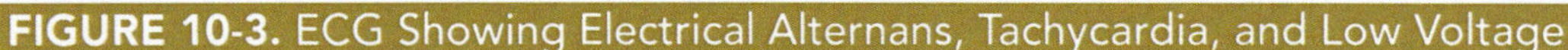

FIGURE 10-3. ECG Showing Electrical Alternans, Tachycardia, and Low Voltage

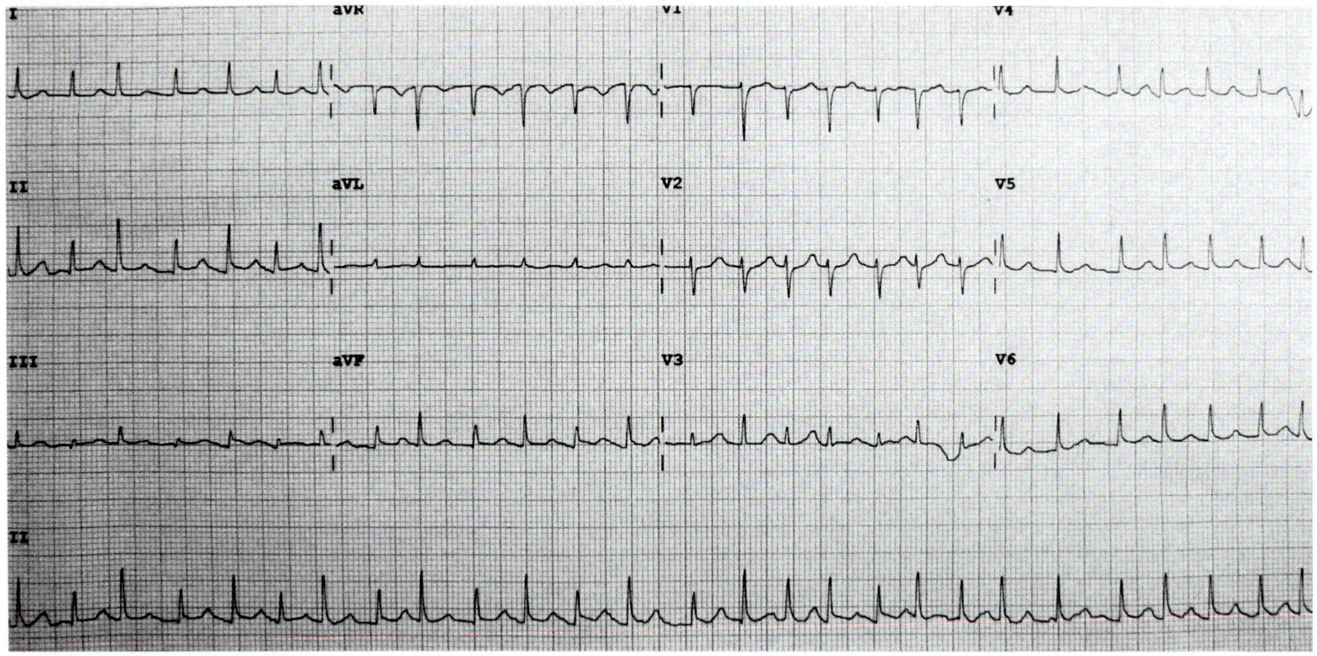

Diagnostic Testing

The initial diagnostic studies obtained for nearly every patient who is experiencing chest pain or dyspnea should include an electrocardiogram (ECG) and a chest radiograph (CXR). Sinus tachycardia is the most common ECG finding, followed to a lesser degree by low voltage.[3,16] If a large effusion is present and the heart is able to swing along its axis, electrical alternans *(Figure 10-3)* might also be manifested.[16] Imaging often will reveal an enlarged cardiac silhouette, commonly called a "water-bottle heart" sign. *(Figure 10-4).*[3,4] Important to note is the lack of pulmonary vascular congestion on the CXR. Clear lungs sounds and an absence of cephalization can help differentiate tamponade from decompensated congestive heart failure.

FIGURE 10-4. Water-Bottle Heart Sign

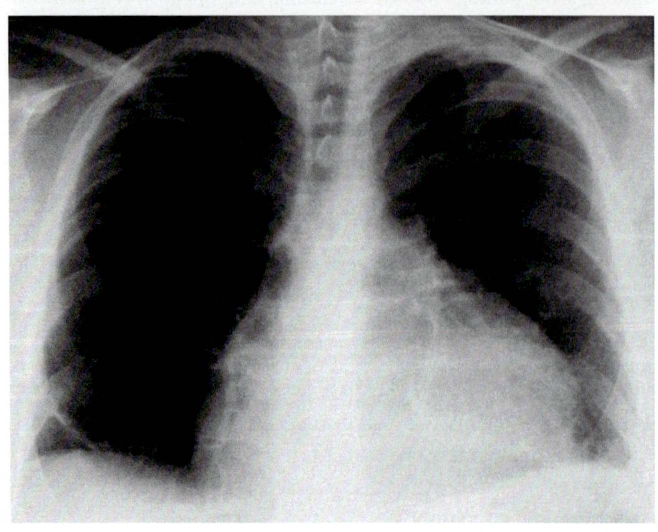

The American Society of Echocardiography/American Heart Association/American College of Cardiology recommends that any suspected pericardial condition, especially tamponade (class I), should be evaluated initially by echocardiography.[8] Echocardiography is widely available, cost effective, noninvasive, and portable. Vital to the care of every critically ill patient with suspected pericardial tamponade, the imaging modality provides essential physiological information that can alter medical therapy and outcomes. Although it has few limitations, it is operator dependent, and patient habitus can preclude acquisition of the anatomical details needed to make a clinical decision.

Other frequently discussed diagnostic imaging modalities for pericardial diseases include computed tomography (CT) and magnetic resonance imaging (MRI). Neither should be part of the initial evaluation of tamponade. CT is relatively rapid and can help distinguish a pericardial fat pad from a true effusion, which can be a point of contention for novice echo operators; however, the test exposes the patient to radiation and contrast media. MRI provides excellent information about soft tissue, but it is very time consuming and not recommended for hemodynamically labile patients.

PEARL

Echocardiography is the diagnostic imaging modality of choice for evaluating cases of suspected tamponade.[6,17,18]

Several echocardiographic findings can be seen with tamponade physiology *(Table 10-3)*. A common misconception is that a large (>2.0 cm) effusion or swinging of the heart is required to make the diagnosis. The most commonly seen signs are right atrial systolic collapse, right ventricular diastolic collapse, septal shifting toward the left, left ventricular pseudohypertrophy, and inferior vena cava (IVC) plethora with decreased respiratory variation.[5,6,8,12,17,18] Sustained right atrial collapse occurring for more than one-third of the cardiac cycle and during late diastole is even more specific.[6,7,18]

Doppler echocardiographic findings most accurately correlate with hemodynamics, specifically the exaggerated respirophasic variation in flow velocities across the tricuspid and pulmonic valves followed by the mitral and aortic valves, respectively.[2,5,11] The synthesis of bedside clinical findings and echocardiographic findings is paramount because the latter can be too sensitive and overdiagnose tamponade in a patient who is fairly asymptomatic.[19] The sensitivity of right atrial collapse varies from 50% to 100% with specificities of 33% to 100%.[20] Echocardiographic quantification alone might be unreliable; it requires a high index of clinical suspicion based on the bedside physical examination and the patient's hemodynamics.

PEARL

Certain patients (eg, those who are mechanically ventilated or who have right heart failure or constrictive pericardial disease) generally have a plethoric IVC, and the inspiratory changes expected with tamponade can be imperceptible.[2,5,6,18]

Traumatic Tamponade

Tamponade secondary to traumatic incidents often is fatal. The prognosis for patients with penetrating injuries is better than for those who have sustained blunt (decelerating) trauma, which often causes aortic dissection. The single most important factor for survival is the presence of vital signs upon arrival at the treatment facility.

In these scenarios, time is of the essence — immediate intervention is required if any signs of life are present. Stabilization can be attempted with pericardiocentesis, allowing the controlled drainage of very small amounts of the hemopericardium, and transfer to a quaternary care institution where subspecialists are readily available. Another option is thoracotomy, followed by opening of the pericardial layers to allow evacuation of the tamponade and repair of any lacerations or crossclamping of the aorta for definitive repair.[5,7,8,17] The latter approach is an ambitious undertaking, requiring immense resources and trained specialists who can immediately repair the defect in the operating room.

TABLE 10-3. Doppler Echocardiographic Signs of Tamponade
Right atrial (late) systolic collapse (highly specific when occurring for >1/3 of the cardiac cycle)
Right ventricular (early) diastolic collapse
IVC plethora with blunted respiratory response
Pericardial effusion with swinging of the heart
Respiratory variations >25% in mitral, aortic, and/or tricuspid flow velocities
Isolated left atrial/ventricular collapse (might be seen with LV compression or pulmonary hypertension)

Hemodynamically Stable Patients

Although hemodynamically stable patients with tamponade fall along the narrow spectrum of tamponade physiology, they have not yet suffered cardiovascular collapse. These cases require resuscitation and continuous cardiac monitoring to thwart impending circulatory failure. These are merely temporary measures until more definitive therapy can be initiated. Management should begin with gentle volume challenges using crystalloids since many patients are intravascularly hypovolemic.[2,12] The judicious administration of fluids often augments blood pressure and cardiac output. Conversely, the administration of excessive amounts of fluid can prove deleterious and worsen the intracardiac pressures, at which point fluids must be discontinued promptly. Patients with more briskly deteriorating hemodynamics despite fluid administration require further pharmacological adjuncts until pericardiocentesis can be performed.

Several studies have listed isoprenaline, dopamine, and dobutamine as suitable and appropriate first-line agents for increasing cardiac output in cases of tamponade.[3,5,9,12] Although no therapy has been demonstrated to be superior, most resources recommend the initial use of dobutamine. Some researchers theorize that vasopressors (eg, norepinephrine) improve blood pressure more than inotrope, but also note their lack of positive effect on cardiac index. Any agents that blunt the endogenous sympathetic and catecholamine surge (eg, beta- and alpha-blockers, anesthetics, or aggressive analgesics) can result in detrimental hemodynamic effects. The initiation of positive-pressure ventilation will further increase intrathoracic pressure and worsen venous return, often resulting in catastrophic circulatory collapse.[2,5,12]

PEARL

Mechanical ventilation can prove deadly in patients with tamponade.

Hemodynamically Unstable Tamponade

Hemodynamically unstable patients require immediate pericardiocentesis or operative repair because of their potentially rapid progression to death. Stability swiftly returns after fluid is evacuated from the pericardial space. Removal of a large amount of pericardial fluid is not necessary to improve hemodynamics and is not advised. Large-volume pericardiocentesis causes abrupt fluid shifts leading to pulmonary edema and rapid respiratory decompensation.[6,7,17] The theory behind these shifts is that the sudden increase in ventricular filling and stroke volume coupled with the lack of time for relaxation in systemic vascular beds results in high afterload and volume overload.[6,7,17] In most cases, the removal of 50 to 100 mL of fluid is sufficient to completely reverse hemodynamics.

Pericardial fluid can be removed using any of several methods, including blind percutaneous drainage, ultrasound-guided percutaneous drainage, percutaneous balloon pericardiotomy, and the surgical creation of a pericardial window.[17,21] For crashing patients in the emergency department or intensive care unit, the latter two options are not feasible. For stable patients whose tamponade is insidious, recurrent, or traumatic, a semielective procedure performed in conjunction with a cardiologist or cardiothoracic surgeon is recommended. The materials needed to perform pericardiocentesis are available in a kit, similar to a central venous catheter kit, which can be used in its stead. In a true emergency, only three tools are essential *(Table 10-4)*. Major complications of the procedure include cardiac chamber perforation, coronary laceration, pneumothorax, intraabdominal laceration, and hollow viscous injury.[5,8,12]

TABLE 10-4. Essential Supplies for Pericardiocentesis

18-gauge spinal needle
20-mL Luer lock syringe
Three-way stopcock

Blind Approach

If ultrasound is unavailable and the patient has a history of tamponade, or if you have a high clinical suspicion that the patient is rapidly deteriorating, approaching arrest, or in PEA, the safest approach is the blind subxiphoid (subcostal) technique *(Figure 10-5)*. A pericardiocentesis kit should be used if available; a central venous catheter kit also can be utilized. If neither is available, any 16- or 18-gauge spinal needle attached to a 20-mL Luer lock syringe is sufficient. Consider using a longer spinal needle for patients with a large body habitus.

FIGURE 10-5. Pericardiocentesis Blind Subxiphoid Approach

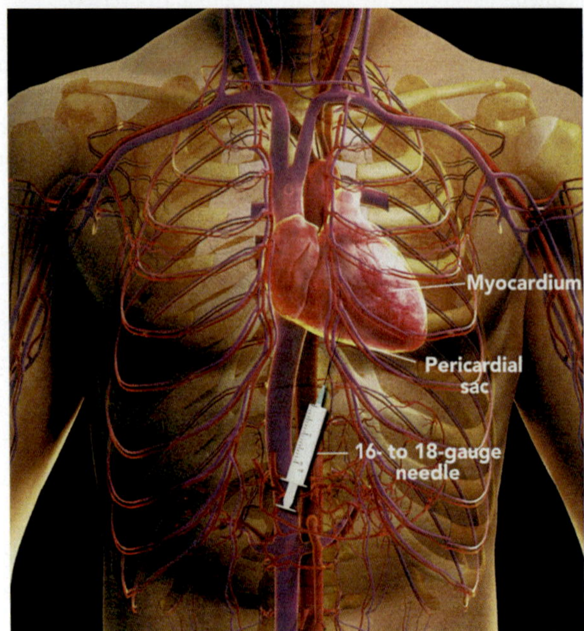

The needle should be inserted between the xiphoid process and left costal margin at a 30° to 45° angle.

Aim for the left midclavicle while directing the needle toward the anterior wall of the right ventricle.

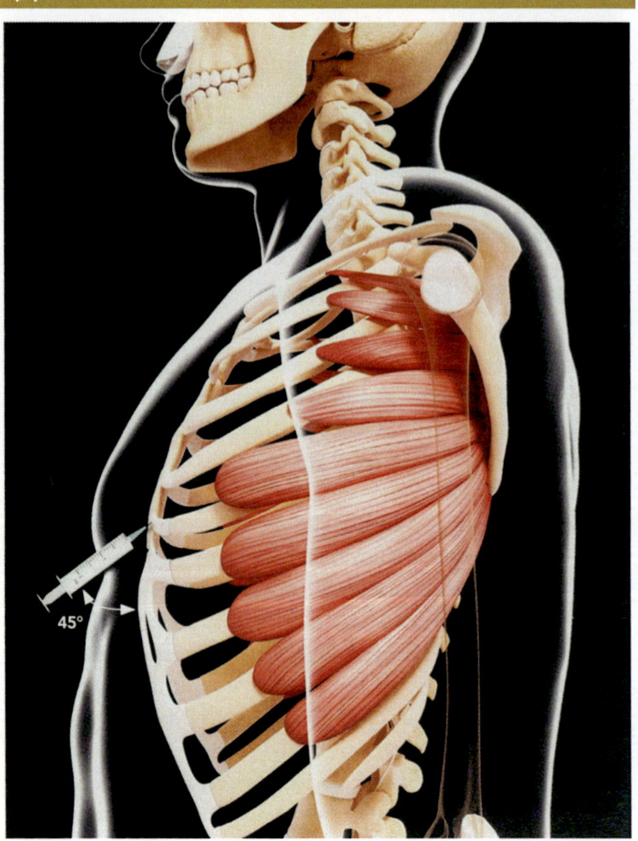

FIGURE 10-6. Ultrasound-Guided Approach

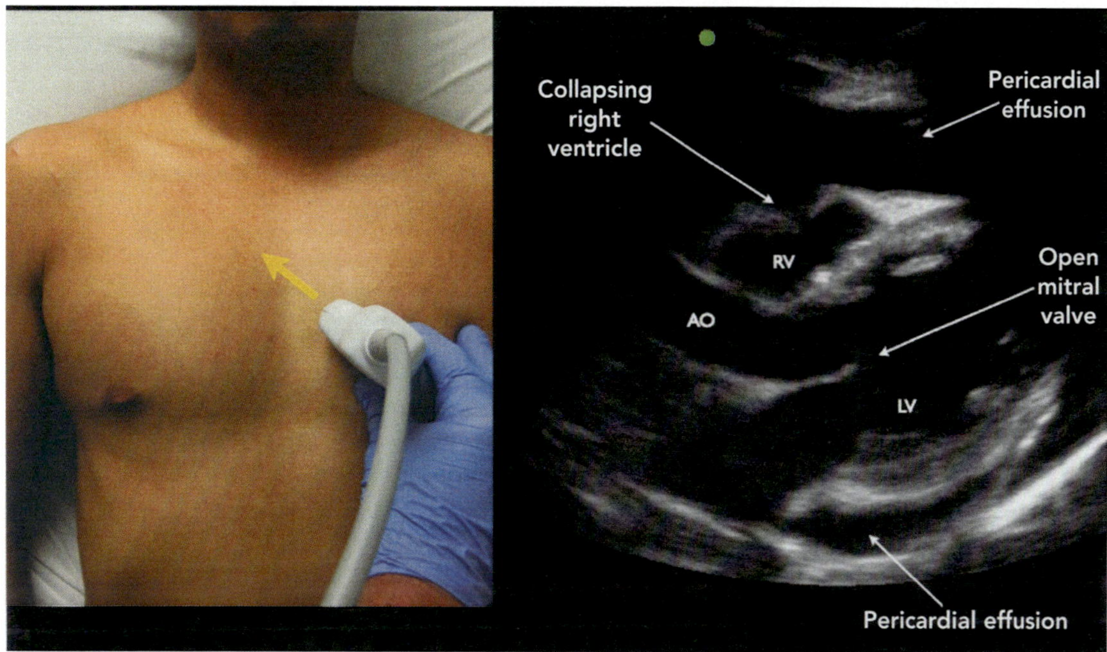

Aspirate where the fluid collection appears to be the largest and closest to the skin/ultrasound transducer. The subxiphoid, apical, and parasternal methods are all viable options.

Insert the needle at the left xiphocostal angle, aiming it toward the left shoulder at a 30- to 45-degree angle. Once a small amount of fluid can be aspirated easily, the hemodynamics should improve dramatically. Remove the syringe and needle while leaving the catheter in place. Then, using a Seldinger technique, insert an indwelling pigtail catheter, which will allow further fluid removal should hemodynamics weaken.

Ultrasound-Guided Approach

If ultrasound is available, it can be used in one of two ways to perform pericardiocentesis. The less experienced sonographer often prefers static guidance. With this approach, imaging is used to identify the largest pocket of fluid and its approximate depth (but not during the aspiration of the effusion). A more precise and safer method is dynamic ultrasound guidance *(Figure 10-6)*.

KEY POINTS

1. Rapidly developing accumulations (as seen in traumatic tamponade) often cause profound hypotension and precipitous death; however, the slow accrual of volume (as seen in non-traumatic forms) allow pericardial distension, remodeling, and gradual transformations without drastic derangements in vital signs.[3,9]
2. In these special populations, the diagnosis of tamponade is even more elusive; so a higher index of suspicion is needed.
3. Pulsus paradoxus can be seen in patients with several conditions: obstructive pulmonary disease, asthma, pulmonary embolism, and right ventricular infarction with shock. It can be absent in certain populations with tamponade: pulmonary hypertension, aortic regurgitation, right heart or regional tamponade, and low-pressure tamponade.[9]
4. Tamponade can develop from a regional/retro-atrial hematoma following cardiac surgery. In this scenario, patients will have vague symptoms similar to those of low-pressure tamponade; a high level of suspicion is needed.[5,6,9,18] Transesophageal echocardiography is favored in this setting.
5. Mechanical ventilation makes the detection of respiratory variations with Doppler technology inaccurate, and therefore impedes the clinician's ability to identify tamponade.
6. Pericardiocentesis should be the first procedure performed in any patient with waning hemodynamics.
7. Tamponade patients should undergo pericardiocentesis prior to mechanical ventilation.

FIGURE 10-7. Three-Step Scoring System for the Diagnosis of Cardiac Tamponade

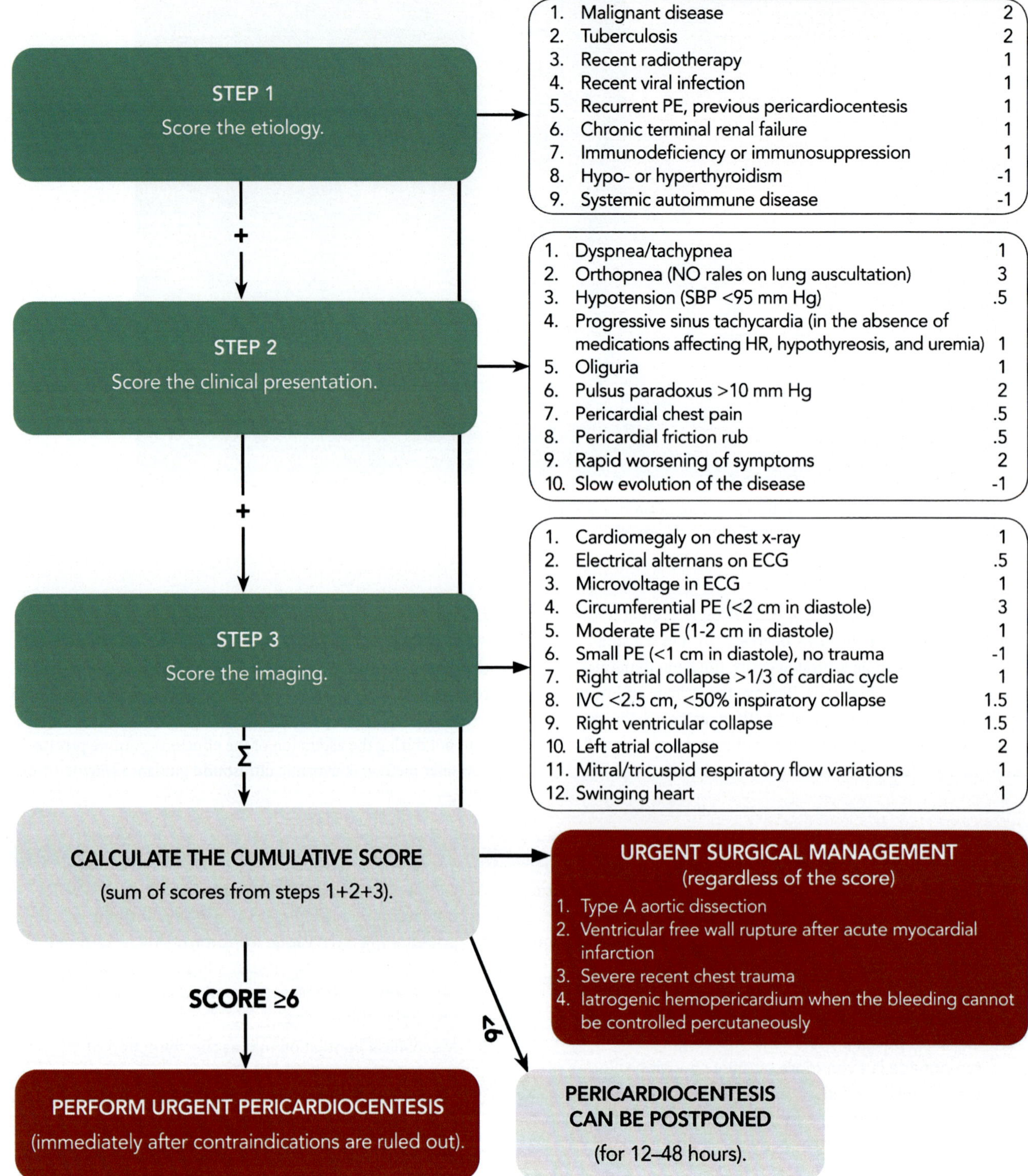

From Ristić AD, Imazio M, Adler Y, et al. Triage strategy for urgent management of cardiac tamponade: a position statement of the European Society of Cardiology Working Group on Myocardial and Pericardial Diseases. *Eur Heart J.* 2014;35:2279-2284.

As with static guidance, the largest fluid pocket is identified and the aspiration is visualized in realtime throughout the entire procedure. This requires good hand-eye coordination and more experience. Unlike in the blind approach — for which only subxiphoid entry is recommended — with ultrasound guidance, apical or parasternal approaches also can be taken. Dynamic ultrasound is associated with a lower incidence of sequelae than pericardiocentesis without visualization.[22] The angle of the needle should follow the transducer trajectory. As with any thoracic procedure, the inferior rib margin should be avoided to prevent neurovascular injury.

The European Society of Cardiology Working Group on Myocardial and Pericardial Diseases recently developed a three-step scoring system for treating patients with cardiac tamponade *(Figure 10-7)*. Based on the integration of clinical symptoms, signs, and echocardiographic findings, the system can be used to identify patients who need immediate pericardiocentesis.[17] A patient who scores a 6 or above requires emergent pericardial drainage; a lower score indicates that drainage can be postponed for up to 48 hours.

Conclusion

Cardiac tamponade is a delicate clinical entity that becomes a ticking time bomb if not identified and treated. With the advent of bedside ultrasound, even novice users can rapidly and easily identify an effusion. Although the signs and symptoms might be nonspecific, echocardiographic findings of right atrial/ventricular diastolic collapse, IVC plethora, and respiratory ventricular interdependence are very suggestive of tamponade. After tamponade physiology has been identified, close cardiac monitoring is warranted, volume resuscitation should be approached carefully, and adjunctive pharmacological agents should be administered if needed. Ultimately, lives are saved when a skilled clinician can rapidly identify tamponade, perform immediate pericardiocentesis in unstable patients, and facilitate stabilization and disposition for definitive therapy.

REFERENCES

1. Shabetai R. Pericardial effusion: haemodynamic spectrum. *Heart.* 2004;90:255-256.
2. Imazio M, Mayosi BM, Brucato A, et al. Triage and management of pericardial effusion. *J Cardiovasc Med (Hagerstown).* 2010;11:928-935.
3. Dudzinski DM, Mak GS, Hung JW. Pericardial diseases. *Curr Probl Cardiol.* 2012;37:75-118.
4. Little WC, Freeman GL. Pericardial disease. *Circulation.* 2006;113:1622-1632.
5. Imazio M, Adler Y. Management of pericardial effusion. *Eur Heart J.* 2013;34:1186-1197.
6. Pepi M, Muratori M. Echocardiography in the diagnosis and management of pericardial disease. *J Cardiovasc Med (Hagerstown).* 2006;7:533-544.
7. Maisch B, Seferović PM, Ristić AD, et al. Guidelines on the diagnosis and management of pericardial diseases. Executive summary [article in Spanish]. *Rev Esp Cardiol.* 2004;57:1090-1114.
8. Cheitlin MD, Armstrong WF, Aurigemma GP, et al. ACC/AHA/ASE 2003 guideline update for the clinical application of echocardiography: summary article: a report of the American College of Cardiology/American Heart Association Task Force on Practice Guidelines (ACC/AHA/ASE Committee to Update the 1997 Guidelines for the Clinical Application of Echocardiography). *Circulation.* 2003;108:1146-1162.
9. Grecu L. Cardiac tamponade. *Int Anesthesiol Clin.* 2012;50:59-77.
10. Spodick DH. Acute cardiac tamponade. *N Engl J Med.* 2003;349:684-690.
11. Bodson L, BouferracheK, Vieillard-Baron A. Cardiac tamponade. *Curr Opin Crit Care.* 2011;17:416-424.
12. Soler-Soler J, Sagrista-Sauleda J, Permanyer-Miralda G. Management of pericardial effusion. *Heart.* 2001;86:235-240.
13. Sagristà-Sauleda J, Angel J, Sambola A, et al. Low-pressure cardiac tamponade: clinical and hemodynamic profile. *Circulation.* 2006;114:945-952.
14. Schiavone WA. Cardiac tamponade: 12 pearls in diagnosis and management. *Cleve Clin J Med.* 2013;80:109-116.
15. Frey B, Butt W. Pulse oximetry for assessment of pulsus paradoxus: a clinical study in children. *Intensive Care Med.* 1998;24:242-246.
16. Seferović PM, Ristić AD, Maksimović R, et al. Pericardial syndromes: an update after the ESC guidelines 2004. *Heart Fail Rev.* 2013;18:255-266.
17. Ristić AD, Imazio M, Adler Y, et al. Triage strategy for urgent management of cardiac tamponade: a position statement of the European Society of Cardiology Working Group on Myocardial and Pericardial Diseases. *Eur Heart J.* 2014;35:2279-2284.
18. Tsang TS, Oh JK, Seward JB, et al. Diagnostic value of echocardiography in cardiac tamponade. *Herz.* 2000;25:734-740.
19. Argulian E, Messerli F. Misconceptions and facts about pericardial effusion and tamponade. *Am J Med.* 2013;126:858-861.
20. Guntheroth WG. Sensitivity and specificity of echocardiographic evidence of tamponade: implications for ventricular interdependence and pulsus paradoxus. *Pediatr Cardiol.* 2007;28:358-362.
21. Loukas M, Walters A, Boon JM, et al. Pericardiocentesis: a clinical anatomy review. *Clin Anat.* 2012;25:872-881.
22. Maggiolini S, Bozzano A, Russo P, et al. Echocardiography-guided pericardiocentesis with probe-mounted needle: report of 53 cases. *J Am Soc Echocardiogr.* 2001;14:821-824.

Aortic Catastrophes

IN THIS CHAPTER

- Thoracic aortic dissections
- Abdominal aortic dissections
- Stable and unstable type A and B dissections
- Complicated and uncomplicated type A and B dissections
- Organ malperfusion
- Surgical indications

George C. Willis and Robert L. Rogers

Thoracic aortic dissection (TAD) and abdominal aortic aneurysm (AAA), two lethal diagnoses that often mimic more benign conditions, can be catastrophic if missed. Frequently heralded by nonspecific symptoms, they can be mistakenly overlooked in the emergency department simply because they are not considered. Most patients with these aortic emergencies are critically ill and must be transported to an operating room or intensive care unit (ICU) after initial resuscitation. With hospital overcrowding, these patients can remain in the emergency department for an indeterminate amount of time, and subsequent complications can result in detrimental outcomes.

Thoracic Aortic Dissection

One of the deadliest causes of chest pain, TAD arises from a tear in the intima of the aorta, which allows blood to enter and travel within the wall of the artery. The intima flap can freely occlude vessels that branch off the aorta and perfuse vital organs. It is the most common catastrophic condition affecting the aorta, occurring 3 times more frequently than ruptured AAA.[1-4]

Several classification schemes for TAD have been developed. Most management options are based on the Stanford system. Stanford type A dissections involve the aortic arch with or without the descending artery, whereas Stanford type B dissections involve only the descending aorta *(Figure 11-1)*.

TAD frequently is misdiagnosed due to its variable clinical presentations; even when recognized early, the path to survival and recovery remains difficult. As many as 40% of patients die immediately, and 20% to 25% die during or after surgery.[5-7] In addition, for every hour the diagnosis of aortic dissection is delayed, the mortality rate increases 1% to 2%.[5,6,8,9]

Diagnosis

The sudden onset of severe chest pain is the most common chief complaint in all patients with TAD.[8,10-12] Classic presentations include anterior chest pain that radiates to the neck or through to the back (for Stanford type A dissections) and back and abdominal pain (for Stanford type B dissections).[8,12,13] Unfortunately, these so-called classic symptoms are found infrequently. Some patients report a resolution of their pain or experience no pain whatsoever, misleading providers into making an incorrect diagnosis.[13-16] High clinical suspicion is key in determining the diagnosis. A family history of aortic dissection or sudden death indicates the possibility of TAD. The physical examination may reveal pulse deficits or a diastolic aortic regurgitation murmur, but these findings are often normal and unhelpful in confirming the diagnosis. Most patients present with a severely elevated blood pressure, often with a systolic blood pressure (SBP) greater than 200 mm Hg and a diastolic blood pressure (DBP) greater than 100 mm Hg; however, they can also be normotensive or hypotensive.[7]

No screening laboratory tests are useful in the diagnosis of TAD. Although a D-dimer test may be adequate in low-risk cases, the results can be falsely negative in patients with chronic dissections, smaller intimal flaps, and thrombosed lumens, and therefore should not be used to exclude the disorder.[17] If TAD is suspected, emergent imaging should be obtained. In such cases, it is common practice to obtain a portable chest radiograph to evaluate for a widened mediastinum. However, this x-ray finding can be seen in only 60% of patients with confirmed dissection; when used alone, it is unreliable for ruling out the diagnosis.[7,8,18-20]

Bedside ultrasound can be used in the emergency department to visualize the aorta. Images can be obtained via transabdominal, parasternal, and suprasternal views.[21-24] Findings suggestive of TAD include a visible intimal flap or aortic root

FIGURE 11-1. Stanford Classification Scheme

Stanford type A dissections involve either the ascending aorta alone (i) or the ascending aorta as well as the descending aorta (ii). Stanford type B dissections involve the descending aorta alone (iii).

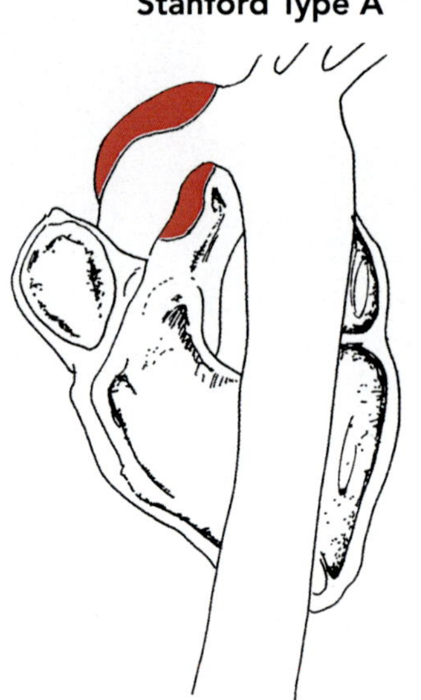

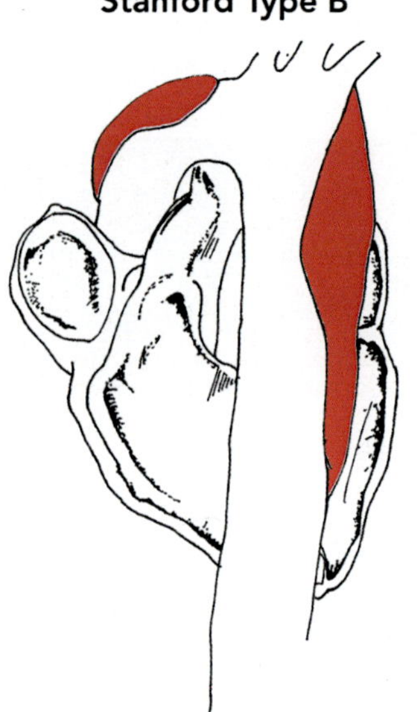

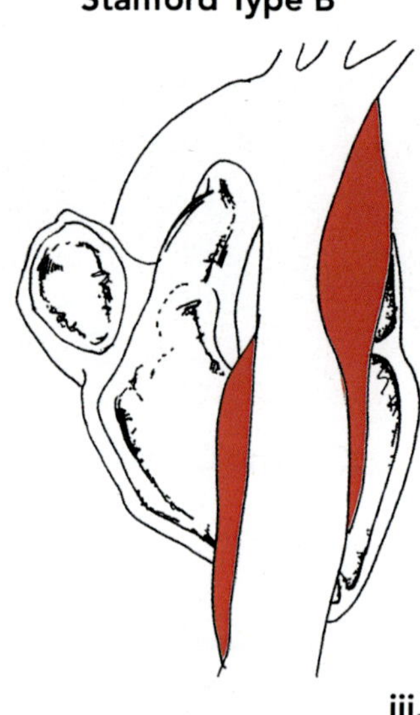

Image courtesy of Miya Hunter-Willis.

FIGURE 11-2. Computed Tomography Scan of a Stanford Type A Aortic Dissection

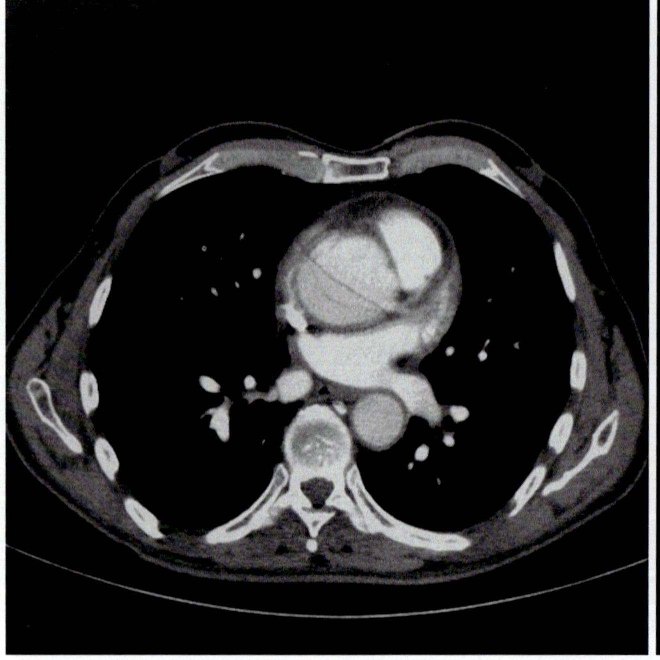

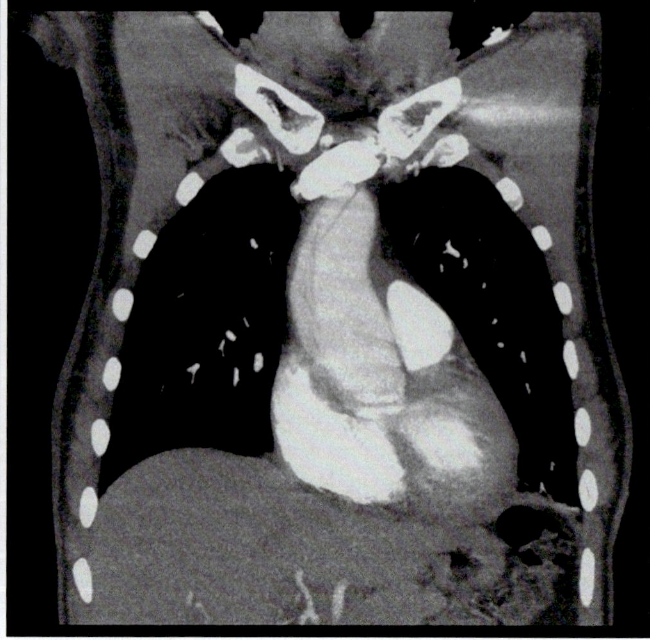

TABLE 11-1. Findings Suggestive of Organ Malperfusion

Area of Malperfusion	Signs and Symptoms
Mesenteric	Abdominal pain, distention, or acute abdomen Elevated lactate level Signs of ischemic bowel on CT scan (eg, thickened bowel wall, pneumatosis intestinalis, perforation)
Renal	Urine output <0.5 mL/kg/hr Elevated serum creatinine Hypertension refractory to afterload reduction Signs of decreased kidney perfusion on CT scan
Carotid/vertebral	Transient ischemic attack or stroke symptoms Altered mental status Paraplegia
Iliac	Pulse deficits Leg discomfort Paresthesias
Coronary	ECG changes Troponin elevation Coronary artery occlusion on angiogram

dilatation; however, confirmatory studies remain necessary.[17] The gold standard for the diagnosis of TAD is multidetector computed tomography (CT) with intravenous contrast *(Figure 11-2)*. If this modality is contraindicated, magnetic resonance imaging (MRI) or transesophageal echocardiography (TEE) is as reliable as CT in making the diagnosis, but their use is limited by their availability.[17,25]

Acute Management

The emergency department management of TAD should proceed using a stepwise approach that remains focused on decreasing shear stress on the aortic wall through blood pressure and heart rate control, identifying and managing complications, and obtaining early surgical consultation.

Continuous blood pressure and heart rate monitoring are critical components of care. Patients should be placed on a continuous cardiac monitor, and an arterial catheter, which provides more accurate data than noninvasive blood pressure cuffs, should be inserted. Blood pressure should be measured in both arms, and the catheter should be placed into the radial artery of the arm that reveals the higher number. Standard laboratory tests should be ordered, including a type and screen, complete blood chemistry, comprehensive metabolic panel, and lactate levels. Patients with TAD should be reassessed frequently for evidence of dissection extension, organ malperfusion *(Table 11-1)*, pulse deficits, and new heart murmurs, all of which portend poorer outcomes.

The primary goal of management is to decrease the shear stress on the aortic wall. To accomplish this goal, both blood pressure and heart rate must be reduced rapidly. The targets are an SBP of 100 to 110 mm Hg and a heart rate below 60 beats per minute. Blood pressure and heart rate reductions are accomplished through the administration of titratable intravenous antihypertensive medications. In contrast to the management of other hypertensive emergencies, where the mean arterial pressure is reduced by no more than 25% in the first 2 hours, patients with aortic dissection require rapid blood pressure and heart rate reductions within minutes. The most commonly used medications and their dosing regimens are listed in Table 11-2.

Heart rate initially can be controlled with intravenous beta-blockers, which also will have a moderate effect on lowering blood pressure. If the patient has a history of asthma or an intolerance to these drugs, nondihydropyridine calcium channel blockers may be used. These agents have negative inotropic effects and do not produce the reflex tachycardia associated with dihydropyridine calcium channel blockers.

PEARL

In the management of aortic dissection, target an SBP <110 mm Hg and a heart rate <60 beats per minute.

If further blood pressure management remains necessary even after the heart rate has been successfully controlled, antihypertensive agents can be initiated. Dihydropyridine calcium channel blockers and nitrates are the standard medications of choice for blood pressure control. These agents should not be used without first reducing the heart rate, as the decrease in blood pressure could result in a reflex tachycardia and worsen shear stress on the damaged aortic wall. Importantly, the use of sodium nitroprusside for blood pressure control in TAD has decreased significantly, primarily because of the risk of cyanide toxicity. Calcium channel blockers such

TABLE 11-2. Blood Pressure and Heart Rate Control Medications for TAD

Drug Class	Agent	Dosing
Heart Rate Control		
Beta-blockers	Esmolol	Load: 500 mcg/kg IV over 1 min Maintenance: 50 mcg/kg/min IV and titrate up to 300 mcg/kg/min IV
	Metoprolol	2.5–5 mg IV every 5 min up to 15 mg IV every 15 min
Calcium channel blockers	Diltiazem	5 mg/hr IV and titrate by 5 mg/hr up to 15 mg/hr IV
	Verapamil	2.5–5 mg IV every 5 min up to 10 mg IV every 15 min
Blood Pressure Control		
Calcium channel blockers	Nicardipine	5 mg/hr IV and titrate up 2.5 mg/hr up to 15 mg/hr IV
Beta-blockers	Labetalol	2 mg/min IV and titrate up 0.5 mg/min up to 8 mg/min IV
Other	Nitroprusside	0.25–0.5 mcg/kg/min IV and titrate to effect up to a maximum dose of 10 mcg/kg/min (cyanide toxicity is associated with rates >4 mcg/kg/min)
	Enalapril	1.25 mg IV every 6 hrs
	Fenoldopam	0.1 mcg/kg/min IV titrate up by 0.05–0.1 mcg/kg/min to a maximum dose of 1.6 mcg/kg/min

as nicardipine are being used much more frequently because of their safety profile.

The acute onset and severity of pain often trigger a catecholamine surge that increases both heart rate and blood pressure. Analgesia should be provided with intravenous narcotics, which can reduce this catecholamine response and provide mild vasodilation to assist with blood pressure control. There is no evidence demonstrating the superiority of any analgesic agent for the comfort of patients experiencing aortic dissection; the authors' preferred analgesic is fentanyl.

Type A Dissections

Type A dissections should be treated as surgical emergencies. These patients have a higher mortality rate than those with type B dissections. Risk factors that portend a poor prognosis are listed in Table 11-3.

Uncomplicated Cases

Even uncomplicated cases (ie, those lacking the risk factors listed in *Table 11-1*) are plagued by a high mortality rate. In addition to receiving aggressive blood pressure and heart rate control, these patients should be monitored and reevaluated frequently for signs of complications. A cardiothoracic surgeon should be consulted for emergent operative intervention; if unavailable, preparations for transfer to the nearest tertiary care center should be made once the patient has been stabilized and heart rate and blood pressure have improved.

Complicated Cases

Most complications arising from type A cases stem from a retrograde extension of the dissection. This occurs when the dissection, which normally extends in an anterograde manner, expands retrograde toward more proximal structures. Common fatal complications include coronary artery malperfusion, carotid artery malperfusion, aortic valve insufficiency, and cardiac tamponade. Management of these complications requires an aggressive approach because of their associated high mortality rates.

Cardiac Complications

Coronary artery malperfusion, which can lead to acute myocardial ischemia or infarction, is one of the most challenging complications of acute aortic dissection. An intimal flap overlying the lumen of a coronary vessel or a dissection of the coronary vessel causes this complication. The right coronary artery is the most commonly affected artery, leading to an inferior ST-segment elevation myocardial infarction (MI). In practice, patients presenting with chest pain often are assumed to have an MI until proved otherwise. Test results such as

TABLE 11-3. Risk Factors Associated with Poor Prognosis

Age >70 years
Abrupt onset of chest pain
Hypotension, shock, or tamponade at presentation
Renal failure at presentation and before surgery
Pulse deficit
Previous aortic valve replacement
Abnormal ECG, particularly ST-segment elevation
Prior MI
Renal and/or visceral ischemia
Underlying pulmonary disease
Preoperative neurological impairment
Massive blood transfusion

diagnostic electrocardiograms (ECGs) or elevated troponin levels can be misleading in patients with coronary artery malperfusion, prompting clinicians to misdiagnosis an isolated MI.[26] The dilemma arises when a cardiac catheterization suite is not available. When patients with MI caused by aortic dissection receive thrombolytic therapy for an assumed acute MI, the outcome tends to be poor.[27]

Patients who receive a diagnosis of coronary malperfusion are at higher risk for postoperative complications if the ischemic myocardium is not urgently revascularized. Any patient with an ECG diagnostic of an ST-segment elevation MI and a low risk for TAD should be treated for acute coronary syndrome (ACS). If the patient's history or risk factor analysis reveals an increased likelihood of TAD, diagnostic imaging of the aorta should be initiated prior to the administration of thrombolytic therapy.

Acute aortic regurgitation occurs in 41% to 76% of patients with type A dissections.[11,28-31] This complication is caused by aortic root dilatation or protrusion of the false lumen into the aortic root, an abnormality that prevents the leaflets from closing completely. Patients can present with a broad spectrum of signs and symptoms, ranging from a hemodynamically insignificant diastolic murmur to frank cardiogenic shock.[32] The acute management of stable patients with acute aortic regurgitation centers on aggressive afterload reduction with intravenous vasodilators until operative repair can be initiated.

Consultation with a cardiothoracic surgeon for early operative management is the next step; in most cases, emergent coronary revascularization must precede the dissection repair to preserve the myocardium. Consulting an interventional cardiologist in concert with a cardiothoracic surgeon often expedites this process. Most surgeons prefer a preoperative angiogram to visualize the anatomy and identify the compromised vessels, although there has been a recent shift toward intraoperative angiograms.[27,33]

Neurological Complications

Central nervous system complications related to acute aortic dissection are common and generally occur as a result of occlusion of the carotid artery or any of the segmental spinal arteries. Classic stroke-like symptoms constitute a well-known presentation of proximal aortic dissection. Neurological manifestations originate from malperfusion of the affected artery secondary to direct occlusion or decreased perfusion from hypotension. Patients with carotid compromise can present with any number of neurological problems with or without chest pain, ranging from hemiparesis to altered mental status or coma. These symptoms are indicative of a dismal prognosis, as brain function rarely improves and patients often die despite operative intervention.[34,35]

Neurological complications require the emergent revascularization of compromised tissue. Unfortunately, beyond operative intervention, therapeutic revascularization treatments are rarely successful. Medical management performed in consultation with a cardiothoracic surgeon and neurologist or neurosurgeon improves the odds of a full recovery.[36] Reducing the time between the initial presentation and intervention also improves patient outcomes.

Unstable Patients

The differential diagnoses for a hypotensive patient with TAD includes cardiac tamponade, myocardial infarction, aortic rupture, and cardiogenic shock from aortic valve insufficiency. Most unstable patients presenting with type A dissections have cardiac tamponade. The pathophysiology involves one of two mechanisms: either the false lumen extends into the pericardium and the hypertensive forces bring about a transudative pericardial effusion, or (less commonly) the dissection ruptures into the pericardium.[37-39] Tamponade is the leading cause of death in patients with type A dissections.[1,11] Hypotensive patients with a type A (proximal) dissection should be assumed to have pericardial tamponade until proved otherwise.

Unstable patients who present with TAD should be intubated for airway protection. Induction agents that have safe and well-established hemodynamic profiles (eg, etomidate) are preferred. After the airway is secured, the next step is to exclude cardiac tamponade. Bedside ultrasonography can be used to evaluate for pericardial effusion, the absence of which rules out tamponade and should trigger consideration of other causes. Clinicians who are particularly adept at ultrasound may be able to evaluate the aortic valve for signs of insufficiency. Surgical intervention is required if an effusion is present.

In most cases of acute cardiac tamponade, pericardiocentesis is warranted. Because this procedure is associated with rebleeding and increased mortality in cases of TAD, it should not be performed unless the patient is acutely decompensating (ie, hypotensive with mental status changes) or in cardiac arrest.[40] Pericardiocentesis should be a last resort, used only as a temporizing measure in patients with proximal aortic dissection complicated by tamponade to offer stability while an operating room is being prepared. If the procedure is to be performed, remove small volumes (10–15 mL) at a time — just enough to restore hemodynamics (ie, SBP >90 mm Hg).[8] Large-volume pericardiocentesis has been associated with worsened outcomes.[40]

Cardiac arrest in patients with type A dissections most commonly is secondary to cardiac tamponade, cardiogenic shock secondary to acute aortic insufficiency, or hypovolemia from rupture and exsanguination. These patients are very difficult to resuscitate without operative intervention. Early consultation with a cardiothoracic surgeon is directly linked to survival. Determination of the cause of the cardiac arrest is paramount when selecting resuscitative measures. The survival rates for patients who present in a hypotensive state or after cardiac arrest are abysmal.

PEARL

Pericardiocentesis should be a last resort in patients who are decompensating or in cardiac arrest with a proximal aortic dissection complicated by tamponade. In such cases, remove only the smallest volume of fluid required to restore hemodynamics.

Fluid resuscitation and vasopressor administration are mainstays of therapy regardless of the cause of shock. This seems counterintuitive to the goal of reducing stress on the aortic wall; however, hemodynamic compromise will decrease overall organ perfusion and potentially worsen outcomes. If the murmur of aortic regurgitation is present or if cardiogenic shock is suspected, inotropes may be required to augment cardiac contractility. Examples of vasopressors and inotropes and their dosing are presented in Table 11-4. If rupture is suspected, packed red blood cells (RBCs) should be the resuscitative fluid of choice. The use of untyped, uncrossmatched blood products is encouraged in this patient population. Once spontaneous circulation has returned, adequate blood pressure must be maintained through careful titration of medications that likely counteract each other. The ultimate goal should be to expeditiously transfer these patients to the nearest operating room, whether in the presenting hospital or a tertiary care facility.

Type B Dissections

Uncomplicated Cases

Uncomplicated type B dissection is most commonly managed medically with blood pressure and heart rate control. Mortality rates associated with medical management alone (10%) are favorable to those associated with primary surgical management (35%).[41] Indications for the operative intervention are listed in Table 11-5. Samples should be drawn for baseline laboratory tests, including a comprehensive metabolic panel for liver enzymes and renal function and a lactate level to assess for mesenteric compromise. Repeat these tests if any suggestion of organ malperfusion arises (see *Table 11-1*). A Foley catheter should be placed to evaluate for decreased urine output as a sign of renal malperfusion. Neurovascular checks should be performed on all extremities to assess pulse deficits and neurovascular compromise every 1 or 2 hours. Finally, after the patient has been stabilized and the blood pressure and heart rate have been optimized, monitoring in an ICU setting is necessary to ensure the frequent reevaluation of potential complications.

TABLE 11-4. Vasopressors and Inotropes for Patients with Unstable TAD

Vasopressors	Dosing
Norepinephrine	Initial dose: 0.05 mcg/kg/min Titrate by 0.02 mcg/kg/min Maximum dose: 0.5 mcg/kg/min
Phenylephrine	Initial dose: 100–180 mcg/min Usual dose range: 0.5–9 mcg/kg/min
Epinephrine	Initial dose: 0.05 mcg/kg/min Titrate by 0.02–0.05 mcg/kg/min Maximum dose: 0.5 mcg/kg/min
Inotropes	
Dobutamine	Initial dose: 2.5 mcg/kg/min Titrate by 2.5 mcg/kg/min Maximum dose: 20 mcg/kg/min

Complicated Cases

The most common complication of type B dissections is organ malperfusion, which is particularly difficult to manage. The organ malperfusion syndromes seen with type A (proximal) aortic dissection also can occur in patients with type B. The mesenteric, renal, and iliac arteries are affected most frequently. In such cases, the intimal flap overlies the branch artery off of the aorta, which places the false lumen in line with the vessel lumen and compromises blood flow to the branch vessel's target organ. In rare instances, the vessel itself also dissects, restricting blood flow. This describes the origin of the phrase "symptoms above and below the diaphragm," as patients can experience chest or upper back pain and symptoms secondary to malperfusion.

Organ malperfusion substantially increases the risk of death. In particular, the mortality rate of patients with mesenteric and renal malperfusion is between 30% and 50%.[35,36,42] Mesenteric malperfusion is the leading cause of death in those with type B dissections.[12] The management of these syndromes often involves operative intervention and urgent revascularization to salvage devitalized tissue. Many cardiothoracic surgeons will not operate on a patient with TAD complicated by organ malperfusion until the specific obstruction has been addressed or corrected.

In addition to aggressive blood pressure and heart rate control, patients require frequent monitoring for signs of worsening organ malperfusion. Serial blood samples for creatinine levels should be obtained if renal malperfusion is suspected. Urine output below 0.5 mL/kg/hr is an ominous sign regardless of the serum creatinine level; this finding is symptomatic of inadequate volume status or impending renal failure. In patients with abdominal pain or diarrhea associated with aortic dissection, mesenteric ischemia should be suspected. In such cases, serial lactate measurements should be obtained, and liver function tests and amylase measurements should be assessed for pancreatic compromise. Bowel ischemia has the highest mortality rate of the malperfusion syndromes. Any complaint of leg discomfort or signs of ischemic compromise of a lower limb should raise suspicion of iliac artery malperfusion. Neurovascular checks should be performed every 1 to 2 hours to assess for pulse deficits.

TABLE 11-5. Indications for Surgical Management of Type B TAD
Rapid progression or decompensation
Intractable chest or back pain
Refractory hypertension
Aortic branch vessel involvement with compromised perfusion to vital organs
Impending aortic rupture

Open aortic repair and revascularization once were the gold standard of care for patients with malperfusion. Recently, however, surgical intervention has been associated with a higher mortality rate; patients die not as a result of the dissection, but from the malperfusion itself. Endovascular procedures such as aortic fenestration performed by an interventional radiologist or cardiologist are being used more often and with promising results. Aortic fenestration is a procedure in which an angiogram is obtained to determine where the artery is compromised. Then several "fenestrations" are created in the dissection flap (the connection between the true and false lumens), using an endovascular device. This allows blood flow through the fenestration and into the malperfused artery and subsequent target organ(s). An interventional radiologist also can place a stent in the artery to maintain patency, especially in cases of branch vessel dissection. These techniques are associated with a much lower mortality rate than open surgical repair of the aorta (12% versus 28%).[35,43,44] Those who undergo branch vessel intervention also appear to have a much lower complication rate than patients who receive open repair alone, who are more likely to require bowel resections for ischemic gut or permanent hemodialysis for renal insufficiency.[45] Surgeons are now delaying surgery for aortic repair, even in cases of type A dissection, allowing an average of 4 days for reperfusion and resolution of symptoms.[45]

Unstable Patients

Several complications can precipitate hypotension in patients with type B dissections; aortic rupture is the most common and fatal cause. It is of primary importance to recognize aortic rupture and provide hemodynamic stabilization. All unstable patients should be intubated for airway protection. Large-bore intravenous access or central catheter placement for large-volume resuscitation is required. Crystalloid can be infused initially, but a rapid switch to packed RBCs to replace lost blood volume is encouraged. Such cases warrant the initiation of a massive transfusion protocol; packed RBCs, platelets, and fresh frozen plasma (FFP) should be administered. Once spontaneous circulation has returned, the patient should be transferred to an operating room for surgical repair, the only definitive treatment for aortic rupture. Although other interventional techniques can be considered, such treatment decisions should be made by the cardiothoracic surgeon.[43,46]

TABLE 11-6. Indications for Surgical Management of AAA
Aortic diameter >5.5 cm in asymptomatic patients
Interval increase of aortic diameter of 0.5 cm in 6 months in asymptomatic patients
Symptomatic patients
Renal malperfusion
Impending or completed rupture

Abdominal Aortic Aneurysm

Most AAAs are diagnosed incidentally on radiographic studies obtained for other reasons.[47] As many as 90% of these ruptures are fatal; the disease kills approximately 13,000 Americans every year. However, the incidence of AAA is on the decline due to a decreasing prevalence of smoking and an increasing number of elective repairs.[48-51] The majority of these aneurysms are caused by atherosclerosis of the aorta, which leads to degenerative changes in aortic elasticity. Patients older than 60 years and those with hypertension, hyperlipidemia, and peripheral vascular disease are most at risk.

Although the vast majority are asymptomatic, the rare patient who presents with signs of an aneurysm presents a real diagnostic dilemma. Frequently misdiagnosed, AAA can manifest in a wide variety of presentations from colicky abdominal or flank pain suggestive of renal colic to altered mental status from hypotension secondary to rupture of the aneurysm.

Diagnosis

Although bedside ultrasonography is an adequate screening tool for AAA and is excellent for measuring the diameter of the aortic lumen, it cannot evaluate for rupture in the retroperitoneal space. AAA should be assumed in any patient with unstable vital signs and ultrasound indications of a rupture regardless of size. An emergent evaluation by a vascular surgeon is paramount. A computed tomography scan without intravenous contrast can evaluate the retroperitoneal space for rupture and measure the diameter of the aortic lumen, whereas intravenous contrast evaluates the aorta for signs of rupture. These modalities should be reserved for stable patients. Any AAA diameter greater than 5 to 5.5 cm requires operative intervention, and any rupture requires repair regardless of the aortic caliber. The risk of rupture increases significantly with diameters greater than 5 cm.[52-54] Other indications for operative intervention are listed in Table 11-6. Once the diagnosis is established, consultation with a vascular surgeon to discuss surgical or medical management is warranted.

Vital signs can remain stable even in cases of ruptured AAA — an incongruity that can make it difficult to assess a patient's true stability. The diagnosis can be particularly puzzling when the rupture is confined to the retroperitoneal space, which fills with blood. In such cases, the blood loss abates secondary to tamponade, allowing the vital signs to restabilize. Patients experience a sudden onset of abdominal or back pain and commonly lose consciousness for a transient period, after which they feel better. However, once the hemorrhage overwhelms that potential space, a precipitous decline ensues. It should never be assumed that a rupture has not occurred simply because the vital signs are stable.

Acute Management

Two large-bore intravenous lines should be placed to enable the infusion of blood products and medications, and cardiac monitoring should be used to evaluate for life-threatening arrhythmias. Any patient with a ruptured AAA should be intubated to protect the airway and maximize oxygenation. Induction agents that maintain hemodynamics are preferred to prevent circulatory compromise.

Laboratory studies, including a complete blood count and basic metabolic panel, should be obtained to evaluate for anemia and renal insufficiency, which can develop if the renal artery is compromised. The lactate level should be measured initially as a baseline and serially every 4 to 6 hours. A type and crossmatch for at least 6 units of packed RBCs should be obtained in case a rupture occurs. A coagulation panel will document any abnormalities that require correction and any anticoagulant medications that warrant reversal. An invasive arterial catheter should be placed to provide the most accurate blood pressure measurements. The targets are an SBP of 100 to 120 mm Hg and a MAP of 60 to 65 mm Hg. Increased blood pressure can exacerbate ongoing blood loss or turn a contained rupture into a free rupture.[55]

As in cases of TAD, blood is the resuscitation fluid of choice for patients with ruptured AAA. A massive transfusion protocol should be initiated, and packed RBCs should be infused until FFP and platelets become available. A ratio of packed RBCs to FFP near 1:1 can reduce the risk of complications and death.[56] Crystalloid is an acceptable alternative until blood products arrive. Once blood pressure goals are met, volume resuscitation can be delayed until operative intervention can begin. The liberal use of fluids or blood products may increase the risk of mortality.[57]

Complications

Patients can present with hypertension, typically attributed to renal artery compromise. The amount of stress on the aortic wall makes the free wall less stable, creating a predisposition toward rupture. Although there is no conclusive evidence to support the benefits of blood pressure reduction, current management goals for hypertension mirror those for hypotension (ie, 100–120 mm Hg). This can be achieved with intravenous antihypertensive medications (*see Table 11-2*), most commonly short-acting beta-blockers. Calcium channel blockers and afterload-reducing agents can be used if a patient is intolerant to beta-blockers.

KEY POINTS

1. Thoracic aortic dissection is 3 times as prevalent as ruptured abdominal aortic aneurysm.
2. Forty percent of patients with TAD die immediately; an additional 20% to 25% die in the hospital even with appropriate management.
3. Delaying the diagnosis increases the mortality rate 1% to 2% per hour after the initial event.
4. A chest radiograph is not sensitive enough to rule out aortic dissection, and a widened mediastinum is seen in only 60% of patients.
5. D-dimer can be falsely negative in patients with chronic dissections, short intimal flaps, and thrombosed false lumens.
6. In hypertensive patients with suspected or confirmed aortic dissection, the blood pressure must be reduced rapidly. Principles of gradual blood pressure reduction for hypertensive emergencies do not apply to the management of acute aortic dissection.
7. To avoid reflex tachycardia, antihypertensive agents should be used only after the heart rate has been controlled.
8. Aortic dissection most commonly involves the right coronary ostium, leading to right coronary artery occlusion and inferior ST-segment elevation MI. The clinician must be prepared to distinguish an MI caused by aortic dissection from an isolated acute MI in patients with chest and back pain.
9. Differential diagnoses for hypotensive type A dissection include:
   - Pericardial tamponade
   - Myocardial infarction
   - Aortic rupture
   - Aortic insufficiency leading to cardiogenic shock
10. Mesenteric malperfusion is the leading cause of death in type B dissections.
11. Acute aortic dissection complicated by organ malperfusion carries a very high mortality rate. Cardiothoracic surgeons, in general, will not operate until the specific malperfusion syndrome has been corrected.
12. Patients with type A acute aortic dissection complicated by organ malperfusion need an aortic fenestration procedure (open or closed) before or at the time of corrective proximal aortic repair. If interventional and surgical resources are unavailable, the patient should be transferred rapidly to a facility that can provide them.
13. Patients with ruptured AAA can have stable vital signs secondary to rupture into the retroperitoneal space and resultant tamponade.
14. Any patient with unstable vital signs and a bedside ultrasound showing an AAA, regardless of size, is experiencing a ruptured AAA until proved otherwise. An emergent evaluation by a vascular surgeon is paramount.
15. If the patient is unstable and has a history of AAA, a vascular surgeon should be consulted early (ie, before imaging) to avoid delays in surgical management.

PEARL

When AAA rupture is suspected, stabilization maneuvers include maintaining the SBP at a maximum of 100 to 120 mm Hg and the MAP at 60 to 65 mm Hg.

Cardiac arrest in a patient with a suspected ruptured AAA likely is the result of hypovolemia caused by exsanguination. The best resuscitation fluid in such cases is blood. A massive transfusion protocol should be initiated; if crossmatched blood is not available, uncrossmatched blood should be given in the interim. If spontaneous circulation returns, the aforementioned protocols of blood pressure management and hemodynamic maintenance are sufficient to stabilize the patient in preparation for the operating room.

What if spontaneous circulation does not return and the patient is still crashing? Case reports have described patients in cardiac arrest secondary to ruptured AAA undergoing open thoracotomy and aortic cross-clamping to stop the exsanguination. This technique preferentially shunts blood to the brain and coronary arteries and away from the rupture to allow enough time for sufficient volume to be infused. Thus the patient is temporary stabilized for transport to the operating room and definitive repair. Thoracotomy should be reserved as a last resort for patients in whom cardiac arrest occurred very early after the emergence of symptoms and for those with witnessed cardiac arrests. Patients who have undergone prolonged resuscitative efforts without return of spontaneous circulation should not be considered for this procedure.

A vascular surgeon should be consulted early regarding the management of any patient presenting with a ruptured AAA regardless of stability. Management options include open repair or endovascular repair, which has a lower mortality rate.[58,59] Most vascular surgeons are willing to proceed even without imaging in an unstable patient with a history of AAA. If a vascular surgeon is not available, the patient should be transported to a tertiary care center after being stabilized.

Conclusion

Aortic aneurysms, dissections, and ruptures are difficult to diagnose and treat. Associated complications further impede the assessment process and therapeutic strategy. Early aggressive management focused on blood pressure control can improve outcomes for these critically ill patients. This group of disorders requires an early team approach, calling on the expertise of multiple medical and surgical specialties.

REFERENCES

1. Meszaros I, Morocz J, Szlavi J, et al. Epidemiology and clinicopathology of aortic dissection. *Chest.* 2000;117:1271-1278.
2. Bickerstaff LK, Pairolero PC, Hollier LH, et al. Thoracic aortic aneurysms: a population-based study. *Surgery.* 1982;92:1103-1108.
3. Clouse WD, Hallett JW Jr, Schaff HV, et al. Acute aortic dissection: population-based incidence compared with degenerative aortic aneurysm rupture. *Mayo Clin Proc.* 2004;79:176-180.
4. Coady MA, Rizzo JA, Goldstein LJ, Elefteriades JA. Natural history, pathogenesis, and etiology of thoracic aortic aneurysms and dissections. *Cardiol Clin.* 1999;17:615-635.
5. Anagnostopoulos CE, Prabhakar MJ, Kittle CF. Aortic dissections and dissecting aneurysms. *Am J Cardiol.* 1972;30:263-273.
6. Masuda Y, Yamada Z, Morooka N, Watanabe S, Inagaki Y. Prognosis of patients with medically treated aortic dissections. *Circulation.* 1991;84(5 suppl):III7-III13.
7. Trimarchi S, Nienaber CA, Rampoldi V, et al. Contemporary results of surgery in acute type A aortic dissection: The International Registry of Acute Aortic Dissection experience. *J Thorac Cardiovasc Surg.* 2005;129:112-122.
8. Hiratzka LF, Bakris GL, Beckman JA, et al. 2010 ACCF/AHA/AATS/ACR/ASA/SCA/SCAI/SIR/STS/SVM guidelines for the diagnosis and management of patients with Thoracic Aortic Disease: a report of the American College of Cardiology Foundation/American Heart Association Task Force on Practice Guidelines, American Association for Thoracic Surgery, American College of Radiology, American Stroke Association, Society of Cardiovascular Anesthesiologists, Society for Cardiovascular Angiography and Interventions, Society of Interventional Radiology, Society of Thoracic Surgeons, and Society for Vascular Medicine. *Circulation.* 2010;121:e266-e369.
9. Hirst AE Jr, Johns VJ Jr, Kime SW Jr. Dissecting aneurysm of the aorta: a review of 505 cases. *Medicine (Baltimore).* 1958;37:217-279.
10. Jex RK, Schaff HV, Piehler JM, et al. Repair of ascending aortic dissection. Influence of associated aortic valve insufficiency on early and late results. *J Thorac Cardiovasc Surg.* 1987;93:375-384.
11. Fann JI, Smith JA, Miller DC, et al. Surgical management of aortic dissection during a 30-year period. *Circulation.* 1995;92(9 suppl):II113-II121.
12. Miller DC, Stinson EB, Oyer PE, et al. Operative treatment of aortic dissections. Experience with 125 patients over a sixteen-year period. *J Thorac Cardiovasc Surg.* 1979;78:365-382.
13. Moon MR. Approach to the treatment of aortic dissection. *Surg Clin North Am.* 2009;89:869-893.
14. Baydin A, Nargis C, Nural M. Painless, acute aortic dissection presenting as an acute stroke. *Mt Sinai J Med.* 2006;73:1129-1131.
15. Ayrik C, Cece H, Aslan O, Karcioglu O, Yilmaz E. Seeing the invisible: painless aortic dissection in the emergency setting. *Emerg Med J.* 2006;23:e24.
16. Young J, Herd AM. Painless acute aortic dissection and rupture presenting as syncope. *J Emerg Med.* 2002;22:171-174.
17. American College of Emergency Physicians Clinical Policies Subcommittee on Thoracic Aortic Dissection, Diercks DB, Promes SB, et al. Clinical policy: critical issues in the evaluation and management of adult patients with suspected acute nontraumatic thoracic aortic dissection. *Ann Emerg Med.* 2015;65:32-42.e12.
18. von Kodolitsch Y, Nienaber CA, Dieckmann C, et al. Chest radiography for the diagnosis of acute aortic syndrome. *Am J Med.* 2004;116:73-77.
19. Hagan PG, Nienaber CA, Isselbacher EM, et al. The International Registry of Acute Aortic Dissection (IRAD): new insights into an old disease. *JAMA.* 2000;283:897-903.
20. Klompas M. Does this patient have an acute thoracic aortic dissection? *JAMA.* 2002;287:2262-2272.
21. Budhram G, Reardon R. Diagnosis of ascending aortic dissection using emergency department bedside echocardiogram. *Acad Emerg Med.* 2008;15:584.
22. Davis CB, Kendall JL. Emergency bedside ultrasound diagnosis of superior mesenteric artery dissection complicating acute aortic dissection. *J Emerg Med.* 2013;45:894-896.
23. Kaban J, Raio C. Emergency department diagnosis of aortic dissection by bedside transabdominal ultrasound. *Acad Emerg Med.* 2009;16:809-810.
24. Rosenberg H, Al-Rajhi K. ED ultrasound diagnosis of a type B aortic dissection using the suprasternal view. *Am J Emerg Med.* 2012;30:2084.e2081-2085.
25. Shiga T, Wajima Z, Apfel CC, Inoue T, Ohe Y. Diagnostic accuracy of transesophageal echocardiography, helical computed tomography, and magnetic resonance imaging for suspected thoracic aortic dissection: systematic review and meta-analysis. *Arch Intern Med.* 2006;166:1350-1356.
26. Hansen MS, Nogareda GJ, Hutchison SJ. Frequency of and inappropriate treatment of misdiagnosis of acute aortic dissection. *Am J Cardiol.* 2007;99:852-856.
27. Kawahito K, Adachi H, Murata S, Yamaguchi A, Ino T. Coronary malperfusion due to type A aortic dissection: mechanism and surgical management. *Ann Thorac Surg.* 2003;76:1471-1476.
28. Mazzucotelli JP, Deleuze PH, Baufreton C, et al. Preservation of the aortic valve in acute aortic dissection: long-term echocardiographic assessment and clinical outcome. *Ann Thorac Surg.* 1993;55:1513-1517.
29. von Segesser LK, Lorenzetti E, Lachat M, et al. Aortic valve preservation in acute type A dissection: is it sound? *J Thorac Cardiovasc Surg.* 1996;111:381-390.
30. Massimo CG, Presenti LF, Marranci P, et al. Extended and total aortic resection in the surgical treatment of acute type A aortic dissection: experience with 54 patients. *Ann Thorac Surg.* 1988;46:420-424.
31. Movsowitz HD, Levine RA, Hilgenberg AD, Isselbacher EM. Transesophageal echocardiographic description of the mechanisms of aortic regurgitation in acute type A aortic dissection: implications for aortic valve repair. *J Am Coll Cardiol.* 2000;36:884-890.
32. Januzzi JL, Eagle KA, Cooper JV, et al. Acute aortic dissection presenting with congestive heart failure: results from the International Registry of Acute Aortic Dissection. *J Am Coll Cardiol.* 2005;46:733-735.
33. Neri E, Toscano T, Papalia U, et al. Proximal aortic dissection with coronary malperfusion: presentation, management, and outcome. *J Thorac Cardiovasc Surg.* 2001;121:552-560.
34. Geirsson A, Szeto WY, Pochettino A, et al. Significance of malperfusion syndromes prior to contemporary surgical repair for acute type A dissection: outcomes and need for additional revascularizations. *Eur J Cardiothorac Surg.* 2007;32:255-262.
35. Lauterbach SR, Cambria RP, Brewster DC, et al. Contemporary management of aortic branch compromise resulting from acute aortic dissection. *J Vasc Surg.* 2001;33:1185-1192.

36. Girardi LN, Krieger KH, Lee LY, Mack CA, Tortolani AJ, Isom OW. Management strategies for type A dissection complicated by peripheral vascular malperfusion. *Ann Thorac Surg.* 2004;77:1309-1314.
37. Garcia-Jimenez A, Peraza Torres A, Martinez Lopez G, Alvarez Dieguez I, Botana Alba CM. Cardiac tamponade by aortic dissection in a hospital without cardiothoracic surgery. *Chest.* 1993;104:290-291.
38. Armstrong WF, Bach DS, Carey LM, Froehlich J, Lowell M, Kazerooni EA. Clinical and echocardiographic findings in patients with suspected acute aortic dissection. *Am Heart J.* 1998;136:1051-1060.
39. Pretre R, Von Segesser LK. Aortic dissection. *Lancet.* 1997;349(9063):1461-1464.
40. Isselbacher EM, Cigarroa JE, Eagle KA. Cardiac tamponade complicating proximal aortic dissection. Is pericardiocentesis harmful? *Circulation.* 1994;90:2375-2378.
41. Umana JP, Lai DT, Mitchell RS, et al. Is medical therapy still the optimal treatment strategy for patients with acute type B aortic dissections? *J Thorac Cardiovasc Surg.* 2002;124:896-910.
42. Shiiya N, Matsuzaki K, Kunihara T, Murashita T, Matsui Y. Management of vital organ malperfusion in acute aortic dissection: proposal of a mechanism-specific approach. *Gen Thorac Cardiovasc Surg.* 2007;55:85-90.
43. Cambria RP, Crawford RS, Cho JS, et al. A multicenter clinical trial of endovascular stent graft repair of acute catastrophes of the descending thoracic aorta. *J Vasc Surg.* 2009;50:1255-1264. e1251-1254.
44. Patel HJ, Williams DM, Meerkov M, Dasika NL, Upchurch GR Jr, Deeb GM. Long-term results of percutaneous management of malperfusion in acute type B aortic dissection: implications for thoracic aortic endovascular repair. *J Thorac Cardiovasc Surg.* 2009;138:300-308.
45. Patel HJ, Williams DM, Dasika NL, Suzuki Y, Deeb GM. Operative delay for peripheral malperfusion syndrome in acute type A aortic dissection: a long-term analysis. *J Thorac Cardiovasc Surg.* 2008;135:1288-1296.
46. Patel HJ, Williams DM, Upchurch GR Jr, Dasika NL, Deeb GM. A comparative analysis of open and endovascular repair for the ruptured descending thoracic aorta. *J Vasc Surg.* 2009;50:1265-1270.
47. Kent KC. Clinical practice. Abdominal aortic aneurysms. *N Engl J Med.* 2014;371:2101-2108.
48. Anjum A, von Allmen R, Greenhalgh R, Powell JT. Explaining the decrease in mortality from abdominal aortic aneurysm rupture. *Br J Surg.* 2012;99:637-645.
49. Mealy K, Salman A. The true incidence of ruptured abdominal aortic aneurysms. *Eur J Vasc Surg.* 1988;2:405-408.
50. Heikkinen M, Salenius J, Zeitlin R, et al. The fate of AAA patients referred electively to vascular surgical unit. *Scand J Surg.* 2002;91:345-352.
51. Johansen K, Kohler TR, Nicholls SC, Zierler RE, Clowes AW, Kazmers A. Ruptured abdominal aortic aneurysm: the Harborview experience. *J Vasc Surg.* 1991;13:240-247.
52. Brown LC, Powell JT. Risk factors for aneurysm rupture in patients kept under ultrasound surveillance. UK Small Aneurysm Trial Participants. *Ann Surg.* 1999;230:289-297.
53. Reed WW, Hallett JW Jr, Damiano MA, Ballard DJ. Learning from the last ultrasound. A population-based study of patients with abdominal aortic aneurysm. *Arch Intern Med.* 1997;157:2064-2068.
54. Brewster DC, Cronenwett JL, Hallett JW Jr, Johnston KW, Krupski WC, Matsumura JS. Guidelines for the treatment of abdominal aortic aneurysms. Report of a subcommittee of the Joint Council of the American Association for Vascular Surgery and Society for Vascular Surgery. *J Vasc Surg.* 2003;37:1106-1117.
55. Arthurs ZM, Sohn VY, Starnes BW. Ruptured abdominal aortic aneurysms: remote aortic occlusion for the general surgeon. *Surg Clin North Am.* 2007;87:1035-1045.
56. Mell MW, O'Neil AS, Callcut RA, et al. Effect of early plasma transfusion on mortality in patients with ruptured abdominal aortic aneurysm. *Surgery.* 2010;148:955-962.
57. Dick F, Erdoes G, Opfermann P, Eberle B, Schmidli J, von Allmen RS. Delayed volume resuscitation during initial management of ruptured abdominal aortic aneurysm. *J Vasc Surg.* 2013;57:943-950.
58. Eliason JL, Clouse WD. Current management of infrarenal abdominal aortic aneurysms. *Surg Clin North Am.* 2007;87:1017-1033.
59. Hirsch AT, Haskal ZJ, Hertzer NR, et al. ACC/AHA 2005 guidelines for the management of patients with peripheral arterial disease (lower extremity, renal, mesenteric, and abdominal aortic): executive summary a collaborative report from the American Association for Vascular Surgery/Society for Vascular Surgery, Society for Cardiovascular Angiography and Interventions, Society for Vascular Medicine and Biology, Society of Interventional Radiology, and the ACC/AHA Task Force on Practice Guidelines (Writing Committee to Develop Guidelines for the Management of Patients With Peripheral Arterial Disease) endorsed by the American Association of Cardiovascular and Pulmonary Rehabilitation; National Heart, Lung, and Blood Institute; Society for Vascular Nursing; TransAtlantic Inter-Society Consensus; and Vascular Disease Foundation. *J Am Coll Cardiol.* 2006;47:1239-1312.

Severe Sepsis and Septic Shock

12

IN THIS CHAPTER

- Sepsis syndromes
- Clinical sepsis identification
- Early cardiovascular resuscitation and hemodynamic optimization
- Early antibiotics and source control
- Adjunctive therapies
- Supportive therapies

Alan C. Heffner

The number of patients hospitalized every year for severe sepsis is skyrocketing; the incidence has doubled in the past decade and is projected to soon surpass 1 million in the US alone.[1,2] More than half of these patients are admitted via the emergency department, highlighting the importance of acute care in sepsis management. The lethality of severe cases often is underestimated; mortality rates range between 25% and 50%, far exceeding those for other common acute conditions such as myocardial infarction and stroke. In addition, sepsis accounts for more aggregate hospital costs (>5%) than any other disease.[3,4]

The Sepsis Syndromes

Infection is classically defined as the microbial invasion of normally sterile tissue or fluid. In practice, confirmation is rare at the time of initial presentation, and infection is presumed based on clinical observations coupled with laboratory and radiological findings. Bacteremia defines the presence of viable bacteria in the blood and is confirmed in fewer than 50% of severe sepsis cases.[5,6] Rarely, clinically important manifestations of infection arise from cytopathic or exotoxin effects in the absence of microbial tissue invasion (eg, *Clostridium difficile* colitis and staphylococcal toxic shock syndrome).

Host response plays a key role in the pathogenesis of many diseases, including sepsis. The term *systemic inflammatory response syndrome* (SIRS) describes the complex activation of the innate immune response, which manifests as systemic inflammation and endothelial dysfunction.[7] SIRS reflects a generalized pathophysiological response to an insult. The resultant cytokine and immunological storm can potentially damage organs remote from the initial injury.

The need for a standardized and practical diagnostic framework for sepsis trials codified the use of SIRS criteria in defining clinical sepsis more than two decades ago.[8] Although SIRS was designed to identify patients at risk of progressing to more severe disease (*Figure 12-1*), it is important to note that it is not specific to infection.[9-11] The generalized immune reaction represents a conserved response to diverse insults, including tissue injury (eg, burns and trauma) and noninfectious inflammatory and immunostimulating diseases. In one epidemiological survey, 17% of adult emergency department patients manifested SIRS, but only 25% of these cases were attributed to infection.[12]

Sepsis is the clinical syndrome of systemic response to microbial infection. In patients with known or suspected infection, SIRS constitutes evidence of sepsis, which encompasses a broad range of diseases — from minor, self-limited infections to life-threatening conditions. These syndromes denote a disease continuum progressing from sepsis (infection with inflammatory response) to severe sepsis (sepsis plus acute organ dysfunction) and septic shock (severe sepsis with cardiovascular failure) *(Table 12-1)*. Although a minority of patients with clinical sepsis present with or progress to severe disease, this group incurs substantial morbidity and mortality.[13]

Clinical Identification

Sepsis is a challenging clinical diagnosis, as signs and symptoms of infection are protean and often subtle and nonspecific. There is no pathognomonic sign or single reliable test to diagnose early disease. Immunocompromised and elderly patients are at greatest risk for severe infection and exhibit an attenuated host response that can hamper bedside detection.

Although the standard diagnosis of sepsis is based on SIRS, the clinical presentation and course of infected patients are rarely as distinct as the definitions suggest. In practice, unexplained SIRS should prompt consideration and investigation for infection *(Figure 12-2)* However, the absence of categorical SIRS (two or more of the four criteria) does not exclude clinically important

FIGURE 12-1. Example of a Severe Sepsis and Septic Shock Treatment Pathway

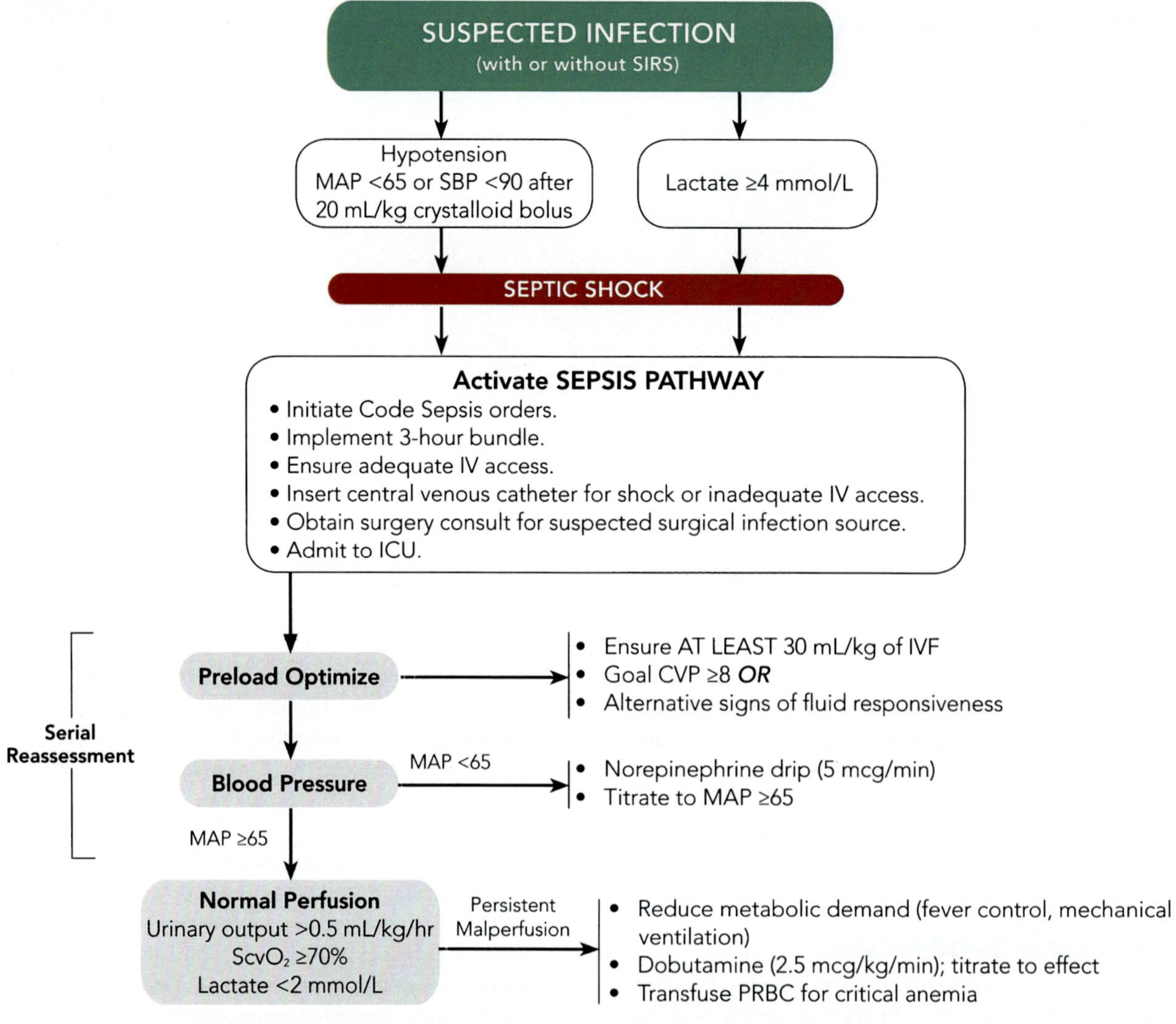

infection.[14] Stated another way, SIRS is neither sensitive nor specific enough to reliably confirm or exclude acute infection or progression to severe disease.[15] Clinical judgment is required.

PEARL

The two markers considered classic for infection — fever and peripheral leukocytosis — are relatively insensitive. One-third of bacteremic patients do not manifest fever at presentation.[16,17] These markers do not reliably distinguish infectious from noninfectious causes of shock.[6]

Severe sepsis should be considered in all patients diagnosed with clinical infection. Specific sources are more commonly associated with progression to severe disease. Pulmonary, urinary, and intraabdominal infections account for half of severe sepsis cases.[18] Other common high-risk sources include the skin and soft tissues and endovascular sites. Any source or agent, including atypical organisms (eg, virus, spirochete, *Rickettsia*, malaria, and yeast) can produce life-threatening disease. The difficulty in clinical identification of sepsis is underscored by the fact that a primary source of infection is not immediately apparent in 33% of patients and remains unidentified in as many as 20% of strongly suspected cases.[5,6] Occult or unidentified infection is associated with an increased risk of death, in part due to delays in recognition and treatment.[13]

Patients must be treated based on suspected or presumed infection because microbiological confirmation is rare early in the course of illness. Given the prevalence and morbidity of severe sepsis, ill-appearing patients and those presenting with unexplained SIRS or shock warrant close surveillance, including expedited diagnostic testing and empiric antibiotics if infection remains a prominent concern.

> **PEARL**
>
> Septic shock develops within 48 hours in approximately 16% of emergency department patients admitted with sepsis.[18,19] It is important to consciously evaluate for early signs of hypoperfusion, end-organ dysfunction, and metabolic stress.

Septic Shock and Severe Sepsis

Shock defines a state of inadequate tissue perfusion in which oxygen delivery does not meet metabolic needs. Contrary to popular belief, the term does not reflect perfusion pressure. As many as 50% of emergency department patients with severe sepsis initially present in compensated shock with normal blood pressure. The difficulty in identifying these cases led to the terms *occult shock* and *cryptic shock*. Since blood pressure alone is insufficient to identify infected patients at high risk, it is important to consciously evaluate for signs of hypoperfusion, end-organ dysfunction, and metabolic stress.

Septic shock is defined by cardiovascular failure manifesting as hypotension or hypoperfusion following initial fluid resuscitation. Transient hypotension often heralds hemodynamic deterioration in infected patients. Physiologically, nonsustained hypotension represents progressive exhaustion of cardiovascular reserve and is the first sign of uncompensated shock. Episodic hypotension is an early warning sign associated with clinical deterioration and increased mortality that should not be dismissed as spurious or inconsequential.[18,20,21]

Uncompensated shock, characterized by sustained hypotension, develops when physiological attempts to maintain normal perfusion pressure are overwhelmed or exhausted. A mean arterial pressure (MAP) less than 65 mm Hg, systolic blood pressure (SBP) less than 90 mm Hg, or SBP more than 40 mm Hg below baseline warrants prompt investigation for cause and comparison with the patient's historical blood pressure.

> **PEARLS**
>
> - ✓ Some patients manifest early septic shock without distress or apparent hypoperfusion. Underappreciation of this presentation is a pitfall in early diagnosis and treatment.
> - ✓ Episodic hypotension is an early warning sign associated with clinical deterioration and should not be dismissed as spurious or inconsequential.

Acute End-Organ Dysfunction

Severe sepsis is marked by the presence of acute organ dysfunction *(Table 12-1)*. Acute kidney and lung injury are most common, followed by cardiovascular, hematological, and neurological dysfunction. Patients with sepsis can be confused, apathetic, or agitated, an association between infection and delirium that often is underappreciated. Laboratory variables such as thrombocytopenia, coagulopathy, hyperbilirubinemia, and elevated lactate concentrations are notable and objective signs of end-organ dysfunction. Acute renal dysfunction is a common early manifestation of organ involvement.[15] Mild elevations of serum creatinine (>0.3 mg/dL from baseline), even in the absence of oliguria, represent acute kidney injury.[22] The severity of disease is directly correlated to mortality.[23] Skin perfusion and mottling are underutilized but insightful markers of organ dysfunction that are linked to outcomes.[24,25]

FIGURE 12-2. Sepsis vs. SIRS

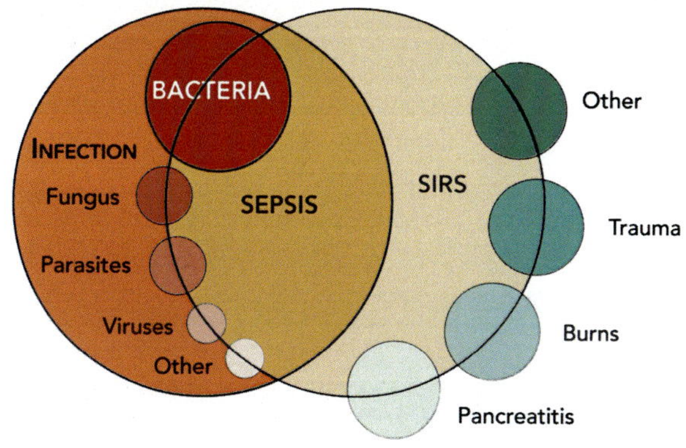

Lactate

Serum lactate is a useful biomarker to grade severity and predict outcomes in a variety of critical illnesses, including sepsis.[26,27] Hyperlactatemia is well recognized in the setting of acute infection and historically has been attributed to anaerobic metabolism linked to tissue hypoxia and hypoperfusion. The source of hyperlactatemia in sepsis is multifactorial, with the contribution of catechol-stimulated aerobic lactate production more considerable than previously appreciated.[28] Hyperlactatemia as a marker of metabolic stress corroborates the clinical observation of elevated levels in normotensive patients without apparent hypoperfusion.

When associated with clinical infection, the serum lactate concentration helps assess the risk of disease progression and outcomes. It stratifies risk independent of hemodynamics and organ dysfunction.[29,30] Supranormal (>2 mmol/L) lactate levels are associated with increased disease severity. Among patients with suspected infection, lactate greater than 4 mmol/L is associated with a 1 in 4 risk of death, a rate that is 10-fold higher than in patients with normal concentrations.[30] This mortality rate holds true even in normotensive patients.[31,32]

Serum lactate should be directly measured because serum bicarbonate, anion gap, and base excess are insensitive screens for clinically important hyperlactatemia. Arterial, venous, and capillary lactate levels are clinically equivalent and unaffected by the infusion of Ringer's lactate.

TABLE 12-1. The Sepsis Syndromes

Infection	Microbial invasion of normally sterile host tissue or fluid
SIRS	The systemic inflammatory response to a variety of insults is manifested by two or more of the following:
	Temperature >38°C (100.4°F) or <36°C (96.8°F)
	Heart rate >90 beats/min
	Respiratory rate >20 breaths/min or $PaCO_2$ <32 mm Hg
	WBC count >12,000/mm³ or <4,000/mm³, or >10% immature bands
Sepsis	The systemic inflammatory response to infection:
	Clinical infection plus SIRS (≥2 of 4 criteria)
Severe sepsis	Sepsis with acute organ dysfunction:
	Acute respiratory failure, including ARDS (PaO_2/FiO_2 <300)
	Acute kidney injury: serum creatinine >0.3 mg/dL from baseline; oliguria (urine output <0.5 mL/kg/hr for 2 consecutive hours)
	Encephalopathy ranging from confusion or apathy to agitation
	Coagulopathy: prothrombin time (PT) >16 sec or activated partial thromboplastin time (aPTT) >60 sec
	Thrombocytopenia: platelet count <100,000/µL
	Hyperbilirubinemia: serum bilirubin >4 mg/dL
	Blood lactate >2 mmol/L
	Clinical malperfusion: cool extremities, mottling, delayed capillary refill
Septic shock	Sepsis with hypotension refractory to initial fluid resuscitation (20 mL/kg):
	SBP <90 mm Hg or >40 mm Hg drop from baseline
	MAP <65 mm Hg or >25 mm Hg drop from baseline

TABLE 12-1a. Sequential (Sepsis-Related) Organ Failure Assessment Score

	Score				
System	0	1	2	3	4
Respiration PaO_2/FiO_2, mm Hg (kPa)	≥400 (53.3)	<400 (53.3)	<300 (40)	<200 (26.7) with respiratory support	<100 (13.3) with respiratory support
Coagulation Platelets, ×10³/µL	≥150	<150	<100	<50	<20
Liver Bilirubin, mg/dL (µmol/L)	<1.2 (20)	<1.2–1.9 (20–32)	2.0–5.9 (33–101)	6.0–11.9 (102–204)	>12.0 (204)
Cardiovascular	MAP ≥70 mm HG	MAP <70 mm HG	Dopamine <5 *OR* dobutamine (any dose)[a]	Dopamine 5.1–15 *OR* epinephrine ≤0.1 *OR* norepinephrine ≤0.1[a]	Dopamine >15 *OR* epinephrine >0.1 *OR* norepinephrine >0.1[a]
Central nervous system GCS[b]	15	13–14	10–12	6–9	<6
Renal Creatinine, mg/dL (µmol/L) Urine output, mL/d	<1.2 (110)	1.2–1.9 (110–170)	2.0–3.4 (171–299)	3.5–4.9 (300–440) <500	>5.0 (440) <200

[a]Catecholamine doses are given as µ g/kg/min for at least 1 hour.
[b]Glasgow Coma Scale (GCS) scores range from 3–15; higher score is favorable.

2016 Revised Sepsis Definitions

The international consensus sepsis definitions were revised in 2016 (*Table 12-1a*).[33] The new guidelines exclude the term *severe sepsis* and propose classifying sepsis by life-threatening organ dysfunction caused by a dysregulated host response to infection. In contrast to the former model, organ dysfunction is standardized as an acute change in total sequential organ failure assessment (SOFA) score of 2 or above, a finding that is associated with hospital mortality greater than 10% in the context of infection.[34,35] Baseline SOFA is assumed to be zero for patients without known preexisting organ dysfunction. In comparison, the diagnosis of *septic shock* is reserved for the subset of patients with profound circulatory, cellular, and metabolic abnormalities that are associated with an even higher risk of death. These patients are clinically identified by persistent hypotension requiring vasopressors to maintain a MAP of 65 or greater and a serum lactate above 2 mmol/L despite adequate fluid resuscitation (a finding associated with a hospital mortality >40%). Although the new definitions aim to provide greater consistency for epidemiological studies and clinical trials, their value in clinical practice remains unclear given the continued use of traditional sepsis definitions for medical coding and billing (as of 2017).

Management

The early recognition of severe sepsis is critical and must be coupled with timely and effective therapy to influence patient survival. The presence of shock, lactate greater than 4 mmol/L, or acute organ dysfunction defines a high-risk patient group with hospital mortality rates ranging from 25% to 50% *(Table 12-2)*. Early structured resuscitation of these patients confers short-term and persistent mortality advantages.[36-39]

Bundling evidence-based practices standardizes multiple interventions that result in improved process and patient outcomes. The utility of this approach is recognized in critical care and is valuable for high-risk diseases with a brief therapeutic window. The *Surviving Sepsis Campaign* and the Institute for Healthcare Improvement advocate a structured resuscitation bundle for patients with severe sepsis *(Table 12-3)*.[40] Bundle compliance generally improves with time, and the highest survival rates are associated with 100% compliance with all care components.[41-43]

Early Cardiovascular Resuscitation and Hemodynamic Optimization

There is no single cardiovascular lesion of sepsis. The disease ignites a complex and dynamic cascade of cardiovascular dysfunction that includes hypovolemia, abnormal vasomotor tone, and primary cardiac dysfunction. These derangements potentiate tissue and organ hypoperfusion and lead to multiorgan dysfunction.[44] Treatment at proximate stages of care affects outcomes and cannot be delayed. The window to reverse critical organ hypoperfusion is measured in hours and often transpires in the emergency department. Acute structured resuscitation influences survival in patients with severe sepsis and septic shock, whereas equivalent but delayed therapy does not yield the same benefit.[39,45] The hemodynamic approach to patients with severe sepsis is similar to the support of patients with any critical illness. A systematic goal-oriented strategy aims to rapidly optimize preload, maintain systemic perfusion pressure, and balance oxygen delivery and perfusion to meet metabolic needs *(Table 12-4)*.

TABLE 12-2. Conditions Linked to Adverse Outcomes
Clinical infection *PLUS*: shock, acute organ dysfunction, or serum lactate ≥4 mmol/L

Fluid Therapy and Optimization

Hypovolemia invoked by transcapillary fluid leak and nitric-oxide–induced vasodilation contributes to absolute and relative hypovolemia in sepsis. Vascular refilling in the form of fluid resuscitation is a central component of early cardiovascular support. Initial volume expansion is achieved through rapid fluid administration. Serial aliquots of crystalloid (15–20 mL/kg) should be infused rapidly over minutes. Sequential boluses should be titrated to perfusion endpoints while monitoring for adverse effects, including pulmonary congestion. The 2012 *Surviving Sepsis Campaign* prioritizes a minimum of 30 mL/kg of crystalloid within the first 3 hours of care.[40] Although total volume requirements are difficult to predict at the onset of resuscitation, empiric crystalloid loading (40-60 mL/kg) within the first hours of care generally is indicated and well tolerated.[46]

Persistent hypoperfusion following initial volume loading of more than 60 mL/kg crystalloid complicates up to 50% of severe sepsis cases.[47] Continuation of additional empiric fluid resuscitation under the assumption of ongoing volume responsiveness risks delaying other appropriate therapy and contributes to unnecessary fluid overload.[48,49] A rational approach to this situation incorporates the selection and titration of subsequent therapy under the guidance of objective cardiovascular monitoring. In the absence of conflicting data, a target central venous pressure (CVP) of 8 to 12 mm Hg is often recommended to optimize preload.[40] Unfortunately, pressure surrogates of preload are poor predictors of fluid response, and there is no consistent threshold of CVP to reliably estimate response to fluid.[50] The optimization of cardiac preload is more complicated than the achievement of a specific CVP goal. Additional bedside tools to ascertain volume responsiveness are described in the chapters on ultrasound and fluid management.

Historically, the targeted endpoint used to guide the dose

TABLE 12-3. Components of the 2015 *Surviving Sepsis Campaign* Bundle
To be completed within 3 hours of arrival:
Measure lactate level.
Obtain blood cultures before giving antibiotics.
Administer broad-spectrum antibiotics.
Administer 30 mL/kg for hypotension or lactate ≥4.
To be completed within 6 hours of arrival:
Apply vasopressors to maintain MAP ≥65 mm Hg.
Remeasure lactate if initial lactate was elevated.
If hypotension persists after initial fluid or initial lactate is ≥4 mmol/L, reassess and document volume status and tissue perfusion via a repeat focused patient examination or two of the following: • CVP measurements • $ScvO_2$ measurements • Bedside ultrasound • Dynamic assessment of fluid responsiveness with passive leg raise or IVF challenge

of resuscitation fluid appeared to be more important than the product chosen (ie, crystalloid versus colloid). Isotonic crystalloids remain the standard initial resuscitation agents due to their widespread availability and cost advantage over colloids. Balanced crystalloid solutions, with a chemical composition approximating that of extracellular fluid, are gaining popularity. This trend follows data indicating the adverse impact of normal saline-induced hyperchloremia on acid-base status, organ function, and patient outcomes.[51] The use of balanced crystalloid solutions in adults with sepsis is associated with reduced mortality.[52,53]

Colloid solutions, composed of electrolyte preparations fortified with large-molecular-weight molecules, provide greater hemodynamic response compared with a given dose of isotonic crystalloid.[54] Although previously considered equally effective when titrated to the same clinical endpoints, crystalloid solutions require 2 to 4 times more volume for equivalent resuscitation. This volume-sparing effect theoretically limits interstitial edema in situations where it could threaten organ function (eg, hypoxemic lung injury, abdominal ascites, or compartment syndrome). Recent meta-analyses demonstrate the safety and improved survival rate associated with albumin use in sepsis resuscitation.[53,55] The early addition of hyperoncotic albumin appears to reduce mortality in patients with spontaneous bacterial peritonitis and end-stage liver disease.[56]

Semisynthetic colloid starch solutions, including hydroxyethyl starch (HES), are under scrutiny; recent trials cast doubt on their safety due to nephrotoxicity and adverse outcomes.[57,58] The routine use of semisynthetic colloids is not recommended, pending additional data.

Vasopressor Support

In patients with sepsis, abnormal vasomotor tone and impaired vascular reactivity manifest as persistent hypotension despite fluid optimization. The goal of vasopressor therapy is to restore blood pressure within the organ autoregulatory range. Fluid optimization ideally should be achieved prior to the initiation of catecholamine support; however, patients with severe hemodynamic compromise can require vasopressors early and in the midst of ongoing volume resuscitation. A MAP target of 65 mm Hg is recommended. Titrating vasopressors to higher targets is not associated with consistent benefit in regional perfusion, but individualized therapy may be indicated to maintain organ blood flow in patients with right-shifted autoregulation.[59] In one randomized trial, targeting MAP at 80 to 85 mm Hg in septic shock patients with chronic hypertension was associated with reduced acute renal failure requiring renal replacement therapy.[60] Invasive arterial monitoring should be considered in patients exhibiting persistent hypotension and requiring catecholamine support.

Norepinephrine is generally considered the vasopressor of choice because of its availability, effectiveness, and wide dosing range. Dopamine is not recommended in the absence of inappropriate bradycardia due to an increased risk of arrhythmia.[61] There is no role for "renal dose" (low-dose) dopamine in attempts to preserve renal function during vasopressor support.[62] Vasodilatory shock is associated with endogenous vasopressin deficiency and is responsive to vasopressin replacement. Vasopressin (0.01–0.04 units/min IV) may be used as an adjunct for hypotension refractory to typical doses of catecholamine therapy, although it does not appear to reduce the risk of death.[63] Dose escalation can trigger ischemic complications and is not recommended.

TABLE 12-4. Prioritized Endpoints of Resuscitation

1. Adequate intravenous access
2. Preload optimization:
   - Serial fluid challenges guided by clinical examination and patient response and tolerance
   - CVP ≥8 mm Hg (≥12 mm Hg if mechanically ventilated)
   - Fluid guided by measures of volume responsiveness
3. Mean arterial pressure ≥65 mm Hg
4. Sustain organ perfusion and match oxygen delivery and consumption. Clinical regional markers include:
   - Cutaneous perfusion
   - Urine output >0.5 mL/kg/hr
   - Mental status

   Global markers:
   - $ScvO_2$ ≥70%
   - Lactate clearance and normalization

Endpoints of Resuscitation

The ultimate goal of resuscitation is to restore oxygen delivery and tissue perfusion to meet global and regional metabolic needs. However, the most appropriate endpoint for resuscitation remains controversial. Although the procedure historically aimed to normalize clinical markers, a growing body of evidence shows that targeting blood pressure, pulse, CVP, and urine output fails to guarantee normal organ perfusion.[36,39] Macrocirculatory markers, especially blood pressure, provide little insight into regional perfusion or the balance of systemic oxygen delivery and utilization, such that resuscitation aimed at these targets risks leaving the patient in compensated shock.[64,65]

Serum lactate concentration and central venous oxygen saturation ($ScvO_2$), two quantifiable objective markers of global perfusion and physiological stress, provide useful gauges for resuscitation. The corollary of serum lactate as a marker of adverse outcomes can be used to corroborate an appropriate response to therapy. Rapid lactate clearance appears to improve survival, whereas persistent hyperlactatemia is associated with organ failure and death. The degree of lactate clearance is inversely related to risk.[66] Lactate clearance greater than 10% per hour is a common goal, although lactate normalization (<2 mmol/L) is most strongly associated with survival.[67,68] In one trial, targeting lactate clearance as a primary resuscitation endpoint was equivalent to targeting the normalization of

$ScvO_2$.[69] The study also revealed a poor correlation between lactate clearance and $ScvO_2$, implying that each measure provides insight into distinct physiological processes.[70]

$ScvO_2$ reflects the systemic balance of oxygen delivery and utilization. Limited oxygen delivery is compensated by enhanced tissue extraction, resulting in a fall in $ScvO_2$ below the normal 70%. In contrast to lactate kinetics, the $ScvO_2$ response is rapid and dynamic, such that monitoring provides immediate feedback on resuscitation efforts (or clinical deterioration).

$ScvO_2$ normalization was a central management target in one pivotal early goal-directed therapy trial.[36] The endpoint's subsequent integration into institutional protocols and the *Surviving Sepsis Campaign* corroborates its value in improving outcomes.[37,71] The maximum $ScvO_2$ achieved during the first 6 hours of care is associated with clinical outcomes. Patients with persistent venous hypoxia have a mortality rate nearly double that of patients in whom normalization is achieved.[72,73]

Despite these data, three recent randomized trials found no systematic outcome difference with early goal-directed septic shock management aimed at normalizing $ScvO_2$.[5,46,74] The early aggressive resuscitation of control patients calls into question the generalizability of these findings to situations in which the same intensity of care is not standard. The results suggest that other endpoints might be comparable gauges of resuscitation and that routine central venous cannulation to facilitate measuring $ScvO_2$ is unnecessary for this sole indication. Currently, $ScvO_2$ remains a pragmatic benchmark of resuscitation when central venous access is available.

Persistent shock, clinical malperfusion, hyperlactatemia, and central venous hypoxia should prompt consideration for intervention, as the normalization of any single endpoint does not guarantee adequate systemic perfusion. A multimodal approach, seeking to normalize a combination of global and regional perfusion and metabolic markers as quickly as possible, is most prudent *(Table 12-4)*.[75] Urine output and clinical perfusion, including skin perfusion, remain legitimate barometers of resuscitation and should be monitored serially.[24,25]

Perfusion Optimization

Treatment targets are inextricably tied to resuscitation and guide therapies that influence clinical outcomes. Persistent malperfusion, as indicated by a failure to restore physiological endpoints of resuscitation despite preload and blood pressure optimization, warrants consideration of additional therapy to reduce metabolic demand or enhance oxygen delivery.

Respiration and hyperthermia are two common sources of enhanced oxygen consumption in infected patients. Even in the absence of hypoxemia, the work and metabolic cost of breathing during acute sepsis can be substantial, diverting blood flow from other vital organs.[76] Persistent malperfusion, including hyperlactatemia and venous hypoxia, often responds to the initiation of mechanical ventilation in this situation.[77] Noninvasive ventilation can help manage evolving respiratory insufficiency; however, this approach should be reserved for awake and cooperative patients without severe hypoxemia.

Cardiac dysfunction is common in patients with severe sepsis as a consequence of chronic disease or acute sepsis-associated cardiomyopathy.[78,79] Elevated cardiac filling pressures are clues to cardiac dysfunction in those who fail to meet resuscitation endpoints. Dobutamine is the preferred inotrope to augment cardiac performance. Low-dose initiation (2.5 mcg/kg/min IV) is recommended to monitor for adverse hypotension or tachycardia, with subsequent titration to clinical effect. Milrinone is an alternative treatment for significant tachycardia or patients using beta-blockers.

A red blood cell transfusion can be used to augment oxygen-carrying capacity in patients with a persistent oxygen delivery-consumption mismatch despite cardiac performance optimization. There is little evidence to declare the optimal

TABLE 12-5. Priorities of Infection Control

1. **Identify source.**
2. **Initiate culture collection. Do not allow this to significantly delay antibiotics.**
3. **Administer antibiotics within 1 hour of recognition of severe sepsis.**
4. **Provide broad-spectrum antibiotics.**
   - Empiric selections should be based on suspected source and risk for drug-resistant organisms.
   - Consider atypical organisms.
   - Choose drug appropriate for host target tissue penetration.
   - Use full loading antibiotic dose.
   - Consider rapid and simultaneous administration of the first antibiotic doses.
5. **Provide decompressive source control when indicated. Minimally invasive procedures are preferred.**

TABLE 12-6. Common Infections Warranting Possible Emergency Source Control

Control Technique	Sources
Device removal	Infected implant
	Infected vascular access
	Urinary catheter
Drainage/ Decompression	Abscess
	Cholangitis
	Pyelonephritis with ureteral obstruction
	Septic arthritis
	Thoracic empyema
Débridement	Complicated soft-tissue infection
	Intestinal infarction
	Mediastinitis
	Small-bowel obstruction

hemoglobin level for cases of acute severe infection. A restrictive transfusion strategy targeting a hemoglobin concentration of 7 to 9 g/dL is not associated with an increased mortality rate in critically ill patients.[80] However, this strategy has not been investigated in patients undergoing acute resuscitation. Transfusion may be considered for cases of critical anemia, defined by persistent hypoperfusion despite measures to reduce metabolic demand and optimize cardiac performance.

Early Antibiotics and Source Control

Source identification and effective infection control are central goals during the early resuscitation of patients with life-threatening infection. Blood and other culture specimens are optimally collected prior to the administration of antibiotics, but sampling should not significantly delay therapy. Time to initiation of effective antimicrobial therapy is an important determinant of outcomes for both pediatric and adult patients.[81] Increased mortality is associated with brief delays in therapy; thus antibiotics should be administered as soon as possible (within 1 hour of severe sepsis recognition is a commonly recommended benchmark).[82-84] Empiric coverage should be broad enough to cover all suspected culprit organisms, as inappropriate therapy is associated with a 5-fold reduction in survival.[85] Patients with resistant and atypical organisms (eg, methicillin-resistant *Staphylococcus aureus*, vancomycin-resistant enterococci, and extended-spectrum, beta-lactamase-producing gram-negative rods) are more likely to suffer the consequences of inappropriate empiric therapy. The initiation of medication should be individualized according to the patient's drug tolerance, recent antibiotic exposure, local microbe resistance patterns, suspected source, and host immune status *(Table 12-5)*.

Anatomical source identification should always be coupled with consideration of definitive infection control measures *(Table 12-6)*. Common foci of infection that are amenable to intervention include peritonitis, intestinal ischemia, cholangitis, pyelonephritis, empyema, indwelling vascular hardware, septic arthritis, necrotizing soft-tissue infection, and other deep cutaneous infections. Drainage, débridement, and removal of these sources often require coordinated multidisciplinary efforts. Source control is an essential component of acute resuscitation and should not be delayed in the hope of improved cardiovascular stabilization. Percutaneous drainage, when available, generally is preferred over open débridement to minimize additional physiological insults.

TABLE 12-7. Adjunctive Therapies for Severe Sepsis

Steroid therapy for refractory septic shock: hydrocortisone (100 mg IV, then 200–300 mg/day in divided doses)
Intravenous immunoglobulin: 1 gm/kg IV

Adjunctive Therapies

A number of adjunctive therapies play potential roles in the management of severe sepsis *(Table 12-7)*. Inadequate adrenal response in the setting of acute critical illness is called *relative adrenal insufficiency*. Steroid supplementation aims to replace physiological hormone function in patients with inadequate reserves. The ability to diagnose this condition is limited because of inconsistencies in proposed criteria and cortisol immunoassays.[86] Adrenocorticotropic hormone testing is not advised to select infected patients for steroid therapy.

TABLE 12-8. Evidence-Based Critical Care Support Therapies

Sterile barrier precautions for all invasive procedures
Safe mechanical ventilation: • Low Vt <7 mL/kg (ideal body weight) • Plateau airway pressure <30 cm H_2O • Endotracheal tube cuff pressure <25 cm H_2O
Aspiration precautions during mechanical ventilation: • Head of bed elevation >30°–45° unless contraindicated • Orogastric or nasogastric tube decompression
Blood sugar control (goal <180 mg/dL)
Prophylaxis: • Gastrointestinal stress ulcer prophylaxis • Deep venous thrombosis prophylaxis

KEY POINTS

1. Lactate is a powerful screening biomarker for infected patients at high risk of complicated disease. Lactate measurements are encouraged in all infected patients considered for hospital admission.
2. The immediate goal of cardiovascular support is to restore and maintain systemic oxygen delivery and end-organ perfusion.
3. Restoration of blood pressure does not guarantee normalized perfusion; additional clinical and laboratory markers should be used to gauge resuscitation adequacy.
4. There is no single best endpoint of resuscitation for all patients or clinical circumstances.
5. Serial single-unit packed cell transfusions are most appropriately guided by resuscitation targets rather than arbitrary hemoglobin goals.
6. Infection control in the form of antibiotics and source control is part of early resuscitation.
7. Antibiotic initiation should be prioritized within 1 hour after the recognition of severe sepsis.
8. Drainage, débridement, and removal of infection sources should not be delayed for anticipated hemodynamic stabilization.

Patients exhibiting vasopressor-refractory shock are candidates for intravenous steroids. Stress-dose steroids are also indicated for patients with severe sepsis and known adrenal dysfunction or chronic steroid dependency even in the absence of shock. Hydrocortisone is the preferred agent and promotes shock reversal, although its mortality benefit remains unclear.[87,88] Dexamethasone is a suboptimal substitute for hydrocortisone, and high-dose corticosteroids are potentially harmful and not indicated for acute infection.

Theoretically, polyvalent intravenous immunoglobulin (IVIG) provides a protective effect in patients with sepsis via several immunomodulating pathways. To date, pooled analyses have failed to provide a clear consensus on the role of various IVIG formulations in the management of severe sepsis and septic shock in adults.[89,90] However, the agent remains a recommended adjunct in the treatment of streptococcal toxic shock syndrome.[91]

Supportive Therapies

The fragility of critically ill patients warrants detailed attention to routine care components. Challenges stemming from delayed ICU admission due to hospital overcrowding reinforce the early implementation of evidence-based support strategies *(Table 12-8)*.

Sepsis is the most common cause of acute respiratory distress syndrome (ARDS); many patients with this condition require mechanical ventilation. Adequate gas exchange and lung protection are the overriding principles of ventilator management. Volume control is the most preferred mode of ventilation unless otherwise indicated. Appropriate mechanical ventilation targets low tidal volume (Vt; Vt <7 mL/kg ideal body weight) and plateau airway pressure less than 30 cm H_2O.[92] Pulmonary shear and strain caused by high Vt contribute to the progression of ARDS. The same low-Vt management strategy should be extrapolated to acute critically ill patients without hypoxemia or abnormal lung compliance.[93]

Derangements of blood glucose concentrations are common during critical illness and are associated with worse outcomes.[94] Diabetic complications, including ketoacidosis and severe hyperglycemia, warrant early treatment to control blood sugar. Maintenance of strict normoglycemia during critical illness is associated with hypoglycemia and does not confer a mortality benefit.[95] Current evidence supports targeting blood sugar levels below 180 mg/dL via intermittent subcutaneous insulin injections or an insulin infusion following stabilization.[96] Patients with severe sepsis are at risk for hypoglycemia even without insulin therapy, so the blood glucose concentration should be monitored serially during resuscitation.

Conclusion

Severe sepsis and septic shock are the most commonly encountered critical illnesses in the emergency department. Emergency physicians are uniquely positioned to affect morbidity and mortality in patients with acute infection. The rapid identification of high-risk patients with suspected infection is the first step. Key components of immediate care focus on early antibiotic administration and cardiovascular resuscitation in the form of fluid therapy and vasopressor support.

REFERENCES

1. Dombrovskiy VY, Martin AA, Sunderram J, Paz HL. Rapid increase in hospitalization and mortality rates for severe sepsis in the United States: a trend analysis from 1993 to 2003. *Crit Care Med.* 2007;35(5):1244-1250.
2. Kumar G, Kumar N, Taneja A, et al. Nationwide trends of severe sepsis in the 21st century (2000-2007). *Chest.* 2011;140(5):1223-1231.
3. Liu V, Escobar GJ, Greene JD, et al. Hospital deaths in patients with sepsis from 2 independent cohorts. *JAMA.* 2014;312(1):90-92.
4. Hall MJ, Williams SN, DeFrances CJ, Golosinskiy A. Inpatient care for septicemia or sepsis: a challenge for patients and hospitals. *NCHS Data Brief.* 2011;(62):1-8.
5. Yealy DM, Kellum JA, Huang DT, et al. A randomized trial of protocol-based care for early septic shock. *N Engl J Med.* 2014;370(18):1683-1693.
6. Heffner AC, Horton JM, Marchick MR, Jones AE. Etiology of illness in patients with severe sepsis admitted to the hospital from the emergency department. *Clin Infect Dis.* 2010;50(6):814-820.
7. Bone RC. Toward an epidemiology and natural history of SIRS (systemic inflammatory response syndrome). *JAMA.* 1992;268(24):3452-3455.
8. Bone RC, Balk RA, Cerra FB, et al. Definitions for sepsis and organ failure and guidelines for the use of innovative therapies in sepsis. The ACCP/SCCM Consensus Conference Committee. American College of Chest Physicians/Society of Critical Care Medicine. *Chest.* 1992;101(6):1644-1655.
9. Rangel-Frausto MS, Pittet D, Costigan M, et al. The natural history of the systemic inflammatory response syndrome (SIRS). A prospective study. *JAMA.* 1995;273(2):117-123.
10. Brun-Buisson C. The epidemiology of the systemic inflammatory response. *Intensive Care Med.* 2000;26 (suppl 1):S64-S74.
11. Sands KE, Bates DW, Lanken PN, et al. Epidemiology of sepsis syndrome in 8 academic medical centers. *JAMA.* 1997;278(3):234-240.
12. Horeczko T, Green JP, Panacek EA. Epidemiology of the systemic inflammatory response syndrome (SIRS) in the emergency department. *West J Emerg Med.* 2014;15(3):329-336.
13. Smith SW, Pheley A, Collier R, et al. Severe sepsis in the emergency department and its association with a complicated clinical course. *Acad Emerg Med.* 1998;5(12):1169-1176.
14. Kaukonen KM, Bailey M, Pilcher D, et al. Systemic inflammatory response syndrome criteria in defining severe sepsis. *N Engl J Med.* 2015;372(17):1629-1638.
15. Dremsizov T, Clemont G, Kellum JA, et al. Severe sepsis in community-acquired pneumonia: when does it happen, and do systemic inflammatory response syndrome criteria help predict course? *Chest.* 2006;129(4):968-978.
16. Seigel TA, Cocchi MN, Salciccioli J, et al. Inadequacy of temperature and white blood cell count in predicting bacteremia in patients with suspected infection. *J Emerg Med.* 2012;42(3):254-259.
17. Lindvig KP, Henriksen DP, Nielsen SL, et al. How do bacteraemic patients present to the emergency department and what is the diagnostic validity of the clinical parameters; temperature, C-reactive protein and systemic inflammatory response syndrome? *Scand J Trauma Resusc Emerg Med.* 2014;22:39.
18. Capp R, Horton CL, Takhar SS, et al. Predictors of patients who present to the emergency department with sepsis and progress to septic shock between 4 and 48 hours of emergency department arrival. *Crit Care Med.* 2015;43(5):983-988.
19. Glickman SW, Cairns CB, Otero RM, et al. Disease progression in hemodynamically stable patients presenting to the emergency department with sepsis. *Acad Emerg Med.* 2010;17(4):383-390.
20. Jones AE, Yiannibas V, Johnson C, Kline JA. Emergency department hypotension predicts sudden unexpected in-hospital mortality: a prospective cohort study. *Chest.* 2006;130(4):941-946.
21. Marchick MR, Kline JA, Jones AE. The significance of non-sustained hypotension in emergency department patients with sepsis. *Intensive Care Med.* 2009;35(7):1261-1264.
22. Bagshaw SM, George C, Bellomo R. Early acute kidney injury and sepsis: a multicentre evaluation. *Crit Care.* 2008;12(2):R47.
23. Joannidis M, Metnitz B, Bauer P, et al. Acute kidney injury in critically ill patients classified by AKIN versus RIFLE using the SAPS 3 database. *Intensive Care Med.* 2009;35(10):1692-1702.
24. Ait-Oufella H, Bige N, Boelle PY, et al. Capillary refill time exploration during septic shock. *Intensive Care Med.* 2014;40(7):958-964.
25. Ait-Oufella H, Lemoinne S, Boelle PY, et al. Mottling score predicts survival in septic shock. *Intensive Care Med.* 2011;37(5):801-807.
26. Smith I, Kumar P, Molloy S, et al. Base excess and lactate as prognostic indicators for patients admitted to intensive care. *Intensive Care Med.* 2001;27(1):74-83.
27. Bakker J, Coffernils M, Leon M, et al. Blood lactate levels are superior to oxygen-derived variables in predicting outcome in human septic shock. *Chest.* 1991;99(4):956-962.
28. Levy B, Gibot S, Franck P, et al. Relation between muscle Na+K+ ATPase activity and raised lactate concentrations in septic shock: a prospective study. *Lancet.* 2005;365(9462):871-875.
29. Trzeciak S, Dellinger RP, Chansky ME, et al. Serum lactate as a predictor of mortality in patients with infection. *Intensive Care Med.* 2007;33(6):970-977.
30. Howell MD, Donnino M, et al. Occult hypoperfusion and mortality in patients with suspected infection. *Intensive Care Med.* 2007;33(11):1892-1899.
31. Shapiro NI, Howell MD, Talmor D, et al. Serum lactate as a predictor of mortality in emergency department patients with infection. *Ann Emerg Med.* 2005;45(5):524-528.

32. Casserly B, Phillips GS, Schorr C, et al. Lactate measurements in sepsis-induced tissue hypoperfusion: results from the surviving sepsis campaign database. *Crit Care Med.* 2015;43(3):567-573.
33. Singer M, Deutschman CS, Seymour CW, et al. The Third International Consensus Definitions for Sepsis and Septic Shock (Sepsis-3). *JAMA.* 2016;315(8):801-810.
34. Shankar-Hari M, Phillips GS, Levy ML, et al. Developing a New Definition and Assessing New Clinical Criteria for Septic Shock. *JAMA.* 2016;315(8):775.
35. Seymour CW, Liu VX, Iwashyna TJ, et al. Assessment of Clinical Criteria for Sepsis. *JAMA.* 2016;315(8):762.
36. Rivers E, Nguyen B, Havstad S, et al. Early goal-directed therapy in the treatment of severe sepsis and septic shock. *N Engl J Med.* 2001;345(19):1368-1377.
37. Rivers EP, Coba V, Whitmill M. Early goal-directed therapy in severe sepsis and septic shock: a contemporary review of the literature. *Curr Opin Anaesthesiol.* 2008;21(2):128-140.
38. Puskarich MA, Marchick MR, Kline JA, et al. One year mortality of patients treated with an emergency department based early goal directed therapy protocol for severe sepsis and septic shock: a before and after study. *Crit Care.* 2009;13(5):R167.
39. Gu WJ, Wang F, Bakker J, et al. The effect of goal-directed therapy on mortality in patients with sepsis–earlier is better: a meta-analysis of randomized controlled trials. *Crit Care.* 2014;18(5):570.
40. Dellinger RP, Levy MM, Rhodes A, et al. Surviving sepsis campaign: international guidelines for management of severe sepsis and septic shock: 2012. *Crit Care Med.* 2013;41(2):580-637.
41. Gao F, Melody T, Daniels DF, et al. The impact of compliance with 6-hour and 24-hour sepsis bundles on hospital mortality in patients with severe sepsis: a prospective observational study. *Crit Care.* 2005;9(6):R764-R770.
42. Nguyen HB, Corbett SW, Steele R, et al. Implementation of a bundle of quality indicators for the early management of severe sepsis and septic shock is associated with decreased mortality. *Crit Care Med.* 2007;35(4):1105-1112.
43. Barochia AV, Cui X, Vitberg D, et al. Bundled care for septic shock: an analysis of clinical trials. *Crit Care Med.* 2010;38(2):668-678.
44. Marshall JC, Cook DJ, Christou NV, et al. Multiple organ dysfunction score: a reliable descriptor of a complex clinical outcome. *Crit Care Med.* 1995;23(10):1638-1652.
45. Jones AE, Brown MD, Trzeciak S, et al. The effect of a quantitative resuscitation strategy on mortality in patients with sepsis: a meta-analysis. *Crit Care Med.* 2008;36(10):2734-2739.
46. Peake SL, Delaney A, Bailey M, et al. Goal-directed resuscitation for patients with early septic shock. *N Engl J Med.* 2014;371(16):1496-1506.
47. Hollenberg SM, Ahrens TS, Annane D, et al. Practice parameters for hemodynamic support of sepsis in adult patients: 2004 update. *Crit Care Med.* 2004;32(9):1928-1948.
48. Michard F, Boussat S, Chemla D, et al. Relation between respiratory changes in arterial pulse pressure and fluid responsiveness in septic patients with acute circulatory failure. *Am J Respir Crit Care Med.* 2000;162(1):134-138.
49. Michard F, Teboul JL. Predicting fluid responsiveness in ICU patients: a critical analysis of the evidence. *Chest.* 2002;121(6):2000-2008.
50. Marik PE, Cavallazzi R, Vasu T, Hirani A. Dynamic changes in arterial waveform derived variables and fluid responsiveness in mechanically ventilated patients: a systematic review of the literature. *Crit Care Med.* 2009;37(9):2642-2647.
51. Yunos NM, Bellomo R, Hegarty C, et al. Association between a chloride-liberal vs chloride-restrictive intravenous fluid administration strategy and kidney injury in critically ill adults. *JAMA.* 2012;308(15):1566-1572.
52. Raghunathan K, Shaw A, Nathanson B, et al. Association between the choice of IV crystalloid and in-hospital mortality among critically ill adults with sepsis. *Crit Care Med.* 2014;42(7):1585-1591.
53. Rochwerg B, Alhazzani W, Sindi A, et al. Fluid resuscitation in sepsis: a systematic review and network meta-analysis. *Ann Intern Med.* 2014;161(5):347-355.
54. Trof RJ, Sukul SP, Twisk JW, et al. Greater cardiac response of colloid than saline fluid loading in septic and non-septic critically ill patients with clinical hypovolaemia. *Intensive Care Med.* 2010;36(4):697-701.
55. Delaney AP, Dan A, McCaffrey J, Finfer S. The role of albumin as a resuscitation fluid for patients with sepsis: a systematic review and meta-analysis. *Crit Care Med.* 2011;39(2):386-391.
56. Sort P, Navasa M, Arroyo V, et al. Effect of intravenous albumin on renal impairment and mortality in patients with cirrhosis and spontaneous bacterial peritonitis. *N Engl J Med.* 1999;341(6):403-409.
57. Perner A, Haase N, Guttormsen AB, et al. Hydroxyethyl starch 130/0.42 versus Ringer's acetate in severe sepsis. *N Engl J Med.* 2012;367(2):124-134.
58. Myburgh JA, Finfer S, Bellomo R, et al. Hydroxyethyl starch or saline for fluid resuscitation in intensive care. *N Engl J Med.* 2012;367(20):1901-1911.
59. LeDoux D, Astiz ME, Carpati CM, Rackow EC. Effects of perfusion pressure on tissue perfusion in septic shock. *Crit Care Med.* 2000;28(8):2729-2732.
60. Asfar P, Meziani F, Hamel JF, et al. High versus low blood-pressure target in patients with septic shock. *N Engl J Med.* 2014;370(17):1583-1593.
61. De BD, Biston P, Devriendt J, et al. Comparison of dopamine and norepinephrine in the treatment of shock. *N Engl J Med.* 2010;362(9):779-789.
62. Kellum JA, Decker M. Use of dopamine in acute renal failure: a meta-analysis. *Crit Care Med.* 2001;29(8):1526-1531.
63. Russell JA, Walley KR, Singer J, et al. Vasopressin versus norepinephrine infusion in patients with septic shock. *N Engl J Med.* 2008;358(9):877-887.
64. Rady MY, Rivers EP, Nowak RM. Resuscitation of the critically ill in the ED: responses of blood pressure, heart rate, shock index, central venous oxygen saturation, and lactate. *Am J Emerg Med.* 1996;14(2):218-225.
65. Poeze M, Solberg BC, Greve JW, Ramsay G. Monitoring global volume-related hemodynamic or regional variables after initial resuscitation: what is a better predictor of outcome in critically ill septic patients? *Crit Care Med.* 2005;33(11):2494-2500.
66. Bakker J, Gris P, Coffernils M, et al. Serial blood lactate levels can predict the development of multiple organ failure following septic shock. *Am J Surg.* 1996;171(2):221-226.
67. Nguyen HB, Rivers EP, Knoblich BP, et al. Early lactate clearance is associated with improved outcome in severe sepsis and septic shock. *Crit Care Med.* 2004;32(8):1637-1642.
68. Puskarich MA, Trzeciak S, Shapiro NI, et al. Whole blood lactate kinetics in patients undergoing quantitative resuscitation for severe sepsis and septic shock. *Chest.* 2013;143(6):1548-1553.
69. Jones AE, Shapiro NI, Trzeciak S, et al. Lactate clearance vs central venous oxygen saturation as goals of early sepsis therapy: a randomized clinical trial. *JAMA.* 2010;303(8):739-746.
70. Puskarich MA, Trzeciak S, Shapiro NI, et al. Prognostic value and agreement of achieving lactate clearance or central venous oxygen saturation goals during early sepsis resuscitation. *Acad Emerg Med.* 2012;19(3):252-258.
71. Levy MM, Dellinger RP, Townsend SR, et al. The Surviving Sepsis Campaign: results of an international guideline-based performance improvement program targeting severe sepsis. *Crit Care Med.* 2010;38(2):367-374.
72. Pope JV, Jones AE, Gaieski DF, et al. Multicenter study of central venous oxygen saturation (ScvO(2)) as a predictor of mortality in patients with sepsis. *Ann Emerg Med.* 2010;55(1):40-46.
73. Castellanos-Ortega A, Suberviola B, Garcia-Astudillo LA, et al. Impact of the Surviving Sepsis Campaign protocols on hospital length of stay and mortality in septic shock patients: results of a three-year follow-up quasi-experimental study. *Crit Care Med.* 2010;38(4):1036-1043.
74. Mouncey PR, Osborn TM, Power GS, et al. Trial of early, goal-directed resuscitation for septic shock. *N Engl J Med.* 2015;372(14):1301-1311.
75. Hernandez G, Pedreros C, Veas E, et al. Evolution of peripheral vs metabolic perfusion parameters during septic shock resuscitation. A clinical-physiologic study. *J Crit Care.* 2012;27(3):283-288.
76. Robertson CH Jr, Pagel MA, Johnson RL Jr. The distribution of blood flow, oxygen consumption, and work output among the respiratory muscles during unobstructed hyperventilation. *J Clin Invest.* 1977;59(1):43-50.
77. Hernandez G, Pena H, Cornejo R, et al. Impact of emergency intubation on central venous oxygen saturation in critically ill patients: a multicenter observational study. *Crit Care.* 2009;13(3):R63.
78. Parrillo JE, Burch C, Shelhamer JH, et al. A circulating myocardial depressant substance in humans with septic shock. Septic shock patients with a reduced ejection fraction have a circulating factor that depresses in vitro myocardial cell performance. *J Clin Invest.* 1985;76(4):1539-1553.
79. Jardin F, Fourme T, Page B, et al. Persistent preload defect in severe sepsis despite fluid loading: A longitudinal echocardiographic study in patients with septic shock. *Chest.* 1999;116(5):1354-1359.
80. Hebert PC, Wells G, Blajchman MA, et al. A multicenter, randomized, controlled clinical trial of transfusion requirements in critical care. Transfusion Requirements in Critical Care Investigators, Canadian Critical Care Trials Group. *N Engl J Med.* 1999;340(6):409-417.
81. Weiss SL, Fitzgerald JC, Balamuth F, et al. Delayed antimicrobial therapy increases mortality and organ dysfunction duration in pediatric sepsis. *Crit Care Med.* 2014;42(11):2409-2417.
82. Kumar A, Roberts D, Wood KE, et al. Duration of hypotension before initiation of effective antimicrobial therapy is the critical determinant of survival in human septic shock. *Crit Care Med.* 2006;34(6):1589-1596.
83. Gaieski DF, Mikkelsen ME, Band RA, et al. Impact of time to antibiotics on survival in patients with severe sepsis or septic shock in whom early goal-directed therapy was initiated in the emergency department. *Crit Care Med.* 2010;38(4):1045-1053.
84. Ferrer R, Artigas A, Levy MM, et al. Improvement in process of care and outcome after a multicenter severe sepsis educational program in Spain. *JAMA.* 2008;299(19):2294-2303.
85. Kumar A, Ellis P, Arabi Y, et al. Initiation of inappropriate antimicrobial therapy results in a fivefold reduction of survival in human septic shock. *Chest.* 2009;136(5):1237-1248.
86. Briegel J, Sprung CL, Annane D, et al. Multicenter comparison of cortisol as measured by different methods in samples of patients with septic shock. *Intensive Care Med.* 2009;35(12):2151-2156.
87. Annane D, Sebille V, Charpentier C, et al. Effect of treatment with low doses of hydrocortisone and fludrocortisone on mortality in patients with septic shock. *JAMA.* 2002;288(7):862-871.
88. Sprung CL, Annane D, Keh D, et al. Hydrocortisone therapy for patients with septic shock. *N Engl J Med.* 2008;358(2):111-124.
89. Laupland KB, Kirkpatrick AW, Delaney A. Polyclonal intravenous immunoglobulin for the treatment of severe sepsis and septic shock in critically ill adults: a systematic review and meta-analysis. *Crit Care Med.* 2007;35(12):2682-2692.
90. Turgeon AF, Hutton B, Fergusson DA, et al. Meta-analysis: intravenous immunoglobulin in critically ill adult patients with sepsis. *Ann Intern Med.* 2007;146(3):193-203.
91. Norrby-Teglund A, Muller MP, Mcgeer A, et al. Successful management of severe group A streptococcal soft tissue infections using an aggressive medical regimen including intravenous polyspecific immunoglobulin together with a conservative surgical approach. *Scand J Infect Dis.* 2005;37(3):166-172.
92. Ventilation with lower tidal volumes as compared with traditional tidal volumes for acute lung injury and the acute respiratory distress syndrome. The Acute Respiratory Distress Syndrome Network. *N Engl J Med.* 2000;342(18):1301-1308.
93. Determann RM, Royakkers A, Wolthuis EK, et al. Ventilation with lower tidal volumes as compared with conventional tidal volumes for patients without acute lung injury: a preventive randomized controlled trial. *Crit Care.* 2010;14(1):R1.
94. Krinsley JS. Association between hyperglycemia and increased hospital mortality in a heterogeneous population of critically ill patients. *Mayo Clin Proc.* 2003;78(12):1471-1478.
95. Griesdale DE, de Souza RJ, van Dam RM, et al. Intensive insulin therapy and mortality among critically ill patients: a meta-analysis including NICE-SUGAR study data. *CMAJ.* 2009;180(8):821-827.
96. Finfer S, Chittock DR, Su SY, et al. Intensive versus conventional glucose control in critically ill patients. *N Engl J Med.* 2009;360(13):1283-1297.

The Crashing Morbidly Obese Patient

13

IN THIS CHAPTER

- Special pharmacological requirements
- Respiratory management
- Predicting the difficult airway
- Patient positioning
- Circulatory management
- Resuscitation and monitoring

Timothy Ellender, Gregory Ruppel, and Brian Oloizia

Obesity is one of the most serious public health crises to emerge in the last century.[1-5] Despite a growing awareness of its risks, including heart disease, type 2 diabetes, obstructive sleep apnea, certain cancers, and osteoarthritis, the number of Americans afflicted by the disease continues to rise.[2,5,7-11] In the United States, obesity is defined by a body mass index (BMI; calculated by dividing weight by the square of the person's height) exceeding 30 kg/m^2.[3,6] On either side of that demarcation is the overweight category (BMI = 25-30 kg/m^2) and the severely or morbidly obese (>40 kg/m^2).[6]

Obesity can shave an estimated 6 to 10 years off a patient's life expectancy and also significant challenges to the American medical system, including increased health care utilization and expenditures.[2,5,11-18] Specifically, it has influenced practice changes in almost all major medical specialties, including adult primary care, pediatrics, surgery, and emergency medicine.[2,12,15,16,19-26] The emergency department resuscitation of the crashing obese patient presents further intellectual, procedural, and technical difficulties that emergency practitioners must be prepared to manage.[26] A thorough understanding of the unique anatomical, hemodynamic, and respiratory requirements of this patient population is vital.

Pharmacological Management

Morbid obesity significantly alters pharmacokinetics as a result of changes in volume of distribution, protein binding, hepatic metabolism, and renal clearance.[27-32] Both direct and indirect methodologies have been used to assess body composition and its effects on drug activity.[29,33] Direct methods are not readily available in most clinical settings, thus indirect measures, which rely on patient attributes such as body weight, height, and sex, are most commonly used.[32] Derivations of these anthropomorphic metrics frequently are employed in the clinical setting.[29] These metrics include adjusted body weight, BMI, body surface area (BSA), ideal body weight (IBW), lean body weight (LBW), percent IBW, and predicted normal weight (PNWT) *(Table 13-1)*. Standard anthropomorphic measures allow calculations for improved patient-specific dosing; however, obesity poses great challenges to these metrics. Because obese patients are predisposed to underdosing and increased toxicity, careful therapeutic drug monitoring is particularly important *(Table 13-2)*.[29]

PEARL

The medication dosing weight (DW = IBW + 0.4 x [TBW – IBW]) commonly is used to guide the administration of hydrophilic drugs in obese patients.

Absorption and Distribution

Decreased gastric emptying in obese patients may increase the absorption of oral medications.[27,29] Conversely, subcutaneous absorption can be diminished by a poor subcutaneous blood supply. Intravenous and intramuscular routes of delivery also are compromised by habitus limitations (access limitations and tissue depth, respectively).

The volume of distribution (Vd) of a drug generally is determined by its lipid solubility.[27,29] Because lipid-soluble agents can be markedly affected by the ratio of adipose tissue to lean body mass, the Vd of lipophilic medications often is higher in the obese patient.[27,33] Many lipid-soluble drugs are dosed on total body weight (TBW) or some combination of IBW plus a percentage of TBW *(Table 13-2)*.[26,29] The impact of obesity on Vd can affect the loading dosing required to obtain the targeted effect (eg, propofol for sedation). With infusions, lipid solubility might alter the agent's duration of action due to its accumulation in fat stores (eg, longer drug half-life).[31,32] Although the effects of obesity on protein binding are minimal, total body water can vary in the obese patient and be altered by resuscitation volume.

TABLE 13-1. Indirect Anthropomorphic Measures

Measure	Formula	Notes
Body mass index (BMI) (kg/m²)	BMI = TBW [kg] / (height [m]²)	Primary method used by WHO to classify obesity; does not distinguish adipose tissue from lean muscle mass.
Body surface area (BSA) (m²)*	BSA (m²) = (TBW [kg] × height [cm] / 3,600)½	The utility of BSA in obesity is unknown. Many assign a BSA of 2 m² when arbitrary limits are exceeded.
Ideal body weight (IBW) (kg)*	IBW (males) = height (cm) – 100 IBW (females) = height (cm) – 110	The addition of gender distinguishes IBW from BMI and BSA. It is not an ideal metric because it does not account for mass composition.
Lean body weight (LBW) (kg)*	LBW (male) = 50 + (2.3 × height [in] – 60) LBW (female) = 45 + (2.3 × height [in] – 60)	
Medication dosing weight (DW) (kg)*	DW = (IBW + 0.4) × (TBW – IBW)	This empiric formula can be used in obese patients for most hydrophilic drugs.
Percentage IBW (%IBW)	(TBW/IBW) × 100	
Predicted normal weight (PNWT) (kg)	Male PNWT = (1.57 × TBW) – (0.0183 × BMI × TBW) – 10.5 Female PNWT = (1.75 × TBW) – (0.0242 × BMI × TBW) – 12.6	
BMI and percentage IBW are used most frequently to classify obesity.		

WHO, World Health Organization
*A simplified formula

Metabolism

Obesity has variable effects on metabolism; critical illness can play a larger role in drug interactions and hepatic blood flow in these patients.[31,32,34] Some studies suggest that obesity increases cytochrome P450 2e1 and phase II conjugation activity, and others suggest the alpha 1-acid glycoprotein decreases the free fraction of active drug.[27,29,31-34] These complex and dynamic changes can affect hepatic metabolism, resulting in increased or decreased clearance rates.[26,29,34]

Elimination

The glomerular filtration rate (GFR) is increased by obesity, which can escalate the clearance rate for drugs that are excreted through the kidneys.[29,30,35] In patients with coexisting renal disease (eg, nephropathy associated with diabetes and hypertension), predicting the renal effects of obesity can be inaccurate due to the poor correlation between formula-based (calculated) and measured creatinine clearance.[30,35] As a result, measured creatinine clearance should be used to determine optimal dosing.[26,36]

Respiratory Management

Physiology

Several derangements of normal respiratory physiology occur with increasing body mass. Functional residual capacity (FRC), expiratory reserve volume, and lung compliance are decreased — a reaction that has a significant impact on the respiratory reserve of the critically ill obese patient.[37] The increased load of adipose tissue, especially around the rib cage and visceral cavity of the abdomen, affects thoracic compliance and mechanical excursion and decreases FRC. The stiffening of the lung parenchyma and the chest wall decreases lung compliance and lung volumes. Lung compliance is further exacerbated by elevated blood volumes and increased alveolar surface tension caused by reduced lung volumes.[37] The combination of increased airway resistance and decreased FRC heightens the risk of expiratory flow limitations and airway closure.[38] These patients will be highly susceptible to obstructive apnea and mild hypoxemia, both of which are aggravated by the supine position.[37] Hypoxia with a widened A-a gradient occurs as ventilation is redistributed from the lower to upper lung zones. The ventilation-perfusion mismatch happens because the area of greatest perfusion remains at the lung bases.[37,38]

The obese patient often adopts a rapid, shallow breathing pattern which, when combined with decreased compliance, leads to respiratory inefficiency and compromised respiratory muscle endurance.[37,39] Resting hypoxemia, increased oxygen requirements associated with rapid breathing, a larger relative dead space, and decreased muscle endurance can predispose the obese patient to respiratory failure even with only minor pulmonary or systemic insults.[37,40,41]

Predicting the Difficult Airway

Obese patients do not tolerate apnea or brief alterations in respiration. Critical desaturation can occur in a relatively short time, making standard intubation difficult and time limited.[42,43]

Many studies have evaluated obesity as a predictor of difficulty with mask ventilation and tracheal intubation.[24,25,44-50] The obstacles that arise with mask ventilation are thought to be secondary to upper airway obstruction caused by tissue redundancy and posterior displacement of the soft palate toward the base of the tongue and epiglottis.[15,50-53] The situation is exacerbated by relaxation during the induction of general anesthesia.[52,54]

There are conflicting data on whether obesity is linked to difficult tracheal intubations or whether BMI is an independent risk factor for failed attempts.[55,56] Either way, airway management preferences are different for morbidly obese patients and lean patients. Operators report favoring fiberoptic bronchoscopy as a first-pass technique in morbidly obese patients and are less likely to choose rapid-sequence intubation.[55]

PEARL

The obese patient is often difficult to ventilate via mask and is at high risk for rapid desaturation and collapse, causing failed early intubation. These factors make airway management a time-sensitive procedure. The prudent operator should assume the patient has a potentially difficult airway while assessing the mouth opening, neck mobility, and Mallampati view. Clinicians should be prepared with airway adjuncts (eg, nasopharyngeal or oropharyngeal airways) and familiar with alternative techniques.

FIGURE 13-1. "Ramped" Patient Position

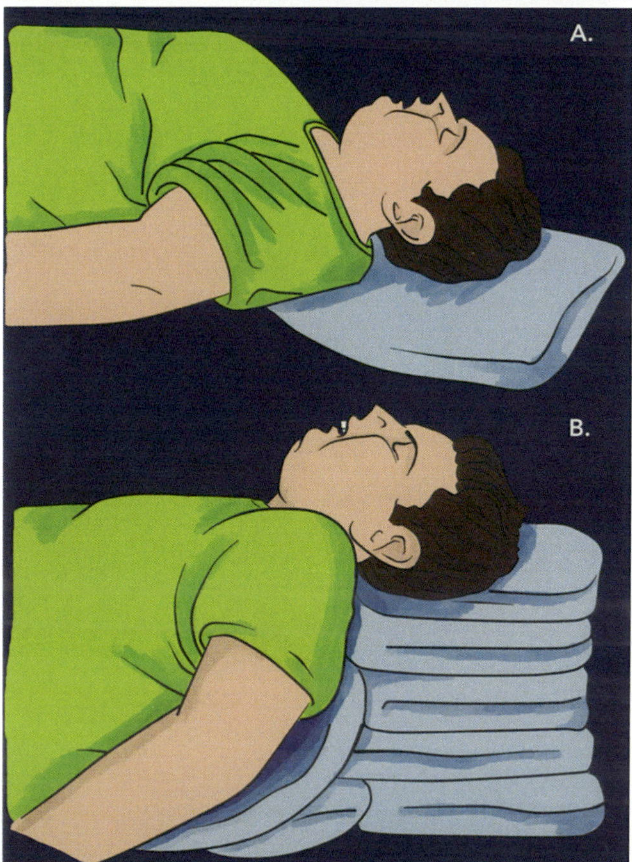

A. Flat, no attempt at achieving best airway position.

B. Ramping improves upper airway patency and decrease work of breathing.

Preoxygenation

Preoxygenation before intubation is an important step toward a safe transition to assisted ventilation. The goal of preoxygenation is to replace the nitrogen within the FRC with oxygen. This exchange increases oxygen stores relative to the size of the FRC. Morbidly obese patients desaturate to a peripheral capillary oxygen saturation (SpO_2) of less than 90% — significantly faster than nonmorbidly obese patients during apnea.[42,57] This shorter time to oxygen desaturation results from reduced FRC, which is exacerbated by induction, paralysis, and supine positioning. Obese patients should remain upright or semirecumbent for as long as possible, and pressure-assistive strategies (eg, positive end-expiratory pressure) should be used to support intubation.[58]

Noninvasive positive pressure ventilation (NPPV) has been studied as a possible intervention for improving preoxygenation in the critically ill patient, but results have been mixed and differ between continuous positive airway pressure (CPAP) and bilevel positive airway pressure (BiPAP). Bilevel support appears to improve SpO_2 values prior to and during intubation compared with simple nonrebreather preoxygenation.[59]

CPAP at 10 cm H_2O prior to tracheal intubation has been shown to favorably affect atelectasis and FRC and increase the duration of nonhypoxic apnea by 1 minute in obese patients undergoing surgery.[60] NPPV via BiPAP using pressure support and positive end-expiratory pressure (PEEP) reaches an end-tidal oxygen concentration (ETO_2) of 95% in a shorter period of time, while also achieving a higher total ETO_2. Interestingly, the use of NPPV does not increase the time to desaturation during a subsequent period of apnea.[61] Similar results have been achieved using CPAP for the preoxygenation of morbidly obese women, in whom the method appears to improve preintubation saturation significantly and reduce desaturation to 90%.[62]

Less is known about BiPAP as an adjunctive therapy for acute respiratory failure in obese patients, as most case reports have focused on the use of positive inspiratory pressure prior to rapid-sequence intubation.[63] While existing evidence seems to support the value of NPPV in improving the efficiency of prexygenation, its ability to prevent rapid oxygen desaturation is less clear.

Patient positioning may address the issue of rapid desaturation.[43] A head-up position eases intubation and preoxygenation effectiveness in airway management.[64] In obese patients, a 25-degree head-up position improves preinduction oxygen tension to 92% and increases time to desaturation during apnea.[65] Preoxygenation in a more upright position may increase oxygen storage and decrease atelectasis, thus improving gas exchange.[65]

TABLE 13-2. General Medication Dosing Guidelines in Obesity

Medication Class	Medication	Loading Dose	
Analgesics	Morphine Remifentanyl Fentanyl	IBW IBW TBW	IBW IBW 0.8 × IBW
Antiarrhythmics	Lidocaine Procainamide Amiodarone	TBW IBW IBW, standard dose	IBW, standard rate IBW, standard rate IBW, standard dose
Antiepileptics	Phenytoin Valproic acid Carbamazepine	IBW + (1.33 × TBW – IBW) NA NA	IBW IBW IBW
Beta-blockers	Propranolol Labetalol Metoprolol Esmolol	IBW IBW IBW IBW	IBW IBW IBW IBW
Calcium channel blockers	Verapamil Diltiazem	TBW TBW	IBW Individualize
Corticosteroids	Methylprednisolone	IBW	IBW
Other cardiac drugs	Digoxin Adenosine Dobutamine	IBW IBW, standard dose NA	IBW IBW, standard dose IBW + 0.4 × (TBW – IBW)
Paralytic agents	Succinylcholine Vecuronium Atracurium Rocuronium	TBW IBW TBW IBW	NA IBW TBW IBW
Sedatives/anesthetics	Benzodiazepines Propofol Thiopental Phenobarbital Ketamine Etomidate	TBW IBW + (0.4 × TBW) TBW TBW IBW TBW	IBW 6 mg/kg/hr IBW IBW IBW NA

IBW, ideal body weight; NA, not applicable; TBW, total body weight

Adapted from Brunette DD. Resuscitation of the morbidly obese patient. *Am J Emerg Med* 2004;22:40-47. Copyright 2004, with permission from Elsevier.

Patient Positioning

The conventional "sniffing" position (ie, 8–10 cm of head elevation) can be suboptimal for performing laryngoscopy in an obese patient and may worsen graded views falsely.[66] A "ramped," head-elevated, or semiseated position can improve preoxygenation and improve visualization of the oral pharynx, larynx, and glottis with less operator effort compared with supine positioning. This technique also gives the clinician greater control over the patient's tongue.[67] Similar laryngeal view enhancements have been achieved using head elevation in fresh human cadavers.[68]

The ramped position can be achieved by placing blankets under the upper body and head until the external auditory meatus and the sternal notch are horizontally aligned (*Figure 13-1*).[66] A table ramp position, which is similar to a head-up position on a standard emergency department bed, is equivalent to the head-up technique achieved with blankets.[45] The use of a standard bed, which makes the routine application of upright positioning more feasible in the clinical encounter, can be achieved by simply lifting the head of the bed more than 25%.

Rapid Sequence Induction Medications

As a result of altered pharmacokinetics in obesity, hydrophilic drugs are generally dosed according to IBW and lipophilic drugs according to TBW.[69] This practice is not completely evidence based, and dosing frequently is calculated on theoretical considerations. Although guidelines for induction agents vary, the dosing of neuromuscular blocking agents is more consistent: TBW is used for calculating the dosing of succinylcholine, and IBW is used for nondepolarizing agents (*Table 13-3*).[69]

Intubation Techniques

Intubation of the obese patient can be challenging, and the optimal technique often is dictated by the skills and experience

FIGURE 13-2. Approach to Airway Management in Obesity

Techniques to improve preoxygenation:[1]
- Head of bed elevated to 25°
- Consider 10 cm H_2O CPAP

Factors that predict difficult intubation in obese patients:[2]
- Short neck
- Thick neck
- Obstructive sleep apnea
- Abnormal upper teeth
- Diabetes mellitus

Techniques to improve RSI:[3]
- Ramped position
- Succinylcholine dosing based on TBW
- Consider advanced techniques (ie, videolaryngoscopy).

Awake technique:[4]
- ≤40 mL of 2% lidocaine for topical anesthesia
- Consider fiberoptic endoscopy or videolaryngoscopy

Technique for BMV:[5]
- Oral/nasal airways
- Two-person technique
- Two-handed jaw thrust
- Ramped position

Confirmation:[6]
- Esophageal detector devices sometimes unreliable

Postintubation management:[7]
- Tidal volume based on IBW
- Consider 10 cm H_2O PEEP
- Reverse Trendelenburg position

Rescue techniques:[8]
- Laryngeal mask airway (eg, Fastrach)

Surgical airway:[9]
- Landmarks may be obscured.
- Longer tracheostomy tube may be required.

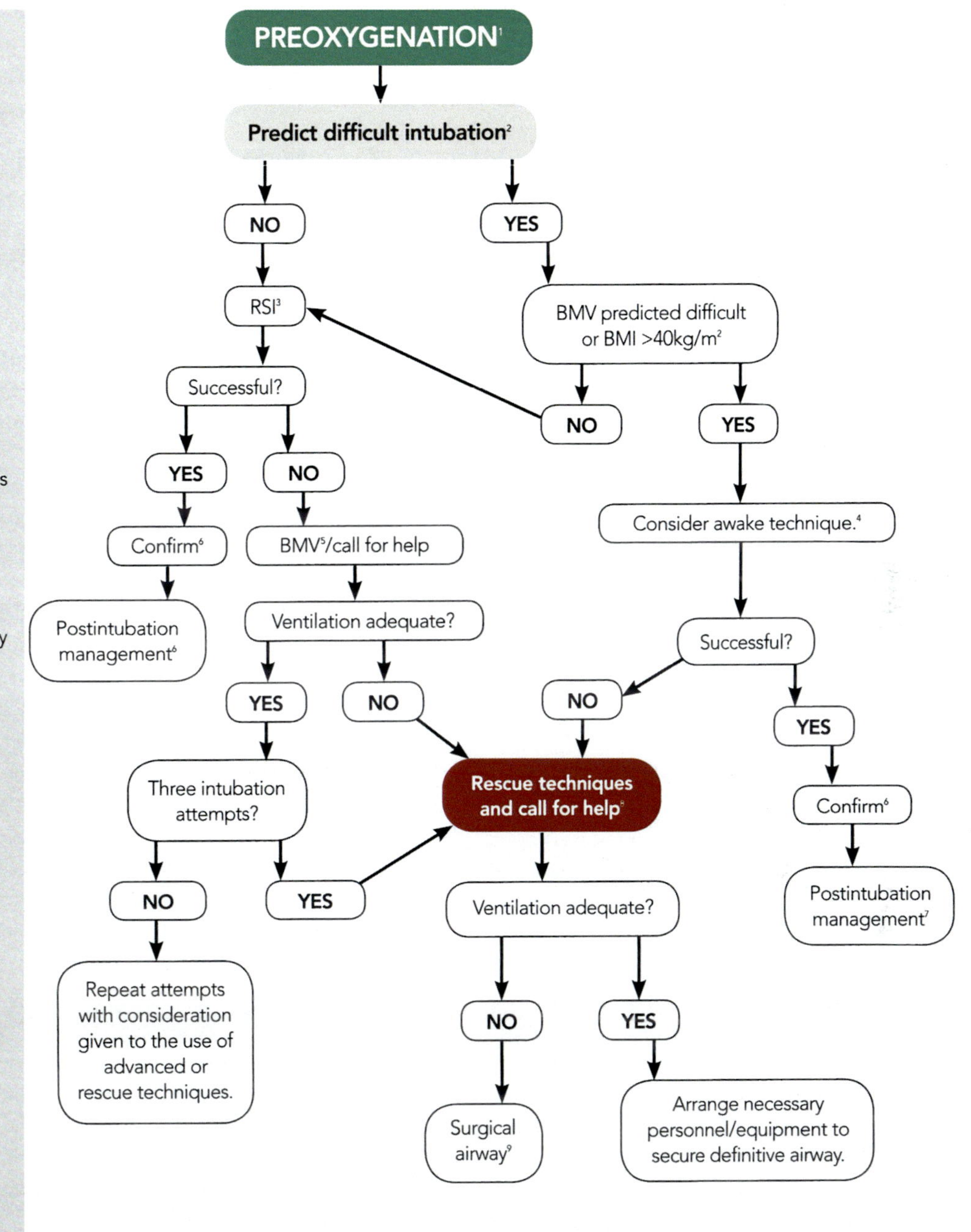

ABBREVIATIONS
RSI = rapid sequence intubation
IBW = ideal body weight
BVM = bag-valve-mask ventilation
TBW = total body weight

of the operator and the resources available *(Figure 13-2)*.[69] When mask ventilation is required, the procedure should be optimized with the use of an oral or nasal airway, an appropriately fitted mask, a two-person technique with a two-handed bilateral jaw thrust, and proper patient positioning.[69] The prudent operator should be prepared for intubation using tools other than direct laryngoscopy. If conditions permit, an awake approach should be considered to limit the risks of difficult mask ventilation and desaturation. Successful rapid sequence intubation can be achieved with skill development and proficiency in the use of video laryngoscopy, supraglottic devices, gum-elastic bougies, and fiberoptic intubation.

The early use of video laryngoscopy should be considered in obese patients, as it has a higher first-attempt success rate than direct laryngoscopy.[48,70-72] In the *Practice Guidelines for Management of the Difficult Airway*, the American Society of Anesthesiologists suggests the use of a supraglottic airway device in patients with failed tracheal intubation and impossible or inadequate mask ventilation.[69,73-75] An inability to oxygenate and ventilate might necessitate a surgical airway, which can be complicated by the distorted landmarks of an obese neck. A nonvisualization Seldinger-type technique, using a small vertical incision and passage of a bougie preloaded with an endotracheal tube, may simplify this procedure.[76]

TABLE 13-3. Calculation of Airway Medication Dosing in Obesity

Total Body Weight	Ideal Body Weight	Lean Body Mass
Etomidate Midazolam Fentanyl Succinylcholine Atracurium	Propofol Vecuronium Rocuronium	Ketamine*

Calculation of drug dosing for the obese patient depends on weight values. Consideration must be given to the pharmacokinetics of the drugs under consideration.[69]

*Adjusted dosing regimen for procedural sedation/rapid sequence intubation.

Mechanical Ventilation

Mechanical ventilation also requires special considerations in obese patients. Tidal volumes should be calculated for IBW rather than TBW, avoiding increased airway pressures and subsequent damage to lung parenchyma. Large tidal volumes have not been shown to significantly improve arterial oxygenation or increase peak inspiratory airway and end-inspiratory pressures.[77] Both PEEP and an upright position have positive effects on respiratory mechanics in the critically ill obese patient.[78]

In a supine position at zero end-expiratory pressure, critically obese patients demonstrate expiratory flow limitations and increased auto-positive end-expiratory pressures (auto-PEEP).[78] Applying PEEP reverses flow limitations without increasing the plateau pressure. However, placing a mechanically ventilated obese patient in a sitting position reverses expiratory flow limitations at zero end-expiratory pressure and creates a drop in auto-PEEP and alveolar pressure (plateau pressure).[78] The level of PEEP required to reverse the expiratory flow limitation is decreased in the sitting position. This sequence is significant from a physiological standpoint. A decreased FRC escalates the risk of expiratory flow limitations, leading to incomplete lung exhalation and air trapping, a complication that can cause patient-ventilator asynchrony. Proper positioning should be considered a lung-protective strategy in the management of mechanically ventilated patients.

KEY POINTS

1. Obese patients are predisposed to underdosing and increased drug toxicity due to changes in the volume of distribution, protein binding, hepatic metabolism, and renal clearance.
2. BMI and percent IBW are the two most frequently used size descriptors to classify obesity.
3. Obesity skews the ratio of adipose tissue to lean body mass, making routine anthropomorphic measures unreliable in medication dosing.
4. Due to an increased volume of distribution in obesity, many lipid-soluble drugs are dosed using a combination of IBW and a percentage of TBW.
5. In the obese patient with renal disease, calculated GFR values are unreliable; measured GFR values should be used in dosing considerations.
6. Pulmonary physiology is altered with increasing body mass, leading to relative hypoxia and fewer physiological reserves. Thus the obese patient often poorly tolerates interruptions in respiration and is prone to exaggerated respiratory collapse even with minor illness.
7. Obese patients can be poor candidates for bag-valve-mask ventilation and are prone to rapid desaturation. The operator should assume the patient has a potentially difficult airway and consider tailored management strategies and alternate approaches.
8. Effective preoxygenation is essential. NPPV has been shown to improve preintubation oxygen saturations and perhaps prolong the time to desaturation. Preoxygenation in an upright positioning (>25 degrees) may reduce atelectasis and improve preoxygenation reserves.

Circulatory Management

Physiological Challenges

Obese patients experience significant cardiovascular alterations. The increased metabolic activity of excess fat increases stroke volume, cardiac output, and left ventricular volume while reducing systemic vascular resistance.[58,79-82] Eventually, the end-diastolic volume may rise significantly and the left ventricular ejection fraction may decrease. These changes may be seen at rest, even in relatively healthy obese patients, and can be a predisposition to early congestive heart failure as a result of obesity cardiomyopathy syndrome.[81-83]

The obese habitus also can present certain challenges to cardiovascular monitoring and access. The use of standard blood pressure sphygmomanometer cuffs often results in artificially elevated readings because of inadequate cuff width and circumference.[58,84] Morbidly obese patients frequently demonstrate classic electrocardiographical changes such as leftward shifts of the P wave, QRS complex, and T-wave axes; low QRS voltage; and conduction delays.[85] This combination of physiological changes and shortfalls in monitoring can skew the prediction of therapeutic endpoints.

PEARL

Although it can be challenging to attain venous access in the obese patient, vascular ultrasound techniques can help. Veins in the antecubital fossa generally are the easiest to cannulate in this population. Standard 1.5-inch needles might be too short to reach all veins; 3- or 4-inch needles might be required even for peripheral venous access.[58]

Resuscitation and Monitoring

The early and aggressive resuscitation of those with severe sepsis or septic shock reduces the risk of organ failure and improves survival.[86] Excessive resuscitation, on the other hand, appears to increase the incidence of complications and death.[87] Thus clinicians are tasked with balancing early aggressive treatment with the deescalation of care in patients who are unlikely to respond to the administration of additional fluid. It can be challenging to predict this responsiveness and identify the interval for a decrease in care; it is important to understand the patient's hemodynamic response to fluids to avoid underdosing or overresuscitation. Methods for guiding resuscitation in the emergency department should be as noninvasive as possible given common resource limitations. These strategies are even more important for obese patients, in whom invasive access can be both technically challenging and time consuming.

One measurement commonly used to assess intravascular volume status is central venous pressure (CVP), obtained by transducing a pressure waveform through either an internal jugular or subclavian central venous line. Two assumptions underlie a resuscitation strategy using CVP: 1) the patient will continue to be fluid responsive and cardiac output will improve until the CVP reaches a theoretical target, and 2) CVP is an accurate predictor of volume responsiveness and status. Because there is a poor correlation between CVP/DeltaCVP and fluid responsiveness, clinician scientists have sought surrogate measurements and physical findings to better guide adequate resuscitation.[88]

Pulse contour analysis, another hemodynamic monitoring method, uses similar principles to determine cardiac performance. Although the requirements for these systems vary, the majority require a central or peripheral arterial catheter and/or a central venous catheter to calculate parameters such

KEY POINTS

9. Elevating the head of the bed or putting the patient in a semi-seated position may enable better tongue control and improve visualization of the oral pharynx, larynx, and glottis with less operator effort compared with the supine position.
10. Early use of videolaryngoscopy in obese patients might enhance first-pass success compared with direct laryngoscopy. Supraglottic devices can assist in cases of failed tracheal intubation and impossible or inadequate mask ventilation.
11. In the mechanically ventilated obese patient, IBW should be used to calculate tidal volumes to avoid excess pressure and barotrauma. A sitting position and adjusted PEEP (8–10 cm H_2O) might reduce expiratory flow limitation, air trapping, and auto-PEEP.
12. Cardiovascular physiology changes with obesity, predisposing the patient to early congestive heart failure as a result of obesity cardiomyopathy syndrome.
13. Routine bedside monitoring such as blood pressure sphygmomanometry and electrocardiac monitoring are prone to error in the obese patient. Blood pressure accuracy can be improved by using a proper ratio of cuff width to arm circumference (2:5).
14. Cardiovascular monitoring is key to resuscitation success. In the morbidly obese patient, noninvasive methods (eg, bedside ultrasound) may be more feasible in a busy emergency department environment.
15. Measurements of changes in vena cava diameter, carotid artery Doppler flow, and cardiac output (as determined by bioreactance) can be used in combination with a passive straight leg raise to determine fluid responsiveness.

as cardiac output, stroke volume variation, and pulse pressure variation based on the arterial pressure waveform. Patients with a large pulse pressure or stroke volume variation are thought to be volume responsive. These methods are limited by certain disease states (eg, arrhythmia and valve disease), however, and become unreliable when beat-to-beat pulse pressure becomes inconsistent. The accuracy of pulse contour analysis remains unclear.[89-95]

Bedside ultrasound may be useful in evaluating fluid responsiveness in the emergency department. In mechanically ventilated septic patients, respiratory changes in inferior vena cava diameter before and after a fluid challenge are good indicators of volume responsiveness independent of changes in central venous pressure.[96-98] However, because inferior vena cava respiratory variation depends on many factors, including patient size, patient positioning, and operator expertise, ultrasound may not be an effective predictor of success.[99] It can be technically difficult to obtain interpretable ultrasound images in morbidly obese patients. Abdominal adipose tissue can increase intraabdominal pressures, thereby affecting vena cava measurements.

A passive leg raise maneuver, accomplished by raising the legs of a supine patient to a 45-degree angle, has been shown to predict fluid responsiveness compared with an empiric fluid bolus.[100-102] This manipulation essentially delivers a reversible endogenous fluid bolus and can be performed while monitoring responses in cardiac output in either the spontaneously breathing or mechanically ventilated patient. It seems to be a reasonable maneuver to predict fluid responsiveness if cardiac output can be assessed simultaneously.[103]

Bioreactance is a noninvasive technology used to monitor cardiac input by tracking the phase of electrical currents that traverse the chest and correlating any shifts to cardiac stroke volume. The most well studied of these devices is the noninvasive cardiac output monitor (NICOM), which uses four electrode pads on the chest wall to gauge changes in pulsatile flow in the thorax. The vast majority of these volume changes stem from the aorta and correlate closely with aortic flow.[103] The technology assumes that changes in aortic blood flow after an intervention are related to alterations in cardiac output. Bioreactance cardiac output measurements, which are similar to those obtained from pulmonary artery catheter thermodilutions, can predictably track these changes when a passive leg raise maneuver is used.[104-109] Although bioreactance provides no mortality benefit and its predictability has been questioned, the technique maintains some appeal in the morbidly obese population, as it can be applied easily in the acute setting.[99]

Transthoracic echocardiography can provide useful information regarding cardiac output; however, it can be difficult to obtain reliable images in obese patients. Changes in cardiac stroke volume after the passive leg raise maneuver and Doppler echocardiography can predict volume responsiveness, as can carotid artery Doppler ultrasound — another exciting alternative.[110] A strong correlation has been demonstrated between increases in the stroke volume index and carotid blood flow when using the bioreactance method as a reference for cardiac output.[111] Though promising, more research is needed to determine whether carotid artery Doppler flow reliably reflects fluid responsiveness. In the morbidly obese population, this method could provide an attractive alternative for assessing fluid responsiveness due to its relative technical ease.

Conclusion

Morbid obesity presents significant clinical challenges; optimal care requires altered strategies at every step of treatment, from medication dosing to physiological monitoring. It is important for the emergency physician to anticipate these difficulties and prepare a resuscitation strategy tailored to the specific needs of this complex patient population.

REFERENCES

1. Haslam D, Rigby N. A long look at obesity. *Lancet.* 2010;376:85-86.
2. Haslam DW, James WP. Obesity. *Lancet.* 2005;366:1197-1209.
3. Haslam D. Obesity: a medical history. *Obes Rev.* 2007;8 (suppl 1):31-36.
4. Obesity: preventing and managing the global epidemic. Report of a WHO consultation. *World Health Organ Techn Rep Ser.* 2000;894:i-xii, 1-253.
5. Muller MJ, Mast M, Langnase K. [WHO warns of obesity epidemic. Are we becoming a society of obese persons?] *MMW Fortschritte der Medizin.* 2001;143:28-32.
6. Wang Y, Wang JQ. Standard definition of child overweight and obesity worldwide. Authors' standard compares well with WHO standard. *BMJ.* 2000;321:1158.
7. Bercault N, Boulain T, Kuteifan K, et al. Obesity-related excess mortality rate in an adult intensive care unit: a risk-adjusted matched cohort study. *Crit Care Med.* 2004;32:998-1003.
8. Smith SC Jr, Haslam D. Abdominal obesity, waist circumference and cardio-metabolic risk: awareness among primary care physicians, the general population and patients at risk-the Shape of the Nations survey. *Curr Med Res Opin.* 2007;23:29-47.
9. Clinical Guidelines on the Identification, Evaluation, and Treatment of Overweight and Obesity in Adults — The Evidence Report. National Institutes of Health. *Obes Res.* 1998;6(suppl 2):51S-209S.
10. Richardson L, Paulis WD, van Middelkoop M, Koes BW. An overview of national clinical guidelines for the management of childhood obesity in primary care. *Prev Med.* 2013;57:448-455.
11. Sturm R, Hattori A. Morbid obesity rates continue to rise rapidly in the United States. *Int J Obes.* 2013;37:889-891.
12. Haslam D. Obesity in primary care: prevention, management and the paradox. *BMC Med.* 2014;12:149.
13. Peeters A, Barendregt JJ, Willekens F, et al. Obesity in adulthood and its consequences for life expectancy: a life-table analysis. *Ann Intern Med.* 2003;138:24-32.
14. Prospective Studies Collaboration, Whitlock G, Lewington S, et al. Body-mass index and cause-specific mortality in 900 000 adults: collaborative analyses of 57 prospective studies. *Lancet.* 2009;373:1083-1096.
15. Grant P, Newcombe M. Emergency management of the morbidly obese. *Emerg Med Australas.* 2004;16:309-317.
16. Bertakis KD, Azari R. The impact of obesity on primary care visits. *Obes Res.* 2005;13:1615-1623.
17. Bertakis KD, Azari R. Obesity and the use of health care services. *Obes Res.* 2005;13:372-379.
18. Thorpe KE, Florence CS, Howard DH, Joski P. The impact of obesity on rising medical spending. *Health Aff (Millwood).* 2004;Suppl Web Exclusives:W4-480-486.
19. Moyer VA, Klein JD, Ockene JK, et al. Screening for overweight in children and adolescents: Where is the evidence? A commentary by the childhood obesity working group of the US Preventive Services Task Force. *Pediatrics.* 2005;116:235-238.
20. Haslam D. What's new — tackling childhood obesity. *Practitioner.* 2006;250:26-27, 29, 31-32 passim.
21. Levi D, Goodman ER, Patel M, Savransky Y. Critical care of the obese and bariatric surgical patient. *Crit Care Clin.* 2003;19:11-32.
22. Brown CV, Velmahos GC. The consequences of obesity on trauma, emergency surgery, and surgical critical care. *World J Emerg Surg.* 2006;1:27.
23. Ogunnaike B. The morbidly obese patient undergoing outpatient surgery. *Int Anesthesiol Clin.* 2013;51:113-135.
24. Levitan RM, Chudnofsky C, Sapre N. Emergency airway management in a morbidly obese, noncooperative, rapidly deteriorating patient. *Am J Emerg Med.* 2006;24:894-896.
25. Holmberg TJ, Bowman SM, Warner KJ, et al. The association between obesity and difficult prehospital tracheal intubation. *Anesth Analg.* 2011;112:1132-1138.
26. Brunette DD. Resuscitation of the morbidly obese patient. *Am J Emerg Med.* 2004;22:40-47.
27. Blouin RA, Kolpek JH, Mann HJ. Influence of obesity on drug disposition. *Clin Pharm.* 1987;6:706-714.

28. Chaput JP, Berube-Parent S, Tremblay A. Obesity and cardiovascular physiology: impact of some pharmacological agents. *Curr Vasc Pharmacol.* 2005;3:185-193.
29. Hanley MJ, Abernethy DR, Greenblatt DJ. Effect of obesity on the pharmacokinetics of drugs in humans. *Clin Pharmacokinet.* 2010;49:71-87.
30. Park EJ, Pai MP, Dong T, et al. The influence of body size descriptors on the estimation of kidney function in normal weight, overweight, obese, and morbidly obese adults. *Ann Pharmacother.* 2012;46:317-328.
31. Brill MJ, Diepstraten J, van Rongen A, et al. Impact of obesity on drug metabolism and elimination in adults and children. *Clin Pharmacokinet.* 2012;51:277-304.
32. Knibbe CA, Brill MJ, van Rongen A, et al. Drug disposition in obesity: toward evidence-based dosing. *Annu Rev Pharmacol Toxicol.* 2015;55:149-167.
33. Blouin RA, Warren GW. Pharmacokinetic considerations in obesity. *J Pharm Sci.* 1999;88:1-7.
34. Kotlyar M, Carson SW. Effects of obesity on the cytochrome P450 enzyme system. *Int J Clin Pharmacol Ther.* 1999;37:8-19.
35. Salazar DE, Corcoran GB. Predicting creatinine clearance and renal drug clearance in obese patients from estimated fat-free body mass. *Am J Med.* 1988;84:1053-1060.
36. Varon J, Marik P. Management of the obese critically ill patient. *Crit Care Clin.* 2001;17:187-200.
37. Salome CM, King GG, Berend N. Physiology of obesity and effects on lung function. *J Appl Physiol.* 2010;108:206-211.
38. Behazin N, Jones SB, Cohen RI, Loring SH. Respiratory restriction and elevated pleural and esophageal pressures in morbid obesity. *J Appl Physiol.* 2010;108:212-218.
39. Biring MS, Lewis MI, Liu JT, Mohsenifar Z. Pulmonary physiologic changes of morbid obesity. *Am J Med Sci.* 1999;318:293-297.
40. Parameswaran K, Todd DC, Soth M. Altered respiratory physiology in obesity. *Can Respir J.* 2006;13:203-210.
41. Ashburn DD, DeAntonio A, Reed MJ. Pulmonary system and obesity. *Crit Care Clin.* 2010;26:597-602.
42. Berthoud MC, Peacock JE, Reilly CS. Effectiveness of preoxygenation in morbidly obese patients. *Br J Anaesth.* 1991;67:464-466.
43. Altermatt FR, Munoz HR, Delfino AE, Cortinez LI. Pre-oxygenation in the obese patient: effects of position on tolerance to apnoea. *Br J Anaesth.* 2005;95:706-709.
44. Brodsky JB, Lemmens HJ, Brock-Utne JG, et al. Morbid obesity and tracheal intubation. *Anesth Analg.* 2002;94:732-736.
45. Rao SL, Kunselman AR, Schuler HG, DesHarnais S. Laryngoscopy and tracheal intubation in the head-elevated position in obese patients: a randomized, controlled, equivalence trial. *Anesth Analg.* 2008;107:1912-1918.
46. Lavi R, Segal D, Ziser A. Predicting difficult airways using the intubation difficulty scale: a study comparing obese and non-obese patients. *J Clin Anesthes.* 2009;21:264-267.
47. Geary B, Collins N. Are we prepared for a growing population? Morbid obesity and its implications in Irish emergency departments. *Eur J Emerg Med.* 2012;19:117-120.
48. Ydemann M, Rovsing L, Lindekaer AL, Olsen KS. Intubation of the morbidly obese patient: GlideScope((R)) vs. Fastrach. *Acta Anaesthesiol Scand.* 2012;56:755-761.
49. Moore AR, Schricker T, Court O. Awake videolaryngoscopy-assisted tracheal intubation of the morbidly obese. *Anaesthesia.* 2012;67:232-235.
50. Duwat A, Turbelin A, Petiot S, et al. [French national survey on difficult intubation in intensive care units.] *Ann Fr Anesth Reanim.* 2014;33:297-303.
51. Collins JS, Lemmens HJ, Brodsky JB. Obesity and difficult intubation: where is the evidence? *Anesthesiology.* 2006;104:6179.
52. Langeron O, Masso E, Huraux C, et al. Prediction of difficult mask ventilation. *Anesthesiology.* 2000;92:1229-1236.
53. Diemunsch P, Langeron O, Richard M, et al. [Prediction and definition of difficult mask ventilation and difficult intubation: question 1. Société Française d'Anesthésie et de Réanimation.] *Ann Fr Anesth Reanim.* 2008;27:3-14.
54. Langeron O, Cuvillon P, Ibanez-Esteve C, et al. Prediction of difficult tracheal intubation: time for a paradigm change. *Anesthesiology.* 2012;117:1223-1233.
55. Dargin JM, Emlet LL, Guyette FX. The effect of body mass index on intubation success rates and complications during emergency airway management. *Intern Emerg Med.* 2013;8:75-82.
56. Sifri ZC, Kim H, Lavery R, et al. The impact of obesity on the outcome of emergency intubation in trauma patients. *J Trauma.* 2008;65:396-400.
57. Jense HG, Dubin SA, Silverstein PI, et al. Effect of obesity on safe duration of apnea in anesthetized humans. *Anesth Analg.* 1991;72:89-93.
58. Brunette DD. Resuscitation of the morbidly obese patient. *Am J Emerg Med.* 2004;22:40-47.
59. Baillard C, Fosse JP, Sebbane M, et al. Noninvasive ventilation improves preoxygenation before intubation of hypoxic patients. *Am J Respir Crit Care Med.* 2006;174:171-177.
60. Gander S, Frascarolo P, Suter M, et al. Positive end-expiratory pressure during induction of general anesthesia increases duration of nonhypoxic apnea in morbidly obese patients. *Anesth Analg.* 2005;100:580-584.
61. Delay JM, Sebbane M, Jung B, et al. The effectiveness of noninvasive positive pressure ventilation to enhance preoxygenation in morbidly obese patients: a randomized controlled study. *Anesth Analg.* 2008;107:1707-1713.
62. Cressey DM, Berthoud MC, Reilly CS. Effectiveness of continuous positive airway pressure to enhance pre-oxygenation in morbidly obese women. *Anaesthesia.* 2001;56:680-684.
63. El-Khatib MF, Kanazi G, Baraka AS. Noninvasive bilevel positive airway pressure for preoxygenation of the critically ill morbidly obese patient. *Can J Anaesth.* 2007;54:744-747.
64. Weingart SD, Levitan RM. Preoxygenation and prevention of desaturation during emergency airway management. *Ann Emerg Med.* 2012;59:165-175 e1.
65. Dixon BJ, Dixon JB, Carden JR, et al. Preoxygenation is more effective in the 25 degrees head-up position than in the supine position in severely obese patients: a randomized controlled study. *Anesthesiology.* 2005;102:1110-1115.
66. Collins JS, Lemmens HJ, Brodsky JB, et al. Laryngoscopy and morbid obesity: a comparison of the "sniff" and "ramped" positions. *Obes Surg.* 2004;14:1171-1175.
67. Fontanarosa PB, Goldman GE, Polsky SS, et al. Sitting oral-tracheal intubation. *Ann Emerg Med.* 1988;17:336-338.
68. Levitan RM, Mechem CC, Ochroch EA, et al. Head-elevated laryngoscopy position: improving laryngeal exposure during laryngoscopy by increasing head elevation. *Ann Emerg Med.* 2003;41:322-330.
69. Dargin J, Medzon R. Emergency department management of the airway in obese adults. *Ann Emerg Med.* 2010;56:95-104.
70. Mosier JM, Stolz U, Chiu S, et al. Difficult airway management in the emergency department: GlideScope videolaryngoscopy compared to direct laryngoscopy. *J Emerg Med.* 2012;42:629-634.
71. Dhonneur G, Abdi W, Ndoko SK, et al. Video-assisted versus conventional tracheal intubation in morbidly obese patients. *Obes Surg.* 2009;19:1096-1101.
72. Andersen LH, Rovsing L, Olsen KS. GlideScope videolaryngoscope vs. Macintosh direct laryngoscope for intubation of morbidly obese patients: a randomized trial. *Acta Anaesthesiol Scand.* 2011;55:1090-1097.
73. Apfelbaum JL, Hagberg CA, Caplan RA, et al. Practice guidelines for management of the difficult airway: an updated report by the American Society of Anesthesiologists Task Force on Management of the Difficult Airway. *Anesthesiology.* 2013;118:251-270.
74. Dhonneur G, Ndoko SK, Yavchitz A, et al. Tracheal intubation of morbidly obese patients: LMA CTrach vs direct laryngoscopy. *Br J Anaesth.* 2006;97:742-745.
75. Frappier J, Guenoun T, Journois D, et al. Airway management using the intubating laryngeal mask airway for the morbidly obese patient. *Anesth Analg.* 2003;96:1510-1515.
76. King DR. Emergent cricothyroidotomy in the morbidly obese: a safe, no-visualization technique. *J Trauma.* 2011;71:1873-1874.
77. Bardoczky GI, Yernault JC, Houben JJ, et al. Large tidal volume ventilation does not improve oxygenation in morbidly obese patients during anesthesia. *Anesth Analg.* 1995;81:385-388.
78. Lemyze M, Mallat J, Duhamel A, et al. Effects of sitting position and applied positive end-expiratory pressure on respiratory mechanics of critically ill obese patients receiving mechanical ventilation. *Crit Care Med.* 2013;41:2592-2599.
79. Alpert MA, Lambert CR, Panayiotou H, et al. Relation of duration of morbid obesity to left ventricular mass, systolic function, and diastolic filling, and effect of weight loss. *Am J Cardiol.* 1995;76:1194-1197.
80. Alpert MA, Lambert CR, Terry BE, et al. Influence of left ventricular mass on left ventricular diastolic filling in normotensive morbid obesity. *Am Heart J.* 1995;130:1068-1073.
81. Alpert MA. Obesity cardiomyopathy: pathophysiology and evolution of the clinical syndrome. *Am J Med Sci.* 2001;321:225-236.
82. Alpert MA, Lavie CJ, Agrawal H, et al. Obesity and heart failure: epidemiology, pathophysiology, clinical manifestations, and management. *Transl Res.* 2014;164:345-356.
83. Ferraro S, Perrone-Filardi P, Desiderio A, et al. Left ventricular systolic and diastolic function in severe obesity: a radionuclide study. *Cardiology.* 1996;87:347-353.
84. Maxwell MH, Waks AU, Schroth PC, et al. Error in blood-pressure measurement due to incorrect cuff size in obese patients. *Lancet.* 1982;2:33-36.
85. Alpert MA, Terry BE, Cohen MV, et al. The electrocardiogram in morbid obesity. *Am J Cardiol.* 2000;85:908-910.
86. Rivers E, Nguyen B, Havstad S, et al. Early goal-directed therapy in the treatment of severe sepsis and septic shock. *N Engl J Med.* 2001;345:1368-1377.
87. Boyd JH, Forbes J, Nakada TA, et al. Fluid resuscitation in septic shock: a positive fluid balance and elevated central venous pressure are associated with increased mortality. *Crit Care Med.* 2011;39:259-265.
88. Marik PE, Baram M, Vahid B. Does central venous pressure predict fluid responsiveness? A systematic review of the literature and the tale of seven mares. *Chest.* 2008;134:172-178.
89. Zimmermann A, Kufner C, Hofbauer S, et al. The accuracy of the Vigileo/FloTrac continuous cardiac output monitor. *J Cardiothorac Vasc Anesth.* 2008;22:388-393.
90. Zimmermann M, Feibicke T, Keyl C, et al. Accuracy of stroke volume variation compared with pleth variability index to predict fluid responsiveness in mechanically ventilated patients undergoing major surgery. *Eur J Anaesthesiol.* 2010;27:555-561.
91. Geerts B, de Wilde R, Aarts L, et al. Pulse contour analysis to assess hemodynamic response to passive leg raising. *J Cardiothorac Vasc Anesth.* 2011;25:48-52.
92. Wiesenack C, Prasser C, Rodig G, et al. Stroke volume variation as an indicator of fluid responsiveness using pulse contour analysis in mechanically ventilated patients. *Anesth Analg.* 2003;96:1254-1257.
93. Donati A, Nardella R, Gabbanelli V, et al. The ability of PiCCO versus LiDCO variables to detect changes in cardiac index: a prospective clinical study. *Minerva Anestesiol.* 2008;74:367-374.
94. Lahner D, Kabon B, Marschalek C, et al. Evaluation of stroke volume variation obtained by arterial pulse contour analysis to predict fluid responsiveness intraoperatively. *Br J Anaesth.* 2009;103:346-351.
95. Davies SJ, Minhas S, Wilson RJ, et al. Comparison of stroke volume and fluid responsiveness measurements in commonly used technologies for goal-directed therapy. *J Clin Anesthes.* 2013;25:466-474.
96. Machare-Delgado E, Decaro M, Marik PE. Inferior vena cava variation compared to pulse contour analysis as predictors of fluid responsiveness: a prospective cohort study. *J Intensive Care Med.* 2011;26:116-1124.
97. Feissel M, Michard F, Faller JP, et al. The respiratory variation in inferior vena cava diameter as a guide to fluid therapy. *Intensive Care Med.* 2004;30:1834-1837.

98. Barbier C, Loubieres Y, Schmit C, et al. Respiratory changes in inferior vena cava diameter are helpful in predicting fluid responsiveness in ventilated septic patients. *Intensive Care Med.* 2004;30:1740-1746.
99. Corl K, Napoli AM, Gardiner F. Bedside sonographic measurement of the inferior vena cava caval index is a poor predictor of fluid responsiveness in emergency department patients. *Emerg Med Australas.* 2012;24:534-539.
100. Maizel J, Airapetian N, Lorne E, et al. Diagnosis of central hypovolemia by using passive leg raising. *Intensive Care Med.* 2007;33:1133-1138.
101. Monnet X, Rienzo M, Osman D, et al. Passive leg raising predicts fluid responsiveness in the critically ill. *Crit Care Med.* 2006;34:1402-1407.
102. Monnet X, Teboul JL. Passive leg raising. *Intensive Care Med.* 2008;34:659-663.
103. Marik PE. Noninvasive cardiac output monitors: a state-of the-art review. *J Cardiothorac Vasc Anesth.* 2013;27:121-134.
104. Raval NY, Squara P, Cleman M, et al. Multicenter evaluation of noninvasive cardiac output measurement by bioreactance technique. *J Clin Monit Comput.* 2008;22:113-119.
105. Marque S, Cariou A, Chiche JD, et al. Comparison between Flotrac-Vigileo and Bioreactance, a totally noninvasive method for cardiac output monitoring. *Crit Care.* 2009;13:R73.
106. Squara P, Denjean D, Estagnasie P, et al. Noninvasive cardiac output monitoring (NICOM): a clinical validation. *Intensive Care Med.* 2007;33:1191-1194.
107. Keren H, Burkhoff D, Squara P. Evaluation of a noninvasive continuous cardiac output monitoring system based on thoracic bioreactance. *Am J Physiol Heart Circ Physiol.* 2007;293:H583-H589.
108. Duus N, Shogilev DJ, Skibsted S, et al. The reliability and validity of passive leg raise and fluid bolus to assess fluid responsiveness in spontaneously breathing emergency department patients. *J Crit Care.* 2015;30:217 e1-e5.
109. Benomar B, Ouattara A, Estagnasie P, et al. Fluid responsiveness predicted by noninvasive bioreactance-based passive leg raise test. *Intensive Care Med.* 2010;36:1875-1881.
110. Levitov A, Marik PE. Echocardiographic assessment of preload responsiveness in critically ill patients. *Cardiol Res Pract.* 2012;2012:819696.
111. Marik PE, Levitov A, Young A, et al. The use of bioreactance and carotid Doppler to determine volume responsiveness and blood flow redistribution following passive leg raising in hemodynamically unstable patients. *Chest.* 2013;143:364-370.

Pulmonary Hypertension

14

IN THIS CHAPTER

- Pathophysiology and classification of pulmonary hypertension
- Evaluation and diagnosis of right ventricular failure
- Management algorithm for pulmonary hypertension
- Special scenarios

James M. Dargin and Lillian Emlet

It is imperative for the emergency care provider to be adept at diagnosing, stabilizing, and managing critically ill patients with pulmonary hypertension and its life-threatening complications.

Pathophysiology and Classification

Pulmonary hypertension (PH), which is defined as an elevated mean pulmonary artery pressure (mPAP) above 25 mm Hg at rest, is caused by restricted blood flow through the arterial circulatory system.[1,2] Increases in right ventricular preload and afterload distend the right ventricle (RV), resulting in reduced contractility and heightened myocardial oxygen demand. Depending on its severity, a distended RV can cause tricuspid regurgitation (TR) and bowing of the interventricular septum into the left ventricle (LV) — complications that can decrease left ventricular preload and cardiac output (CO).[3,4] Clinically, right ventricular failure can manifest as dyspnea, chest pain, palpitations, lower extremity edema, and syncope.[5-7]

A number of conditions cause PH, which is classified by the World Health Organization (WHO) in five groups *(Table 14-1)*.[8] Pulmonary arterial hypertension (PAH) (WHO Group 1) is an uncommon disease with a pathophysiology that is distinct from other forms of PH. It is a progressive disorder caused by dysfunction of the endothelium in the small pulmonary arteries, resulting in increased arterial resistance; symptoms typically are severe at the time of diagnosis (WHO functional class II or III *[Table 14-2]*).[9-11]

The most prevalent form of PH (WHO Group 2) can result from valvular heart disease or, more commonly, heart failure with preserved ejection fraction (HFpEF).[12,13] About half of all heart failure patients have HFpEF, and the presence of PH or right ventricular dysfunction is associated with poor outcomes.[14] A combination of postcapillary PH (hydrostatic pressure from elevated left ventricular end-diastolic pressure) and precapillary PH (pulmonary vascular remodeling and vasoconstriction from endothelial dysfunction) contribute to WHO Group 2. Patients with PH caused by HFpEF are likely to be older, female, and suffer from additional comorbidities such as hypertension, obesity, coronary artery disease, diabetes mellitus, atrial fibrillation, and hyperlipidemia.[15,16]

WHO Group 3 includes pulmonary diseases that cause hypoxia such as interstitial lung disease, chronic obstructive pulmonary disease (COPD), acute respiratory distress syndrome, alveolar hypoventilation, and high altitude exposure. As many as 25% of patients with sleep apnea syndromes suffer from PH.[17,18] COPD is responsible for more than 50% of chronic cor pulmonale cases in the United States; 5% to 20% of these patients eventually develop severe PH.[19] Patients with thromboembolic disease involving more than 40% of the pulmonary circulation tend to develop PH (WHO Group 4) and have associated RV dysfunction.[20]

Diagnosis

PH can be confirmed during right heart catheterization by an mPAP greater than 25 mm Hg and a pulmonary capillary wedge pressure less than 15 mm Hg. Increased resistance in the pulmonary arteries and capillaries is confirmed when the mPAP is elevated and the wedge pressure is normal. In cases of left heart failure, the wedge pressure is elevated, indicating increased resistance in the pulmonary veins. Echocardiography remains the initial method of evaluating for PH and associated RV dysfunction. A comprehensive echocardiographical analysis is beyond the scope of practice for most emergency physicians and intensivists. However, a focused cardiac ultrasound (FoCUS) can be a helpful adjunct to the emergency department examination of patients with PH.[21-23] Echocardiographic changes suggestive of *acute* right ventricular failure include

TABLE 14-1. WHO Classification of Pulmonary Hypertension[8]

GROUP 1 (Pulmonary Arterial Hypertension)
Idiopathic
Heritable
Drug and toxin induced
Associated with connective tissue disease, HIV, portal hypertension, congenital heart disease, schistosomiasis, chronic hemolytic anemia, pulmonary venoocclusive disease
GROUP 2 (Left-Sided Heart Disease)
Systolic dysfunction
Diastolic dysfunction
Valvular heart disease
GROUP 3 (Chronic Lung Disease)
COPD
Interstitial lung disease
Sleep-disordered breathing
Alveolar hypoventilation disorders
Chronic exposure to high altitude
Developmental abnormalities
GROUP 4 (Chronic Thromboembolic Disease)
GROUP 5 (Unclear Multifactorial Mechanisms)
Hematological disorders: chronic hemolytic anemia, myeloproliferative disorders, splenectomy
Systemic disorders: sarcoidosis, pulmonary Langerhans cell histiocytosis, lymphangioleiomyomatosis, neurofibromatosis, vasculitis
Metabolic disorders: glycogen storage disease, Gaucher's disease, thyroid disease
Other: tumor obstruction, fibrosing mediastinitis, chronic renal disease

TABLE 14-2. WHO Functional Classification of Pulmonary Hypertension[11]

Class I: Ordinary physical activity does not cause undue dyspnea, fatigue, chest pain, or near syncope.
Class II: Comfortable at rest. Ordinary physical activity causes undue dyspnea, fatigue, chest pain, or near syncope.
Class III: Comfortable at rest. Less than ordinary physical activity causes undue dyspnea, fatigue, chest pain, or near syncope.
Class IV: Unable to carry out any physical activity without symptoms. Dyspnea and/or fatigue may occur at rest.

right ventricular dilation, right ventricular hypokinesis, and septal dyskinesis (flattening with paradoxic movement toward the free wall of the LV). Patients with *chronic* right ventricular failure, as can be seen in chronic cor pulmonale, manifest right ventricular hypertrophy and right atrial dilation. Dilation of the inferior vena cava, superior vena cava, and hepatic veins also may be seen in patients with severe PH, as can pericardial effusion. Doppler ultrasonography may over- or underestimate PA pressure and is recommended primarily as a screening tool prior to right heart catheterization, which ultimately is necessary for the definitive diagnosis of PH, assessment of disease severity, and potential response to vasodilator therapy.[24]

Treatment

The management of PH includes treatment of the underlying cause (eg, obstructive sleep apnea) and the administration of diuretics, supplemental oxygen, and PH-specific medications. These agents include calcium channel blockers, endothelin antagonists, phosphodiesterase-5 inhibitors, and a soluble guanylate cyclase stimulator *(Table 14-3)*.[24] Confirmation of the specific WHO group is important since treatment algorithms differ between them. PH-specific drugs generally are reserved for those in WHO Group 1. Epoprostenol and endothelin antagonists have been shown to be ineffective and potentially harmful for patients in WHO Group 2, in whom the drugs can increase pulmonary edema without providing a mortality benefit.[26] The use of PDE-5 inhibitors (eg, sildenafil) is promising for these patients, as it has been associated with improved symptoms and hemodynamics.[2] For patients in Group 3, management should be focused on treating the underlying lung disease and preventing hypoxia. No studies have shown convincing evidence to warrant pulmonary vasodilator treatment in this group.

If an initial screening echocardiogram suggests PH, right heart catheterization must be performed to properly diagnose and categorize the hypertension. For those in Group 1, vasoreactivity testing with inhaled nitric oxide (iNO) during right heart catheterization determines the potential benefit of vasodilatory therapy. A positive vasoreactivity response is defined as a decrease in mPAP of at least 10 mm Hg, with the overall mPAP decreasing to 40 mm Hg or less. This pattern of response is seen in fewer than 10% of patients with PH; these cases generally are managed with calcium channel blockers.[27] PAH is a rare and complicated disease that often necessitates collaborative treatment at a tertiary care center where specialists in pulmonary medicine, cardiology, and rheumatology are available.

For patients presenting to the emergency department with acute right ventricular failure caused by severe PH, the administration of iNO and prostacyclins (inhaled or intravenous) can be considered. iNO rapidly diffuses across the alveolar-capillary membrane and functions as endogenous NO, which vasodilates the pulmonary vasculature, causes bronchodilation, and provides antiinflammatory and antiproliferative effects. The inhaled route provides greater effect in the lungs and minimizes systemic side effects. iNO is delivered in a dose range of 5 to 80 ppm continuously through a ventilator circuit or nasal cannula adaptors. Methemoglobinemia and systemic hypotension are the primary side effects when iNO is administered at high doses for long periods. Rebound PH can occur when the agent is discontinued abruptly; however, this side effect is mitigated by slow weaning.[28]

Response to Therapy

A patient's clinical course and response to treatment can be measured by evaluating right heart function using a number of modalities. Although there appears to be no clear benefit to the *routine* use of the pulmonary artery (PA) catheter in ICU patients, it is often used to guide therapy in those with PH who are critically ill. Alternatively, the PA pressure and right ventricular function can be estimated in select cases using echocardiography, which reduces the need for repeat right heart catheterization. Echocardiography appears to be more accurate in cases of severe PH and less reliable in those with borderline disease.

Tricuspid regurgitation is required to obtain the measurements needed to estimate the PAP.[29] Monitoring trends in the brain natriuretic peptide level can have prognostic value and also may serve as a useful adjunct when assessing changes in right ventricular function. Other measures for evaluating the response to therapy include the 6-minute walk test and additional biomarkers (eg, troponin, uric acid, and endothelin-1).

The Stable Patient

If the patient with PH is deemed stable after a rapid assessment of airway, breathing, and circulation, the diagnostic evaluation and treatment should be approached in a systematic manner *(Figure 14-1)*. Patients with PH often present to the emergency department with an acute illness that is related to their PH, a side effect of a medication used to treat it, or

TABLE 14-3. Pulmonary Arterial Hypertension-Specific Medications[24]

Category	Typical Dose	Indication	Side Effects
Calcium channel blockers			
Amlodipine	20–30 mg/days PO	Absence of RV failure and positive vasoreactivity	Hypotension, RV dysfunction, peripheral edema, reflex tachycardia
Nifedipine	180–240 mg/days PO	Absence of RV failure and positive vasoreactivity	Hypotension, RV dysfunction, peripheral edema, reflex tachycardia
Diltiazem	720–960 mg/days PO	Absence of RV failure and positive vasoreactivity	Hypotension, RV dysfunction, bradycardia
Endothelin receptor antagonists			
Bosentan	62.5–125 mg PO BID	FC II or III without evidence of rapid disease progression	Peripheral edema, palpitations, chest pain, hepatotoxicity
Ambrisentan	5–10 mg/days PO	FC II or III without evidence of rapid disease progression	Peripheral edema, headache, nasal congestion
Macicentan	10 mg/days PO	FC II or III without evidence of rapid disease progression	Headache, anemia
PDE-5 inhibitors			
Sildenafil	5–20 mg PO TID	FC II or III without evidence of rapid disease progression	Visual changes, hypotension
Tadalafil	40 mg/days PO	FC II or III without evidence of rapid disease progression	Visual changes, hypotension
Prostanoids			
Epoprostenol	25–40 ng/kg/min IV	FC III with rapid progression or FC IV	Rebound PH (half-life = minutes), flushing, headache, jaw pain, diarrhea
Treprostinil	1.25–40 ng/kg/min SQ or IV infusion	FC III with rapid progression or FC IV	Rebound PH (half-life = hours), flushing, headache, diarrhea
Iloprost	2.5–5 mcg/dose inhaled 6–9 times/day	FC III with rapid progression or FC IV	Cough, headache, flushing, syncope, rebound PH
Soluble guanylate cyclase stimulator			
Riociguat	1–2.5 mg PO TID	CTEPH	Hypotension, headache

RV, right ventricular; FC, functional class; PH, pulmonary hypertension; CTEPH, chronic thromboembolic pulmonary hypertension

FIGURE 14-1. Managing the Stable Patient with Pulmonary Hypertension

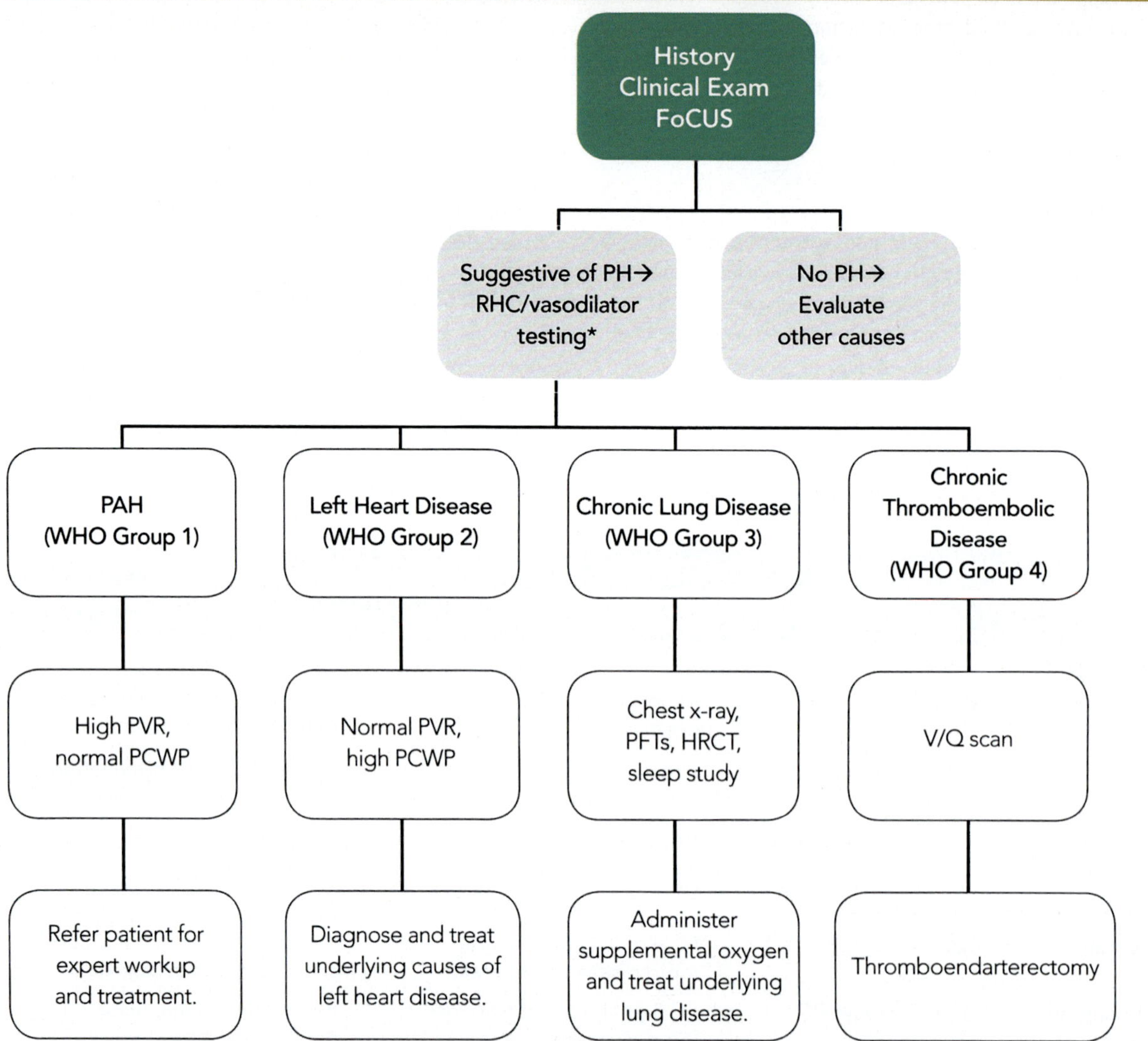

Abbreviations: FoCUS = Focused cardiac ultrasound, PH = pulmonary hypertension, RHC = right heart catheterization, PAH = pulmonary arterial hypertension, PVR = pulmonary vascular resistance, PCWP = pulmonary capillary wedge pressure, PFTs = pulmonary function tests, HRCT = high-resolution CT

WHO Group 5: Miscellaneous causes (hematological, systemic sclerosis disorders, metabolic disorders, other)

*Pulmonary hypertension is defined as a mean pulmonary artery pressure >25 mm Hg, pulmonary capillary wedge pressure <15 mm Hg, and pulmonary vascular resistance >3 WU. Positive vasodilator testing is a decrease in mean pulmonary artery pressure by >10 mm Hg to reach a mean pulmonary artery pressure <40 mm Hg with the administration of inhaled nitric oxide or intravenous epoprostenol.

another condition that has exacerbated their symptoms. It is critical to obtain a detailed history regarding the underlying cause and current treatment of the patient's PH. Dyspnea often is the presenting symptom; patients also may show signs of right ventricular failure, including peripheral edema, jugular venous distension, and hepatomegaly. A TR murmur (a low-pitched systolic murmur over the lower midsternum that increases on inspiration), a pulmonary regurgitation murmur (a diastolic murmur at the left sternal edge that increases on expiration), or an accentuated pulmonic component of the second heart sound (P_2) might be detected on cardiac examination. Evidence of right ventricular hypertrophy and right axis deviation can be seen on the electrocardiogram, along with prominent v waves on a central venous pressure tracing.[30]

PEARL

If patient stability permits, obtain a history to determine the classification of PH (WHO Group) and gather information about the patient's baseline functional status and symptoms.

PEARLS

- ✓ The timely diagnosis and treatment of the underlying cause of acute illness may prevent further deterioration in patients with PH.
- ✓ Provide oxygen support to prevent further hypoxemia and pulmonary vasoconstriction.
- ✓ Consider gentle diuretic therapy to unload the RV and therefore improve left ventricular function.

Acute Right Ventricular Failure

Severe illness (eg, sepsis), hypoxemia, or pulmonary embolism (PE) can cause a sudden elevation in PA pressure in patients with PH. This can precipitate a rapid deterioration of right ventricular function, leading to shock, cardiovascular collapse, and death. The following conditions should be considered in the PH patient with acute ventricular failure.

Sepsis

Clinicians should maintain a high index of suspicion for sepsis in those with PH who become acutely ill. Patients with severe disease often have indwelling central venous catheters, a common site of infection. Chronic right ventricular failure can lead to bowel edema, disruption of the intestinal barrier, and translocation of bacteria. Furthermore, certain treatments for PH and connective tissue diseases require immunosuppressive therapy, which increases the risk of infection.

Sepsis can have dramatic effects on right ventricular function. Peripheral vasodilation, reduced venous return to the right heart, increased vascular permeability, and hypovolemia decrease right ventricular preload, and cytokines released during sepsis can impair right ventricular contractility.[31] Although vasodilation and a drop in systemic vascular resistance occur with sepsis, the pulmonary circulation tends to experience the opposite effect, with an *increase* in vascular resistance as a result of alterations in circulating levels of vasoactive agents in the lungs. Acidosis from sepsis can cause pulmonary vasoconstriction and increase PA pressures. Without proper treatment, right ventricular failure and cardiovascular collapse can quickly ensue.

Clinicians should administer early broad-spectrum empiric antibiotics if sepsis is suspected. Fluid resuscitation, particularly when administered early, will improve right ventricular function in the setting of hypovolemia. However, overfilling the RV can worsen cardiac function; fluid resuscitation often is guided with the use of echocardiography or a PA catheter. Aggressively correcting acidosis and hypoxia can reduce PA pressures and right ventricular afterload in patients with sepsis. Norepinephrine is the vasopressor of choice for cases of septic shock and has been shown to increase mPAP and pulmonary vascular resistance (PVR) without adversely affecting right ventricular function. Dobutamine, a common inotrope, can be added to norepinephrine to improve cardiac contractility after adequate fluid resuscitation.[32] Dobutamine improves CO better than norepinephrine, increasing contractility while reducing left ventricular afterload; however, the drug's effectiveness is limited by systemic hypotension.[34] Vasopressin also can be used in conjunction with norepinephrine in patients with septic shock.[33]

Fluid resuscitation in patients with severe PH and right ventricular dysfunction can be difficult. High right-sided filling pressures can impede left ventricular diastolic filling, particularly when right ventricular end-diastolic pressure begins to exceed left ventricular end-diastolic pressure.[3] Serial reexaminations of the patient and follow-up echocardiograms often are required to determine when further fluid resuscitation will be detrimental to right ventricular function. Monitoring through PA catheterization might be necessary to determine the optimal filling pressures that correlate with an improvement in CO.

Hypoxia

Multiple factors affect blood flow to the lungs, the most important being hypoxic pulmonary vasoconstriction. The smooth muscle cells in pulmonary arterioles are sensitive to changes in alveolar oxygen levels. As the alveolar partial pressure of oxygen (PO_2) drops, vasoconstriction occurs and blood flow is redistributed to areas with higher PO_2. The elevation in PA pressure from hypoxic vasoconstriction increases right ventricular afterload and can lead to right ventricular failure. The correction of hypoxemia is critical to preventing acute elevations in PA pressure. Supplemental oxygen should be provided to improve the oxygen saturation; if the patient remains hypoxemic, noninvasive positive pressure or mechanical ventilation may be required.

Tachyarrhythmias

Atrial tachyarrhythmias frequently occur in patients with PH; atrial fibrillation and atrial flutter are the most common arrhythmias. Patients with PH may have a dilated RV due to pressure and volume overload, and the septum can bow into the left ventricular cavity, impairing its filling. Reduced right ventricular compliance often occurs with PH and also can hinder right ventricular filling. Atrial contraction becomes important to both right and left ventricular filling during diastole in those with severe disease. Atrial tachyarrhythmias are poorly tolerated in patients with PH and right ventricular dysfunction. Rate control is often ineffective in improving hemodynamics, so treatment should be aimed at maintaining and restoring sinus rhythm using antiarrhythmics (eg, amiodarone) or electrical cardioversion for patients with new-onset arrhythmias or hemodynamic instability.[35] Agents with negative inotropic properties (eg, calcium channel blockers and beta-blockers) can trigger right ventricular decompensation and should be avoided in patients with significant right ventricular dysfunction. Digoxin is often used for rate control in chronic atrial fibrillation. Radiofrequency ablation also can be used for refractory atrial flutter.

Pulmonary Embolism

Patients with PH are at high risk of venous thromboembolic disease, owing to a sedentary lifestyle from poor functional status and sluggish blood flow through the right-sided circulation. Even a small PE can cause critical elevations in PA pressure; the diagnosis should be considered in any PH patient who experiences a sudden clinical deterioration. Anticoagulation treatments should be initiated, and thrombolytic therapy should be considered if there are signs of hemodynamic instability. In patients with worsening chronic thromboembolic PH that is refractory to medical therapy, pulmonary endarterectomy can be performed at specialized centers.

TABLE 14-4. Management of the Crashing Patient with Pulmonary Hypertension

A. Airway
Provide noninvasive pulmonary support for right ventricular unloading and correction of hypoxia.
Preoxygenate.
Reduce sedative doses to prevent cardiovascular collapse during tracheal intubation.
Consider the early use of inotropes and vasopressors (eg, dobutamine, milrinone, norepinephrine, epinephrine) for right ventricular support.
B. Breathing
Use relatively high concentrations of oxygen and low levels of positive end-expiratory pressure to correct hypoxia during mechanical ventilation.
Correct hypercapnia using relatively high respiratory rates while maintaining low tidal volumes.
Administer adequate sedation for ventilator synchrony.
Consider the use of prone positioning for ARDS and right ventricular failure.
C. Circulation
Obtain serial FoCUS examinations to evaluate acute vs chronic right ventricular failure.
Use echocardiography as a noninvasive means of monitoring fluid resuscitation.
Use inotropes (milrinone, dobutamine) and vasopressors (norepinephrine, epinephrine) as required to treat shock from right ventricular failure.
Consider IV epoprostenol or treprostinil for patients with PAH (WHO Group 1) and severe disease.
Consider inhaled nitric oxide for right ventricular failure with hemodynamic instability and hypoxia.
Avoid the abrupt withdrawal of pulmonary vasodilating medications such as epoprostenol.

Medication Withdrawal

The abrupt withdrawal of pulmonary vasodilating medications can result in rebound PH and sudden clinical deterioration. The risk of this occurrence is highest with prostanoids. Epoprostenol has an extremely short half-life (<6 minutes) and is provided as a continuous intravenous infusion, typically from a portable infusion pump administered through a tunneled catheter. An abrupt interruption of the infusion caused by a pump or catheter malfunction can result in rebound PH — a life-threatening complication. Treprostinil, which can be administered either intravenously or through a continuous subcutaneous infusion, has a longer half-life of approximately 3 hours. This benefit provides a better window of opportunity for providing a replacement infusion in the event of an unexpected disruption. Any patient who presents with an inadvertently interrupted prostanoid infusion (particularly epoprostenol) should be treated as a medical emergency, and priority should be given to delivering the medication promptly to prevent rebound PH.

PEARL

Patients with PH may experience acute right ventricular failure in the setting of an severe illness such as sepsis, hypoxemia, arrhythmias, or PE.

The Critically Ill Patient

Airway Management

Patients with PH who are in a near-cardiac-arrest state should undergo a rapid evaluation of airway, breathing, and circulation. Hypoxia can cause an acute rise in the pulmonary artery pressure and precipitate a rapid deterioration in right ventricular function as well as cardiovascular collapse. If the patient remains hypoxemic despite high-flow supplemental oxygen and noninvasive ventilator support, intubation might be required.

Patients with severe PH and right ventricular dysfunction are at high risk of adverse events during emergency airway management, including hypotension, hypoxia, and cardiac arrest. Cardiovascular collapse can occur in response to systemic hypotension triggered by induction agents, a sudden increase in PA pressures from positive-pressure ventilation, or worsening hypoxemia and hypercapnic acidosis during intubation attempts. While equipment is being prepared for intubation, preparations should be made to optimize hemodynamics, including a small intravenous fluid bolus for hypovolemic or vasodilated patients. Vasopressors should be prepared in anticipation of hypotension. The patient should be optimally preoxygenated, receiving high-flow oxygen through the demand valve of a bag-valve-mask system. Maintaining the patient in the upright position while preparing for intubation can aid in preoxygenation. Assuming the patient does not have an anticipated difficult airway, rapid sequence intubation is generally the most effective method of securing the airway.

PEARL

The initial step in managing the crashing PH patient is a rapid assessment of airway, breathing, and circulation (*Figure 14-2*).

Induction agents used for rapid sequence intubation in patients with severe PH and right ventricular dysfunction must be chosen carefully, with particular attention to dosing. Pretreating with agents that cause sympatholysis (eg, opioids or benzodiazepines) is not advised, as they can reduce sympathetic tone and precipitate marked hypotension. Etomidate and ketamine are good choices for induction due to their relative hemodynamic stability, particularly compared with alternative agents such as midazolam and propofol. Etomidate or ketamine should be given at a reduced dose to prevent hypotension (etomidate: 0.1–0.15 mg/kg, or ketamine: 0.5–0.75 mg/kg). Neuromuscular blocking agents should be given at normal doses. In select cases, awake fiberoptic intubation with airway topical anesthetics and minimal sedation should be considered.

Postintubation Management

In the period immediately following intubation, blood pressure should be monitored every 3 to 5 minutes. In the event of life-threatening hypotension, vasopressors should be initiated and titrated rapidly. Auto-positive end-expiratory pressure (PEEP; also referred to as intrinsic PEEP, breath stacking, and dynamic hyperinflation) is caused by progressive air trapping in the lungs. This postintubation complication can be triggered by rapid ventilation with a resuscitation bag if the time allowed for exhalation is insufficient. Auto-PEEP is particularly deleterious in the patient with severe PH and right ventricular failure, as the increase in intrathoracic pressure not only will exacerbate the pulmonary artery pressure but reduce CO from decreased venous return to the heart.

If auto-PEEP is suspected, the endotracheal tube should be immediately disconnected from any form of ventilation (resuscitation bag or mechanical ventilation). A rapid rush of air or a prolonged expiration of trapped air from the endotracheal tube suggests the presence of this complication. Patients with significant auto-PEEP often experience a rapid return of hemodynamic stability after being disconnected from mechanical ventilation and completing exhalation. Slow ventilation (10–12 breaths/min) using single-hand ventilation with the resuscitation bag (tidal volume of approximately 500 mL) should be provided immediately following intubation to avoid this complication.

Following intubation, the lowest effective dose of sedatives and analgesic agents should be used to avoid hemodynamic instability. Small bolus doses of opioids such as fentanyl (25-mcg IV boluses) can be used for analgesia. Likewise, low doses of midazolam (1–2 mg IV) can be used for anxiolysis. These agents are preferable over propofol, which has significant vasodilatory and myocardial suppressive effects.

Mechanical Ventilation

Both hypoxemia and hypercapnia can elevate pulmonary artery pressures and should be corrected. High levels of PEEP and relatively large tidal volumes (common ventilation strategies for managing hypoxia and hypercapnia, respectively) will result in high airway pressures and compression of pulmonary capillaries, further elevating the PA pressure. A strategy for mechanical ventilation that balances the need to correct hypoxia and hypercapnia with the need to avoid elevations in PA pressure is critical. Hypoxia should be corrected using relatively high concentrations of oxygen rather than aggressive PEEP, with a goal of maintaining an oxygen saturation above 92%. Hypercapnia should be corrected by using relatively high respiratory rates, rather than high tidal volumes, with a goal tidal volume less than 8 mL/kg of ideal body weight. Both the PEEP and tidal volume should be adjusted to achieve a goal plateau pressure less than 30 cm H_2O, which will help avoid elevations in the PA pressure. It can be difficult to maintain adequate oxygenation with relatively low levels of PEEP, particularly in acute respiratory distress syndrome (ARDS). High-frequency oscillation and prone ventilation can be useful modalities for managing severe ARDS and right ventricular failure.[36,37]

Fluid Resuscitation

Many patients with PH have right ventricular volume overload requiring diuresis; however, others present with hypovolemic shock that necessitates fluid resuscitation. The RV is thin walled and does not deliver the same force of contraction as the muscular LV. The classic teaching is that the RV is more dependent on preload than the LV, and aggressive fluid resuscitation should be administered for the failing RV. However, when the RV becomes overfilled with aggressive fluid resuscitation, it will dilate and the interventricular septum will bow into the left ventricular cavity. Bowing of the septum effectively reduces the size of that cavity and limits its filling and output. Continually assessing the response to fluid resuscitation is critical in the patient with PH and right ventricular dysfunction. Overaggressive fluid resuscitation can *worsen* cardiac function.

Determining volume status can be difficult in patients with underlying PH and baseline right ventricular dysfunction. Central venous pressure (CVP) is a poor predictor of volume status in the critically ill and often is relatively high at baseline in cases of PH.[38] These patients can be hypovolemic despite relatively high filling pressures. Placement of a PA catheter can be useful to evaluate the hemodynamic response to fluid resuscitation in patients with shock. Echocardiography can be useful as a noninvasive means of monitoring for signs of right ventricular overload during fluid resuscitation.

The primary goal of resuscitation in patients with right ventricular failure and cardiogenic shock is to maintain enough coronary perfusion pressure to improve perfusion of the RV. Reductions in right ventricular afterload, wall tension, and end-diastolic pressures, and improved systemic hypotension are the hallmarks of right ventricular resuscitation. Reductions in the overdistension, ischemia, and failure of the RV improve left ventricular preload and CO.[1,39] Counterintuitively, aggressive diuresis — combined with transfusion to correct anemia and restore the sinus rhythm (arrhythmia prevention and resynchronization) — are key to improving right ventricular function.

Vasoactive Agents

Once adequate fluid resuscitation has been achieved, vasopressor medications can be administered to restore systemic blood pressure, and inotropes may be employed to bolster right ventricular output in patients with shock. Dobutamine is an inotrope that augments cardiac contractility and causes vasodilation, reducing right ventricular afterload. Similarly, milrinone augments cardiac contractility and dilates the systemic and pulmonary vasculature. It is often considered the first-line inotropic agent for PH and right ventricular failure because it appears to cause less tachycardia and more pulmonary vasodilation than dobutamine.[40] Milrinone has a relatively long half-life of 2 hours (compared with minutes for dobutamine) and should be used with caution in hypotensive patients. In addition, hypotensive patients often require vasopressors to maintain adequate blood pressure and coronary perfusion and counteract the systemic vasodilation associated with the use of inotropic agents.

All vasopressors increase pulmonary artery resistance to some extent due to their vasoconstricting effects. Evidence suggests that norepinephrine may increase systemic blood pressure with fewer deleterious effects on pulmonary resistance than other vasopressor agents.[41-43] Norepinephrine only modestly augments right ventricular contractility and often is used in conjunction with the inotrope dobutamine. Epinephrine also improves blood pressure and cardiac contractility and can be used as a single agent instead of a dobutamine-norepinephrine combination treatment for patients with shock. Vasopressin may *reduce* pulmonary resistance through the release of NO in the lungs, causing pulmonary vasodilation.[44,45] This agent can be used in conjunction with norepinephrine in cases of septic shock. Caution should be used when prescribing phenylephrine in patients with severe PH and right ventricular dysfunction. The drug causes a pure increase in afterload without improving cardiac contractility and can impair right ventricular function. Even at large centers with experience in managing PH, the in-hospital mortality rate remains high for patients with right heart failure who decompensate acutely.[46,47]

Pulmonary Vasodilators

The RV is thin walled and unable to effectively pump when faced with a sudden increase in PA pressure caused by severe hypoxemia or PE; however, a *reduction* in PA pressure can significantly improve RV function. In hemodynamically unstable patients, PAH-specific therapies tend to cause systemic vasodilation and can be difficult to initiate or up-titrate owing to systemic hypotension. Selective vasodilation of the pulmonary vasculature with treatments such as NO can be useful in hemodynamically unstable patients with PH. Inhaled NO is typically delivered through a face mask or an endotracheal tube.

KEY POINTS

1. Important questions to ask when assessing a patient with PH:
   - What is the WHO Group classification?
   - What is the patient's baseline PA pressure and right ventricular function (based on echocardiography and right heart catheterization results)?
   - What PAH-specific treatment is the patient receiving?
2. Any acute illness that increases the PA pressure or impairs right ventricular function can result in the sudden clinical deterioration of a patient with underlying PH.
3. Treat sepsis in patients with PH with the goal of improving systemic tissue perfusion. This includes providing adequate oxygenation and ventilation, reducing metabolic demand, and improving hemodynamics.
4. Optimize right ventricular preload, reduce right ventricular afterload, and improve contractility.
5. Maintenance and restoration of sinus rhythm are key to preserving hemodynamic stability in patients with arrhythmias.
6. The disruption of prostanoid infusions can be life-threatening and should be treated as a medical emergency.
7. Etomidate or ketamine should be used at reduced doses to prevent hemodynamic instability during rapid sequence intubation.
8. Avoid auto-PEEP to prevent postintubation hemodynamic instability.
9. Hypoxia should be corrected using relatively high concentrations of oxygen rather than high PEEP.
10. Hypercapnia should be corrected using relatively high respiratory rates while maintaining low tidal volumes.
11. Inhaled NO might improve hypoxia and right ventricular function in patients with severe cardiopulmonary compromise.
12. Overaggressive fluid resuscitation can worsen right ventricular failure.
13. Mechanical support might be required when medical therapy fails to achieve hemodynamic stability.
14. Outcomes from cardiac arrest in patients with PH are poor.

The drug, which directly causes vasodilation of the pulmonary vasculature and "unloads" the failing right heart, enters ventilated portions of the lungs and amplifies blood flow — a mechanism that improves ventilation-perfusion mismatching in hypoxic patients.

Intravenous prostanoids (eg, espoprostenol or treprostinil) remain the first-line therapy for WHO Class 1 patients with PAH.[48] When parenterally administered, they improve exercise tolerance, hemodynamics, quality of life, and survival rates. These medications usually are initiated at low doses in the inpatient setting and titrated slowly over days *(Table 14-3)*, often with the use of invasive hemodynamic monitoring (PA catheter) to gauge the response to therapy. Patients must be monitored closely for side effects such as systemic hypotension, jaw pain, flushing, and diarrhea.

PEARL

Hemodynamic instability should be anticipated in PH patients requiring intubation.

Heart Failure

Consideration 1: Mechanical Support

In the event that medical therapy cannot achieve hemodynamic stability in a patient with PH and a failing right heart, multiple options for mechanical support are available. Right ventricular assist devices (RVADs), which circulate blood from the vena cava or right atrium to the pulmonary artery, have been used successfully to treat right and left ventricular failure. RVADs tend to be less effective in treating right ventricular failure stemming from severe PH, as the rise in pulmonary blood flow increases PA pressures. This further damages the pulmonary circulation and does not provide adequate blood flow to the LV. Venoarterial extracorporeal membrane oxygenation (VA-ECMO) removes deoxygenated blood from the venous system and circulates oxygenated blood to the arteries, treating both cardiogenic shock and hypoxemia. VA-ECMO can be used to manage massive PE, support patients with chronic thromboembolic PH treated with pulmonary thromboendarterectomy, and act as a bridge to lung transplantation.

Consideration 2: Cardiac Arrest

The patient with PH who experiences cardiac arrest should be treated using standard advanced cardiac life support protocols. The outcomes for those with PH and right ventricular failure who develop cardiac arrest are poor; unfortunately, resuscitation efforts are generally unsuccessful.[49] The high PVR in this population makes it difficult to generate adequate circulation with chest compressions. High-dose epinephrine (1-mg IV) used during cardiopulmonary resuscitation likely will further elevate the PA pressure. There is some evidence that vasopressin causes the release of NO in the lungs, potentially reducing pulmonary artery pressure. Although there are no clinical data to support or refute this practice, it is reasonable to consider the use of vasopressin (40 units IV) as an alternative to epinephrine during cardiac arrest. Given the poor outcomes from cardiac arrest in these patients, timely discussions about advance directives are essential. Discussions regarding "do not resuscitate" orders should be broached in those with acute decompensation, particularly when the deterioration is rapid and a reversible process cannot be identified.

REFERENCES

1. Agarwal R, Gomberg-Maitland M. Current therapeutics and practical management strategies for pulmonary arterial hypertension. *Am Heart J.* 2011;162:201-213.
2. Humbert M, Evgenov O, Stasch JP. *Handbook of Experimental Pharmacotherapy: Pharmacotherapy of Pulmonary Hypertension.* Springer: New York; 2013.
3. Chan CM. Klinger JR. The right ventricle in sepsis. *Clin Chest Med.* 2008;29:661-676.
4. Wiedemann HP, Matthay RA. Acute right heart failure. *Crit Care Clin.* 1985;1:631-661.
5. Haddad F, Doyle R, Murphy D, et al. Right ventricular dysfunction in cardiovascular disease, part II. *Circulation.* 2008;117:1717-1731.
6. Simon MA. Assessment and treatment of right ventricular failure. *Nat Rev Cardiol.* 2013;10:204-218.
7. Green EM, Givertz EM. Management of acute right ventricular failure in the intensive care unit. *Curr Heart Fail Rep.* 2012;9:228-235.
8. Simoneau G, Gatzoulis MA, Adatia I, et al. Updated clinical classification of pulmonary hypertension. *J Am Coll Cardiol.* 2013;62:D34-D41.
9. Ling Y, Johnson MK, Condliffe R, et al. Changing demographics, epidemiology, and survival of incident pulmonary arterial hypertension: results from the pulmonary hypertension registry of the United Kingdom and Ireland. *Am J Resp Crit Care Med.* 2012;186:790-796.
10. Hubert M, Sitbon O, Yaici A, et al. Survival in incident and prevalent cohorts of patients with pulmonary arterial hypertension. *Eur Resp J.* 2010;36:549-555.
11. Rubin LJ. Diagnosis and management of pulmonary arterial hypertension: ACCP evidence-based clinical practice guidelines. *Chest.* 2014;126:7S-10S.
12. Oudiz RJ. Pulmonary hypertension associated with left heart disease. *Clin Chest Med.* 2007;28:233-241.
13. Melenovsky V, Hwang SJ, Lin G, et al. Right heart dysfunction in heart failure with preserved ejection fraction. *Eur Heart J.* 2014;35:3452-3462.
14. Dhingra A, Garg A, Kaur S, et al. Epidemiology of heart failure with preserved ejection fraction. *Curr Heart Fail Rep.* 2014;11:354-365.
15. Chen M. Heart failure with preserved ejection fraction in older adults. *Am J Med.* 2009;122:713-723.
16. Lam CSP, Roger VL, Rodeheffer RJ, et al. Pulmonary hypertension in heart failure with preserved ejection fraction. *J Am Coll Cardiol.* 2009;53:1119-1126.
17. Alchanatis M, Tourkohirit G, Kakouros S, et al. Daytime pulmonary hypertension in patients with obstructive sleep apnea: the effect of continuous positive airway pressure on pulmonary hemodynamics. *Respiration.* 2001;68:566-572.
18. Owan TE, Hodge DO, Herges RM, et al. Trends in prevalence and outcome of heart failure with preserved ejection fraction. *N Engl J Med.* 2006;355:251-259.
19. Chaouat A, Naieje R, Weitzenblum E. Pulmonary hypertension in COPD. *Eur J Resp.* 2008;32:1371-1385.
20. Fedullo PF, Auger WR, Kerr KM, et al. Chronic thromboembolic pulmonary hypertension. *N Engl J Med.* 2001;345:1465-1472.
21. Spencer KT, Kimura BJ, Korcarz CE, et al. Focused cardiac ultrasound: recommendations from the American Society of Echocardiography. *J Am Soc Echocardiogr.* 2013;26:567-581.
22. Rudski LG, Lai WW, Afilalo J, et al. Guidelines for the echocardiographic assessment of the right heart in adults: a report from the American Society of Echocardiography. *J Am Soc Echocardiogr.* 2010;23:685-713.
23. Via G, Hussain A, Wells M, et al. International evidence-based recommendations for focused cardiac ultrasound. *J Am Soc Echocardiogr.* 2014;27:683.
24. Taichman DB, Ornelas J, Chung L, et al. Pharmacologic therapy for pulmonary arterial hypertension in adults. *Chest* 2014;146:449-475.
25. Fisher MR, Forfia PR, Chamera E, et al. Accuracy of Doppler echocardiography in the hemodynamic assessment of pulmonary hypertension. *Am J Resp Crit Care Med.* 2009;179:615-621.
26. McClaughlin VV, Archer SL, Badesch DB, et al. ACCF/AHA 2009 Expert consensus document on pulmonary hypertension. *J Am Coll Cardiol.* 2009;53:1573-1619.
27. Sitbon O, Humbert M, Jais X, et al. Long-term response to calcium channel blockers in idiopathic pulmonary hypertension. *Circulation.* 2005;111:3105-3111.
28. Christension J, Lavoie A, Bhorade S, et al. The incidence and pathogenesis of cardipulmonary deterioration of abrupt withdrawal of inhaled nitric oxide. *Am J Resp Crit Care Med.* 2000;161:1443-1449.
29. Kuppahally SS, Michaels AD, Tandar A, et al. Can echocardiographic evaluation of cardiopulmonary hemodynamics decrease right heart catheterizations in end-stage heart failure patients awaiting transplantation? *Am J Cardiol.* 2010;106:1657-1662.
30. Ahearn GS, Tapson VF, Rebeiz A, et al. Electrocardiography to define clinical status in primary pulmonary hypertension and pulmonary arterial hypertension secondary to collagen vascular disease. *Chest.* 2002;122:524-527.
31. Parker MM, McCarthy KE, Ognibene FP, et al. Right ventricular dysfunction and dilatation, similar to left ventricular changes, characterization the cardiac depression of septic shock in humans. *Chest.* 1990;97:126-131.

32. Dellinger RP, Levy MM, Rhodes A, et al. Surviving Sepsis Campaign: international guidelines for the management of severe sepsis and septic shock. *Crit Care Med.* 2013;41:580-637.
33. Russell JA, Walley KR, Singer J, et al. Vasopressin versus norepinephrine infusion in patients with septic shock. *N Engl J Med.* 2008;358:877-887.
34. Kerbaul F, Rondelet B, Motte S, et al. Effects of norepinephrine and dobutamine on pressure load-induced right ventricular failure. *Crit Care Med.* 2004;32:1035-1040.
35. Tongers J, Schwerdtfeger B, Klein G, et al. Incidence and clinical relevance of supraventricular tachyarrhythmias in pulmonary hypertension. *Am Heart J.* 2007;153:127-132.
36. David M, von Bardeleben RS, Weiler N, et al. Cardiac function and haemodynamics during transition to high frequency oscillatory ventilation. *Eur J Anaesthesiol* 2004;21:944-952.
37. Vieillard-Baron A, Charron C, Caille V, et al. Prone positioning unloads the right ventricle in severe ARDS. *Chest* 2007;132:1440-1446.
38. Marik P, Cavallazi R. Does the central venous pressure predict fluid responsiveness? An updated meta-analysis and a plea for some common sense. *Crit Care Med.* 2013;41:1774-1781.
39. Zamanian RT, Haddad F, Doyle R et al. Management strategies for patients with pulmonary hypertension in the intensive care unit. *Crit Care Med.* 2007;35:2037-2050.
40. Price LC, Wort SJ, Finey SJ, et al. Pulmonary vascular and right ventricular dysfunction in adult critical care: current and emerging options for management: a systematic literature review. *Crit Care.* 2010;14:R169.
41. Kwak YL, Lee CS, Park YH, et al. The effect of phenylepherine and norepineprhine in patients with chronic pulmonary hypertension. *Anaesthesia.* 2002;57:9-14.
42. Ghignone M, Girling L, Prewitt RM. Volume expansion versus norepinephrine in treatment of a low cardiac output complicating an acute increase in right ventricular afterload in dogs. *Anesthesiology.* 1984;60:132-135.
43. Angle MR, Molloy DW, Penner B, et al. The cardiopulmonary and renal hemodynamic effects of norepinephrine in canine pulmonary embolism. *Chest.* 1989;95:1333-1337.
44. Russ RD, Walker BR. Role of nitric oxide in vasopressinergic pulmonary vasodilation. *Am J Physiol.* 1991;262:H743-747.
45. Tayama E, Ueda T, Shojima T, et al. Arginine vasopressin is an ideal drug after cardiac surgery for the management of low systemic vascular resistance hypotension concomitant with pulmonary hypertension. *Interact Cardiovasc Thorac Surg.* 2007;6:715-719.
46. Sztrymf B, Souza L, Bertolleti X, et al. Prognostic factors of acute heart failure in patients with pulmonary arterial hypertension. *Eur Resp J.* 2010;36:1286-1293.
47. Campo A, Mathal SC, Le Pavec J, et al. Outcomes of hospitalisation of right heart failure in pulmonary arterial hypertension. *Eur Resp J.* 2011;38:359-367.
48. Badesch DB, McLaughlin VV, Delcroix M, et al. Prostanoid therapy for pulmonary arterial hypertension. *J Am Coll Cardiol.* 2004;43:56S-61S.
49. Hoeper MM, Galie N, Murali S, et al. Outcome after cardiopulmonary resuscitation in patients with pulmonary arterial hypertension. *Am J Resp Crit Care Med.* 2002;165:341-414.

Left Ventricular Assist Devices

15

IN THIS CHAPTER

- Centrifugal versus axial continuous-flow devices
- Resuscitation and stabilization
- Diagnostic testing
- LVAD complications

John C. Greenwood, Daniel L. Herr, and Nicholas J. Hiivala

In the past decade, the number of patients with left ventricular assist devices (LVADs) has risen exponentially.[1,2] These devices can be used as a temporizing measure in patients with advanced chronic heart failure awaiting transplantation and as a bridge to recovery and destination therapy. Permanent LVAD implantation (destination therapy) can be performed in certain patients with advanced heart failure and a low likelihood of successful transplantation.[3,4] Continuous-flow pumps are used in all patients receiving destination therapy and in the vast majority of those for whom the LVAD is being used as a primary treatment.[1] Pulsatile pumps are rarely used today but can be implanted for right ventricular (RV) support in cases of RV failure.

For patients with continuous-flow LVADs, the 1- and 2-year survival rates are approximately 80% and 70%, respectively.[1] Unfortunately, these patients have a high risk of outpatient complications, including bleeding, right heart failure, arrhythmia, infection, stroke, and thrombosis. As the number of patients receiving mechanical support for advanced heart failure continues to increase, it is imperative that emergency physicians are able to recognize potential complications and rapidly resuscitate the crashing patient with an LVAD *(Figure 15-1)*.

Centrifugal versus Axial Continuous-Flow Devices

First-generation LVADs provided circulatory support using a pneumatic pump to generate pulsatile blood flow. Modern LVADs maintain continuous flow with a centrifugal or axial flow pump. These devices have a number of advantages over the older models, including smaller size, increased durability, increased energy efficiency, and lower thrombogenicity.[5,6] These devices are surgically implanted and have minimal external hardware. The centrifugal pumps are directly connected to the patient's left ventricle and lie within the pericardium (above the diaphragm). Blood returns to the ascending aorta by way of a separate outflow cannula. Axial flow pumps have a left ventricular (LV) inflow cannula that is connected in series to an intracorporeal pump located either above or below the diaphragm *(Figure 15-2)*.

Commercial brands include HeartWare HVAD, Jarvic 2000, Thoratec HeartMate II, and Heart Assist 5. The centrifugal flow HeartWare HVAD and the axial flow HeartMate II are the most common LVADs in use today *(Figure 15-3)*.[1]

Resuscitation and Stabilization

The emergency physician should be aware of common complications that can occur with LVAD patients as well as the laboratory and diagnostic tests that should be considered. During the initial evaluation, a brief history should be obtained, including contact information for the patient's LVAD coordinator and cardiothoracic surgeon, who may be able to help coordinate care and disposition from the emergency department. The clinician must determine whether the patient is stable or unstable, identify the type of device, and search for life-threatening complications. A focused history should include the type of device, when it was placed, previous complications, and the contact information for the patient's LVAD care team.

The control box, or system controller, acts as the interface between the patient and the LVAD and should be closely inspected. This device displays the battery power and indicates information about any recent alarms, which can help identify the cause of the patient's presentation *(Table 15-1)*. For patients being assessed at an LVAD center, a larger console that displays specific data points, including power, flow, speed, and pulsatility, may be available *(Figure 15-4)*. This additional information should help identify the cause of the patient's decompensation.

A thorough physical examination should be performed next; however, obtaining vital signs can be challenging in the

FIGURE 15-1. LVAD Patient Management

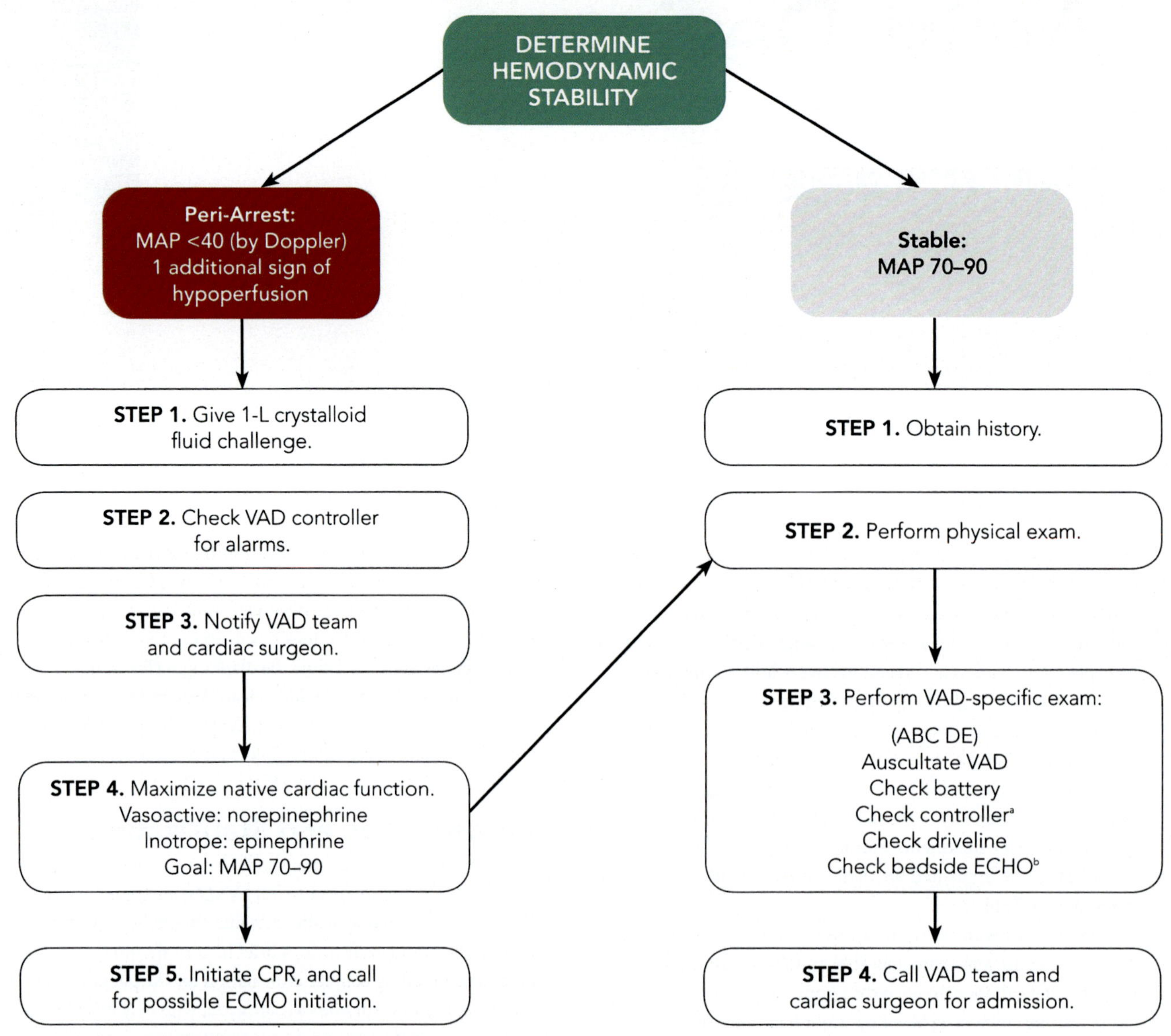

[a]For controller algorithm and differential, see Figure 15-4.
[b]For bedside ECHO algorithm and differential, see Figure 15-7.

patient with a continuous-flow device. Patients often lack central or peripheral pulses unless their native heart function has recovered (eg, a patient with myocarditis who received an LVAD as a bridge to recovery). Circulation can be assessed by simply reviewing the flow data, which are often recorded on the system controller.

The patient's blood pressure can be measured with a manual cuff and an arterial Doppler device. The mean arterial pressure (MAP) can be measured by locating either the brachial or radial artery with the Doppler device. The manual cuff should be inflated until the auditory flow can no longer be heard and then slowly released. The patient's MAP is recorded when the sound of arterial flow returns through the Doppler device. The target MAP is between 70 and 80 mm Hg, with a maximum of 90 mm Hg. Elevations in MAP significantly increase the risk of stroke.

TABLE 15-1. System Controller Functions
Controls the LVAD motor power and speed
Performs diagnostic assessments
Records and stores data
Indicates battery levels
Alerts the user to advisory and hazard alarms

FIGURE 15-2. Flow Pumps

A. Chest radiograph showing a HeartWare centrifugal flow pump
B. Chest radiograph with HeartMate II axial flow pump located below the diaphragm

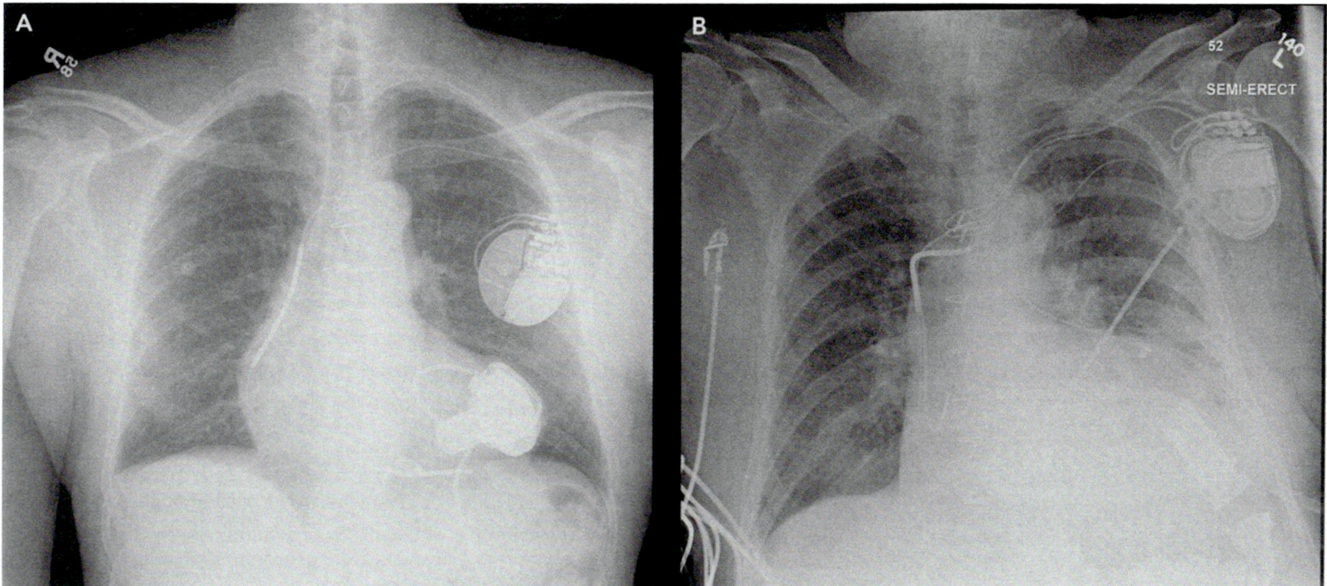

FIGURE 15-3. System Controllers

A. HeartMate II system controller

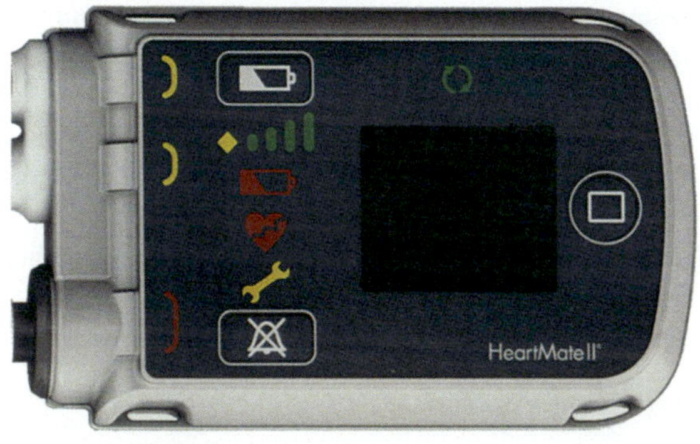

B. The HeartWare HVAD system controller

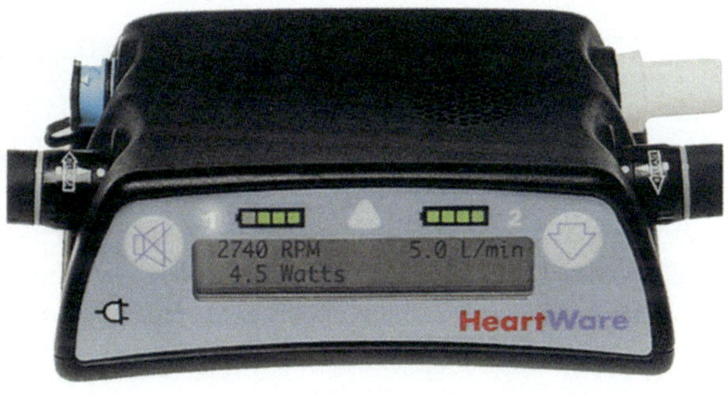

Consider early placement of an arterial line, which will provide continuous, accurate measurements of the MAP.

For an LVAD to efficiently run, the patient's intravascular volume must be filled appropriately. Continuous-flow LVADs are highly dependent on adequate preload. If the MAP is below 70 mm Hg, a bolus of crystalloid solution should be promptly administered. Hypovolemia can lead to a significant change in the LVAD's flow secondary to reduced blood volume.

These devices also are afterload sensitive. Uncontrolled increases in MAP above 90 mm Hg often reduce power, flow, cardiac output, and distal perfusion. Any patient with a MAP greater than 90 mm Hg is at increased risk of cerebral vascular events (ie, hemorrhage, ischemia) and should be promptly treated with afterload-reducing medications.[7] A flow diagram for the differential diagnosis based on common VAD alarms is presented in Figure 15-5. Pulse oximetry readings can be difficult to obtain and might be unreliable in these patients. Because most LVADs provide continuous blood flow, a pulsatile pulse oximetry waveform may be absent. It is important to confirm low oxygen values with a rapid arterial blood gas sample.

After the primary assessment, the next step should be to auscultate the patient's chest; a characteristic "hum" ensures the device is running. A faint knocking sound can indicate motor obstruction from suckdown or rotor thrombus. Signs of

FIGURE 15-4. Thoratec HeartMate II Inpatient Console

Simultaneously displays LVAD flow, speed, power, and pulsatility index in addition to other device-specific data.

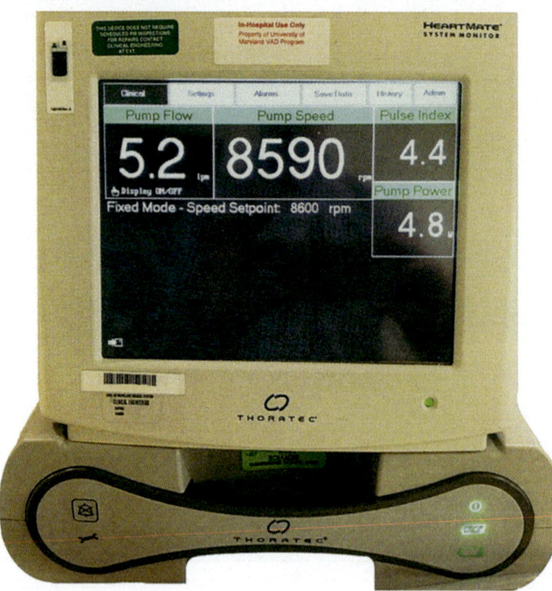

cardiogenic shock such as cool extremities, pulmonary edema, jugular venous distention, or cor pulmonale can be present if the LVAD is not functioning properly.

PEARL

A knocking sound can be indicative of a motor obstruction from suckdown or rotor thrombus.

The power cord or driveline, which usually exits from the patient's abdomen *(Figure 15-6)*, should be closely inspected for damage, fractures, and signs of infection around the exit site. In some patients, the driveline is tunneled under the skin to the scalp. Scalp pedestals have a lower risk for infection than abdominal ports, but they are prone to crack with direct trauma.[8]

TABLE 15-2. Important Laboratory Tests

Complete blood count
Comprehensive metabolic panel
Coagulation studies: PT/PTT/INR, thrombelastogram (TEG) if available
Hemolysis studies: lactate dehydrogenase (LDH), plasma free hemoglobin if available
Urinalysis
Consider: bacterial cultures/blood cultures (if concerned for infection), platelet function tests, and type and screen (if concerned for bleeding)

Diagnostic Testing

When assessing and stabilizing a crashing patient with an LVAD, a number of diagnostic tests should be rapidly performed. Laboratory tests can be used to assess for signs of active bleeding, hemolysis, infection, and electrolyte abnormalities *(Table 15-2)*. Although LVADs operate independently of the intrinsic cardiac conduction pathway, dysrhythmias can significantly impair right ventricular function; an electrocardiogram should be performed.

A chest radiograph should be obtained to look for signs of heart failure, worsening cardiomegaly, pulmonary edema, pneumonia, and driveline damage. Several LVAD pump configurations can be seen on an x-ray *(Figure 15-7)*. A bedside transthoracic echocardiogram is among the most valuable diagnostic tools for the acute evaluation of any patient with an LVAD. The test can be used to quickly assess for the presence of pericardial tamponade or RV and LV dysfunction. Most abnormalities can be visualized using standard echocardiography techniques. Parasternal long axis, apical four-chamber, and subxiphoid views can provide a large amount of information

FIGURE 15-5. Differential Diagnosis for the Patient with an LVAD

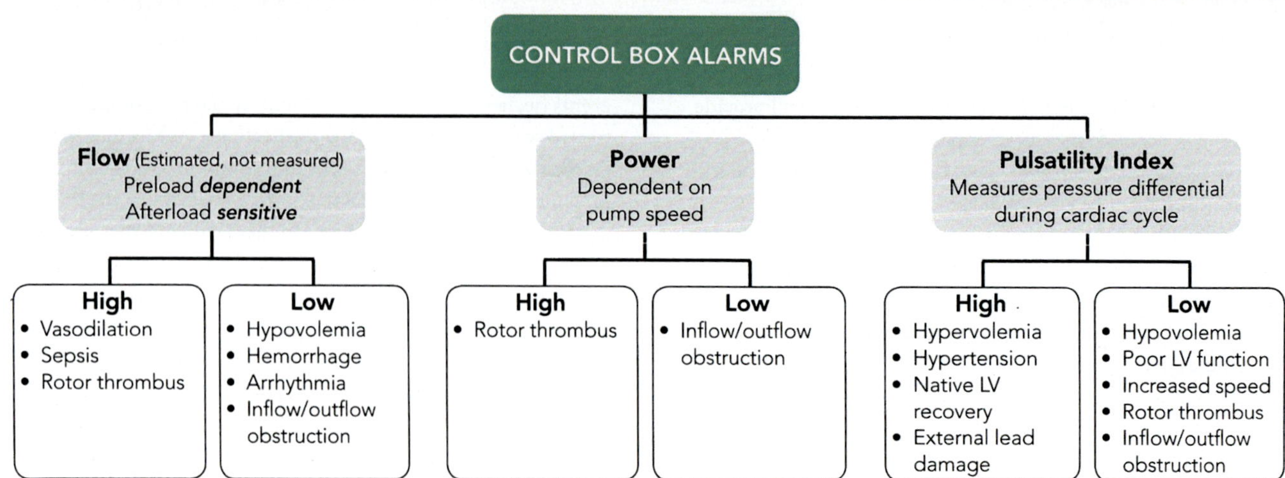

regarding the functional status of the device *(Figure 15-8)*.

During insertion, the LVAD inflow cannula is directed toward the mitral valve. Over time, it can migrate toward the intraventricular septum or simply to an off-axis position. Continuous-flow devices provide regular LV unloading, so the size of the LV cavity generally remains stable at end systole in these patients.[9] An overdistended left ventricle with rightward shift of the intraventricular septum may indicate pump malfunction, a pump thrombus, or severe aortic regurgitation *(Figure 15-9)*. If a pump thrombus is present, a hypoechoic mass often can be visualized near the inflow cannula. An underfilled left ventricle will be seen in patients with hypovolemia, excessive pump speeds, or severe RV failure *(Figure 15-10)*. There should be a high suspicion for suckdown in the patient with an arrhythmia or hypotension if the LV cavity appears to have a volume similar to the size of the LVAD inflow cannula *(Figure 15-11)*.

PEARL

An overdistended left ventricle with rightward shift of the intraventricular septum is indicative of pump malfunction, a pump thrombus, or severe aortic regurgitation.

It is important to visualize and examine both the right and left ventricles. An overdistended right ventricle will be seen in patients with RV failure, usually as a result of severe tricuspid regurgitation. RV dysfunction can present months to years after the LVAD is placed.[10] An underfilled right ventricle should raise suspicion for hypovolemia or tamponade even if an effusion is not well visualized. Because effusions can be difficult to see in an LVAD patient, clinicians should consider this complication if evidence of an underfilled right- or left-sided heart chamber is detected. Hemopericardium should be suspected if a pericardial effusion is visualized, as all LVAD patients are undergoing therapeutic anticoagulation. After the patient has been stabilized, a formal transthoracic echocardiogram should be obtained.

PEARL

Suspect hemopericardium if a pericardial effusion is visualized.

LVAD Complications

Hemorrhage

Gastrointestinal bleeding, epistaxis, and intracranial hemorrhage have been reported in LVAD patients.[11] Common causes include a supratherapeutic international normalized ratio (INR), intestinal arteriovenous malformations, and bleeding dyscrasias such as acquired von Willebrand disease.[12,13] Patients usually are undergoing long-term systemic anticoagulation (eg, Coumadin) and antiplatelet therapy (eg, aspirin, dipyridamole), which is important to consider during resuscitation. Patients commonly have an INR of 2.0 to 3.0 (those with a HeartWare device usually have a slightly higher INR target of 2.5–3.5).

FIGURE 15-6. HeartWare HVAD

A power cable is shown exiting the patient's abdomen.

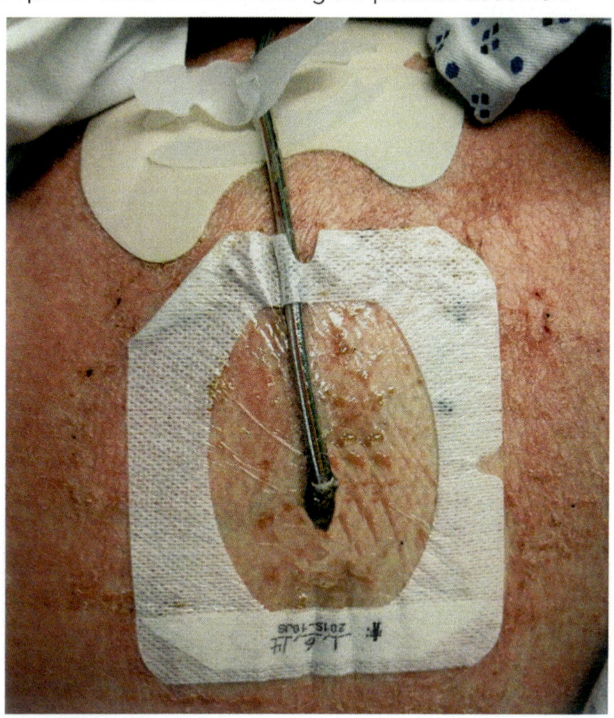

The resuscitation of a bleeding patient should begin with standard therapy to reverse an elevated INR with fresh frozen plasma or prothrombin complex concentrate, if available. Platelet dysfunction associated with acquired von Willebrand disease is common and believed to be the result of platelet exposure to the mechanical sheer stress that occurs with continuous-flow devices.[13,14] Treatment with DDAVP or cryoprecipitate can be effective. Platelet transfusions may be necessary in those taking antiplatelet medications. Rapid thrombelastography and platelet function assays can assist targeted blood component therapy in reversing coagulopathy.[15]

PEARL

Correction of coagulopathy in a patient with an LVAD often requires warfarin reversal, the administration of DDAVP, and platelet transfusions.

Pump Thrombosis

LVAD pump thrombosis should be considered in any patient presenting with cardiac arrest, cardiogenic shock, decreased pump flow, pump power spikes, recurrent heart failure, or echocardiographic findings of abnormal LV unloading.[16] Thrombosis is a life-threatening, long-term complication that can result in stroke, peripheral embolism, heart failure, and death.[17,18] Thromboembolic events have been reported in 2.7% to 35% of all patients with LVADs.[19] HeartMate devices were once

FIGURE 15-7. Chest Radiographs of Different LVAD Models

A. Jarvic 2000 with postauricular power cord placement **B.** Jarvic 2000 with abdominal power cord placement **C.** HeartWare HVAD **D.** Thoratec HeartMate II.

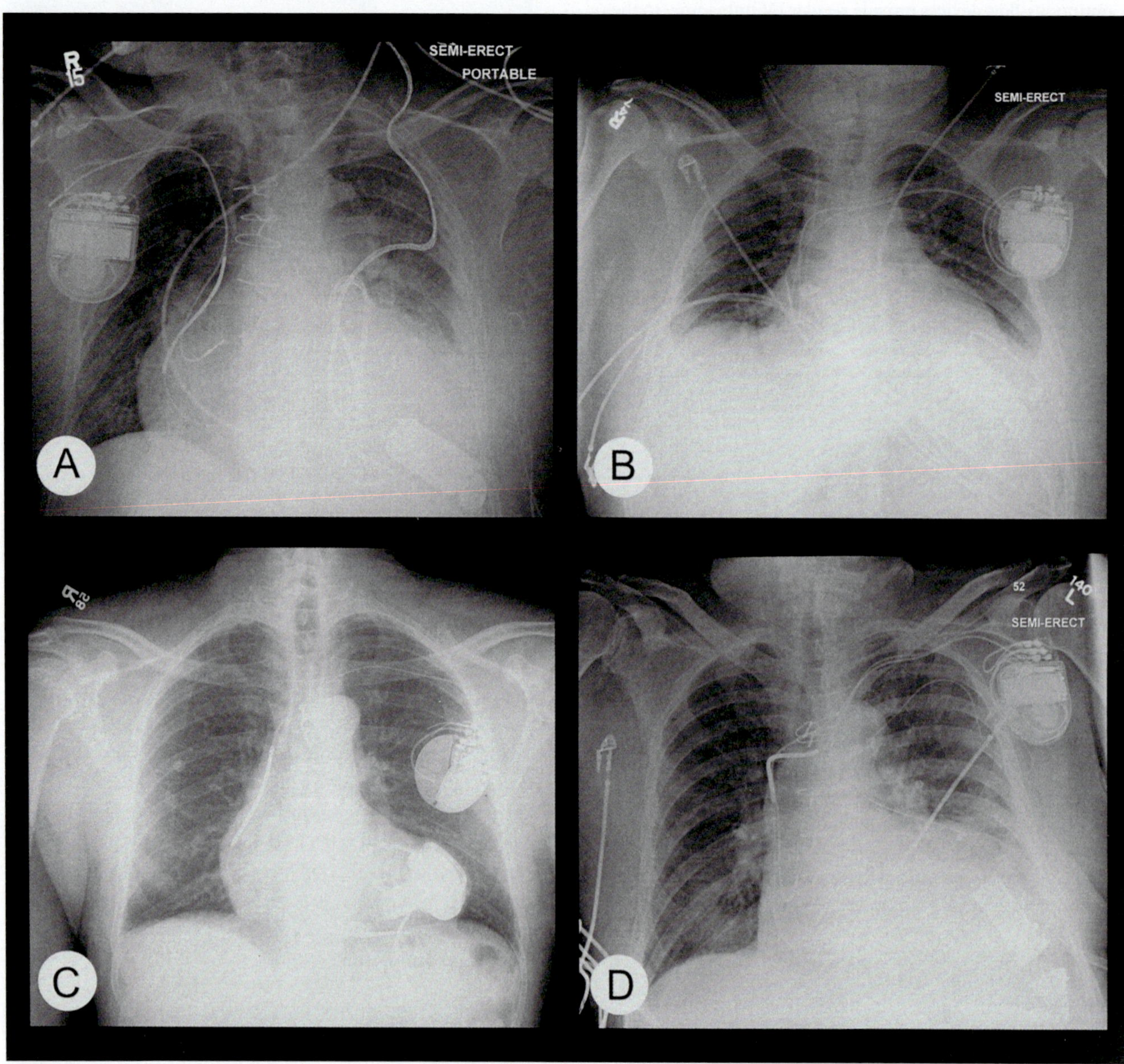

thought to have a low (3%) incidence of thrombosis due to their specific mechanical design.[20,21] However, a recent study detected an elevated risk for this complication among patients with HeartMate II devices implanted after 2011.[22] The reason for this increase is unclear.

Pump thrombus should be suspected if the lactate dehydrogenase is above 1,500 mg/dL (2.5 to 3 times the upper limit of normal), if the patient has hemoglobinuria, or if there is an elevation in the plasma-free hemoglobin.[11,16,23] If thrombosis is suspected, systemic anticoagulation with a continuous heparin infusion should be initiated. Consult the LVAD team to discuss emergent treatment options, including thrombolytic agents, antiplatelet therapy, and the need for emergent surgical pump replacement or explantation.

Suction Events

Suction (or suckdown) occurs when the patient's intraventricular septum (or another area within the myocardium) is sucked into the inflow cannula of the LVAD. This can result from decreased LV filling caused by RV failure, restrictive or hypertrophic cardiomyopathies, arrhythmias, outflow cannula migration, or hypovolemia.[11,24] Suction events reduce flow and cause diminished power (in centrifugal-flow devices) or power spikes (in axial-flow devices). Patients can

FIGURE 15-8. Differential Diagnosis Based on Various Transthoracic Echocardiography Findings

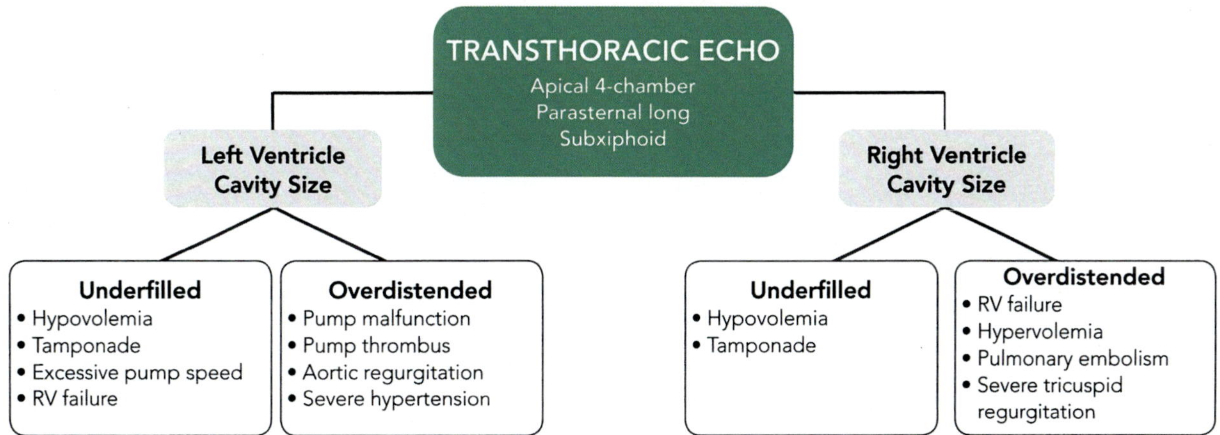

present with hypotension, intermittent syncope, or an arrhythmia. Rapid correction of this mechanical problem requires prompt recognition and treatment with an intravenous fluid bolus.

Infectious Complications

Infections are the most common cause of death among patients who require LVADs for long-term mechanical circulatory support.[25] Driveline, pump pocket, and device infections can be devastating and most frequently occur within the first 3 months after placement.[25,26] The most common location of infection is the driveline exit site, which is usually located in the abdomen. Patients with infected hardware often present with symptoms of malaise, low-grade fever, and mild tenderness around the driveline.

Ventricular assist devices are commonly placed within the pericardium, in an anatomical "pocket" within the abdominal cavity, or in the peritoneal space below the lateral rectus muscle. Pump pocket infection should be considered in LVAD patients presenting with fever, leukocytosis, and abdominal pain, especially in the setting of a driveline infection.[26,27] Additional diagnostic imaging should include abdominal ultrasound or computed tomography (CT) to identify an LVAD-related fluid collection or abscess.

It is possible for the pump itself to become colonized with bacterial pathogens, commonly referred to as "pump endocarditis." Signs and symptoms that should increase suspicion for this complication include low-grade fever, peripheral septic emboli, and pump thrombus. In any patient with an LVAD, it is critically important to search for causes of transient bacteremia or fungemia, consider health care-associated infections, and closely inspect the driveline for signs of cellulitis.[28] Hardware infections carry a particularly high mortality rate.[29,30]

The most common infecting organisms are skin and gastrointestinal pathogens: *Staphylococcus aureus*; *S. epidermidis*; and *Enterococcus*, *Pseudomonas*, *Enterobacter*, and *Klebsiella* species.[31-34] Fungal infections are estimated to occur in approximately 9% of LVAD patients. *Candida* infections are less common than bacterial infections but are responsible for the highest mortality rates.[35-37]

Resuscitation of the patient with a suspected LVAD infection should begin with aggressive intravenous fluid administration to maintain adequate preload. Early broad-spectrum antibiotic administration should include treatment for both methicillin-resistant *S. aureus* (MRSA) and gram-negative bacterial infections. Empiric antifungal therapy should be strongly considered, as fungal infections are not uncommon and can have devastating consequences. Definitive source control with surgical drainage of the localized fluid collection, device exchange, or explantation for transplant is often required.

Arrhythmias

Patients with LVADs may present with cardiac arrhythmias classified as either primary or secondary based on the underlying cause. Primary arrhythmias are intrinsic to the electrical conduction pathways of the heart and occur independent of the LVAD itself. Ventricular arrhythmias are common and can be caused by electrical remodeling, secondary scarring, or myocardial fibrosis. Because the patient's cardiac output is supported by the LVAD and the pump's flow settings are *independent* of intrinsic cardiac conduction, primary arrhythmias such as supraventricular tachycardia or ventricular tachycardia are often tolerated without clinical signs or symptoms.[38] Many patients present with the automatic implantable cardioverter defibrillator in place and may report feeling it fire prior to arrival. In the case of frequent ICD firing, a magnet can be placed over the AICD to prevent additional firing.

FIGURE 15-9. Transthoracic Echocardiographical Findings of LVAD Rotor Thrombus

Note the distended LV, even with increased speed settings.

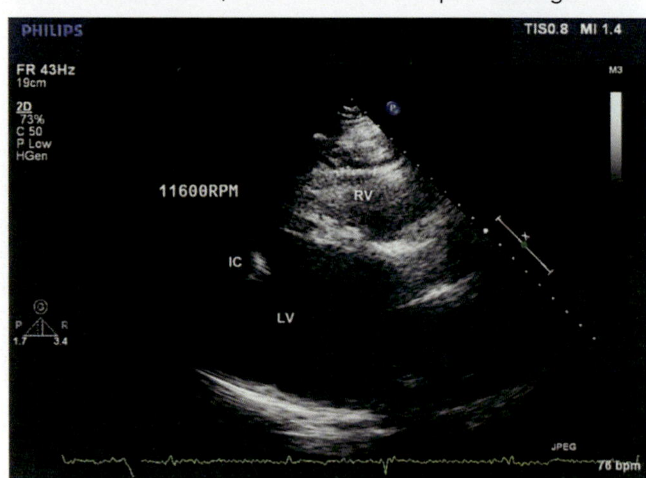

FIGURE 15-10. Bedside Echocardiogram Showing RV Failure

Note the distended RV with an RV:LV ratio approaching 1:1.

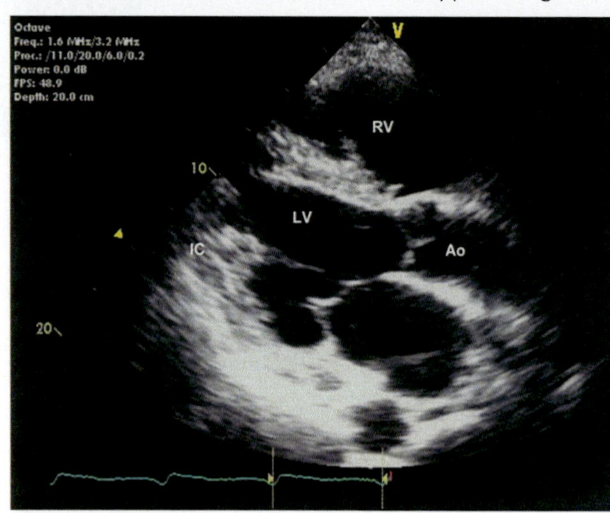

FIGURE 15-11. Bedside Echocardiogram Revealing Suckdown from Hypovolemia

A. Unedited parasternal long (PSL) view. **B.** Same PSL view; note the LV cavity size is equal to the LVAD's inflow cannula (*).

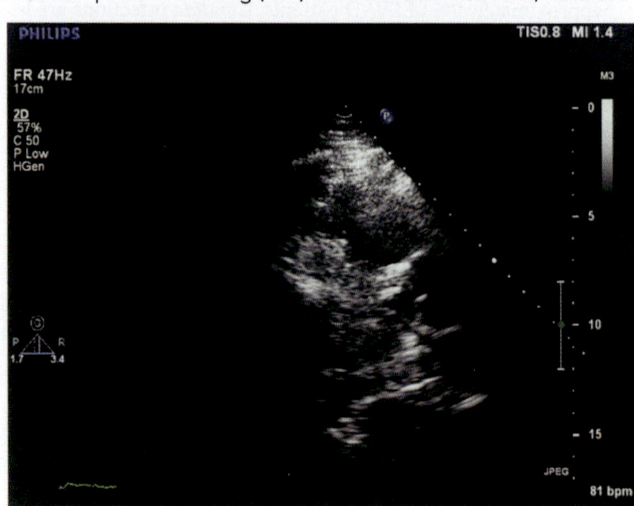

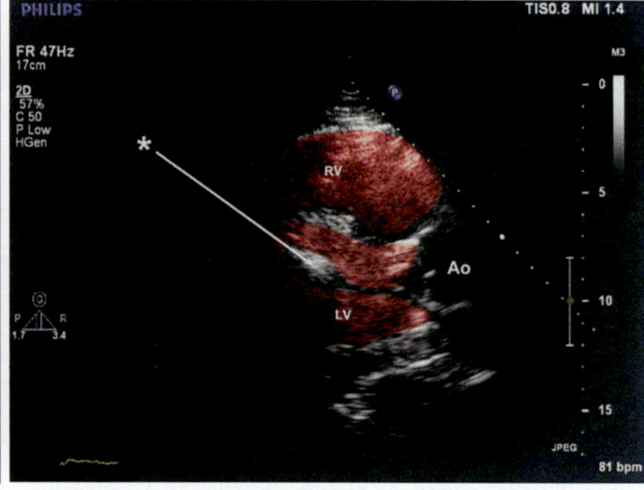

PEARL

Arrhythmias such as supraventricular and ventricular tachycardia are often tolerated without clinical signs or symptoms in LVAD patients.

Secondary causes of cardiac arrhythmias can occur if the LV septum or free wall is sucked into the inflow conduit (suckdown) of the device. Hypovolemia, inadequate pulmonary venous return, and inflow conduit migration are common causes of a secondary arrhythmia.[39]

In the emergency department, it is often difficult to determine whether the arrhythmia has a primary or secondary cause. The management of any LVAD patient presenting with an arrhythmia should begin with a prompt fluid challenge followed by an emergent bedside echocardiogram to assess if the patient would benefit from more aggressive volume resuscitation or adjustments of the device settings.

RV failure and reduced LV filling can occur if a primary arrhythmia is left untreated; therefore, primary arrhythmias should be managed in a timely manner with cardioversion or antiarrhythmic medications. There is limited evidence to guide the choice of antiarrhythmic drugs when managing a primary arrhythmia. Amiodarone is often used as a first-line agent, although beta-blockers can also be considered. Mexiletine can be given during in-patient management for refractory ventricular tachycardia.[40,41]

Mechanical Failure

Mechanical pump failure is one of the most feared LVAD complications. Signs of this malfunction include the inability to detect blood pressure with a Doppler device, the absence of sounds of a running motor on auscultation, and the absence of power indicators on the LVAD control box. If pump failure is suspected, it is important to contact the patient's cardiothoracic surgeon, LVAD engineer, and on-call nurse immediately to obtain vital information about the device.

In any patient without evidence of perfusion (MAP <40 mm Hg plus at least one other sign of hypoperfusion [eg, loss of consciousness or cyanosis]), treatment should begin promptly with aggressive volume resuscitation and standard advanced cardiac life support interventions. An epinephrine infusion should be started to maximize intrinsic cardiac output, and a heparin infusion should be strongly considered if there is any suspicion for pump thrombosis. The rapid initiation of venoarterial extracorporeal membrane oxygenation may be required as a bridge to definitive therapy.

First-generation pulsatile LVADs can be manually pumped to provide adequate blood flow (60–90 pumps per minute). However, most newer-generation devices do not have manual hand pumps or pneumatic drives. One of the biggest misperceptions about patients with LVADs is that CPR should never be performed in the setting of mechanical pump failure. Although the procedure theoretically increases the risk of device dislodgement, CPR is not contraindicated; the fear of dislodgement appears to be overstated.[42] If the patient's MAP remains unidentifiable after 1 minute despite maximal medical therapy, the manual hand pump should be connected or chest compressions should be initiated right away.

Conclusion

The use of LVADs for both temporary and permanent treatment of advanced heart failure is rapidly increasing. Emergency physicians should maintain a high degree of suspicion for the most feared complications associated with these devices: thrombosis, infection, hemorrhage, arrhythmias, and mechanical failure. Any time a patient with an LVAD presents to the emergency department, the patient's surgeon and device coordinator should be contacted immediately, as they will be able to provide invaluable information about the medical history and help with disposition planning.

REFERENCES

1. Kirklin JK, Naftel DC, Pagani FD, et al. Sixth INTERMACS annual report: a 10,000-patient database. *J Heart Lung Transplant.* 2014;33:555-564.
2. Khazanie P, Hammill BG, Patel CB, et al. Trends in the use and outcomes of ventricular assist devices among medicare beneficiaries, 2006 through 2011. *J Am Coll Cardiol.* 2014;63:1395-1404.

KEY POINTS

1. Most ventricular assist devices provide support through continuous flow. As a result, LVAD patients usually lack palpable peripheral pulses.
2. Circulation can be assessed by reviewing the LVAD flow data reported on the system controller.
3. LVADs are preload *dependent* and afterload *sensitive*. When resuscitating crashing patients, it is critical to monitor the intravascular fluid status and MAP.
4. Bedside echocardiography should be rapidly performed to evaluate for the following:
   - Hypovolemia/suckdown
   - RV dysfunction
   - Pulmonary embolism
   - Tamponade
   - LVAD dysfunction
   - Pump thrombus
5. Correction of coagulopathy in a patient with an LVAD often requires warfarin reversal, the administration of DDAVP, and platelet transfusions.
6. HeartMate II LVADs implanted after 2011 appear to have an increased risk of thrombosis (about 8% at 3 months), much higher than originally reported.
7. Strongly consider thrombosis in the patient presenting with power alarms, clinical signs of cardiogenic shock, or indications of hemolysis (eg, elevated lactate dehydrogenase or plasma-free hemoglobin).
8. Intravenous fluids are the initial treatment for suction events.
9. Driveline infections are a medical emergency and necessitate evaluation for deeper soft tissue and hardware infections.
10. The septic patient with an LVAD requires aggressive fluid resuscitation to maintain adequate preload for the pump to maintain adequate forward flow.
11. Empiric antibiotic coverage should be given for MRSA and for gram-negative, gram-positive, and fungal organisms.
12. Because their cardiac output is independent of the electrical conduction of the heart, patients with LVADs often can tolerate arrhythmias (eg, supraventricular and ventricular tachycardia) without showing clinical signs of distress.
13. Maintain a high suspicion for hypovolemia (suckdown) in the LVAD patient presenting with a new ventricular arrhythmia.
14. In the unstable LVAD patient presenting with an arrhythmia, consider early cardioversion to improve RV output.
15. Chest compressions may be performed in the event of mechanical pump failure and prolonged signs of hypoperfusion.

3. Kirklin JK, Naftel DC, Kormos RL, et al. Third INTERMACS annual report: The evolution of destination therapy in the United States. *J Heart Lung Transplant.* 2011;30:115-123.
4. Kirklin JK, Naftel DC, Pagani FD, et al. Long-term mechanical circulatory support (destination therapy): on track to compete with heart transplantation? *J Thorac Cardiovasc Surg.* 2012;144:584-603.
5. Wieselthaler GM, Schima H, Hiesmayr M, et al. First clinical experience with the DeBakey VAD continuous-axial-flow pump for bridge to transplantation. *Circulation.* 2000;101:356-359.
6. Schmid C, Tjan TD, Etz C, et al. First clinical experience with the Incor left ventricular assist device. *J Heart Lung Transplant.* 2005;24:1188-1194.
7. Slaughter MS, Pagani FD, Rogers JG, et al. Clinical management of continuous-flow left ventricular assist devices in advanced heart failure. *J Heart Lung Transplant.* 2010;29(4 suppl):S1-S39.
8. Jarvik R, Westaby S, Katsumata T, et al. LVAD power delivery: a percutaneous approach to avoid infection. *Ann Thorac Surg.* 1998;65:470-473.
9. Ammar KA, Umland MM, Kramer C, et al. The ABCs of left ventricular assist device echocardiography: a systematic approach. *Eur Heart J Cardiovasc Imaging.* 2012;13:885-899.
10. Kormos RL, Teuteberg JJ, Pagani FD, et al. Right ventricular failure in patients with the HeartMate II continuous-flow left ventricular assist device: Incidence, risk factors, and effect on outcomes. *J Thorac Cardiovasc Surg.* 2010;139:1316-1324.
11. Slaughter MS, Rogers JG, Milano CA, et al. Advanced heart failure treated with continuous-flow left ventricular assist device. *N Engl J Med.* 2009;361:2241-2251.
12. Letsou GV, Shah N, Gregoric ID, et al. Gastrointestinal bleeding from arteriovenous malformations in patients supported by the Jarvik 2000 axial-flow left ventricular assist device. *J Heart Lung Transplant.* 2005;24:105-109.
13. Geisen U, Heilmann C, Beyersdorf F, et al. Non-surgical bleeding in patients with ventricular assist devices could be explained by acquired von Willebrand disease. *Eur J Cardiothorac Surg.* 2008;33:679-684.
14. Klovaite J, Gustafsson F, Mortensen SA, et al. Severely impaired von Willebrand factor-dependent platelet aggregation in patients with a continuous-flow left ventricular assist device (HeartMate II). *J Am Coll Cardiol.* 2009;53:2162-2167.
15. Ashbrook M, Walenga JM, Schwartz J, et al. Left ventricular assist device-induced coagulation and platelet activation and effect of the current anticoagulant therapy regimen. *Clin Appl Thromb Hemost.* 2013;19:249-255.
16. Goldstein DJ, John R, Salerno C, et al. Algorithm for the diagnosis and management of suspected pump thrombus. *J Heart Lung Transplant.* 2013;32:667-670.
17. Aaronson KD, Slaughter MS, Miller LW, et al. Use of an intrapericardial, continuous-flow, centrifugal pump in patients awaiting heart transplantation. *Circulation.* 2012;125:3191-3200.
18. Pagani FD, Miller LW, Russell SD, et al. Extended mechanical circulatory support with a continuous-flow rotary left ventricular assist device. *J Am Coll Cardiol.* 2009;54:312-321.
19. Piccione W Jr. Left ventricular assist device implantation: short and long-term surgical complications. *J Heart Lung Transplant.* 2000;19(8 suppl):S89-S94.
20. Rose EA, Levin HR, Oz MC, et al. Artificial circulatory support with textured interior surfaces: a counterintuitive approach to minimizing thromboembolism. *Circulation.* 1994;90(5 Pt 2):II87-II91.
21. Frazier OH, Rose EA, Macmanus Q, et al. Multicenter clinical evaluation of the HeartMate 1000 IP left ventricular assist device. *Ann Thorac Surg.* 1992;53:1080-1090.
22. Starling RC, Moazami N, Silvestry SC, et al. Unexpected abrupt increase in left ventricular assist device thrombosis. *N Engl J Med.* 2014;370:33-40.
23. Shah P, Mehta VM, Cowger JA, et al. Diagnosis of hemolysis and device thrombosis with lactate dehydrogenase during left ventricular assist device support. *J Heart Lung Transplant.* 2014;33:102-104.
24. Topilsky Y, Pereira NL, Shah DK, et al. Left ventricular assist device therapy in patients with restrictive and hypertrophic cardiomyopathy. *Circ Heart Fail.* 2011;4:266-275.
25. Holman WL, Park SJ, Long JW, et al. Infection in permanent circulatory support: Experience from the REMATCH trial. *J Heart Lung Transplant.* 2004;23:1359-1365.
26. Holman WL, Kirklin JK, Naftel DC, et al. Infection after implantation of pulsatile mechanical circulatory support devices. *J Thorac Cardiovasc Surg.* 2010;139:1632-1636.
27. Chinn R, Dembitsky W, Eaton L, et al. Multicenter experience: prevention and management of left ventricular assist device infections. *ASAIO J.* 2005;51:461-470.
28. Holman WL, Skinner JL, Waites KB, et al. Infection during circulatory support with ventricular assist devices. *Ann Thorac Surg.* 1999;68:711-716.
29. Argenziano M, Catanese KA, Moazami N, et al. The influence of infection on survival and successful transplantation in patients with left ventricular assist devices. *J Heart Lung Transplant.* 1997;16:822-831.
30. Monkowski DH, Axelrod P, Fekete T, et al. Infections associated with ventricular assist devices: epidemiology and effect on prognosis after transplantation. *Transpl Infect Dis.* 2007;9:114-120.
31. Gordon RJ, Weinberg AD, Pagani FD, et al. Prospective, multicenter study of ventricular assist device infections. *Circulation.* 2013;127:691-702.
32. Kalya AV, Tector AJ, Crouch JD, et al. Comparison of Novacor and HeartMate vented electric left ventricular assist devices in a single institution. *J Heart Lung Transplant.* 2005;24:1973-1975.
33. Sivaratnam K, Duggan JM. Left ventricular assist device infections: three case reports and a review of the literature. *ASAIO J.* 2002;48:2-7.
34. Sinha P, Chen JM, Flannery M, et al. Infections during left ventricular assist device support do not affect posttransplant outcomes. *Circulation.* 2000;102(19 suppl 3):III194-III199.
35. Aslam S, Hernandez M, Thornby J, et al. Risk factors and outcomes of fungal ventricular-assist device infections. *Clin Infect Dis.* 2010;50:664-671.
36. Shoham S, Shaffer R, Sweet L, et al. Candidemia in patients with ventricular assist devices. *Clin Infect Dis.* 2007;44:e9-e12.
37. Bagdasarian NG, Malani AN, Pagani FD, et al. Fungemia associated with left ventricular assist device support. *J Card Surg.* 2009;24:763-765.
38. Oz MC, Rose EA, Slater J, et al. Malignant ventricular arrhythmias are well tolerated in patients receiving long-term left ventricular assist devices. *J Am Coll Cardiol.* 1994;24:1688-1691.
39. Vollkron M, Voitl P, Ta J, et al. Suction events during left ventricular support and ventricular arrhythmias. *J Heart Lung Transplant.* 2007;26:819-825.
40. Boyle A. Arrhythmias in patients with ventricular assist devices. *Curr Opin Cardiol.* 2012;27:13-18.
41. Pedrotty DM, Rame JE, Margulies KB. Management of ventricular arrhythmias in patients with ventricular assist devices. *Curr Opin Cardiol.* 2013;28:360-368.
42. Shinar Z, Bellezzo J, Stahovich M, et al. Chest compressions may be safe in arresting patients with left ventricular assist devices (LVADs). *Resuscitation.* 2014;85:702-704.

The Critically Ill Poisoned Patient

16

IN THIS CHAPTER

- Assessment, physical examination, and monitoring
- Gastrointestinal decontamination
- Cardiopulmonary support
- Neuromuscular excitation

Daniel M. Lugassy, Fermin Barrueto, Jr., and Bryan D. Hayes

Caring for the critically ill poisoned patient in the emergency department can be extremely challenging, gratifying, and frustrating all at once. The sickest patients often arrive unaccompanied and without the ability to communicate details about recent events or provide a medical history. The clinician must rely on the physical examination, electrocardiographical analysis, and laboratory interpretation to piece together a unified diagnosis. Although most poisoned patients do well with general supportive care, in some instances this approach is inadequate or potentially harmful.

Evaluation and Monitoring

The approach to all critically ill poisoned patients begins with aggressive care. Establishing intravenous access, providing supplemental oxygen, monitoring vital signs and pulse oximetry, stabilizing the ABCs, and obtaining a bedside glucose measurement and electrocardiogram (ECG) are all critical actions. A thorough but brief physical examination should be performed and must include a close evaluation of the skin (color, dry, diaphoretic), oral and respiratory secretions, reflexes, eyes (ocular clonus or nystagmus), muscle tone, bowel sounds, and bladder size. A constellation of symptoms can point to a toxidrome and lead to a diagnosis.

For routine, low-risk exposures, a minimal laboratory assessment includes a basic metabolic panel and measurement of liver enzyme levels. The serum acetaminophen concentration should be checked in any patient who reports ingestion of that compound. Even among those who report no ingestion of products containing acetaminophen, 1 in 500 will have a concentration warranting antidotal therapy.[1] Although urine toxicology screens can be ordered, they often yield false positives and negatives and seldom alter patient management.[2] No clinical scenario discussed in this chapter will benefit from a routine urine drug screen. When assessing a critically ill poisoned patient, early consultation with a poison control center or local medical toxicologist can provide useful guidance regarding current management strategies.

Gastrointestinal Decontamination

Not long ago, patients with toxic ingestions routinely received syrup of ipecac, gastric lavage, and activated charcoal. Syrup of ipecac is no longer indicated and has been removed from almost all clinical settings.[3] Furthermore, the American Academy of Pediatrics recommends that the drug no longer be used as a home treatment strategy.[4] Single-dose activated charcoal has yet to show a significant ability to improve morbidity or mortality rates. Furthermore, its use can be complicated by aspiration and lead to life-threatening chemical pneumonitis.[5] Charcoal is contraindicated in caustic ingestions, as it will obscure the visualization of the esophagus and gastrointestinal (GI) tract during endoscopy. Data regarding the benefit of orogastric lavage in poisoned patients are limited and controversial.[6,7] There may be a benefit if the procedure is performed within 1 hour after ingestion for severe or potentially severe exposures.[6] Gastric lavage should not be routinely performed for the treatment of poisoned patients. In the rare instance the procedure is indicated, it should be performed only by individuals with proper training and expertise with the consultation of a poison center or medical toxicologist.

Despite limited clinical evidence, GI decontamination should be considered when the suspected toxicity carries a high risk of morbidity and mortality and in critically ill patients with severe and life-threatening symptoms. This chapter focuses on poisonings associated with the highest mortality — the patients who have the greatest potential to benefit from GI decontamination. Early consultation with a medical toxicologist will assist with decision making regarding the administration of charcoal and the use of gastric lavage or whole bowel irrigation.[8]

Cardiopulmonary Management

When evaluating a critically ill poisoned patient, the ECG can provide vital clues and indicate the need for emergent antidotal treatment. Several key features of the ECG must be examined closely: QRS prolongation (wide complex tachycardia) caused by sodium channel blockade, torsade de pointes/QT interval prolongation from a multitude of medications, and dysrhythmias induced by digoxin/cardioactive steroids.

QRS Prolongation/Wide Complex Tachycardia

Widened QRS complexes and a rightward axis on an ECG can represent cardiotoxicity from drugs with Vaughan Williams class IA antidysrhythmic properties or quinidine like effects (eg, amantadine, cocaine, diphenhydramine, quinine, tricyclic antidepressants).[9] Through blockade of fast-acting sodium channels of the His-Purkinje system and ventricular myocardium, a delay in depolarization (at phase 0 of the action potential) results in widening of the QRS complex. Clinically, these patients have decreased inotropy and cardiac output, which manifests as severe hypotension or life-threatening dysrhythmias.[10] The hypotension from tricyclic antidepressants, specifically, is exacerbated by concurrent alpha blockade.

Wide complex tachycardias caused by toxins can be difficult to distinguish from true ventricular tachycardia (VT) and other mimics such as hyperkalemia, atrial fibrillation with bundle-branch block, and supraventricular tachycardia (SVT) with aberrancy.[11] Figure 16-1 demonstrates the following electrocardiographic findings suggestive of cardiotoxicity from class IA drugs: tachycardia, a QRS complex greater than 100 msec, terminal 40-msec changes (R in aVR, S in I, and aVL), right bundle-branch block, and right axis deviation. These cardiotoxic effects are often seen in patients with tricyclic antidepressant overdose.[12] A variety of other toxins produce similar sodium channel-blocking effects, and each displays unique clinical symptoms. For example, acute cocaine intoxication and diphenhydramine overdose present with contrasting sympathomimetic and anticholinergic toxidromes, respectively, but they both carry class IA cardiotoxicity that causes wide complex tachycardia.

Emergent treatment is indicated for patients who manifest electrocardiographic signs of class IA toxicity along with hypotension or life-threatening dysrhythmias *(Table 16-1)*. Toxin-induced wide complex dysrhythmias can be refractory to traditional therapies such as electrical cardioversion, adenosine, and amiodarone.[13] Sodium bicarbonate provides extracellular sodium that can overcome the sodium channel blockade. A bolus of sodium bicarbonate at a dose of 1 or 2 mEq/kg should be administered.[11] The ECG must be continuously monitored for narrowing of the QRS complex, which can suddenly lengthen within moments of the initiation of treatment. The endpoint of treatment should be QRS narrowing, with improvement in blood pressure and cessation of dysrhythmia. Patients who respond to a bolus of sodium bicarbonate may be placed on a continuous infusion. Severely poisoned patients receiving a continuous infusion of sodium bicarbonate can require additional boluses if the QRS widening persists. The serum pH must be monitored to maintain a safe level of less than 7.55.[10,11]

FIGURE 16-1. Tricyclic Antidepressant Poisoning

Widened QRS, deep S wave in I and aVL, and R in aVR.

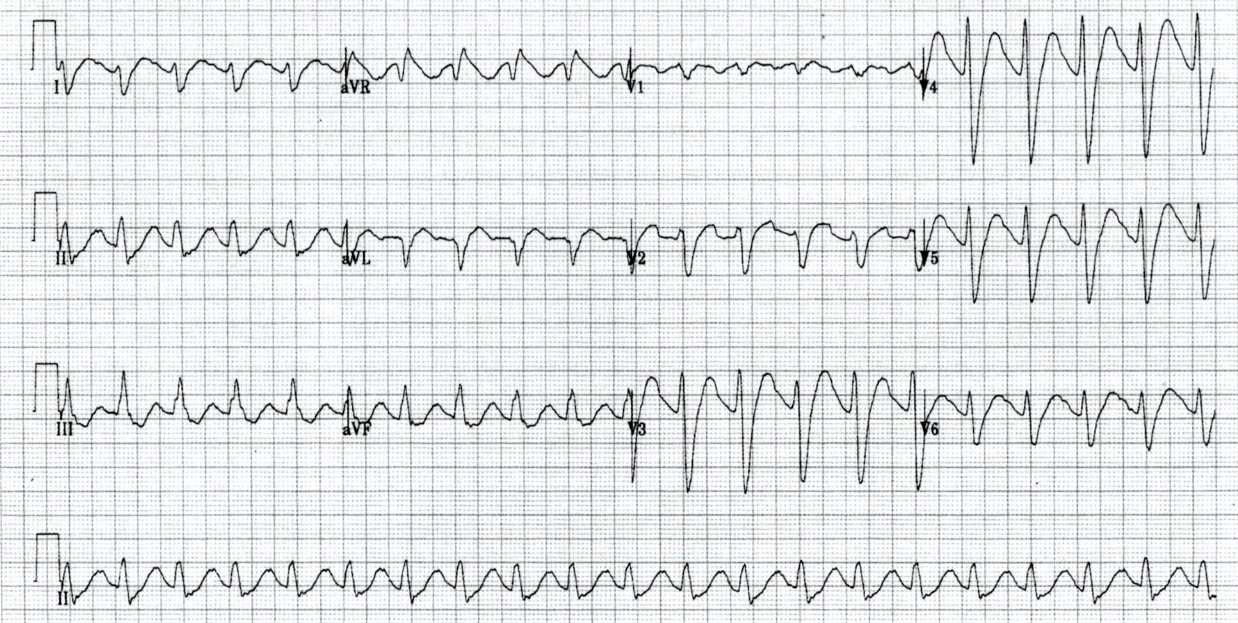

Image courtesy of lifeinthefastlane.com

PEARL

Toxin-induced wide complex dysrhythmias can be refractory to traditional therapies such as electrical cardioversion, adenosine, and amiodarone.[13]

Sodium bicarbonate ampules are commonly packaged in 50-mL vials at a concentration of either 8.4% or 7.5% (50 or 44 mEq of sodium bicarbonate, respectively). Therefore, when treating a 100-kg patient, four ampules (200 mL of 8.4% solution) would be needed to achieve a bolus dose of 2 mEq/kg. A continuous sodium bicarbonate infusion can be made by placing three ampules (150 mL of either 8.4% or 7.5% solution) of sodium bicarbonate into a 1-liter bag of D5W run at two or three times the maintenance rate.[11] The medication should be diluted with water rather than with a sodium-containing fluid, which would create a dangerously hypertonic and hypernatremic solution. Other complications of the therapy include excessive alkalemia, hypervolemia, hypokalemia, and hypernatremia. Frequent monitoring of electrolytes and serum pH (avoiding values >7.55) is warranted.

If the QRS interval does not narrow with a bolus of sodium bicarbonate, ensure that an appropriate weight-based bolus was administered. If a repeat bolus fails to correct the dysrhythmia, lidocaine may be used.[13] Although the administration of this class IB agent might seem counterintuitive given its sodium channel-blocking properties, it has high affinity for inactivated sodium channels and therefore does not cause additional QRS interval widening. In fact, some data demonstrate that lidocaine can competitively bind at the same site on cardiac sodium channels as tricyclic antidepressants.[14] Class IA and class IC antiarrhythmics (eg, procainamide and flecainide) are always contraindicated in the treatment of wide complex arrhythmias. Human and animal data have demonstrated the safety and benefit of lidocaine in treating cocaine-induced wide complex tachycardia, but its use in countering other class IA toxins is still unclear. Beta-blockers and calcium channel blockers should be avoided, as they can further blunt cardiac conduction. Amiodarone, which blocks beta-receptors as well as sodium, potassium, and calcium channels, has no defined role in the management of toxin-induced wide complex tachycardias. Its use presents potential harm and should be avoided until the causative agent has been clearly identified.[10]

TABLE 16-1. Treatment of Class IA Poisoning Manifesting as QRS Prolongation, Hypotension, or Arrhythmias

Fluid resuscitation: normal saline or lactated Ringer's solution

Sodium bicarbonate:

- 1-2 mEq/kg as a bolus over 1-2 min
- Monitor response with continuous ECG to observe for narrowing of the QRS complex.
- If patient responds, initiate a sodium bicarbonate infusion.
- Repeat bolus as needed.

Vasopressors: norepinephrine is the preferred agent, but others may be used (eg, epinephrine, vasopressin).

For refractory arrhythmias: lidocaine (1-1.5 mg/kg IV bolus over 2-3 min followed by 1-4 mg/min IV infusion)

PEARLS

- ✓ When treating a poisoned patient who has QRS prolongation (>100 msec) and signs of cardiovascular toxicity, consider the administration of sodium bicarbonate if traditional interventions such as cardioversion and defibrillation have been ineffective.
- ✓ Amiodarone, which blocks beta-receptors as well as sodium, potassium, and calcium channels, should not be used in patients with toxin-induced wide complex tachycardias.

Prolonged QT Interval/Torsade de Pointes

The QT interval represents the period of ventricular depolarization and repolarization. Measured from the onset of the QRS complex to the end of the T wave, the length of the interval shortens in the presence of tachycardia and lengthens with bradycardia. The controversial Bazett formula, which takes heart rate into account, commonly is accepted as an accurate measure of the QT interval, known as the "corrected QT" or "QTc."[15,16] It is calculated by measuring the longest QT interval and dividing it by the square root of the preceding R-R interval. Computer analysis of QTc measurements is reliable if the rhythm is regular and T waves are clear; if those conditions are not present, the interval should be manually calculated.

The normal range of the QTc interval varies with age, sex, and race. Values below 440 msec are considered normal.[17] Accepted upper limits are 440 to 460 msec in men and 440 to 470 msec in women.[16,17] When considering the approval of a new drug, the US Food and Drug Administration (FDA) meticulously assesses its effect on the QT interval.[18] The prolongation of this interval represents an increased risk of polymorphic VT, which can degenerate to torsade de pointes (TdP). Literally a "twisting of the points," TdP describes the characteristic undulating pattern that the QRS complexes undergo in a sinusoidal-type pattern. The ECG of a patient on methadone who presented for treatment of syncope is shown in Figure 16-2. It illustrates an extremely prolonged QTc with runs of polymorphic VT and a characteristic slow-fast-slow pattern seen with QTc prolongation. An electrocardiographical analysis for TdP and assessment of QTc should be performed in patients presenting with cardiovascular complaints such as lightheadedness, dizziness, syncope, palpitations, or even cardiac arrest. Intermittent episodes of apparent VT should prompt close investigation of the QTc.

Fortunately, the number of patients in whom TdP develops after drug-induced prolongation of the QT interval is small. TdP is a nonperfusing rhythm that can degenerate into ventricular fibrillation and therefore must be identified and rapidly managed. Specific therapy is necessary because the traditional approach to the management of VT can be unsuccessful.

Although there is clinical evidence that an abnormally prolonged QTc interval (>500 msec) significantly increases the risk for TdP, some patients with QTc values well above normal (500–600 msec) never develop the complication, while others with minimal elevation (<500 msec) do.[15-17] In patients with acquired or drug-induced QT prolongation, bradycardia can increase the propensity to convert to TdP. Hundreds of common medications, including as many as 3% of noncardiac drugs, can cause QT prolongation in both therapeutic and toxic doses *(Table 16-2)*.[15-17] Several online resources (eg, www.crediblemeds.org) list medications confirmed to induce this abnormality.

Risk Factors

Patients with a congenital long QT interval are at higher risk for TdP when exposed to drugs that cause QT prolongation.[17] Electrolyte abnormalities such as hypokalemia, hypomagnesemia, and hypocalcemia can independently prolong the QT interval.[16] The risk of TdP is also increased with the concurrent use of multiple QT-prolonging drugs and interactions between drugs that alter their metabolism.[17] Alterations in liver or kidney function can affect the metabolism of certain medications, leading to abnormally elevated serum concentrations. Other recognized risk factors include bradycardia, female sex, and atrioventricular blockade.[15-17]

Treatment

Emergency physicians should be prepared to perform immediate electrical cardioversion in any patient with a TdP rhythm, which can degenerate into ventricular fibrillation and unstable VT. An immediate bolus of intravenous magnesium (1–2 g over 1–2 min) should be the first-line treatment.[17] Magnesium acts as a calcium channel blocker, preventing spontaneous depolarization during the ventricular repolarization that is responsible for causing TdP. An infusion of magnesium should be initiated after the bolus to suppress TdP until the QTc interval shortens. The aggressive repletion of potassium, magnesium, and calcium may help shorten the interval. The magnesium bolus may be repeated.

If the patient remains in refractory TdP, the heart rate may be stimulated to beat faster by one of two interventions — overdrive pacing (cutaneous or transvenous) or the administration of isoproterenol. Once electrical and mechanical capture have been obtained, the target heart rate should be 90 to 110 beats/min. This increased rate decreases the QTc interval. Isoproterenol, a $beta_1$-agonist, also increases the heart rate. The infusion should be titrated to achieve a heart rate of more than 90 beats/min. Once the patient has been stabilized, the next step is to identify the offending agent and consider GI decontamination or another form of removal. Hemodialysis can be used for medications that are cleared via the kidneys (eg, sotalol).[16,17]

FIGURE 16-2. Severe QTc Prolongation with Polymorphic VT Caused by Methadone

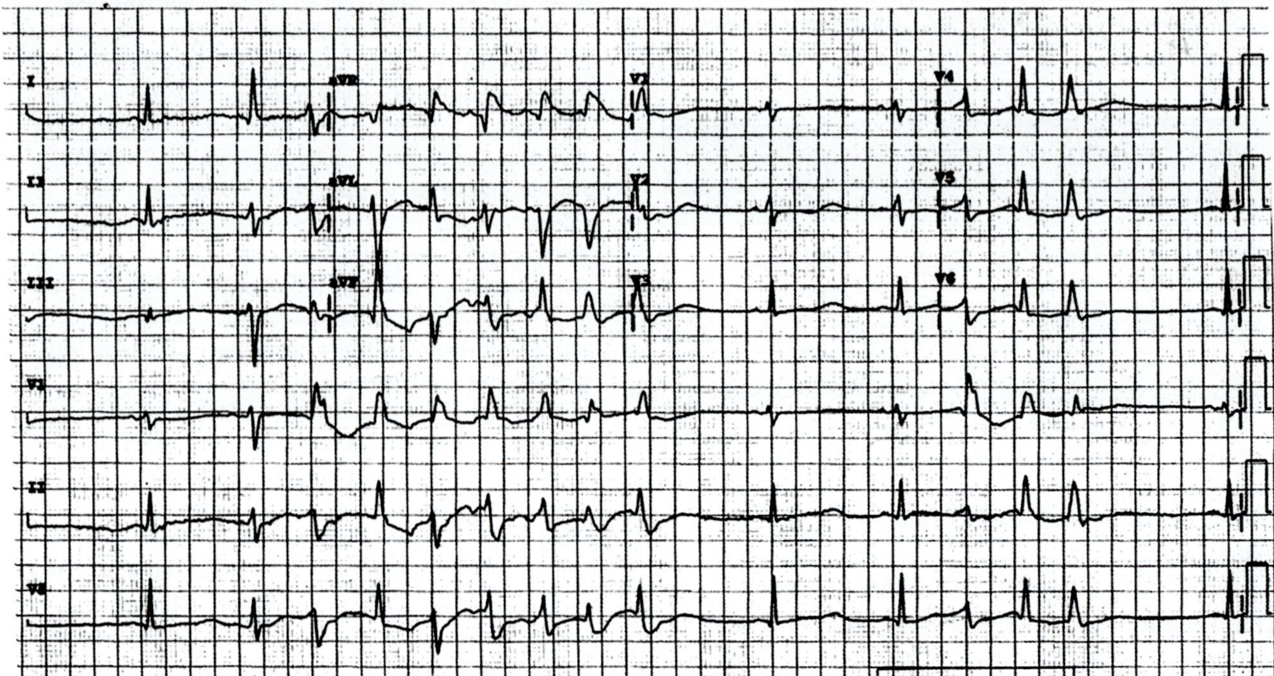

Antihypertensive Overdose

High blood pressure afflicts nearly 30% of American adults, 68% of whom are prescribed an antihypertensive medication; many of these patients take more than one class of drug.[19] Although most of these agents can cause low blood pressure in overdose, calcium channel blockers and beta-blockers are associated with significant morbidity and mortality because they can induce severe hypotension that is refractory to traditional therapies.

Calcium channel blockers, which prevent calcium from entering the cells of the heart and blood vessel walls, are used to treat hypertension, arrhythmias, angina, and migraine headaches. They are further broken down into two subsets: the nondihydropyridines (which act on the peripheral vasculature and the myocardium) and the dihydropyridines (which are selective for the peripheral vasculature). In the periphery, these agents cause smooth-muscle relaxation and vasodilation; in the myocardium, channel blockade decreases contractility and conduction. At therapeutic doses, calcium channel blockers decrease blood pressure and serve as an antiarrhythmic. Beta-blockers impede beta-adrenergic surface receptors throughout the body (in the heart, eye, peripheral vascular smooth muscle, and liver). They vary in their selectivity of $beta_1$-, $beta_2$-, and $beta_3$-receptor activities, and some have additional alpha-receptor-blocking properties (eg, labetalol and carvedilol).

Only a few medications cause hypotension and bradycardia. Calcium channel blocker, beta-blocker, digoxin, and clonidine toxicity should be considered in the differential diagnosis of a poisoned patient with those clinical signs. Given their effect on the heart, nondihydropyridines will induce hypotension with paradoxic bradycardia. Dihydropyridines, on the other hand, will manifest hypotension with reflex tachycardia, although in a large overdose they may lose selectivity and behave like a nondihydropyridine.[20] Individuals with beta-blocker overdose are also likely to present with hypotension and bradycardia.[21]

The difference between the clinical manifestations of overdoses of calcium channel blockers and beta-blockers is subtle. We address the management of them concurrently because, in acute overdose, it can be impossible to distinguish them and the treatments overlap.

After aggressive intravenous fluid resuscitation, atropine, glucagon, and calcium may be administered to patients experiencing persistent hypotension and bradycardia *(Table 16-3)*. Atropine can be used to treat bradycardia and thereby improve cardiac output and blood pressure, but it is often ineffective.

TABLE 16-2. Drugs that Can Cause QTc Prolongation and Torsade de Pointes

Amiodarone	Ibutilide
Clarithromycin	Methadone
Disopyramide	Procainamide
Erythromycin	Quinidine
Fluconazole	Sotalol
Fluoxetine	Terfenadine
Haloperidol	Terodiline

Glucagon

Glucagon is a specific antidote for beta-blocker poisoning. It bypasses beta-blockade and leads to the activation of adenyl cyclase, the very action of a beta-agonist. If the glucagon bolus elicits a favorable response, then a continuous infusion must follow at a rate based on that initial reaction. For example, if a response is observed at 5 mg, then the infusion should begin at 5 mg/hr. Most patients who receive large doses of glucagon will experience emesis; pretreatment with an antiemetic can help avoid this side effect. This reaction can preclude its use in a severely ill patient with depressed mental status and an unprotected airway. Glucagon is a tachyphylactic drug: its clinical effect diminishes over a short time.

Calcium

Intravenous boluses of calcium should be administered for refractory hypotension in patients with confirmed or suspected overdose of a calcium channel blocker or beta-blocker. Increasing the extracellular calcium concentration elevates the gradient across the cell membranes, allowing more calcium to enter the cell. This improves MAP more than the negative chronotropy. Recommendations for the management of patients suspected of calcium channel blocker poisoning call for the administration of 13 to 25 mEq of calcium *(Table 16-3)* in the form of either calcium gluconate or calcium chloride salts. As with glucagon, patients should receive a continuous infusion of calcium after the bolus.

Aggressive administration is warranted for severe refractory hypotension, but there are no clear guidelines on total measured serum calcium limits. In a case report of a severe calcium channel blocker overdose, the serum calcium concentration peaked at 15 mg/dL.[22] Permissive hypercalcemia is not without risk: it can cause nausea, vomiting, flushing, and constipation. Rigorous monitoring of the serum calcium and phosphorus levels for calculation of the calcium-phosphate product can help predict the likelihood of crystallization. Medical toxicology consultation can guide continued management.

Hyperinsulinemia Euglycemia Therapy

Despite maximal therapy with intravenous fluids, atropine, glucagon, and vasopressors, patients with severe calcium channel blocker or beta-blocker overdose can remain profoundly hypotensive. For years, insulin has been known to have beneficial inotropic and chronotropic effects. Hyperinsulinemia euglycemia therapy (HIET) uses high-dose insulin infusions while maintaining serum glucose within normal limits. The dosing protocol is presented in Table 16-4.

The exact mechanism of action for this therapy is unclear. One theory suggests that the poisoned myocardium is in a stressed state, preferring glucose as a substrate instead of the free fatty acids that it normally uses.[23,24] There is convincing animal

TABLE 16-3. Dosing in Calcium Channel and Beta-Blocker Toxicity

Atropine
Adults: 0.5–1 mg IV
Children: 0.02 mg/kg (≥0.1 mg) IV (may be repeated every 2–3 min; total maximum 3 mg)
Glucagon
Adults: 2–5 mg slow IV push repeated every 5–10 mins (up to a total dose of 10 mg), followed by an infusion at the hourly rate of response (ie, if 5 mg provided a response, start a continuous infusion at 5 mg/hr)
Children: 50–150 mcg/kg slow IV push, then 50 mcg/kg/hr up to the maximum adult dose
Calcium (bolus with 13–25 mEq)
1 g of calcium gluconate (4.3 mEq of calcium)[a,b]
1 g of calcium chloride (13.4 mEq of calcium)[a,b]
Adults: Slow IV push over 5–10 minutes of 30–60 mL of 10% of calcium gluconate *OR* 10–20 mL of 10% calcium chloride
Children: 0.1 mL/kg of 10% calcium gluconate Continuous infusions of 0.5 mEq/kg/hr of calcium may be initiated after 3–4 bolus doses (described above) but should be preceded by checking calcium and phosphorus concentrations.

[a]*One ampule usually contains 10 mL of a 10% solution of either calcium chloride or calcium gluconate; confirm before administering.*
[b]*Calcium chloride has about three times the molar amount of calcium as calcium gluconate but is associated with a significant risk of sclerosis.*

evidence and anecdotal human case reports that HIET improves hemodynamic function.[21,24-27] Given the grave nature of these poisonings, HIET should be considered with the initiation of vasopressors (or even earlier in patients who do not respond to fluids, glucagon, and calcium).

PEARL

High-dose boluses and infusions of insulin can be safe in the treatment of refractory calcium channel blocker or beta-blocker overdose. This therapeutic approach is associated with a low incidence of clinically significant hypoglycemia and hypokalemia.

In a 100-kg person, a bolus of 100 units of insulin followed by 50 to 100 units/hour is an appropriate starting regimen.[25] Although often questioned, the safety of this therapy has been well demonstrated and does not induce significant episodes of hypoglycemia. While the quantity may seem intimidating, a dose response relationship appears to exist and the benefits of these high insulin doses far outweigh the risks. Low-dose insulin does not provide an inotropic or chronotropic benefit.[26]

Once the peripheral insulin receptors are saturated, the risk of hypoglycemia is reduced.

Many patients can be maintained on HIET alone without vasopressors, thus avoiding the severe complications associated with vasopressor therapy, including tachyarrhythmias or ischemic injury to the bowel, limbs, or vital organs. If the patient responds to HIET, hemodynamic monitoring will show an increase in ejection fraction and cardiac function.[21] HIET might not increase the heart rate. In cases of severe peripheral vasodilation, vasopressors may be required to augment decreased systemic vascular resistance.

Despite adequate boluses and infusion of dextrose, recurrent episodes of hypoglycemia can signal resolution of calcium channel blocker poisoning. Calcium channels facilitate exocytosis in beta-islet cells and are thus responsible for baseline-mediated insulin release.[25] This is why patients without underlying diabetes can display hyperglycemia in calcium channel blocker overdose. It also may be a clue to the nature of the initial exposure. Improved hemodynamics and decreased vasopressor requirements are other indications that the insulin infusion may be titrated down.

Vasopressors

After interventions with intravenous fluids, atropine, glucagon, and calcium, the management of refractory hypotension may require an infusion of catecholamines. No specific evidence-based recommendations have been formulated; however, norepinephrine offers a theoretical advantage over other vasopressors because it provides myocardial stimulation at $beta_1$-receptors of the heart. In

TABLE 16-4. HIET Dosing

Begin with an IV bolus of regular insulin (1 unit/kg). If serum glucose <250 mg/dL, concurrently administer a bolus of dextrose (25–50 g or 0.5–1 g/kg IV).
After bolus, initiate regular insulin (0.5–1 unit/ kg/hr) plus a continuous infusion of dextrose (0.5 g/kg/hr), and titrate to maintain glucose levels of 110–150 mg/dL.
Monitor serum glucose every 30 minutes for the first 1–2 hours until euglycemia is maintained.
Potassium should also be monitored closely and repleted to maintain within normal limits.
The insulin bolus and infusion can take 20–30 minutes to induce a clinical inotropic/chronotropic effect. Increase insulin infusion by 0.5–1 unit/kg/hr every 60 minutes (similar to administration of a pressor to maintain desired hemodynamic effect).
Optimal insulin dosing is unknown, but patients have been maintained on insulin infusion rates as high as 2–5 units/kg/hr.

addition, it has potent $alpha_1$-adrenergic effects on the peripheral vasculature. Vasopressin, phenylephrine, dopamine, and dobutamine have all been used to treat overdoses of calcium channel blockers and beta-blockers with varying degrees of success. Invasive monitoring and echocardiography will provide insight into which vasopressors might provide optimal hemodynamic function.

PEARL

One way to differentiate a beta-blocker overdose from a calcium channel-blocker overdose is that beta-blockers typically do not affect blood glucose or cause hypoglycemia. Calcium channel blockers cause hyperglycemia.

Intralipid Infusion

The use of 20% intravenous lipid emulsion therapy in calcium channel blocker or beta-blocker overdose is still experimental, but limited data suggest that it can improve hemodynamic function in this clinical scenario.[28,29] The therapy first was discovered as an antidote to cardiac arrest after the unintentional injection of intravenous bupivacaine.[30] Two theories about its action have been postulated. One is that intralipid acts as a "lipid sink," providing an alternate binding site for lipophilic drugs such as bupivacaine. The other theory proposes that intralipid increases the free fatty acid concentration, providing the heart with its normally preferred energy source.[28,29] Intralipid preparations and recommended dosing regimens are presented in Table 16-5.[31,32]

Intralipid can be found on many anesthesia carts because of its benefit in cases of acute bupivacaine toxicity. The agent currently is reserved for the most severe cases of calcium channel blocker/beta-blocker overdose that are refractory to all other therapies and involve impending or current cardiac arrest. There is limited human experience with intralipid. Although the rate and extent of complications are unknown, hypersensitivity reactions, pancreatitis, acute lung injury, and deep vein thrombosis have been reported in human case reports and series.[33-35] Lipid emboli have been observed in animal trials. Poison control centers and medical toxicologists are good sources of information about the use of this compound.

Alternative Therapies

Phosphodiesterase inhibitors such as milrinone and amrinone have been employed to improve myocardial inotropy, but they can cause hypotension.[36] Extracorporeal membrane oxygenation has been used successfully in some pediatric poisonings.[37] Cardiopulmonary bypass, transvenous pacemakers, and intraaortic balloon pumps have also been used. Despite limited evidence about the efficacy of these adjuncts, they may be life-saving measures for bridging patients through acute toxicity. Early discussion with consultants can expedite such heroic measures.

Neuromuscular Excitation

Toxin-Induced Seizures/Status Epilepticus

The main inhibitory neurotransmitter is gamma-aminobutyric acid (GABA), which binds to the GABA receptor that is linked to a chloride channel. The opening of this channel by GABA binding allows an influx of chloride into the cell, resulting in inhibitory hyperpolarization. Other drugs that affect chloride influx or attenuate the GABA receptor are ethanol, benzodiazepines, barbiturates, and propofol. The primary excitatory neurotransmitter is glutamate, which binds to kainate, AMPA, and NMDA receptors. Additional neurotransmitters and channels (eg, adenosine and sodium channels) are also involved in the pathology of toxin-induced seizures. A wide range of drugs and toxins can cause acute seizures *(Table 16-6)* or lower the seizure threshold, uncovering underlying epileptic disease.

The emergency department management of seizures is the same regardless of their cause. The patient should be stabilized, intravenous access should be established, and the airway should be protected. Alterations in glucose, electrolytes, oxygen, blood pressure, and temperature should be addressed, and eclampsia should be considered until a woman's pregnancy status is known. Severe hyponatremia, toxin-induced or primary metabolic, must be considered in patients experiencing seizures and can be caused by a variety of toxins (eg, MDMA and other amphetamines). Withdrawal syndromes associated with the abrupt cessation of ethanol or benzodiazepines use in adults can present as seizures. Opioid withdrawal usually does not trigger seizures in adults, but it can cause them in neonates.

Management of Seizures

Patients who are actively seizing should receive rapidly escalating doses of benzodiazepines to terminate the convulsions. If the seizures do not respond to treatment or are recurrent and meet clinical criteria for status epilepticus, pyridoxine (vitamin B_6) should be emergently given as an intravenous push.

TABLE 16-5. Intralipid Therapy for Calcium Channel Blocker/Beta-Blocker Overdose

Standard treatment
Obtain a prepared infusion if possible, or request an infusion from the pharmacy that is made from IV lipid preparations used in total parenteral nutrition.
For patients with severe refractory cardiovascular collapse or impending or current cardiac arrest
Bolus: 1–1.5 mL/kg over 1 minute using a 20% intravenous lipid emulsion solution.
Repeat every 3–5 minutes (maximum dose 3 mL/kg).
Some clinicians begin an infusion after the initial bolus at a rate of 0.25 mL/kg/min until hemodynamic recovery is achieved.
Discuss the latest indications with your local poison control center or medical toxicologist.

There are very few causes of true toxin-induced convulsive status epilepticus, and fewer that are benzodiazepine resistant. Isoniazid, *Gyromitra* mushroom species, and rocket fuel are hydrazines that produce benzodiazepine-resistant seizures requiring pyridoxine therapy to terminate status epilepticus.[38]

PEARL

Isoniazid, *Gyromitra* mushroom species, and rocket fuel are hydrazines that produce benzodiazepine-resistant seizures requiring pyridoxine therapy to terminate status epilepticus.[38]

Hydrazines inhibit the metabolic pathway responsible for the normal production of GABA metabolized from glutamate. This generates an excess of glutamate, increases excitation, and decreases GABA and inhibition — an imbalance that ultimately produces severe acute convulsions. Although pyridoxine therapy is specific to this group of toxins, it is prudent to empirically administer at least 1 dose to patients with status epilepticus when any of the following conditions applies: a toxin-induced seizure is suspected, the patient has a history of tuberculosis (TB) or resides in an area of endemic TB, or the cause of the seizures cannot be explained. The dose of pyridoxine for seizures is extremely high compared with routine replacement *(Table 16-7)*, but its adverse-effect profile is low, and complications are expected only with chronic continuous elevated dosing regimens. Because they share a primary mechanism of action, drug-induced hyponatremia and inappropriate antidiuretic hormone secretion usually can be approached the same way. In patients with toxin-induced seizures, phenytoin will be unsuccessful at terminating convulsions and can harm patients poisoned by cocaine, tricyclic antidepressants, or theophylline.[38]

Hyperthermic Syndromes

Several syndromes and exposures can lead to toxicologically induced hyperthermia. Emergency physicians should be familiar with the clinical presentations of serotonin syndrome, neuroleptic malignant syndrome, malignant hyperthermia, and sympathomimetic overdose *(Table 16-8)*. Although each entity has a different mechanism of action, they share the ability to cause excess neuromuscular activity. This can lead to increased heat production and spur a rapid rise in the patient's core temperature.

Toxin-induced hyperthermia can be difficult to distinguish from temperature elevations caused by infection.[39] One of the key differences is that infection produces an inflammatory response, causing the endogenous release of cytokines and interleukins; this mechanism resets the thermoregulation center of the hypothalamus, raising the body's temperature. Hyperthermia resulting from exposure to a toxin is frequently caused by extreme muscular rigidity or activity. Until an infectious process is definitively ruled out, it is most appropriate to empirically treat the patient for a potential poisoning along with standard measures for infection-related hyperthermia.

Obtain a rectal temperature or core body temperature immediately on any patient suspected of hyperthermia, as oral and axillary temperatures are unreliable. A common pitfall is to assume that a normal core body temperature rules out these toxin-induced hyperthermic syndromes. All of these syndromes (except malignant hyperthermia) can present with a wide spectrum of clinical severity. The early recognition of neuroleptic malignant syndrome and cessation of neuroleptic therapy are likely to decrease morbidity and mortality.[40]

The complications associated with toxin-induced hyperthermia include rhabdomyolysis, seizures, disseminated intravascular coagulopathy, arrhythmias, multisystem organ failure, and death.[39] The length of time a patient spends in a hyperthermic state correlates with the likelihood of complications; as little as 30 minutes at temperatures above 39°C (102.2°F) increases morbidity and mortality.[41]

The most critical action when patients are significantly hyperthermic is to aggressively sedate and cool them *(Table 16-9)*. Muscular rigidity and agitation can be halted with appropriate benzodiazepine administration. If this does not lower the core temperature, the patient must be intubated, paralyzed, and cooled rapidly. Active cooling must be initiated immediately

TABLE 16-6. Seizure-Inducing Toxins

Amphetamines	Isoniazid
Antihistamines	Lidocaine
Antipsychotics	Lindane
Bupropion	MDMA (ecstasy)
Caffeine	Organophosphate
Camphor	Phencyclidine (PCP)
Carbon monoxide	Theophylline
Cocaine	Tramadol
Hydrazines	Tricyclic antidepressants

TABLE 16-7. Treatment of Toxin-Induced Seizures

First line — benzodiazepines
Diazepam may offer slight benefit and synergy with pyridoxine in isoniazid-induced seizures; otherwise, no specific agent is preferred.
Second line — pyridoxine (vitamin B_6)
Adults: Empirically treat with a 5-g slow IV push; if seizure terminates before completion of bolus, allow remainder to be infused over the next 30 minutes.
Children: 70 mg/kg (maximum 5 g) In isoniazid overdose, pyridoxine can be given in an amount equal to the dose of isoniazid ingested.
Third line — barbiturates and propofol
Both will likely require intubation.

Special consideration: tricyclic antidepressants in overdose can cause acute seizures that may be responsive to benzodiazepines, but special consideration must be given to administering sodium bicarbonate.

to bring the core temperature below 39°C (102.2°F) within 15 to 20 minutes. In patients with heat stroke, ice water bath immersion is the superior method of cooling. The most practical method is to pack the patient in ice from head to toe, posteriorly and anteriorly. New technologies such as endovascular coils used to control hypothermia after cardiac arrest have not been studied in the treatment of heat stroke or toxin-induced hyperthermia, but they might have benefit.

Other toxins (eg, cyanide, carbon monoxide, and even salicylate) can cause hyperthermia by poisoning mitochondria and uncoupling oxidative phosphorylation. This side effect results from the inefficiency of normal ATP production and usually is a very late or preterminal finding.[42]

TABLE 16-8. Clinical Features of Several Toxin-Induced Hyperthermic Syndromes

Serotonin syndrome (caused by excess serotonin stimulation)
Develops within minutes to hours after a combination, initiation, or increase of pro-serotonergic drugs (eg, selective serotonin reuptake inhibitors, monoamine oxidase inhibitors, dextromethorphan, meperidine, lithium, linezolid)
Tremor, spontaneous or inducible clonus of extremities or eyes, hyperreflexia (may be greater in lower extremities than in upper)
Neuroleptic malignant syndrome (caused by excess blockade of dopamine or withdrawal from dopaminergic agents)
Insidious onset, developing over days to weeks of chronic or high-dose neuroleptics (eg, haloperidol, phenothiazines, or withdrawal from dopaminergic medications for Parkinsonism)
Early symptoms can be mistaken for psychiatric illness, as facial muscles may portray a flat affect and patients might move more slowly than usual.
Tremor, trismus, drooling, "lead pipe" muscle rigidity, hyperreflexia caused by severe muscle rigidity, elevated creatine kinase
Malignant hyperthermia (inherited disorder affecting intracellular calcium release from the sarcoplasmic reticulum)
Typically develops in the operating room within minutes to hours after exposure to succinylcholine and inhalation anesthetics (halothane)
An early finding in an intubated patient may be increased end-tidal CO_2 and difficulty ventilating because of chest wall rigidity.
Severe muscle rigidity and masseter spasm during intubation are associated with the development of malignant hyperthermia.
Sympathomimetic excess (severe agitation caused by drug-induced excess catecholamine release)
Cocaine, amphetamines, MDMA (ecstasy)
Severe agitation, diaphoresis, mydriasis

Cholinergic Crisis

Organophosphates and carbamates are compounds that can cause acute and life-threatening cholinergic toxicity. Most commonly used as insecticides and pesticides, they have also been used as a means of suicide, as agents of terrorism, and in chemical warfare.[43] The compounds bind to cholinesterases, preventing the metabolism of acetylcholine and resulting in significant cholinergic excess. The classic features of this crisis can be broken down by the effect of excess acetylcholine at three receptors *(Table 16-10)*. Unlike organophosphates, carbamates do not "age," meaning they can reversibly bind and spontaneously release cholinesterases. In addition, carbamates are less toxic to the central nervous system. Exposure to organophosphates and carbamates can occur via inhalation, ingestion, and dermal, ocular, and parenteral routes. Clinicians caring for patients who have been exposed to these compounds must ensure their own safety by appropriately decontaminating the patient and using personal protective equipment.

Atropine is the mainstay of treatment, inducing competitive antagonism of acetylcholine at muscarinic sites. The defined clinical endpoint is the achievement of adequate atropinization through aggressive treatment of bronchorrhea *(Table 16-11)*.

TABLE 16-9. Critical Actions for Managing Toxin-Induced Hyperthermia

STOP all drugs and refrain from administering any agents that could exacerbate current hyperthermic syndrome (eg, haloperidol to sedate the patient with possible neuroleptic malignant syndrome).
CALM with benzodiazepines; endpoint should be control of agitation and muscular rigidity; intubate and paralyze if needed.
COOL patient immediately if the above interventions fail to decrease core temperature. Cooling is best achieved by packing the patient in ice from head to toe, anteriorly and posteriorly.
Antidotes
Serotonin syndrome: cyproheptadine, serotonin antagonist
Neuroleptic malignant syndrome: bromocriptine, dopamine agonist
Malignant hyperthermia: dantrolene, a direct skeletal muscle relaxant, decreases calcium release from the sarcoplasmic reticulum
Note: Of all these antidotes, only dantrolene for malignant hyperthermia is warranted for emergent use that could be lifesaving. Cyproheptadine and bromocriptine are available only in oral preparations, have not been shown to improve outcomes, and do not replace the principles of aggressive sedation and cooling.

Pralidoxime should be administered to all patients with suspected or confirmed organophosphate exposure who present with severe signs of toxicity, neuromuscular weakness, or who require a significant amount of atropine. Although pralidoxime may not be beneficial in all types of organophosphate poisonings (eg, those caused by carbamates), the associated morbidity/mortality of such exposures warrants its continued use.[44]

PEARL

Seizures after organophosphate exposure should be emergently treated with benzodiazepines, as they might not be halted by atropine and pralidoxime.

Severe Metabolic Acidosis

In all critically ill poisoned patients, the anion gap must be measured quickly. The gap is calculated using the following formula:

$$[Na^+] - [Cl^- + HCO_3^-]$$

Depending on laboratory technique, the normal range for the anion gap is 6 to 14 mEq/L. An increase in the gap beyond the accepted normal range, accompanied by metabolic acidosis, represents an increase in unmeasured endogenous (eg, lactate) or exogenous (eg, salicylates) anions.[45] Several toxins produce an elevated anion gap. Although the mnemonic CAT MUDPILES is incomplete, it can be used to consider toxicological causes of an increased anion gap *(Table 16-12)*.

A thorough history accompanied by a careful analysis of laboratory data often provides the information necessary to confirm the suspected diagnosis; however, routine laboratory testing can be insufficient in some cases. Clues to the diagnosis can be ascertained from additional laboratory assessments: measurements of arterial and/or venous blood gases; serum/urine ketone concentrations; blood urea nitrogen; and creatinine, lactate, and salicylate levels. Normal renal function and an undetectable salicylate concentration quickly exclude uremia and salicylate toxicity, respectively. The absence of ketones does not rule out diabetic/starvation/alcoholic ketoacidosis but makes it less likely. Lactic acidosis is responsible for elevated anion gaps in carbon monoxide, cyanide, metformin, propylene glycol, iron, and isoniazid (seizures) toxicity. Toluene is a rare toxin that causes anion gap elevation by hippuric acid formation.

Three important and relatively common causes of elevated anion gap metabolic acidosis are cyanide toxicity, toxic alcohol ingestion, and severe salicylate toxicity. Even with adequate airway support, oxygenation, and fluid resuscitation, patients with these types of poisonings might not survive without toxin-specific management.

Cyanide

Cyanide is a mitochondrial toxin that inhibits the function of cytochrome oxidase at the α_3 portion. This disrupts the electron transport chain at a critical step in the utilization of oxygen. Despite adequate oxygenation, the element cannot be used, resulting in cellular hypoxia. A shift toward anaerobic metabolism produces metabolic acidosis with an increase in the serum lactic acid concentration.[46]

Cyanide is known for inducing extremely rapid neurological and cardiovascular collapse. Neurological symptoms can quickly progress from headache to agitation, seizures, and coma. Cyanide poisoning can initially produce the cardiovascular

TABLE 16-10. Features of Cholinergic Toxicity

Muscarinic
SLUDGE: salivation, lacrimation, urination, diarrhea, GI cramps, emesis
Killer B's: bronchorrhea, bronchospasm, bradycardia
Some patients have miosis.
Nicotinic (autonomic ganglia)
Diaphoresis, tachycardia, hypertension, mydriasis
Nicotinic (neuromuscular junction)
Muscle fasciculation, weakness, and paralysis
Depending on the stage of toxicity and the location and chemical binding features of each specific agent, the patient could exhibit tachycardia or bradycardia, so no single symptom should rule in or rule out clinical suspicion of organophosphate or carbamate toxicity.

TABLE 16-11. Initial Dosing for Cholinergic Toxicity

Atropine
IVP: 0.5–2 mg in adults, and 0.02 mg/kg in children, depending on severity
Minimum doses (0.5 mg in adults and 0.1 mg in children) should be given to avoid paradoxic bradycardia.
Aggressively repeat dose every 3–5 minutes, doubling each subsequent dose in severe cases.
Titrate to drying of bronchial secretions.
Tachycardia is not a contraindication and should not suppress aggressive therapy.
Pralidoxime (2-PAM)
Adults: 1–2 g in 100 mL of normal saline over 15–30 minutes
Children: 20–40 mg/kg (maximum 2 g) of normal saline over 15–30 minutes
These doses may be repeated in 1 hour if muscle weakness and fasciculation are not relieved.
Initial dose may be repeated every 3–6 hours as needed for severe poisoning *OR* continuous infusion may be initiated for severe cases. **Adults and children:** 10–20 mg/kg/hr (maximum 500 mg/hr)
Expert medical consultation should be sought to direct appropriate dosing.

effects of hypertension and bradycardia, but most patients present with hypotension and tachycardia. Bradycardia can represent a preterminal event. Diagnostically, cyanide concentrations usually are not available quickly enough to aid in management. Increased anion gap metabolic acidosis and an elevated lactate (>8 mmol/L) should raise suspicion of cyanide poisoning.[46] Given the patient's inability to use oxygen, "arterialization" of venous blood can be indicated by elevated venous (>90%) oxygenation.

Patients can be exposed to cyanide through inhalation, ingestion, or via dermal and parenteral routes. The rate of onset of symptoms is related to the route of exposure. The inhalation of gaseous hydrogen cyanide results in nearly immediate collapse, while ingestion of a cyanide salt such as sodium cyanide can induce clinical effects in 20 minutes. Cyanide salts are commonly found in chemical laboratories, photo processing chemicals, and jewelers' supplies. A history of such occupations or exposure should raise clinical suspicion for cyanide toxicity. Fire victims can be exposed to hydrogen cyanide gas liberated from the burning of the wool, plastics, nylon, and polyurethane found in automobiles, carpets, home furniture, and appliances. A lactate concentration higher than 10 mmol/L on arrival in fire victims without significant cutaneous burns is a sensitive marker for an elevated blood cyanide concentration.[46] These patients tend to suffer from concurrent carbon monoxide poisoning, asphyxia, trauma, and thermal injury — all of which can be indistinguishable from cyanide poisoning.

PEARL

A lactate concentration above 10 mmol/L on arrival in fire victims without significant cutaneous burns is a sensitive marker for elevated blood cyanide.[46]

The "original" cyanide antidote kit contains amyl nitrite, sodium nitrite, and sodium thiosulfate *(Table 16-13)*. The amyl and sodium nitrites cause the production of a small amount of methemoglobin, which removes cyanide from the mitochondria. Sodium thiosulfate provides cofactors for rhodanese, an enzyme that assists in metabolizing cyanide to thiocyanate, a relatively nontoxic metabolite that is eliminated via the kidneys. Importantly, fire victims suspected to have elevated carboxyhemoglobin concentrations should not receive amyl and sodium nitrite. The production of a small amount of methemoglobinemia in these patients is potentially devastating, as neither carboxyhemoglobin nor methemoglobin can deliver oxygen to the tissues.

Hydroxocobalamin, which is FDA-approved for the treatment of cyanide poisoning, is a precursor to cyanocobalamin (vitamin B_{12}). The agent binds cyanide and displaces the hydroxyl radical to form the vitamin, which is rapidly eliminated in the urine.[47] In fire victims, hydroxocobalamin appears to be safer than the traditional cyanide antidote kit.[48] It may be used in conjunction with sodium thiosulfate, but the two drugs should not be concurrently administered through the same intravenous line.[49] Transient hypertension and prominent red discoloration of the skin and urine should be anticipated following hydroxocobalamin administration (which can last up to 7 days).[50]

Toxic Alcohol Ingestion

Methanol and ethylene glycol are "toxic" alcohols because their degradation leads to extremely poisonous metabolites that produce significant metabolic acidosis and specific end-organ damage. Methanol is used as a denaturant for ethanol, a solvent, a fuel (eg, buffet can heaters), and an ingredient in windshield wiper fluid. Ethylene glycol is found in antifreeze, solvents, de-icers, and air conditioning units. Both chemicals produce inebriation similar to and often mistaken for ethanol intoxication; however, the absence of central nervous system depression does not exclude a potentially life-threatening exposure. Methanol is metabolized to formic acid, an ocular toxin that produces a spectrum of changes from blurred vision to blindness and the pathognomonic "snowfield vision." Ethylene glycol's toxic metabolites include oxalic acid, which causes renal failure, hypocalcemia, and calcium oxalate crystalluria.[51]

Poisoning should be suspected with any known ingestion of a product containing toxic alcohols, and in any patient who shows signs of unexplained metabolic acidosis or a significantly elevated osmolar gap (>50) *(Table 16-14)* or fails to respond to treatment for another presumed cause of an elevated anion gap acidosis (eg, thiamine and dextrose for alcoholic ketoacidosis).[52] The serum lactate concentration can be falsely elevated in patients with ethylene glycol poisoning given that one of its metabolites, glycolic acid, can be misinterpreted as lactate.[53]

PEARL

The serum lactate concentration can be falsely elevated in patients with ethylene glycol poisoning given that one of its metabolites, glycolic acid, can be misinterpreted as lactate.[53]

TABLE 16-12. MUDPILES Mnemonic

C = Carbon monoxide, cyanide
A = Aspirin (salicylate), alcoholic ketoacidosis, acetaminophen
T = Toluene
M = Methanol, metformin
U = Uremia
D = Diabetic ketoacidosis
P = Propylene glycol, propofol
I = Iron, isoniazid, ibuprofen
L = Lactic acidosis
E = Ethylene glycol
S = Salicylates (aspirin), starvation ketoacidosis

TABLE 16-13. Cyanide Antidote Kit

Amyl Nitrite Pearls
Crack open and place under patient's nose; may use while IV line is being established.
Do NOT give this portion of kit to fire victims.
Sodium Nitrite (infuse over 3–5 minutes)
Adult: 10 mL (300 mg)
Children: 0.33 mL/kg (maximum 10 mL)
Do NOT give this portion of kit to fire victims.
Sodium Thiosulfate (infuse over 3–5 minutes)
Adult: 50 mL (12.5 g)
Children: 1.65 mL/kg (maximum 50 mL)
Hydroxocobalamin (infuse over 15 minutes)
Adult: 5 g (2 vials lyophilized)
Children: 70 mg/kg (maximum 5 g)

Special consideration: Sodium thiosulfate and hydroxocobalamin may be given together for possible synergistic effect, but they should never concurrently run through the same intravenous line.

Although the parent compounds of ethylene glycol and methanol are osmotically active, their metabolites (oxalic acid and formic acid) are not.[54] Therefore, as time passes and metabolism occurs, the osmolar gap will fall and the metabolites will cause the anion gap to rise.[55]

Patients who present very early after exposure theoretically will demonstrate osmolar gap elevations, with or without elevations in the anion gap. Conversely, late presenters who have metabolized the alcohol will display an elevated anion gap and a very low to normal osmolar gap.[56] This progression will be halted in the presence of ethanol because alcohol dehydrogenase preferentially metabolizes ethanol over ethylene glycol or methanol. This "protective" effect is the reason ethanol can be used to treat toxic alcohol ingestions, but it should be used only when fomepizole is not readily available.[57]

PEARL

Without treatment and with no concurrent ethanol intoxication, the natural progression of toxic alcohol ingestions, despite resuscitation, is a declining osmolar gap mirrored by an increasing anion gap.

Fomepizole (4-methyl-pyrazole, Antizol [Paladin Labs, Quebec, Canada]) is an alcohol dehydrogenase inhibitor that prevents the metabolism of ethylene glycol and methanol from creating toxic metabolites. The agent, which might be the only therapy needed for mild to moderate exposures, should be administered as soon as possible in all suspected or confirmed cases of ethylene glycol or methanol poisoning *(Table 16-15)*. Critically ill patients warrant immediate nephrology consultation because emergent hemodialysis is indicated in cases of severe metabolic acidosis, end-organ toxicity, renal

TABLE 16-14. Osmolar Gap Calculation and Clinical Utility for Toxic Alcohol Ingestion

Osmolar gap = measured osmolarity – calculated osmolarity:
Measured osmolarity is obtained from clinical laboratory analyses.
Calculated osmolar gap = (2 × Na^+) + (glucose/18) + (BUN/2.8) + (ethanol/4.6)
Units: Na^+ (mEq/L), glucose (mg/dL), BUN (mg/dL), ethanol (mg/dL)
Osmolar gap >50 is highly specific for alcohol toxicity.
Note: A "normal" osmolar gap never rules out a toxic alcohol ingestion.[45]

TABLE 16-15. Fomepizole Dosing Regimen

Administer a loading dose of 15 mg/kg IV, followed by 10 mg/kg every 12 hours for 4 doses.
Each dose is infused over 30 minutes.
If the patient requires dialysis, increase the dosing frequency to every 4 hours.

failure, and methanol or ethylene glycol concentrations greater than 25 mg/dL. Unfortunately, this intervention is not readily available.[51]

Conclusion

We have discussed some of the more common and complex medications and chemicals that can cause severe toxicity. Consultation with a medical toxicologist or poison control center can assist with management. Treatment of the critically poisoned patient requires immediate identification of the toxicant, anticipation of the toxicity, and the administration of antidotal therapy when appropriate.

REFERENCES

1. Ashbourne JF, Olson KR, Khayam-Bashi H. Value of rapid screening for acetaminophen in all patients with intentional drug overdose. *Ann Emerg Med.* 1989;18:1035-1038.
2. Tenenbein M. Do you really need that emergency drug screen? *Clin Toxicol.* 2009;47:286-291.
3. Höjer J, Troutman WG, Hoppu K, et al. Position paper update: ipecac syrup for gastrointestinal decontamination. *Clin Toxicol (Phila).* 2013;51(3):134-139.
4. American Academy of Pediatrics Committee on Injury Violence, and Poison Prevention. Poison treatment in the home. *Pediatrics.* 2003;112:1182-1185.
5. Chyka PA, Seger D, Krenzelok EP, et al. Position paper: single-dose activated charcoal. *Clin Toxicol.* 2005;43:61-87.
6. Kulig K, Bar-Or D, Cantrill SV, et al. Management of acutely poisoned patients without gastric emptying. *Ann Emerg Med.* 1985;14:562-567.
7. Benson BE, Hoppu K, Troutman WG, et al. Position paper update: gastric lavage for gastrointestinal decontamination. *Clin Toxicol.* 2013;51:140-146.
8. Thanacoody R, Caravati EM, Troutman B, et al. Position paper update: whole bowel irrigation for gastrointestinal decontamination of overdose patients. *Clin Toxicol (Phila).* 2015;53(1):5-12.
9. Sharma A, Hexdall A, Chang E, et al. Diphenhydramine-induced wide complex dysrhythmia responds to treatment with sodium bicarbonate. *Am J Emerg Med.* 2003;21:212-215.
10. Kalimullah EA, Bryant SM. Case files of the medical toxicology fellowship at the toxikon consortium in Chicago: cocaine-associated wide-complex dysrhythmias and cardiac arrest — treatment nuances and controversies. *J Med Toxicol.* 2008;4:277-283.
11. Hollowell H, Mattu A, Perron AD, et al. Wide-complex tachycardia: beyond the traditional differential diagnosis of ventricular tachycardia vs supraventricular tachycardia with aberrant conduction. *Am J Emerg Med.* 2005;23:876-889.

KEY POINTS

1. Despite limited clinical evidence, GI decontamination should be considered when the suspected toxicity carries a high risk of morbidity and mortality and in critically ill patients who are displaying severe and life-threatening symptoms.
2. The endpoint of treatment is QRS narrowing, with improvement in blood pressure and cessation of dysrhythmia. Patients who respond to a bolus of sodium bicarbonate may be placed on a continuous infusion.
3. For a patient presenting with TdP, an immediate bolus of intravenous magnesium, 1 to 2 grams over 1 to 2 minutes, is the first-line agent.[18]
4. Recommendations for the management of patients suspected of calcium channel blocker poisoning call for the administration of 13 to 25 mEq of calcium *(Table 16-3)* in the form of either calcium gluconate or calcium chloride salts.
5. Patients who are actively seizing should receive rapidly escalating doses of benzodiazepines to terminate the convulsions.
6. It is critical to aggressively sedate and cool patients who are significantly hyperthermic.

12. Thanacoody HKR, Thomas SHL. Tricyclic antidepressant poisoning: cardiovascular toxicity. *Toxicol Rev.* 2005;24:205-214.
13. Wood D, Dargan P, Hoffman R. Management of cocaine-induced cardiac arrhythmias due to cardiac ion channel dysfunction. *Clin Toxicol.* 2009;47:14-23.
14. Foianini A, Joseph Wiegand T, Benowitz N. What is the role of lidocaine or phenytoin in tricyclic antidepressant-induced cardiotoxicity? *Clin Toxicol (Phila).* 2010;48:325-330.
15. Roden D. Clinical practice. Long-QT syndrome. *N Engl J Med.* 2008;358:169-176.
16. Yap Y, Camm AJ. Drug induced QT prolongation and torsades de pointes. *Heart.* 2003;89:1363-1372.
17. Gupta A, Lawrence A, Krishnan K, et al. Current concepts in the mechanisms and management of drug-induced QT prolongation and torsade de pointes. *Am Heart J.* 2007;153:891-899.
18. Yap YG, Camm J. Risk of torsades de pointes with non-cardiac drugs. Doctors need to be aware that many drugs can cause QT prolongation. *BMJ Br Med J (Clin Res).* 2000;320:1158-1159.
19. Ostchega Y, Dillon C, Hughes J, et al. Trends in hypertension prevalence, awareness, treatment, and control in older U.S. adults: data from the National Health and Nutrition Examination Survey 1988 to 2004. *J Am Geriatr Soc.* 2007;55:1056-1065.
20. Smith S, Ferguson K, Hoffman R, et al. Prolonged severe hypotension following combined amlodipine and valsartan ingestion. *Clin Toxicol.* 2008;46:470-474.
21. Mgarbane B, Karyo S, Baud F. The role of insulin and glucose (hyperinsulinaemia/ euglycaemia) therapy in acute calcium channel antagonist and beta-blocker poisoning. *Toxicol Rev.* 2004;23:215-222.
22. Hung YM, Olson KR. Acute amlodipine overdose treated by high dose intravenous calcium in a patient with severe renal insufficiency. *Clin Toxicol.* 2007;45:301-303.
23. Kline JA, Leonova E, Raymond RM. Beneficial myocardial metabolic effects of insulin during verapamil toxicity in the anesthetized canine. *Crit Care Med.* 1995;23:1251-1263.
24. Kline JA, Tomaszewski CA, Schroeder JD, et al. Insulin is a superior antidote for cardiovascular toxicity induced by verapamil in the anesthetized canine. *J Pharmacol Exp Ther.* 1993;267:744-750.
25. Greene S, Gawarammana I, Wood D, et al. Relative safety of hyperinsulinaemia/ euglycaemia therapy in the management of calcium channel blocker overdose: a prospective observational study. *Intensive Care Med.* 2007;33:2019-2024.
26. Nickson C, Little M. Early use of high-dose insulin euglycaemic therapy for verapamil toxicity. *Med J Aust.* 2009;191:350-352.
27. Yuan TH, Kerns WP, Tomaszewski CA, et al. Insulin-glucose as adjunctive therapy for severe calcium channel antagonist poisoning. *J Toxicol Clin Toxicol.* 1999;37:463-474.
28. Cave G, Harvey M. Intravenous lipid emulsion as antidote beyond local anesthetic toxicity: a systematic review. *Acad Emerg Med.* 2009;16:815-824.
29. Jamaty C, Bailey B, Larocque A, et al. Lipid emulsions in the treatment of acute poisoning: a systematic review of human and animal studies. *Clin Toxicol.* 2010;48:1-27.
30. Weinberg G. Lipid infusion therapy: translation to clinical practice. *Anesth Analg.* 2008;106:1340-1342.
31. American College of Medical Toxicology. ACMT position statement: interim guidance for the use of lipid resuscitation therapy. *J Med Toxicol.* 2011;7:81-82.
32. Vanden Hoek TL, Morrison LJ, Shuster M, et al. Part 12: cardiac arrest in special situations: 2010 American Heart Association Guidelines for Cardiopulmonary Resuscitation and Emergency Cardiovascular Care. *Circulation.* 2010;122(18 suppl 3):S829-S861.
33. Levine M, Skolnik AB, Ruha AM, et al. Complications following antidotal use of intravenous lipid emulsion therapy. *J Med Toxicol.* 2014;10:10-14.
34. Abdelmalek D, Schwarz ES, Sampson C, et al. Life-threatening diphenhydramine toxicity presenting with seizures and a wide complex tachycardia improved with intravenous fat emulsion. *Am J Ther.* 2014;21:542-544.
35. Shenoy U, Paul J, Antony D. Lipid resuscitation in pediatric patients — need for caution? *Paediatr Anaesth.* 2014;24:332-334.
36. Love JN, Leasure JA, Mundt DJ, et al. A comparison of amrinone and glucagon therapy for cardiovascular depression associated with propranolol toxicity in a canine model. *J Toxicol Clin Toxicol.* 1992;30:399-412.
37. Hendren WG, Schieber RS, Garrettson LK. Extracorporeal bypass for the treatment of verapamil poisoning. *Ann Emerg Med.* 1989;18:984-987.
38. Wills B, Erickson T. Drug- and toxin-associated seizures. *Med Clin North Am.* 2005;89:1297-1321.
39. Boyer E, Shannon M. The serotonin syndrome. *N Engl J Med.* 2005;352:1112-1120.
40. Strawn J, Keck P, Caroff S. Neuroleptic malignant syndrome. *Am J Psychiatr.* 2007;164:870-876.
41. Dematte JE, O'Mara K, Buescher J, et al. Near-fatal heat stroke during the 1995 heat wave in Chicago. *Ann Intern Med.* 1998;129:173-181.
42. Temple AR. Pathophysiology of aspirin overdosage toxicity, with implications for management. *Pediatrics.* 1978;62:873-876.
43. Roberts D, Aaron C. Management of acute organophosphorus pesticide poisoning. *BMJ Br Med J (Clin Res).* 2007;334:629-634.
44. Nelson LS, Perrone J, DeRoos F, et al. Aldicarb poisoning by an illicit rodenticide imported into the United States: *Tres Pasitos. J Toxicol Clin Toxicol.* 2001;39:447-452.
45. Chabali R. Diagnostic use of anion and osmolal gaps in pediatric emergency medicine. *Pediatr Emerg Care.* 1997;13:204-210.
46. Baud FJ, Barriot P, Toffis V, et al. Elevated blood cyanide concentrations in victims of smoke inhalation. *N Engl J Med.* 1991;325:1761-1766.
47. Forsyth JC, Mueller PD, Becker CE, et al. Hydroxocobalamin as a cyanide antidote: safety, efficacy and pharmacokinetics in heavily smoking normal volunteers. *J Toxicol Clin Toxicol.* 1993;31:277-294.
48. Borron SW, Baud FJ, Barriot P, et al. Prospective study of hydroxocobalamin for acute cyanide poisoning in smoke inhalation. *Ann Emerg Med.* 2007;49:794-801.
49. Shepherd G, Velez LI. Role of hydroxocobalamin in acute cyanide poisoning. *Ann Pharmacother.* 2008;42:661-669.
50. Uhl W, Nolting A, Golor G, et al. Safety of hydroxocobalamin in healthy volunteers in a randomized, placebo-controlled study. *Clin Toxicol.* 2006;44(suppl 1):17-28.
51. Brent J. Fomepizole for ethylene glycol and methanol poisoning. *N Engl J Med.* 2009;360:2216-2223.
52. Hoffman RS, Smilkstein MJ, Howland MA, et al. Osmol gaps revisited: normal values and limitations. *J Toxicol Clin Toxicol.* 1993;31:81-93.
53. Morgan TJ, Clark C, Clague A. Artifactual elevation of measured plasma L-lactate concentration in the presence of glycolate. *Crit Care Med.* 1999;27:2177-2179.
54. Glaser DS. Utility of the serum osmol gap in the diagnosis of methanol or ethylene glycol ingestion. *Ann Emerg Med.* 1996;27:343-346.
55. Hovda KE, Hunderi OH, Rudberg N, et al. Anion and osmolal gaps in the diagnosis of methanol poisoning: clinical study in 28 patients. *Intensive Care Med.* 2004;30:1842-1846.
56. Soghoian S, Sinert R, Wiener S, et al. Ethylene glycol toxicity presenting with non-anion gap metabolic acidosis. *Basic Clin Pharmacol Toxicol.* 2009;104:22-26.
57. Mgarbane B, Borron S, Baud F. Current recommendations for treatment of severe toxic alcohol poisonings. *Intensive Care Med.* 2005;31:189-195.

The Crashing Trauma Patient

17

IN THIS CHAPTER

- Identifying and managing life- and limb-threatening injuries
- Managing the trauma airway
- Managing traumatic brain injury
- Optimizing resuscitation
- Preparing the patient for definitive treatment or transfer

Michael A. Gibbs and David W. Callaway

The emergency clinician often is confronted simultaneously with multiple life-threatening conditions requiring divergent diagnostic and therapeutic pathways. It is essential to correctly prioritize imaging and laboratory studies and interventions to avoid critical delays in treatment. By following a simple algorithm that adheres to basic principles and adapts to changes in clinical status, clinicians can maximize patient outcomes.

The management of acutely injured patients demands a collaborative approach. Each member of the team must understand his specific role, the constantly changing resuscitative priorities, and the overall management plan in the context of multiple coincident injuries. Every effective team has a clearly identified leader who must remain vigilant while receiving input from other clinicians, reassessing the patient's clinical status, and prioritizing the next steps in care.

Although a comprehensive, succinct description of the evaluation and management of this patient population is challenging to articulate, a simple set of goal-directed recommendations can guide care for the crashing trauma patient:

1. Develop a rapid and effective method of identifying and prioritizing critical injuries.
2. Employ rational resuscitative strategies that address critical physiological derangements.

These actions are driven by the answers to two very basic questions: *What do I need to know? What do I need to do?*

TABLE 17-1. Injury Identification: The Basic Approach
Step 1: Effectively manage the airway.
Step 2: Identify and control immediate threats to maintaining central perfusion.
Step 3: Identify and address severe intracranial injuries.
Step 4: Identify and control other potentially life-threatening thoracic and abdominal injuries.
Step 5: Identify and control potentially limb-threatening injuries.
Step 6: Identify and treat noncritical injuries.

Injury Identification

The Basic Approach

The initial resuscitation of the critically injured patient can be reduced to a straightforward strategy: problems must be identified and treated in the order of their immediate threat to life, followed by the immediacy of their threat to functional outcome. The stepwise process listed in Table 17-1 can be applied regardless of the specific injuries involved. It is important for the resuscitation team to strictly adhere to these priorities and not be distracted by noncritical diagnostic studies or therapeutic interventions.

Step 1. Control the airway immediately.

Control of the airway is the first and most critical component of resuscitation. The decision to intubate is complex and influenced by several factors *(Table 17-2)*. The general dictum to intubate early applies more often than not to the acutely injured patient. This is particularly true when the injuries are likely to cause abrupt anatomical distortions of the airway and for patients whose overall physiological reserves are threatened. The one mitigating factor that must be considered is the intravascular volume status. Rapid sequence intubation (RSI) and institution of positive-pressure ventilation can cause severe and refractory hypotension in the hypovolemic patient. This risk must be weighed against the potential benefits of delaying intubation to allow fluid resuscitation or prepare for surgical intervention.

TABLE 17-2. Indications for Intubation of the Trauma Patient
Loss of airway or inability to protect the airway due to facial and/or neck injuries
Severe head injury with a GCS score ≤8 (higher if head injury is obvious and the patient is combative)
Significant chest injury with inadequate oxygenation/ventilation
Insufficient ventilatory effort
Low preexisting physiological reserve
Significant inhalation injury
Note: the patient's *anticipated course* should contribute to the decision to intubate early.

Consider the patient with a small stab wound to the neck, stable vital signs, and no overt clinical evidence of airway compromise. Although this seemingly innocuous initial presentation might reassure the clinician at the bedside, airway obstruction can develop rapidly with little warning. As a second example, consider the patient with a severe displaced pelvic ring fracture who is being prepared for transfer. As hemorrhage remains uncontrolled, the patient is likely to abruptly decompensate in the back of the ambulance. Finally, consider the elderly patient with blunt chest trauma and multiple rib fractures. Increased work of breathing, hypercarbia, and progressive respiratory failure are almost unavoidable. In each of these cases, early airway management is both prudent and protective and allows the treating clinician to approach the intervention when the patient's physiology is at its best, not its worst.

Step 2. Identify and control immediate threats to central perfusion.

The clinical picture of impending cardiovascular collapse is seldom subtle; it typically is heralded by profound hypotension and clear signs of inadequate perfusion. If the patient fails to respond to initial volume resuscitation and external hemorrhage control, a rapid assessment must be performed to find the most likely cause of bleeding; immediate (often surgical) intervention is required. A physical examination may be sufficient, as is the case with penetrating injuries, and can be augmented by rapid diagnostic tests (eg, a focused assessment with sonography for trauma [FAST] and plain films of the chest and pelvis). Control of hemorrhage and stabilization of perfusion outweigh all other concerns.

The diagnostic approach varies based on the mechanism of injury. In the crashing patient with blunt multisystem trauma, shock may stem from any source or a combination of sources *(Table 17-3)*. The assessment of penetrating trauma is different and based on an understanding of trajectory *(Table 17-4)*. The location of a stab wound generally can be pinpointed with accuracy. However, the trajectory of bullets or other missiles is much less predictable, so it is wise to cast a wide diagnostic net.

Step 3. Identify and address severe intracranial injuries.

If the patient has evidence of adequate perfusion with resuscitation, the next step is to assess the likelihood of an intracranial lesion requiring neurosurgical intervention. Initial triage includes a physical examination and assessment of the Glasgow Coma Scale (GCS) score. Any patient with a GCS score below 8, especially in the presence of lateralizing signs, must be presumed to have a surgical lesion. Computed tomography (CT) of the head should be prioritized in these cases even over interventions targeted at ongoing but manageable hemorrhage, a presumed intraabdominal injury, or compromise of an extremity. Patients with GCS scores above 13 have a slight probability of requiring neurosurgical intervention, so CT of the head may be delayed, depending on the clinical situation. Patients with GCS scores between 8 and 13 should be triaged based on individual circumstances. Pitfalls in the evaluation of patients with suspected intracranial injury are listed in Table 17-5.

Step 4. Identify and control potentially life-threatening intrathoracic and intraabdominal injuries.

After establishing sustainable perfusion and determining the presence of intracranial pathology, potentially life-threatening intrathoracic and intraabdominal injuries should be diagnosed and managed *(Table 17-6)*. This is the primary phase for obtaining more sophisticated diagnostic imaging studies. Potential problems include:

- Ongoing hemorrhage in the chest, abdomen, or pelvis
- Hollow viscus injuries
- Contained aortic injuries
- Other contained major vascular injuries

TABLE 17-3. Causes of Shock in the Critically Ill Trauma Patient
Hemorrhagic Causes
Intraabdominal
Intrathoracic
Retroperitoneal
Long-bone fractures
External
Scalp (infants and small children)
Nonhemorrhagic Causes
Tension pneumothorax
Pericardial tamponade
Myocardial contusion
Spinal cord transection
Coexistent medical conditions (eg, acute myocardial infarction, gastrointestinal bleed, medications)

Step 5. Identify and control potentially limb-threatening injuries.

Once life-threatening injuries have been addressed, injuries threatening limb function can be addressed *(Table 17-7)*. This is another area in which specific diagnostic testing will be necessary. Injuries in this category include:

- Injuries associated with neurovascular compromise
- Open fractures
- Massive soft-tissue injuries
- Compartment syndrome

Step 6. Identify and treat noncritical injuries.

Injuries of a noncritical nature should be addressed last *(Table 17-8)*. Examples include:

- Simple long-bone fractures
- Facial fractures
- Lacerations

The Diagnostic Toolbox

With advances in technology, the number of diagnostic options for the evaluation of trauma patients is growing. When time is of the essence, emergency physicians must be able to select the right tool to get the right information. Each approach and modality has strengths and weaknesses, which are reviewed below.

Physical Examination

A crashing trauma patient requires a careful, targeted physical examination; however, it is important to recognize that while valuable, such assessments have limitations. The challenge is to understand when the physical examination is enough and when additional diagnostic tests are warranted. Studies report a 5% to 10% rate of occult abdominal injuries when patients are evaluated with a physical examination alone.[1-3] These findings are especially common in patients with neurological impairments and multiple coincident or severe distracting injuries and those at the extremes of age. It is logical that the same pitfalls apply to other organ systems.

Laboratory Testing

Although laboratory tests are easy to obtain and relatively inexpensive, the information they provide seldom provokes a change in the acute management plan.[4] These data are more useful in establishing trends rather than pinpointing a diagnosis or swaying a course of action. In the crashing trauma patient, it is reasonable to obtain laboratory studies, acknowledging that they will be most useful for downstream providers. The serum lactate level is a useful marker of global perfusion. In the critically ill patient, serial measurements every 2 to 4 hours can be used to assess the adequacy of resuscitation.[5,6]

Plain Film Imaging

As experience with CT imaging grows, many centers have questioned the need for plain film imaging. Chest film is favored by some providers because it is fast and simple and provides valuable information,[7] but other providers have challenged the need for routine chest radiography and cited overall low yield of chest CT,[8] favoring clinically based test selection.[9]

As the debate on imaging continues, it is useful to return to the critical question: *How will the information obtained affect patient management?* A chest film that reveals a massive hemothorax or a pelvic radiograph that shows an "open-book" injury with 5 cm of pubic diastasis can be acted upon immediately. It should be determined whether plain films will provide information that the clinician must know *before* leaving the trauma room.

TABLE 17-4. Key Points in the Evaluation of the Patient with Penetrating Trauma
Step 1. Find all the holes and mark them prior to radiography.
Step 2. Consider the trajectory of the injury.
Neck wound • Is there a major vascular injury? • Is the airway compromised? • Has the chest cavity been penetrated (see below)? • Tests: chest x-ray, strongly consider CT angiography in injuries involving zone I or zone III; consider surgical exploration.
Chest wound • Is there a major vascular injury? • Does the patient have pericardial tamponade? • Does the patient have a tension pneumothorax? • Has the abdominal cavity or neck been penetrated (see below)? • Tests: chest x-ray, FAST; consider surgical exploration.
Abdominal/flank wound • Is there a major vascular injury? • Has the chest cavity been penetrated (see above)? • Tests: FAST (limited sensitivity for abdominal injury), DPL, chest x-ray; consider surgical exploration.
Extremity wound • Is there a major vascular injury? • Has the chest or abdominal cavity been penetrated (see above)? • Tests: ankle-brachial index; consider surgical exploration.

TABLE 17-5. Pitfalls in the Evaluation of Patients with Suspected Intracranial Injury
Failure to consider reversible causes such as hypoglycemia, hypoxia, shock
Failure to manage overall patient with respect to perfusion and oxygenation
Attribution of neurological dysfunction to intoxication
Delays in transfer to obtain a head CT in the patient with severe neurological dysfunction
Failure to consider cerebrovascular disease in the at-risk patient

In general, plain films of the spine or extremity are of very little value in the crashing trauma patient. Obtaining these images may waste precious time, especially if transfer to a tertiary center is imminent. Instead, maintain spinal immobilization at all times, and reduce and splint obvious extremity fractures.

Bedside Ultrasonography

Bedside ultrasonography can be a very useful adjunct in the management of the injured patient.[10] Correctly applied, it serves as an extension of the physical examination.[11] Thus it is important for clinicians to understand the following caveats to maximize effectiveness and avoid false-negative FAST studies:

- The FAST detects free fluid as a surrogate for injury, not the injury itself. The detection of fluid is the first step, with the second step being better definitive characterization of specific injuries (ie, using CT, angiography, or laparotomy).
- Ultrasonography provides the highest yield in patients who are in shock. A positive (or negative) FAST in the hypotensive blunt trauma patient injury (eg, chest asymmetry, crepitus, seatbelt sign) provides valuable information regarding the next step. In this population, sensitivities and specificities exceed 95%.[10-13]
- Ultrasonography is highly sensitive for detecting hemopericardium and should be used early in the evaluation of patients with penetrating torso trauma.[14,15] Exceptions include patients with large pericardial lacerations that can evacuate into the left chest. Hemopericardium should be considered in patients with penetrating chest trauma, a negative FAST, and fluid in the left hemithorax. Serial FAST examinations can increase diagnostic accuracy.[16]
- In patients with bladder rupture, the detection of free intraabdominal fluid can reflect the presence of urine, not blood.[16] This is especially likely in patients with anterior pelvic ring fractures.[17] Diagnostic peritoneal lavage (DPL) or CT imaging can help in these cases.
- Thoracic ultrasonography may provide higher sensitivity for detecting pneumothorax compared to a single anteroposterior chest film (see *Chapter 22*). As is the case for the abdominal and cardiac examinations, sonographic evaluation of the chest relies on surrogate measures of the disease (ie, the presence or absence of lung sliding and comet tails).[18,19]

Computed Tomography Imaging

The use of CT imaging in trauma has flourished. Third- and fourth-generation multidetector technology boasts superior image quality, rapid acquisition time, and impressive reformatting capabilities. Injuries for which CT imaging was previously thought to be insensitive (eg, pancreas, bowel, diaphragm) can now be interrogated with a high degree of precision. In many large trauma centers, the use of routine CT scanning of the head, neck, chest, abdomen, and pelvis has been promoted.[20,21] However, this approach has not been well studied in critically ill trauma patients. In this population, the question is less "Will I get enough information?" and more "Is the patient stable enough to travel to radiology?"

Diagnostic Peritoneal Lavage

DPL is a rapid method of detecting intraperitoneal hemorrhage and is especially useful in the hemodynamically unstable patient.[22-24] Although largely supplanted by bedside

TABLE 17-6. Evaluation of Potentially Life-Threatening Thoracic and Abdominal Injuries

Physical Examination
External signs of injury (eg, chest asymmetry, crepitus, seatbelt sign)
Penetrating injuries
Signs of decreased ventilation
Peritoneal signs
Pelvic instability or deformity
Diagnostic Strategy
Bedside testing options: • Chest film • Pelvic film • FAST
Definitive testing options: • CT • CT or plain film angiography

TABLE 17-7. Evaluation of Potentially Limb-Threatening Extremity Injuries

Physical Examination
Limb deformity
Evidence of inadequate perfusion
Hard signs of vascular injury: • Expanding hematoma • Loss of distal pulses • Active arterial bleeding
Soft signs of vascular injury: • Proximity of penetrating wounds or high-risk fractures • Nonexpanding hematoma • Evidence of associated peripheral nerve injury
Open wounds, especially in proximity to fractures
Tight compartments, especially lower leg
Diagnostic Strategy
Bedside testing options: • Ankle-brachial index • Bedside assessment of compartment pressure • Plain films
Definitive testing options: • CT • CT or plain film angiography • Surgical exploration

ultrasonography, it remains a valuable tool in the evaluation of unstable patients.[25] In the crashing patient with suspected abdominal injury, DPL should be considered when ultrasonography is not available, FAST results are equivocal, or a positive FAST result is likely to render a false positive (eg, pelvic trauma with possible bladder rupture and uroperitoneum).[16,17]

Clinical Decision Rules

Clinical decision rules have been developed to guide imaging of the spine, brain, and pelvis injury in stable patients. These processes have been incorporated into the most recent ATLS guidelines.[26-30] Preliminary studies also have explored the use of clinical decision rules to guide management of chest and abdominal injury in stable patients.

There currently are no formal clinical rules to support imaging decisions in the crashing trauma patient. It is logical to assume that the sicker the patient, the less room there is for error. Therefore, diagnostic imaging should be used liberally in this population.

Resuscitation Essentials

Managing the Trauma Airway

Failure to manage the airway is one of the most common preventable causes of death in trauma patients.[31-33] Once the decision to intubate has been made, a successful strategy will combine sophisticated assessment skills, the ability to predict physiological derangements, and technical proficiency with multiple airway management devices. The clinician must plan quickly and rapidly to answer two related questions:

1. Will the procedure be difficult?
2. What is the best airway management strategy?

Predicting the Difficult Airway

The "LEMON" mnemonic represents a validated, practical, systematic assessment that can be performed rapidly at the bedside to predict difficult laryngoscopy and intubation.[34-35] The mnemonic refers to assessing five predictors of difficulty: external features, geometry of the airway, the Mallampati score, obstruction, and neck mobility. The approach is endorsed in the most recent ATLS guidelines (see *Chapter* 2).[36]

Choosing an Airway Management Strategy

An effective airway management strategy combines two independent predictive steps: *anticipating* the technically difficult airway and selection of the most appropriate technique to overcome it, and *anticipating* the physiological response to intubation and the drugs used to facilitate the procedure.

Once the airway has been assessed for potential technical difficulty, questions about physiology can be guided by the "trauma ABCs."[37]

A — Airway Injury?

Injury to the airway mandates that the clinician recognize the inherent risk of neuromuscular blockade. In this situation, a number of alternatives may be considered, including sedative-assisted awake orotracheal intubation, fiberoptic or videolaryngoscopic intubation with topical anesthesia and sedation, surgical cricothyroidotomy, or a double setup technique (RSI with surgical airway equipment at the ready).

B — Brain Injury?

The overriding priorities during intubation of the patient with severe head injury are avoiding hypotension and/or hypoxia and resultant secondary injuries and employing a neuroprotective pharmacological regimen. RSI is the standard in this population unless it is contraindicated by airway trauma or anatomical difficulties.

There are no studies demonstrating improved outcomes with premedication strategies (eg, lidocaine, fentanyl, and defasciculation) to decrease the sympathetic response to laryngoscopy. Therefore, a simple strategy using a neuroprotective induction agent and a short-acting neuromuscular blocking drug is logical, practical, and safe.

C — Cervical Injury?

All blunt trauma patients have cervical injury until proven otherwise. Because a single cross-table lateral cervical spine radiograph has limited sensitivity for fracture, interrupting the resuscitation to obtain this image should be avoided. The spine should be held in line at all times during airway management, and compliance with this practice should be documented in the medical record.

C — Chest Injury?

Acute chest injury markedly limits respiratory reserve and virtually ensures rapid desaturation when paralysis is induced. Decompensation should be anticipated in patients with significant blunt or penetrating chest trauma. An airway rescue plan should be ready, and deliberate steps should be taken to maximally preoxygenate the patient and rapidly perform RSI.

Risks persist after successful laryngoscopy, when positive-pressure ventilation can rapidly convert a simple pneumothorax into a tension pneumothorax. Should this injury be known or suspected, the team should be prepared to perform an immediate needle chest decompression or chest tube thoracostomy.

S — Shock?

In the hemodynamically compromised patient, multiple factors can worsen shock during airway management. Induction agents decrease vascular tone and cardiac output. A loss of muscle tone following paralysis and initiation of positive-

TABLE 17-8. Evaluating Noncritical Injuries
Physical Examination
Once life-threatening injuries have been identified and stabilized, a thorough, head-to-toe secondary survey should be performed.
Diagnostic Strategy
Definitive imaging of facial fractures
Plain film imaging of extremity fractures

pressure ventilation decrease venous return and cardiac output.

When patients are in shock, several steps can be taken to avoid decompensation. If time permits, fluids should be rapidly administered to augment preload. Induction drugs with the most favorable hemodynamic profiles (eg, etomidate, ketamine) should be selected over those more likely to decrease vascular tone and cardiac output (eg, thiopental, propofol, midazolam). When a patient is in frank shock, dosing should be reduced by *50% regardless of the drug selected.*

Etomidate is, at this time, the induction agent of choice for trauma intubations. Although recent data suggest a risk of transient adrenal suppression with etomidate use, the favorable hemodynamic profile in the hemodynamically compromised patient may offset that risk.[38-41] Until a clear detrimental effect is demonstrated, it is difficult to ignore the superiority of this drug in this setting.[42]

Ketamine is an attractive alternative to etomidate in the injured patient.[40] Because the drug augments sympathetic outflow and therefore increases heart rate and blood pressure, it is frequently used in hypotensive trauma patients without brain injury. The common reservation with using ketamine in brain-injured patients is that increases in cerebral blood flow and cerebral metabolic rates will increase intracranial pressure (ICP). However, recent data challenge this assertion, demonstrating reductions in ICP in children with brain trauma after ketamine administration.[43]

Optimizing Resuscitation

General Principles

Failure to recognize and adequately treat shock is an important problem during the early phases of trauma management, and is one of the leading causes of preventable death.[44] Clinicians must develop a unique resuscitative strategy for each case based on known or suspected injuries, the evolving clinical status, and the patient's preinjury condition. This strategy must be fluid, changing in tandem with careful reassessment.

The physical examination can be insensitive for the detection of ongoing hemorrhage and subclinical shock. This is especially true in elderly trauma patients, who generally have decreased physiological reserves.[45,46] The addition of serum markers (eg, lactate, base deficit) significantly improves the ability to assess tissue perfusion and hypoxia across all age groups.[6,47] Serial measurements of these markers will help guide the resuscitation. Bedside ultrasound assessment of the diameter of the inferior vena cava also can help evaluate preload and response to fluid therapy (see *Chapter 22*).[48]

Fluid and Transfusion Therapy

Normal saline and lactated Ringer's solution remain the fluids of choice for initial trauma resuscitation, and there is no compelling evidence that colloid therapy offers any benefit.[49] A growing body of literature supports limiting crystalloid therapy in the actively bleeding patient and employing damage control resuscitation (DCR) to improve patient outcomes.[50] The ninth edition of the Advanced Trauma Life Support (ATLS) manual has incorporated this principle, now recommending only 1 liter of crystalloid before transitioning to blood products in traumatic shock patients.[51]

DCR is an evolving concept in trauma resuscitation and was developed in a battlefield setting.[50] Its key principles are early mechanical hemorrhage control, hemostatic resuscitation (ie, limited crystalloid administration coupled with immediate coagulation factor replacement), prevention of hypothermia, and avoidance of acidosis.[50,51] The importance of DCR is highlighted in the most critically ill trauma patients and in those undergoing massive transfusion, defined as the administration of 10 or more units of packed red blood cells (PRBCs) within 24 hours. Because massive transfusion is required in only 1% to 3% of civilian trauma patients, institutional protocols should be developed to facilitate effective execution of this low-frequency intervention.

When the need for massive transfusion is evident or anticipated, it should immediately begin in the emergency department and be continued while the patient is moved to an operating room, angiography suite, or intensive care unit (ICU). When massive transfusion is employed, use of a 1:1:1 ratio of fresh frozen plasma, platelets, and PRBCs lowers overall transfusion requirements, forestalls coagulopathy, and decreases mortality (see *Chapter 18*).[52-58]

Trauma patients receiving transfusion should be considered for early administration of tranexamic acid (TXA), a lysine analogue that binds plasminogen and prevents the formation of plasmin and slowing the degradation of fibrin clots. Hyperfibrinolysis is suspected to be a major contributor to the acute coagulopathy seen in severe injury. TXA, which reduces all-cause mortality and death due to bleeding, has the greatest benefit if administered within 1 hour and sustained up to 3 hours after injury.[59]

The treatment also has a mortality advantage as a component in the DCR strategy, with an important caveat that the survival benefit was greatest in patients receiving massive transfusion.[60] Many trauma centers have protocols for the empirical administration of TXA for patients receiving blood transfusions within 3 hours after injury. The drug should be administered as a 1-gram bolus followed by a 1-gram infusion over 8 hours.

PEARL

Use a 1:1:1 ratio of platelets, plasma, and PRBCs in massive transfusion protocols.

Hypovolemic Resuscitation

The resuscitation of a crashing patient with penetrating torso wounds should follow a unique resuscitative paradigm. Overzealous fluid administration with the aim of achieving a normal blood pressure increases intracavitary bleeding and mortality. The practice of hypovolemic resuscitation is based on the Houston experience, wherein immediate transport to the operating room with minimal fluid therapy was associated with increased survival and fewer complications.[61] A target systolic blood pressure of 80 to 90 mm Hg is reasonable, assuming rapid surgical control of bleeding can be achieved. This strategy should not be applied to patients with coincident brain injuries or blunt multisystem trauma.

PEARL

A hypovolemic resuscitation strategy should not be used in patients with brain trauma, as it may decrease cerebral perfusion pressure and worsen neurological injuries.

Neuroresuscitation

Early resuscitation of the patient with severe traumatic brain injury (TBI) can have a profoundly beneficial effect on survival. Hypotension plays a critical role in morbidity and mortality; even a single episode of hypotension has been associated with a 150% increase in the risk of death.[62] During the early management of these cases, the primary objective should be to maintain adequate central nervous system (CNS) perfusion at all times to minimize secondary brain injury.[63]

In the emergency department, this translates into a diligent search for hemorrhagic and nonhemorrhagic causes of shock, adequate fluid and transfusion therapy, careful drug selection to avoid iatrogenic hypotension (eg, during RSI), and planning for the definitive control of bleeding. These decisions must be made in close collaboration with neurosurgery colleagues.

Management of Severe Traumatic Brain Injury

Severe TBI is the primary cause of death and serious disability after trauma. Each year, 50,000 patients die from head injuries and another 80,000 are left with permanent neurological disabilities.[63,64] It is critical to have a sophisticated understanding of the imperatives of early TBI care. Adherence to published evidence-based guidelines decreases variability and improves outcomes.[65,66] The initial management of these patients should focus on the following:

- Effective management of the airway
- Careful maintenance of adequate tissue perfusion
- Medical treatment of clinically evident intracranial hypertension
- Timely consultation with and transfer to a trauma center

At the center of an effective TBI management strategy is the prevention of secondary injury brought on by hypotension and/or hypoxemia. At the bedside, this translates into early airway management and fluid resuscitation, cautious administration of vasoactive medications, and prompt hemorrhage control.

Once the airway is secure, the clinician can assess whether the patient has intracranial hypertension and, if so, what should be done to manage it. In the hemodynamically stable patient with clear signs of impending herniation (ie, rapid neurological decline, pupillary asymmetry, motor posturing), medical therapy to reduce elevated ICP is indicated. In such cases, Brain Trauma Foundation (braintrauma.org) guidelines recommend early mannitol therapy (1–1.5 g/kg) as the initial approach. Consistent with the goal of avoiding secondary injury, mannitol should be given with caution or withheld from hypotensive patients and those with significant ongoing hemorrhage.[63]

The role of hyperventilation in the management of severe TBI has evolved considerably. Once a mainstay of early therapy, the approach is now known to cause considerable morbidity in patients with severe TBI. Hyperventilation reduces ICP at the expense of cerebral blood flow. In an acutely injured patient, in whom CNS perfusion is already threatened, the treatment further impairs regional blood flow and causes significant tissue ischemia.[67,68] Hyperventilation should be reserved for patients with signs of impending herniation who fail to respond to mannitol and for those with significant hypotension, in whom the drug is contraindicated. Aggressive hyperventilation should be as brief as clinically possible, typically with a target rate above 30 mm Hg.[63]

The anticoagulated patient with TBI deserves special mention. When controlled for injury severity, studies have demonstrated markedly worse outcomes for patients taking warfarin.[69,70] Anticoagulation reversal should be initiated early, if possible, preferably before transfer. Although the use of prothrombin concentrate complex (PCC) products is increasingly popular in TBI patients, no clinical trials have compared this therapy with fresh frozen plasma (FFP) in this population. There is no demonstrated benefit of PCC over conventional therapy with FFP.[71] Prospective, randomized trials are urgently needed in this domain.

The timely transfer of severely brain-injured patients to centers capable of providing operative and intensive care is essential. When severe TBI is clinically evident, time should not be wasted obtaining a head CT scan. Sound clinical judgment, early communication, and regional referral protocols will bring efficiency to the process.

Preparing for Definitive Management

After initial resuscitation and rapid diagnostic evaluation in the emergency department, the injured patient may be transferred to an operating room or ICU for definitive care. However, patients might remain in the resuscitation space while therapeutic decisions are made and resources marshaled. During this time, the intensity of care may decrease as providers shift their perception of the situation or their role in patient care. It is imperative that the resuscitative team maintains active management of the injured patient until definitive hand-off to another clinical provider team. In many emergency departments, this means providing ICU-level care in the resuscitation space, with attention to neurological care, medications, active warming, correction of coagulopathy and metabolic derangements, and preparations for surgical intervention.

Preparing for Transfer

For the majority of injured patients, care begins outside a regional trauma center. Trauma systems that connect community and regional hospitals have superior patient outcomes, especially for the critically injured.[72-74] Decisions to transfer are based primarily on local resources and involve complex processes unique to each institution. The challenge is to provide stabilizing care without delaying transfer and definitive therapy unnecessarily. Although the solution is not always self-evident or easy to achieve, a minimalistic approach is logical.

Once the decision to transfer has been made, clinicians should do only what must be done and request tests only if the results will be acted upon. A study of 249 consecutive adult trauma patients transferred to a regional Canadian trauma center over a 2-year period illustrates the second point. Roughly one-third of these patients underwent CT imaging prior to transport. In no case was the CT result used to determine the need for transfer, and in no case did it lead to a decision to perform surgery before transfer.[75] Interventions that should and should not be done prior to transfer are listed in Key Points.

Another essential element of the transfer process hinges on effective communication. This is grounded on basic principles such as establishing transfer policies and procedures ahead of time, communicating early, ensuring that all relevant documents and test results are available for downstream care providers, and participating in the ongoing regional quality assurance process.

Conclusion

Emergency department management of the crashing trauma patient is complex, challenging, and stressful. Injury identification begins by determining the need for immediate airway control and evaluating central perfusion deficits, severe intracranial injuries, intrathoracic and intraabdominal trauma, and limb-threatening injuries. Successful resuscitation strategies must include airway management, appropriate fluid and transfusion therapy, and management of traumatic brain injury. Many critically ill trauma patients require transfer to a regional trauma center. Interventions only should be performed prior to transport if they will contribute to the transfer decision and have no impact on the timing of the transfer.

REFERENCES

1. Schurink GW, Bode PJ, van Luijt PA, et al. The value of physical examination in the diagnosis of patients with blunt abdominal trauma: a retrospective study. *Injury.* 1997;29:261-265.
2. American College of Emergency Physicians. Clinical policy: critical issues in the evaluation of adult patients presenting to the emergency department with acute blunt abdominal trauma. *Ann Emerg Med.* 2004;43:278-290.
3. Holmes J, Nguyen H, Jacoby RC, et al. Do all patients with left costal margin injuries require radiographic evaluation for abdominal injury? *Ann Emerg Med.* 2005;46:232-236.
4. Asimos A, Gibbs MA, Marx JA, et al. Value of point-of-care blood testing in emergent trauma management. *J Trauma.* 2000;48:1101-1108.
5. Paladino L, Sinert R, Wallace D, et al. The utility of base deficit and arterial lactate in differentiating major from minor injury in trauma patients with normal vital signs. *Resuscitation.* 2008;77:363-368.

KEY POINTS

1. **Airway management in the crashing trauma patient**
   - Preparation
     - Perform a focused airway assessment to predict difficulty.
     - Identify surgical airway landmarks ahead of time.
     - Place appropriate airway rescue equipment nearby.
     - Perform a brief neurological examination before intubation.
     - Maximize preload in hypotensive patients and those with traumatic brain injury.
   - Drug selection
     - Choose neuroprotective agents for patients with brain injury.
     - Be cautious with agent selection and dosage to avoid hypotension.
     - Provide appropriate postintubation analgesia and sedation.
   - Rescue
     - Choose the approach/device that is most likely to be successful in your hands.
     - Know when to call for help.
2. **Even transient hypoxemia dramatically worsens outcomes; therefore, intubate early.**
   - Rapid-sequence intubation is the preferred technique.
   - Use a neuroprotective sedative (eg, etomidate).
   - Pretreatment with lidocaine, fentanyl, or a defasciculating dose of a neuromuscular blocking agent is controversial.
3. **Even transient hypotension dramatically worsens outcomes; therefore, resuscitate aggressively.**
   - Rapid identification of coincident hemorrhage is crucial.
   - Maintain CNS perfusion.
   - Be cautious with medications that can precipitate hypotension.
4. **Mannitol**
   - Can reduce elevated ICP
   - Recommended dose: 1–1.5 g/kg
   - Can precipitate hypotension:
     - Withhold if blood pressure is ≤90 mm Hg.
     - Use with caution if blood pressure is >90 mm Hg and tenuous and/or if there is ongoing hemorrhage.
     - Administer small sequential boluses (0.25–0.5 g/kg) if hypotension is a risk.

6. Callaway DW, Shapiro NI, Donnino MW, et al. Serum lactate and base deficit as predictors of mortality in normotensive elderly blunt trauma patients. *J Trauma.* 2009;66:1040-1044.
7. Wisbach GG, Sise MJ, Sack DI, et al. What is the role of chest X-ray in the initial assessment of stable trauma patients? *J Trauma.* 2007;62:74-79.
8. Cyer HM. Chest radiography in blunt trauma patients: is it necessary? *Ann Emerg Med.* 2006;47:422-423.
9. Plurad D, Green D, Demetriades D, et al. The increased use of chest computed tomography for trauma: is it being over utilized? *J Trauma.* 2007;62:631-635.
10. Shackford SR, Rogers FB, Osler TM, et al. Focused abdominal sonography for trauma: the learning curve of nonradiologist clinicians in detecting hemoperitoneum. *J Trauma.* 1999;46:553-556.
11. Rozycki GS, Root D. The diagnosis of intraabdominal injury. *J Trauma.* 2010;68:1019-1023.
12. Lee BC, Ormasby EL, McGahan JP, et al. The utility of sonography for the triage of blunt abdominal trauma patients to exploratory laparotomy. *Am J Roentgenol.* 2007;188:415-421.
13. Rozycki GS, Ballard R, Feliciano DV, et al. Surgeon-performed ultrasound for assessment of truncal injuries: lessons learned from 1,540 patients. *Ann Surg.* 1998;228:16-28.
14. Rozycki GS, Feliciano DV, Ochsner MG, et al. The role of ultrasound with possible penetrating cardiac wounds: a prospective multicenter study. *J Trauma.* 1999;46:543-552.
15. Rozycki GS, Feliciano DV, Schmidt JA, et al. The role of surgeon-performed ultrasound in patients with possible cardiac wounds. *Ann Surg.* 1996;223:737-746.
16. Jones AE, Mason P, Tayal VT, et al. Uroperitoneum presenting as a positive FAST in a patient with bladder rupture. *Am J Emerg Med.* 2003;25:373-377.
17. Tayal VS, Nielsen A, Jones AE, et al. Accuracy of trauma ultrasound in major pelvic injury. *J Trauma.* 2006;61:1453-1457.
18. Knudtson JL, Dort JM, Helmer SD, et al. Surgeon-performed ultrasound for pneumothorax in the trauma suite. *J Trauma.* 2004;56:527-530.
19. Wilkerson RG, Stone MB. Sensitivity of bedside ultrasound and supine anteroposterior chest radiography for the identification of pneumothorax after blunt trauma. *Acad Emerg Med.* 2010;17:11-17.
20. Salim A, Sangthong B, Martin M, et al. Whole body imaging in blunt multisystem trauma patients without signs of injury: results of a prospective study. *Arch Surg.* 2006;141:468-473.
21. Deunk J, Brink M, Dekker HM, et al. Routine versus selective multidetector-row computed tomography (MDCT) in blunt trauma patients: level of agreement on the influence of additional findings on management. *J Trauma.* 2009;67:1080-1086.
22. Root HD, Hauser CW, McKinley CR, et al. Diagnostic peritoneal lavage. *Surgery.* 1965;57:633-637.
23. Henneman PL, Marx JA, Moore EE, et al. Diagnostic peritoneal lavage: accuracy in predicting necessary laparotomy following blunt and penetrating trauma. *J Trauma.* 1990;30:1345-1355.
24. Blow O, Bassam D, Butler K, et al. Speed and efficiency in the resuscitation of blunt abdominal trauma patients with multiple injuries: the advantage of diagnostic peritoneal lavage over abdominal computerized tomography. *J Trauma.* 1998;44:287-290.
25. Cha JY, Kashuk JL, Sarin EL, et al. Diagnostic peritoneal lavage remains a valuable adjunct to modern imaging techniques. *J Trauma.* 2009;67:330-336.
26. Hoffmann JR, Mower WR, Wolfson AB, et al. Validity of a set of clinical criteria to rule out injury to the cervical spine in patients with blunt trauma. *N Engl J Med.* 2000;343:94-99.
27. Stiell IG, Clement CM, McKnight RD, et al. The Canadian C-spine rule versus the NEXUS low-risk criteria in patients with trauma. *N Engl J Med.* 2003;349:2510-2518.
28. Stiell IG, Wells GA, Vandemheen K, et al. The Canadian CT Rule for patients with minor head injury. *Lancet.* 2001;357:1391-1396.
29. Duane TM, Tan BB, Golay D, et al. Blunt trauma and the role of routine pelvic radiographs: a prospective analysis. *J Trauma.* 2002;53:463-468.
30. Gonzalez RP, Fried PQ, Bukhalo M. The utility of clinical examination in screening for pelvic fractures in blunt trauma. *J Am Coll Surg.* 2002;194:121-125.
31. Dunham MC, Barraco RD, Clark DE, et al. Guidelines for emergency tracheal intubation immediately after trauma injury. *J Trauma.* 2003;55:162-179.
32. Esposito TJ, Sanddal ND, Hansen JD, et al. Analysis of preventable trauma deaths and inappropriate trauma care in a rural state. *J Trauma.* 1995;39:955-962.
33. Esposito TJ, Sanddal TL, Reynolds SA, et al. Effect of a voluntary trauma system on preventable death and inappropriate care in a rural state. *J Trauma.* 2003;54:662-670.
34. Murphy MF, Walls RM. Identification of the difficult and failed airway. In: Walls RM, Murphy MF, eds. *Manual of Emergency Airway Management.* 3rd ed. Philadelphia, PA: Lippincott Williams & Wilkins; 2008:81-93.
35. Reed MJ. Can an airway assessment score predict difficulty at intubation in the emergency department? *Emerg Med J.* 2005;22:99-110.
36. Kortbeek JB, Al Turki SA, Jameel A, et al. Advanced Trauma Life Support, 8th ed, the evidence for change. *J Trauma.* 2008;64:1638-1650.
37. Gibbs MA. Trauma. In: Walls RM, ed. *Manual of Emergency Airway Management.* 2nd ed. Philadelphia, PA: Lippincott Williams & Wilkins; 2004:251-261.

5. **Hyperventilation**
   - Can reduce elevated ICP
   - Presents the potential for local CNS hypoperfusion
   - Mild hyperventilation ($Paco_2$ of 35–40 mm Hg) for all patients with TBI
   - Use aggressive hyperventilation only as a temporizing measure if clear clinical signs of herniation are present (ie, blown pupil, motor posturing, rapid neurological decline + coma) or signs of herniation are visible on CT.
   - Use in conjunction with other measures (eg, mannitol, sedation) whenever possible.
   - Use for the shortest duration possible.
6. **Interventions that should be done BEFORE transfer**
   - Manage the airway.
   - Secure adequate intravenous access.
   - Control external bleeding.
   - Begin PRBC transfusion if the patient is persistently hypotensive after administration of 2 liters of crystalloid with the potential for continued hemorrhage.
   - Reverse anticoagulant medications in patients with intracranial, major intracavitary, or external hemorrhage.
   - Perform tube thoracostomy for symptomatic pneumothorax or hemothorax.
   - Stabilize grossly displaced pelvic ring fractures and provide external compression.
   - Reduce dislocations with clear vascular compromise.
   - Splint extremity fractures.
   - Protect the patient from hypothermia.
7. **Interventions that should NOT delay transfer**
   - Once the decision to transfer has been made, further diagnostic imaging is unlikely to be of benefit and is likely to be repeated at the receiving institution.
   - The following tests can be considered only if they will cause absolutely no delay in transfer:
     - Head CT
     - Abdominal CT
     - Plain films of the extremities for obvious fractures
     - Cervical imaging after the spine is immobilized properly
     - Specific laboratory testing
8. **Communication and the transfer process**
   - When clinical instability or the nature of the injuries mandates transfer, communicate early. Do not wait for test results.
   - Ensure the transfer of all notes, images, test results, and summary of interventions.

38. Hildreth AN, Mejia VA, Maxwell RA, et al. Adrenal suppression following a single dose of etomidate for rapid sequence intubation: a prospective randomized trial. *J Trauma.* 2008;65:573-579.
39. Warner KJ, Cuschieri J, Jurkovich GJ, et al. Single-dose etomidate for rapid sequence intubation may impact outcome after severe injury. *J Trauma.* 2009;67:45-50.
40. Fields AM, Rosbolt MB, Cohn SM. Induction agents for intubation of the trauma patient. *J Trauma.* 2009;67:867-869.
41. Andrade FM. Postintubation hypotension: the "etomidate paradox." *J Trauma.* 2009;67:417.
42. Oglesby AJ. Should etomidate be the induction agent of choice for rapid sequence intubation in the emergency department? *Emerg Med J.* 2004;21:655-659.
43. Bar-Joseph G, Guilburd Y, Tamir A, et al. Effectiveness of ketamine in decreasing intracranial pressure in children with intracranial hypertension. *J Neurosurg Pediatr.* 2009;4:40-46.
44. Teixeira PFR, Inaba K, Hadjizacharia P, et al. Preventable or potentially preventable mortality at a mature trauma center. *J Trauma.* 2007;63:1338-1347.
45. Jacobs DG, Plaisier BR, Barie PS, et al. EAST Practice Management Guidelines Work Group. Practice management guidelines for geriatric trauma: the EAST Practice Management Guidelines Work Group. *J Trauma.* 2003;54:391-416.
46. Callaway DW, Wolfe R. Geriatric trauma. *Emerg Med Clin North Am.* 2007;25:837-860.
47. Paladino L, Sinert R, Wallace D, et al. The utility of base deficit and arterial lactate in differentiating major from minor injury in trauma patients with normal vital signs. *Resuscitation.* 2008;77:363-368.
48. Yanagawa Y, Sakamoto T, Odaka Y. Hypovolemic shock evaluated by sonographic measurement of the inferior vena cava during resuscitation in trauma patients. *J Trauma.* 2007;63:1245-1248.
49. Perel P, Roberts I. Colloids versus crystalloids for fluid resuscitation in critically ill patients. *Cochrane Database Syst Rev.* 2007;(4):CD000567.
50. Holcomb JB, Jenkins D, Rhee P, et al. Damage control resuscitation: directly addressing the early coagulopathy of trauma. *J Trauma* 2007;62(2)307-310.
51. American College of Surgeons Committee on Trauma. Advanced trauma life support program of doctors, 9th edition. Chicago: American College of Surgeons; 2004.
52. Gonzalez EA, Moore FA, Holcomb JB, et al. Fresh frozen plasma should be given early to patients requiring massive transfusion. *J Trauma.* 2007;62:112-119.
53. Teixeira PGR, Inaba K, Shulman I, et al. Impact of plasma transfusion in massively transfused trauma patients. *J Trauma.* 2009;66:693-697.
54. Dente CJ, Shaz BH, Nicholas JM, et al. Improvements in early mortality and coagulopathy are sustained better in patients with blunt trauma after institution of a massive transfusion protocol in a civilian Level I trauma center. *J Trauma.* 2009;66:1616-1624.
55. Perkins JG. An evaluation of the impact of apheresis platelets used in the setting of massively transfused trauma patients. *J Trauma.* 2009;26:S77.
56. Cotton BA, Reddy N, Hatch QM, et al. Damage control resuscitation is associated with reduction in resuscitation volumes and improvement in survival in 390 damage control laparotomy patients. *Ann Surg.* 2011;254(4):598-605.
57. Holcomb JB, del Junco, DJ, Fox EE, et al; PROMMITT Study Group. The prospective, observational, multicenter, major trauma transfusion (PROMMITT) study: comparative effectiveness of a time-varying treatment with competing risks. *JAMA Surg.* 2013;148(2): 127-136.
58. Holcomb JB, Tilley BC, Baraniuk S, et al. Transfusion of plasma, platelets, and red blood cells in a 1:1:1 vs a 1:1:2 ratio and mortality in patients with severe trauma. The PROPPR randomized clinical trial. *JAMA.* 2015;313(5):471-482.
59. CRASH-2 trial collaborators. Effects of tranexamic acid on death, vascular occlusive events, and blood transfusion in trauma patients with significant haemorrhage (CRASH-2): a randomized, placebo-controlled trial. *Lancet.* 2010;376(9734):23-32.
60. Morrison JJ, Dubose JJ, Rasmussen TE, et al. Military Application of Tranexamic Acid in Trauma Emergency Resuscitation (MATTERs) study. *Arch Surg.* 2012;147(2):113-119.
61. Bickell WH, Wall MJ, Pepe PE, et al. Immediate versus delayed fluid resuscitation for hypotensive patients with penetrating torso injuries. *N Engl J Med.* 1994;331:1105-1109.
62. Chesnut RM, Marshall LF, Klauber MR, et al. The role of secondary brain injury in determining outcome from severe head injury. *J Trauma.* 1993;34:216-221.
63. Brain Trauma Foundation. Guidelines for the management of severe traumatic brain injury, 3rd edition. *J Neurotrauma.* 2007;24(suppl 1).
64. Langlois JA, Rutland-Brown W, Wald MM, et al. The epidemiology and impact of traumatic brain injury: a brief overview. *J Head Trauma Rehabil.* 2006;21:375-378.
65. Hesdorgger DC, Ghajar J. Marked improvement in adherence to traumatic brain injury guidelines in United States trauma centers. *J Trauma.* 2007;63:841-848.
66. Fakhry SM, Trask AL, Waller MA, et al. Management of brain-injured patients by an evidence-based medicine protocol improves outcomes and decreases hospital charges. *J Trauma.* 2004;54:492-500.
67. Coles JP, Minhas PS, Fryer TD, et al. Effect of hyperventilation on cerebral blood flow in traumatic head injury: clinical relevance and monitoring correlates. *Crit Care Med.* 2002;30:1950-1959.
68. Marion DW, Puccio A, Wisiniewski SR, et al. Effect of hyperventilation on extracellular concentrations of glutamate, lactate, pyruvate, and local cerebral blood flow in patients with severe traumatic brain injury. *Crit Care Med.* 2002;30:2619-2625.
69. Franko J, Kish KJ, O'Connell BG, et al. Advanced age and preinjury warfarin anticoagulation increase the risk of mortality after head trauma. *J Trauma.* 2006;61:107-110.
70. Pieracci FM, Eachempate SR, Shou J, et al. Degree of anticoagulation, but not warfarin use itself, predicts adverse outcomes after traumatic brain injury in elderly trauma patients. *J Trauma.* 2007;63:525-530.
71. Johansen M, Wikkelso A, Lunde J, et al. Prothrombin complex concentrate for reversal of vitamin K antagonist treatment in bleeding and non-bleeding patients. *Cochrane Database of Systematic Rev.* 2015;7:CD010555.
72. Cudnik MT, Newgard CD, Sayre M, et al. Level I versus level II trauma centers: an outcomes-based assessment. *J Trauma.* 2009;66:1321-1326.
73. Hedges JR, Newgard CD, Veum-Stone J, et al. Early neurosurgical procedures enhance survival in blunt head injury: propensity score analysis. *J Emerg Med.* 2009;37:115-123.
74. Newgard CD, McConnell KJ, Hedges JR, et al. The benefit of higher level of care transfer of injured patients from nontertiary hospital emergency departments. *J Trauma.* 2007;63:965-971.
75. Onzuka J, Worster A, McCreadie B. Is computerized tomography of trauma patients associated with a transfer delay to a regional trauma centre? *Can J Emerg Med.* 2008;10:205-208.

Emergency Transfusions

18

IN THIS CHAPTER

- Red blood cell transfusions
- Massive transfusion protocols
- Platelet transfusions
- Plasma transfusions
- Adverse effects of blood product transfusions

Joseph R. Shiber

The transfusion of blood products is a common intervention in critical care practice. More than 1.4 million units of red blood cell (RBC) concentrates and 1.6 million units of platelets are administered in the United States every year.[1] Although the lifesaving treatment's popularity has grown in the last decade, the number of transfusions given in the intensive care setting has declined, as physicians have begun to adopt more conservative transfusion policies.[2-4]

Transfusions are used to prevent and treat shock, hypovolemia, and coagulopathy; maintain oxygen-carrying capacity; and stabilize vascular oncotic pressure without causing adverse effects.[5-8] Whole blood was commonly given in the early stages of transfusion medicine, with a preference for "fresh" whole blood (stored for <24 hours at 22°C).[6] In the US, a unit of whole blood (450 mL at collection with 60 mL of anticoagulant added) has a shelf life of 35 days, but the platelet function and coagulant factor quickly degrade. Modern blood banking practices, including the separation of whole blood into distinct components, can dramatically lengthen the viability of these products.[7] Whole blood transfusion is rarely given outside combat hospital situations.[7,9]

A single unit of packed RBCs will raise the hemoglobin (Hgb) level by 1 g/dL and the hematocrit (Hct) by 3% in a 70-kg patient without ongoing blood loss.[3,7] The average half-life of a transfused RBC is 57.7 days. Patients with pure RBC aplasia require a 2-unit transfusion approximately every 2 weeks.[7]

The North American population has the following blood types: O, 44%; A, 43%; B, 9%; and AB, 4%. Eighty-four percent of the population is Rh positive, and the other 16% is Rh negative. For a critically ill or injured patient, "emergency release" blood is typically type O, the universal RBC donor. Blood type O that is Rh negative is a precious resource and is reserved for women with childbearing potential in order to prevent Rh(D) antibody complications.[1] Type-specific blood is usually available within 15 minutes after the specimen is received in the blood bank and should be given for ongoing hemorrhage or uncorrected shock after the emergency release blood. Crossmatching will take 45 to 60 minutes if no antibodies are detected.[1,3] Platelets, plasma, and cryoprecipitate must be ABO compatible but do not require crossmatching. AB plasma is the universal plasma donor since it does not contain anti-A or anti-B antibodies. Platelets usually are available in 5 to 15 minutes, and plasma and cryoprecipitate in 5 to 30 minutes.[1,9]

Red Blood Cell Transfusion

RBC transfusion can increase oxygen delivery, expand blood volume, alleviate symptoms of acute blood loss anemia, and relieve cardiac ischemia *(Table 18-1)*.[10,11] A clear distinction needs to be made between chronic anemia, which can be well tolerated by otherwise healthy individuals, and acute hemorrhage, which represents loss of red cell mass and intravascular volume. The initial Hgb and Hct in acute blood loss do not reflect the actual extent of hemorrhage since the recruitment of interstitial and intracellular fluid into the intravascular space is not immediate. Unless crystalloid or colloid is given to replace the volume lost, the Hgb and Hct levels will underestimate the extent of the hemorrhage.[7,12]

The degree of acute blood loss should be clinically evaluated using vital signs and physical examination findings such as tachycardia, orthostasis, decreased pulse pressure, pallor, cool extremities, and delayed capillary refill. Frank arterial hypotension is a late finding in acute blood loss.[3] In hypovolemic shock, the systolic pressure is decreased as a result of falling cardiac output caused by lowered filling pressures, and the diastolic pressure rises in response to increased systemic vascular resistance. This compensatory effect is only temporary and goes away with frank cardiovascular collapse.

PEARL

The initial Hgb and Hct in acute blood loss do not reflect the actual extent of hemorrhage since the recruitment of interstitial and intracellular fluid into the intravascular space is not immediate. Unless crystalloid or colloid is given to replace the volume lost, the Hgb and Hct will underestimate the extent of the hemorrhage.[7,12]

In a healthy person at rest, oxygen delivery is 4 times greater than tissue utilization. Even with an isolated decrease in Hgb to 10 g/dL, oxygen delivery will be twice that needed for resting consumption.[13] Signs and symptoms of anemia are unlikely to be evident at Hgb values above 7 or 8 g/dL in healthy patients. Even critically ill patients with chronic anemia can tolerate a Hgb of 7 g/dL, except those with preexisting coronary, pulmonary, or cerebrovascular disease.[5,7,11] The anemic patient has a diminished arterial oxygen content but is able to increase oxygen delivery by escalating cardiac output and coronary blood flow through vasodilation.

Myocardial oxygen extraction increases from 25% at baseline; at approximately 50%, the anaerobic threshold is reached and myocardial lactate levels increase.[7] Therefore, the current recommendations for packed RBC transfusions are more liberal in patients with coronary artery disease, particularly those with acute myocardial ischemia.[1,6,13,14] The likelihood of benefit from the transfusion of packed RBCs to nonbleeding patients is summarized in Table 18-2. Clinical judgment and data (such as lactate levels and central venous oxygen saturation) should be used to individually assess each case and weigh the benefits and risks of transfusion against the dangers of ongoing anemia.[1,12,14]

PEARL

In a healthy person at rest, oxygen delivery is 4 times greater than tissue utilization. Even with an isolated decrease in Hgb to 10 g/dL, the oxygen delivered will still be twice that needed for resting consumption.[13]

In a previously healthy patient with blood loss of less than 20% to 25% and no ongoing hemorrhage, only volume restoration with crystalloid or colloid is needed.[3,6] If the total blood volume loss exceeds 20% to 25% (with a normal blood volume of 70 mL/kg), regardless of the presenting blood indices, RBC transfusion may be indicated. Transfusion can be indicated at lower percentages of blood volume loss if there is a high risk of ongoing hemorrhage (eg, patients with trauma, postpartum hemorrhage, or gastrointestinal bleeding, particularly with concomitant cirrhosis). In such situations, group O packed RBCs are given because this is the most expedient blood product available. Type ABO-specific blood may be given next if more is required, but eventually crossmatched blood should be administered. Patients with sickle cell anemia might require RBC transfusion upon arrival in the emergency department. In those who are critically ill, particularly with acute chest syndrome, a Hct of 30% and a Hgb-sickle of less than 30% should be the goal.[8]

PEARL

TBV estimation of actual body weight (mL/kg):

	OBESE	THIN	NORMAL
Male	60	65	70
Female	55	60	65

For example, a 70-kg man would have a TBV of ~5 L (70 × 70 = 4,900), which is 10 units of whole blood.

Massive Transfusion

The term *massive transfusion* traditionally describes the administration of more than 10 units of blood, or an amount equal to the patient's total blood volume (TBV) within 24 hours.[3] Updated definitions include replacement of more than 50% of TBV within 3 hours and transfusion of more than 4 RBC units within 1 hour, with anticipated need for ongoing blood products.[15-17] Massive transfusion is warranted in 1% to 3% of civilian trauma patients and has been used in those with gastrointestinal bleeding, ruptured abdominal aortic aneurysm, ruptured ectopic pregnancy, and obstetrical or postpartum hemorrhage.[9,18] Risk factors that predict the need for massive transfusion in trauma patients include abnormal vital signs on presentation (tachycardia and hypotension), pH levels below 7.25, Hct less than 32%, a penetrating mechanism of trauma, and evidence of free fluid on bedside ultrasonography.[18]

TABLE 18-1. General Indications for Red Blood Cell Transfusion

Evidence of hemorrhagic shock
Acute blood loss of >20%–25% estimated blood volume
Symptomatic anemia in a euvolemic patient
Hgb <7 g/dL in a critically ill patient
Hgb <8 g/dL in a patient with an acute coronary syndrome
Hgb <9 g/dL preoperatively with expected blood loss of >500 mL
Hgb <10 g/dL in a possibly euvolemic patient with evidence of tissue hypoxemia
Sickle cell acute chest syndrome if Hgb <10 g/dL or Hgb-SS >30%

TABLE 18-2. Likelihood of Benefit From Transfusion of Packed RBCs[7,10,13]

Hgb	Is transfusion beneficial?
>10 g/dL	Unlikely
7–10 g/dL	Potentially beneficial if other deficits in oxygen transport are present
<7 g/dL	Likely

Critically ill or injured patients who have sustained significant blood loss are likely to present with coagulopathy resulting from platelet and clotting factor consumption. They also are likely to present with tissue hypoperfusion, acidosis, and hypothermia, all of which cause dysfunction of the remaining coagulation factors and platelets.[3,9,18] Resuscitation with crystalloid, colloid, or packed RBCs can cause further dilutional coagulopathy. Early trauma-induced coagulopathy (ETIC) develops in up to 50% of severely injured patients within 30 minutes of injury, even prior to packed RBC and fluid resuscitation. In addition to the factors mentioned above, coagulopathy involves increased thrombomodulin expression on endothelial cells due to hypoperfusion, which leads to protein C activation and inhibition of factors V and VIII. Fibrinolysis also is enhanced by accelerated plasmin formation and depletion of plasminogen activator inhibitor-1 (PAI-1), leading to hyperfibrinolysis and subsequent fibrinogen depletion. Development of ETIC is a predictor of death independent of injury severity.[15,19-21]

Hemostatic resuscitation *(Table 18-3)* is a strategy that uses all blood components to provide the equivalent of whole blood in an effort to prevent or treat the coagulopathy associated with massive transfusions.[15] An equal ratio of packed RBC units, FFP, and platelet units (1:1:1 resuscitation) is associated with decreased mortality in trauma patients receiving massive transfusion.[3,9,18] A transfusion of this 1:1:1 solution would have a volume of 645 mL, an Hct of 29% to 30%, a platelet count of 80 to 90 × 10^9/L, and approximately 60% to 65% of coagulation factor activity, which is clearly not equal to whole blood.[9] For this reason, crystalloid and colloid infusions should be limited in patients requiring massive transfusion to prevent further dilutional coagulopathy and thrombocytopenia while allowing permissive hypotension until definitive hemorrhage control has been achieved. The strategy of hemostatic resuscitation includes the early administration of plasma and platelets to prevent hemorrhagic exacerbation.[9,18]

Because of their slow turnaround times, conventional coagulation assays such as prothrombin time (PT) and partial thromboplastin time (PTT) are not useful for predicting the need for a massive transfusion protocol (MTP) or for directing blood component therapy during resuscitation. Point-of-care testing of hemostasis using thromboelastography (TEG) might be better at identifying coagulopathy and guiding the blood products used within the MTP.[15,16,22] TEG results can be available more rapidly and provide quantitative measurements of the individual components involved in hemostasis. Unlike PT and PTT, which gauge secondary hemostasis, TEG allows measurement of all of the phases necessary for adequate clot formation, including platelet function in primary hemostasis, coagulation factor activity (VII, VIII, X), and cross-linking of the fibrin to strengthen the clot. The modality also detects hyperfibrinolysis, a main contributor to ETIC, which is not pinpointed by conventional coagulation assays.

TABLE 18-3. Hemostatic Resuscitation Guidelines

Expedite control of hemorrhage to reduce the need for blood products and prevent consumptive coagulopathy and thrombocytopenia.
Limit crystalloid infusion to prevent dilutional coagulopathy.
Maintain a goal systolic blood pressure of 80–100 mm Hg until definitive hemorrhage control is achieved.
Transfuse at 1:1:1 ratio of packed RBCs/FFP/platelets (1 apheresis unit = 5 platelet units).
Frequently monitor potassium, ionized calcium, lactate, and blood gas values.

Importantly, TEG can be used to distinguish "medical" from "surgical" bleeding in postoperative patients. If abnormalities are noted (*Figures 18-1* and *18-2*), the appropriate component can be given and the test can be repeated to verify correction. If the patient is still bleeding when all aspects of hemostasis are normal, the source of hemorrhage is vascular and requires surgical or mechanical intervention. Since TEG can be checked and then repeated until clinical improvement is seen, it can be considered part of goal-directed hemostatic resuscitation, much like serum lactate in the management of a shock patient. Although TEG has demonstrated benefits in guiding blood product administration and reducing transfusion requirements and the need for MTP activation, it has not been found to reduce the mortality rate in these patients.[15,16,21,23,24]

Platelet Transfusion

Platelet units are obtained by separating them from single donor units of whole blood or, more commonly, apheresis. An apheresis platelet unit contains 4.2 × 10^{11} platelets and is equivalent to 4 to 6 individual platelet units.[2,12] Each unit also contains approximately 50 mL of plasma.[7] Platelets are stored at room temperature (22°C) for up to 5 days. Each unit can increase the platelet count of a 75-kg patient by 5,000 to 10,000/µL, and an apheresis unit will raise the count by 20,000 to 40,000/µL.[8,16] Approximately one-third of all circulating platelets, whether transfused or released from the marrow, are pooled in the spleen; this number is larger in patients with splenomegaly. The *in vivo* lifespan of a platelet is 9 to 10 days.[26]

Maintaining the integrity of the vascular endothelium by filling the gaps in the junctions between endothelial cells requires approximately 7,000 platelets per microliter. When the number of circulating platelets falls below 7,000 /µL, mucosal surfaces start to bleed and measured blood in the stool increases.[7,26] The platelet count should be kept above 50,000/µL in patients who are actively bleeding and even higher (>100,000/µL) in those with microvascular bleeding, particularly involving the central nervous system or retina.[6,7] To decrease the chance of hemorrhage in a patient without recognized risk factors for bleeding, platelets should be transfused when the count is below 10,000/µL.[27] Platelet transfusion thresholds for other clinical scenarios are listed in Table 18-4.

Platelet transfusions are contraindicated in certain groups

FIGURE 18-1. Normal Thromboelastogram Tracing

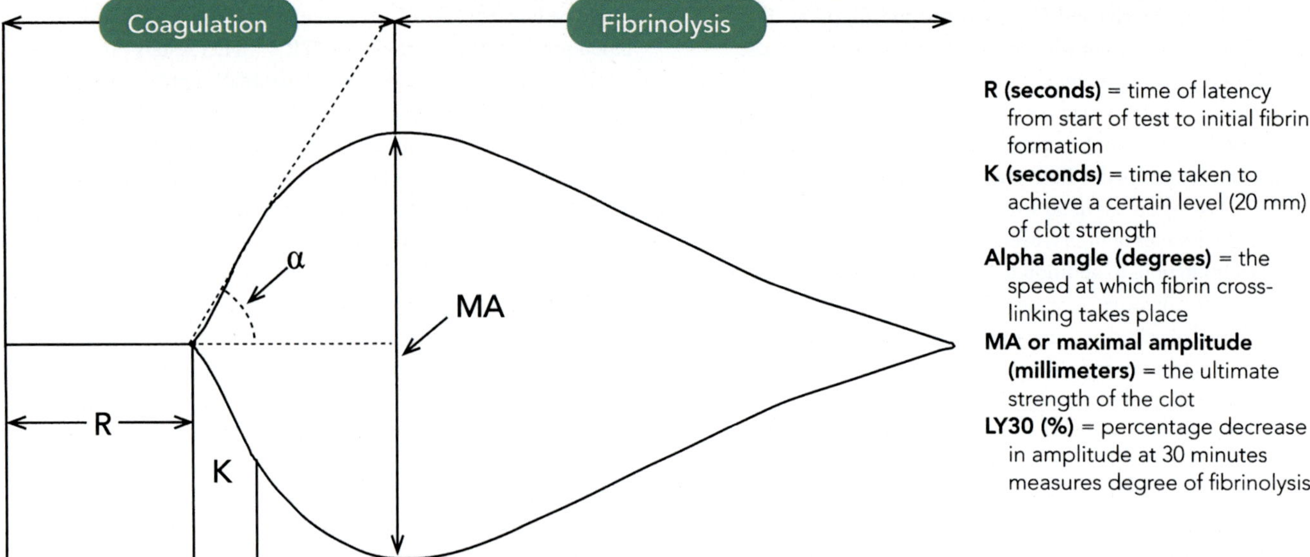

Adapted from: Teodoro de Luz L, Nascimento B, Rizoli S. Thromboelastography (TEG): practical considerations on its clinical use in trauma resuscitation. *Scan J Trauma Resusc Emerg Med.* 2013;21:29-37.

FIGURE 18-2. Examples of Normal and Abnormal TEG Tracings

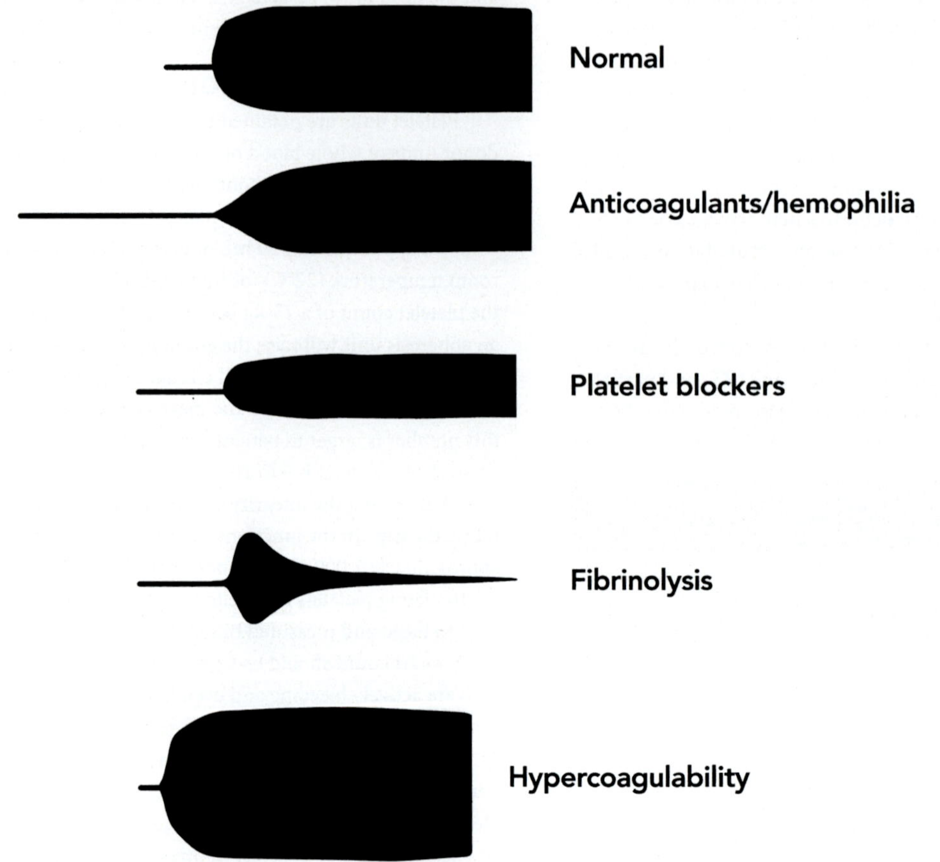

Adapted from: Teodoro de Luz L, Nascimento B, Rizoli S. Thromboelastography (TEG): practical considerations on its clinical use in trauma resuscitation. *Scan J Trauma Resusc Emerg Med.* 2013;21:29-37.

of patients with thrombocytopenia. Giving platelets to patients with thrombotic thrombocytopenic purpura, hemolytic uremic syndrome, or heparin-induced thrombocytopenia will worsen the microvascular thrombosis. The treatment might not be deleterious but is unlikely to be effective in patients with thrombocytopenia caused by immune-mediated platelet destruction.[6,8,26]

Plasma Transfusion

One unit of plasma contains between 200 and 280 mL of fluid volume. After separation from whole blood, it can be frozen for up to 1 year but must be used within 24 hours after thawing (hence the name fresh frozen plasma).[7] Each milliliter of FFP contains approximately 1 unit of each coagulation factor and 2 mg of fibrinogen. One unit of FFP should increase clotting factors by 5% and contains about 500 mg of fibrinogen, twice as much as is in a unit of cryoprecipitate but in a much larger volume.[28] Optimally, plasma should be ABO compatible, but it does not require crossmatching. A critically ill hemorrhaging patient initially should receive AB plasma, which often is immediately accessible. Due to the limited supply of this universal plasma, however, subsequent units from group A can be given if type-specific plasma is unavailable. It takes 25 to 30 minutes to thaw frozen plasma, so it is necessary to keep a thawed supply immediately available for critically ill or injured patients.[15,17]

A plasma transfusion used to prevent bleeding is different than one initiated to treat it. Bleeding does not usually occur until the PT, PTT, or international normalized ratio (INR) is more than 1.5 times higher than normal; therefore, there is little benefit in prophylactic plasma transfusion in a nonbleeding patient with coagulation function test results below these levels. The exception is patients in need of neurosurgical or ophthalmological procedures, who may be at increased risk for devastating results of hemorrhage. In such cases, a value of 1.3 times higher than normal is the threshold for transfusion.[8]

Hemostasis commonly can be achieved with doses of 10 to 20 mL/kg, which can raise clotting factor levels by 15% to 30%; however, 30 mL/kg should be given to bleeding patients who are critically ill.[7,8,28] This dose may be repeated in 4 to 6 hours to maintain adequate factor levels, or a constant infusion can be given until hemostasis is achieved. Prothrombin complex concentrate (PCC) has been used for congenital bleeding disorders and for reversal of warfarin-induced coagulopathy, but has not been fully evaluated in critically hemorrhaging patients. It contains factors II, VII, IX, and X, and provides effects similar to those of FFP but in a smaller volume. It can be infused quickly, does not need to be thawed, and has been used as an adjunct to MTP. Although more studies are needed to fully establish benefits and safety, there is increasing evidence favoring the use of coagulation factor concentrates over FFP.[29,30]

The common clinical indications for plasma transfusion are listed in Table 18-5. Although vitamin K is indicated, it can take 12 to 18 hours to correct the factor deficiency (II, VII, IX, X) induced by warfarin. FFP tranfusion is indicated for faster reversal in symptomatic or high-risk patients. If a single-factor deficiency is confirmed, it is preferable to use specific replacement factors, which are purified and standardized in activity and carry an extremely low risk of infectious disease transmission (or no risk if they are made by a recombinant process).[7,8]

Plasma transfusion is indicated for the treatment of thrombotic thrombocytopenic purpura, hemolytic uremic syndrome, and the syndrome of hemolysis, elevated liver enzymes, and low platelets. Although plasmapheresis also may be required, delays in obtaining vascular access and appropriate staff may necessitate plasma administration in the emergency department, which can be lifesaving.[7,8] Acute angioedema, particularly if caused by C1 esterase inhibitor deficiency, is another indication for transfusion. FFP transfusion also may be necessary for disseminated intravascular coagulation if bleeding is the clinical feature causing the most concern.

A newly recognized but important benefit of plasma transfusion is its impact on endothelial cell function. Through effects on endothelial cells and the extracellular matrix, plasma reduces endothelial permeability and improves thrombin

TABLE 18-4. Guidelines for Platelet Transfusions in Various Clinical Scenarios
Stable patient without increased bleeding risk: <10,000/μL
Patient with increased bleeding risk: <20,000/μL
For bedside procedure: <20,000 μL (eg, central venous catheters, tube thoracostomy)
For most surgery: <50,000/μL (except neurological/ophthalmological surgery: <100,000/μL)
For bleeding: <50,000/μL (except central nervous system or retinal bleeding: <100,000/μL)

Adapted from: Kaufman RM, Djulbegovic B, Gernsheimer T, et al. Platelet transfusion: a clinical practice guideline from the AABB. *Ann Intern Med.* 2015;162:205-213.

TABLE 18-5. Indications for Plasma Transfusion
Massive transfusion protocol
Hemorrhage in liver disease
Disseminated intravascular coagulation
Multiple coagulation factor deficiency
Thrombotic thrombocytopenic purpura
Rapid reversal of warfarin effect
Prevention of bleeding if PT/PTT/INR >1.5 x normal (except for central nervous system or retinal bleeding, then >1.3 x normal)
Acute angioedema caused by C1 esterase inhibitor deficiency

generation and vascular vasomotor stability. These favorable effects decrease vascular space loss into the interstitial tissue, help maintain arterial blood pressure, and support hemostasis.[28]

Cryoprecipitate Transfusion

Cryoprecipitate is obtained when a unit of frozen plasma is thawed at 4°C (39.2°F). The resultant 10 to 15 mL of plasma contains fibrinogen, factor VIII, von Willebrand factor, and factor XIII. Each unit of cryoprecipitate contains 80 to 100 units of factor VIII activity and 150 to 200 mg of fibrinogen.[6,8,14] This is a smaller amount of fibrinogen than is contained in plasma, but it is more concentrated, so cryoprecipitate can be a better choice when volume overload is a concern. As with FFP, cryoprecipitate requires ABO compatibility but not crossmatching.

A dose of 2 to 4 units/kg is expected to increase the fibrinogen level by 60 to 100 mg/dL.[7] A fibrinogen level above 150 to 200 mg/dL is the goal of cryoprecipitate transfusion for any bleeding patient. Below this level, PT and PTT values will be elevated despite sufficient clotting factors, and perioperative and postoperative bleeding increases.[29] Cryoprecipitate transfusion is indicated for any deficient fibrinogen state such as massive transfusion, disseminated intravascular coagulation, congenital hypofibrinogenemia, or reversal of thrombolytic therapy. It is also indicated for factor XIII deficiency.[7,8]

Transfusion of cryoprecipitate is an option for factor VIII deficiency and von Willebrand disease if the respective factor concentrates are unavailable. Although it also has been given for bleeding abnormalities associated with uremia, desmopressin is the preferred treatment for this disorder.[7,8] Fibrinogen concentrates are currently approved in the United States only for the treatment of congenital fibrinogen deficiency, but their use has reduced mortality and transfusion requirements in trauma patients during an MTP.[15]

Albumin Transfusion

Albumin provides 80% of intravascular oncotic pressure. Patients with disease states associated with low albumin levels (eg, cirrhosis and nephrotic syndrome) can require albumin transfusions to maintain intravascular volume (*Table 18-6*). The protein is derived from human sources but is heat-treated and does not transmit viruses. It is available as a 5% solution, which is oncotically equivalent to normal plasma, and a 25% solution, which is hyperoncotic and can pull 3 to 4 times the volume administered from the interstitial space into the vascular space.[8]

TABLE 18-6. Indications for Albumin Transfusion[8]

Indication
Nephrotic syndrome resistant to diuretics
Volume replacement with plasmapheresis
Fluid resuscitation for sepsis or burns associated with interstitial edema
Prevention of vascular collapse after large-volume paracentesis

The typical dose is 50 to 100 mL; however, if the patient does not have adequate extravascular hydration, additional isotonic fluids should be given. After 4 hours, 50% of infused albumin is lost to the extravascular space.

PEARL

After 4 hours, 50% of infused albumin is lost to the extravascular space.

Adverse Effects of Transfusions

Complications from blood component therapy include acute immunological transfusion reactions, allergic reactions, volume overload, viral or bacterial transmission, acute lung injury, and immunomodulating effects associated with an increased risk of nosocomial infection and multiorgan failure (*Table 18-7*).[11,14,26,31,32] The risk of a transfusion-related adverse event is 10%, and the risk of it being a serious event is 0.5%.[1] Transfusion-related acute lung injury (TRALI) is the leading cause of transfusion-related morbidity and mortality.[33] The third most common cause of serious transfusion-related complications, including death, is bacterial contamination of blood products.[1]

Hemolytic transfusion reactions occur when preformed IgM against ABO antigens causes complement activation and intravascular hemolysis. Patients experience fever, chills, dyspnea, hypotension, tachycardia, and diffuse myalgias along with hemoglobinemia and hemoglobinuria. The haptoglobin level will be low, and bilirubin will be elevated. These complications most commonly are the result of patient misidentification and clerical errors.

Nonhemolytic transfusion reactions are caused by an amnestic response against non-ABO erythrocyte antigens that was not identified by crossmatch testing. Complement is not activated, but RBCs are cleared by the reticuloendothelial system 2 to 10 days later. The clinical picture is less severe than with hemolytic transfusion reactions, and there is modest elevation

TABLE 18-7. Clinical Presentation of Transfusion Reaction Types

Type	Presentation
Acute hemolytic	Fever, chills, dyspnea, tachycardia, hypotension, back/flank pain
Febrile	Fever, chills (patient not ill appearing)
Mild allergic	Urticaria, pruritus
Anaphylactic	Bronchospasm, dyspnea, angioedema, tachycardia, hypotension
TRALI	Dyspnea, decreased arterial oxygen saturation, fever, hypotension, normal/low central venous pressure
Hypervolemic	Dyspnea, headache, tachycardia, hypertension, elevated central venous pressure
Septic	Fever, chills, hypotension, tachycardia, vomiting

of bilirubin without hemoglobinemia and hemoglobinuria.[1,8] Allergic reactions are common, occurring in about 1% of all transfusions. Most are mild, consisting of pruritus and hives; frank anaphylaxis is rare.

The risk of disease transmission per unit of blood transfused is 1:2 million for HIV, 1:500,000 for hepatitis B, and 1:2 million for hepatitis C.[8,26] The risk for bacterial infection transmission (which is highest for platelets since they are stored at room temperature to keep their activity) is 1:2,000 to 3,000 platelet units. Fortunately, only 1 in 5,000 contaminated units causes sepsis.[16,34] Bacteria can be transferred if the skin preparation at the phlebotomy site was unsterile, the donor had transient bacteremia, a blood banking procedure was not sterile, or the integrity of the bag or tubing was breached. Gram-negative rods (*Serratia*, *Pseudomonas*, *Yersinia*, *Enterobacter*, and *Salmonella*) and gram-positive cocci (*Staphylococcus* and *Streptococcus*) are the most common organisms.[7]

TRALI occurs following 1 in 1,000 to 5,000 units of transfused blood products, the highest risk being associated with plasma-containing transfusions.[7,35,36] These injuries can result when the recipient has neutrophils that are already primed by a prior stimulus (eg, trauma, infection, malignancy) and adherent to the pulmonary endothelium, which are then stimulated by donor antileukocyte antibodies in the blood product.[37] The activated neutrophils cause diffuse pulmonary capillary leaks and lead to noncardiogenic pulmonary edema. Dyspnea, decreased oxygen saturation, and bilateral fluffy pulmonary infiltrates with a normal left ventricular end-diastolic pressure occur within 6 hours after transfusion. TRALI typically resolves within 72 hours but has a mortality rate as high as 20%.[38,39]

The crucial prevention of adverse effects begins with scrupulous adherence to blood bank policies to avert incompatibility reactions. Irradiation of blood products, which prevents donor leukocytes from replicating, should be ordered for patients at risk for graft-versus-host disease as follows: those with severe cellular immunodeficiency (but not AIDS), those on potent chemotherapeutic regimens, and those receiving transfusions from biological relatives. Graft-versus-host disease has no effective treatment and a 90% mortality

TABLE 18-8. Treatment of Transfusion Reactions

Reaction	Treatment
General • Fever (≥1°C increase in temperature) • Chills • Rigors • Urticaria • Dyspnea • Tachycardia • Hyper/hypotension • Chest/abdominal/back pain • Unwell feeling	Stop transfusion immediately. Rapidly assess patient. Verify compatibility of blood product with patient. Notify blood bank of possible problem. Maintain crystalloid infusion. Support respiratory function.
Mild allergic reaction (most common)	Diphenhydramine IV Acetaminophen Consider slowly restarting transfusion once patient is asymptomatic.
Anaphylaxis	Epinephrine IM/IV Albuterol nebulizer Isotonic fluids Diphenhydramine
ABO incompatibility	Isotonic fluids Diuretics to maintain urine output >100 mL/hr Bicarbonate infusion to keep urine pH above 7
TRALI	Oxygen and mechanical ventilation strategies as in acute respiratory distress syndrome
Fluid overload	Diuretics IV Oxygen Continuous positive airway pressure Slower rate for further transfusion
Bacterial infection	Culture all remaining blood products. Administer broad-spectrum antibiotics. Provide supportive care.

rate.[6-8] All blood products should be given with an isotonic noncalcium-containing solution such as normal saline to prevent hemolysis and clotting.[8] Except in cases of hemorrhagic shock, the transfusion should be started at a slow rate for the first 15 minutes while the patient is monitored closely for signs of a reaction, the severity of which primarily is determined by the volume of blood transfused.[7]

If any symptoms of a transfusion reaction emerge *(Table 18-7)*, the blood product should be immediately halted while the patient is assessed and the blood bank is notified. If the allergic reaction is mild, the patient should be treated with acetaminophen and diphenhydramine, and the transfusion can be safely continued. An anaphylactic reaction should be appropriately treated, and the patient should not be rechallenged by continuing the transfusion. The management of hemolytic transfusion reactions includes intravenous volume expansion and diuretics to maintain urine output at more than 100 mL/hr, and bicarbonate to raise the urinary pH above 7.0. The treatment of TRALI is supportive; oxygen and positive-pressure ventilation are effective, but there is no role for diuretics or steroids.[38,39]

Each blood product should be given over a maximum of 4 hours to decrease bacterial contamination.[7,8] If the patient's volume status is labile or if there is concern about congestive heart failure, each unit can be split by the blood bank and given even more slowly. Diuretics also may be administered.[24] As in MTPs, rapid transfusion can be associated with hypothermia if more than 100 mL/min of volume is given for more than 30 minutes without using a blood-warming device. Other complications of rapid transfusion include hypocalcemia due to citrate toxicity, alkalosis due to citrate conversion, and hyperkalemia due to potassium release from stored erythrocytes.[6-8] Each 1 mL of blood contains 1 mg of iron, so there are about 250 mg in a unit of packed RBCs.[7] Although this iron load may be helpful in a patient with iron deficiency, it can be deleterious to a patient who requires frequent transfusions.

Transfusions activate an inflammatory cascade and have immunomodulating effects associated with immunosuppression, increased risk of nosocomial infections, acute lung injury, and increased mortality. Intensive care patients who receive fewer units of blood products have fewer serious infections, shorter lengths of stay, and a lower mortality rate than those who receive more transfusions.[2,13,14,31]

Adjunctive Therapies

Several nonblood products may augment or replace a transfusion strategy. Recombinant activated factor VII (rFVIIa) initiates the extrinsic coagulation pathway when complexed with tissue factor at sites of injury. Currently, rFVIIa is approved by the US Food and Drug Administration (FDA) only for the treatment of hemophilia and factor VII deficiency; however, it has been used with some success in coagulopathic trauma patients and has decreased the need for massive transfusion, reduced the total amount of blood products required, and decreased the incidence of organ failure. An increase in vascular thromboembolic events in patients treated with rFVIIa has been documented. Importantly, rFVIIa does not improve outcomes in trauma or surgical patients.[9,18]

Desmopressin increases the endothelial cell release of von Willebrand factor molecules. It is FDA approved for the treatment of hemophilia A and von Willebrand disease type 1 but also can be used clinically to control uremic bleeding. Aminocaproic acid inhibits plasmin and is approved by the FDA for the enhancement of hemostasis in any hyperfibrinolytic state (eg, certain acute leukemias) or after fibrinolytic therapy.[9,18] The dose is 0.3 µg/kg administered intravenously.[28] Tranexamic acid (TXA), another antifibrinolytic, has been shown to reduce mortality in military and civilian trauma patients, particularly if administered early (<3 hours from injury but preferably within the first hour).[40] If ETIC is confirmed by hyperfibrinolysis on TEG, then TXA should be administered regardless of time since injury: it will still have benefits and appears to pose minimal risk. Additionally, the agent should be given whenever a MTP is initiated. The dose is a 1-g load followed by an infusion of 1 g over 8 hours.[15,40]

KEY POINTS

1. Risk factors that predict the need for massive transfusion include abnormal vital signs on presentation with tachycardia (heart rate >120 beats/min) and hypotension (SBP <90 mm Hg), pH <7.25, initial Hct <32%, a penetrating mechanism of trauma, and evidence of free fluid on bedside ultrasonography.[15,16,18]
2. A common initial MTP package includes 6 PRBC units (O- for women and O+ for men), 4 plasma units (AB initially but A can be safely administered), and 1 apheresis platelet unit. Cryoprecipitate can be given on an individual basis. The implementation of an MTP generally is believed to improve the speed by which blood products are available by optimizing coordination between the blood bank, laboratory services, and clinical team.[25]
3. The platelet count should be kept >50,000/µL in a patient who is actively bleeding and even higher (>100,000/µL) for microvascular bleeding involving the central nervous system or retina.[6,7]
4. If symptoms of a transfusion reaction emerge, the blood product should be immediately halted while the patient is assessed and the blood bank is notified. If the allergic reaction is mild, the patient should be treated with acetaminophen and diphenhydramine, and the transfusion may be continued. An anaphylactic reaction should be appropriately treated; the patient should not be rechallenged by continuing the transfusion.

Conclusion

As many critically ill patients remain in the emergency department for exceedingly long periods awaiting an intensive care unit bed, it is imperative that emergency physicians understand the indications for the transfusion of blood products. Equally important is the ability to recognize and manage the complications associated with this lifesaving treatment, namely allergic reactions (including anaphylaxis), hemolytic reactions, and TRALI.

REFERENCES

1. Despotis GJ, Zhang L, Lublin DM. Transfusion risks and transfusion-related pro-inflammatory responses. *Hematol Oncol Clin North Am.* 2007;21:147-161.
1. Chung, K-W, Basavaraju SV, Mu Y, et al. Declining blood collection and utilization in the United States. *Transfusion.* 2016;doi: 10.1111/trf.13644. [Epub ahead of print]
2. Brandt MM, Rubinfeld I, Jordan J, et al. Transfusion insurgency: practice change through education and evidence-based recommendations. *Am J Surg.* 2009;197:279-283.
3. Peterson SR, Weinberg JA. Transfusions, autotransfusions, and blood substitutes. In: Feliciano DV, Mattox KL, Moore EE, eds. *Trauma.* 6th ed. New York, NY: McGraw-Hill; 2008:235-242.
4. American Association of Blood Banks. National Blood Bank Data Resource Center. Available at: www.aabb.org. Accessed on July 21, 2015.
5. Hebert PC, Tinmouth A. Anemia and red blood cell transfusion in critically ill patients. In: Fink MP, ed. *Textbook of Critical Care.* 5th ed. Philadelphia, PA: Elsevier Saunders; 2005:1421-1426.
6. Isbister JP. Blood component therapy. In: Fink MP, ed. *Textbook of Critical Care.* 5th ed. Philadelphia, PA: Elsevier Saunders; 2005:1427-1435.
7. Cushing MM, Ness PM. Blood cell components. In: Hoffman R, ed. *Hematology: Basic Principles and Practice.* 5th ed. Philadelphia, PA: Churchill Livingstone; 2008:146-154.
8. McPherson M, Pincus P. Transfusion administration. In: Henry S, ed. *Clinical Diagnosis and Management by Laboratory Methods.* 21st ed. Philadelphia, PA: W.B. Saunders; 2006:486-499.
9. Perkins JG, Cap AP, Weiss BM, et al. Massive transfusion and nonsurgical hemostatic agents. *Crit Care Med.* 2008;36:S325-S339.
10. Napolitano LM, Corwin HL. Efficacy of red blood cell transfusion in the critically ill. *Crit Care Clin.* 2004;20:255-268.
11. Napolitano LM, Kurek S, Luchette FA, et al. Clinical practice guideline: red blood cell transfusion in adult trauma and critical care. *Crit Care Med.* 2009;37:3124-3139.
12. Isbister JP. Decision making in perioperative transfusion. *Transfus Apheresis Sci.* 2002;27:19-28.
13. Aronson D, Dann EJ, Bonstein L, et al. Impact of red blood cell transfusion on clinical outcomes in patients with acute myocardial infarction. *Am J Cardiol.* 2008;102:115-119.
14. Marik PE, Corwin HL. Efficacy of red blood cell transfusion in the critically ill: a systematic review of the literature. *Crit Care Med.* 2008;36:1654-1667.
15. Pham HP, Shaz BH. Update on massive transfusion. *Br J Anaesthe.* 2013;111(S1):71-82.
16. Johansson PI, Sørensen AM, Larsen CF, et al. Low hemorrhage-related mortality in trauma patients in a Level I trauma center employing transfusion packages and early thromboelastography-directed hemostatic resuscitation with plasma and platelets. *Transfusion.* 2013;53:3088-3099.
17. Sorenson B, Fries D. Emerging treatment strategies for trauma-induced coagulopathy. *Br J Surg.* 2012;99(S1):40-50.
18. Sihler KC, Napolitano LM. Massive transfusion: new insights. *Chest.* 2009;136:1654-1667.
19. Kashuk JL, Moore EE, Sawyer M, et al. Primary fibrinolysis is integral in the pathogenesis of the acute coagulopathy of trauma. *Ann Surg.* 2010;252:434-442.
20. Ives C, Inaba K, Branco BC, et al. Hyperfibrinolysis elicited via thromboelastography predicts mortality in trauma. *J Am Coll Surg.* 2012;215:496-502.
21. Rugeri L, Levrat A, David JS, et al. Diagnosis of early coagulation abnormalities in trauma patients by rotation thrombelastography. *J Thromb Haemost.* 2007;5:289-295.
22. Cotton BA, Faz G, Hatch QM, et al. Rapid thromboelastography delivers real-time results that predict transfusion within 1 hour of admission. *J Trauma.* 2011;2:407-414.
23. Teodoro de Luz L, Nascimento B, Rizoli S. Thromboelastography (TEG): practical considerations on its clinical use in trauma resuscitation. *Scan J Trauma Resusc Emerg Med.* 2013;21:29-37.
24. Bollinger D, Seeberger MD, Tanaka KA. Principles and practice of thromboelastography in clinical coagulation management and transfusion practice. *Transfusion Med Rev.* 2012;26:1-13.
25. del Junco DJ, Holcomb JB, Fox EE, et al. Resuscitate early with plasma and platelets or balance blood products gradually: PROMMTT study. *J Trauma Acute Care Surg.* 2013;75:S24-S30.
26. Slichter SJ. Platelet transfusion therapy. *Hematol Oncol Clin North Am.* 2007;21:697-729.
27. Kaufman RM, Djulbegovic B, Gernsheimer T, et al. Platelet transfusion: a clinical practice guideline from the AABB. *Ann Intern Med.* 2015;162:205-213.
28. Seghatchian J, Samama MM. Massive transfusion: an overview of the main characteristics and potential risks associated with substances used for correction of a coagulopathy. *Transfus Aphes Sci.* 2012;47:235-243.
29. Fries D. The early use of fibrinogen, prothrombin complex concentrate, and recombinant-activated factor VIIa in massive bleeding. *Transfusion.* 2013;53:91S-95S.
30. Frontera JA, Gordon E, Zach V, et al. Reversal of coagulopathy using prothrombin complex concentrates is associated with improved outcome compared to fresh frozen plasma in warfarin-associated intracranial hemorrhage. *Neurocrit Care.* 2014;21:397-406.
31. Wahl WL, Hemmila MR, Maggio PM, Arbabi S. Restrictive red blood cell transfusion: not just for the stable intensive care unit patient. *Am J Surg.* 2008;195:803-806.
32. Beale E, Zhu J, Chan L, et al. Blood transfusion in critically injured patients: a prospective study. *Injury.* 2006;37:455-465.
33. Chaiwat O, Lang JD, Vavilala M, et al. Early packed red blood cell transfusion and acute respiratory distress syndrome after trauma. *Anesthesiology.* 2009;110:351-360.
34. MacLennan S, Williamson LM. Risks of fresh frozen plasma and platelets. *J Trauma.* 2006;60:S46-S50.
35. Marik PE, Corwin HC. Acute lung injury following blood transfusion: expanding the definition. *Crit Care Med.* 2008;36:3080-3084.
36. Benson AB, Moss M. Trauma and acute respiratory distress syndrome: weighing the risks and benefits of blood transfusions. *Anesthesiology.* 2009;110:216-217.
37. Silliman CC. The two-event model of transfusion-related acute lung injury. *Crit Care Med.* 2006;34:S124-S131.
38. Skeate RC, Eastlund T. Distinguishing between transfusion related acute lung injury and transfusion associated circulatory overload. *Curr Opin Hematol.* 2007;14:682-687.
39. Triulzi DJ. Transfusion-related acute lung injury: current concepts for the clinician. *Anesth Analg.* 2009;108:770-776.
40. The CRASH-2 collaborators. The effects of tranexamic acid on death, vascular occlusive events, and blood transfusion in trauma patients with significant haemorrhage: a randomized placebo-controlled trial. *Lancet.* 2010;376:23-32.

Intracerebral Hemorrhage

19

IN THIS CHAPTER

- Airway management and mechanical ventilation
- Blood pressure control
- Hemostatic therapy
- Management of increased intracranial pressure
- Surgical therapy

Dale S. Birenbaum and Justin D. Britton

Spontaneous intracerebral hemorrhage (ICH) is a devastating disease with high rates of death and disability despite continued advances in medical treatment. Chronic hypertension, cerebral amyloid angiopathy, and the use of anticoagulants are important factors associated with the occurrence of ICH. These patients generally present with symptoms that include headache, vomiting, altered mental status, and neurological deficits. The disorder accounts for approximately 10% to 15% of all cerebral vascular accidents (CVAs) and has a 30-day mortality rate as high as 50%.[1,2] Importantly, half of all deaths occur within the first 48 hours.[1-5]

Patient outcomes ultimately depend on several factors such as age, initial Glasgow Coma Scale (GCS) score, and the cause, location, and size of the hemorrhage. The presence of intraventricular hemorrhage (IVH), hematoma expansion, and hydrocephalus substantially increases morbidity and mortality. In fact, patients with an ICH volume above 60 mL and an initial GCS score of less than 8 have a 30-day mortality rate of 91%, whereas patients with an initial hematoma volume less than 30 mL and an initial GCS score greater than 9 have a 30-day mortality rate of 19%.[1-5] Factors closely related to mortality are listed in Table 19-1.

Pathophysiology

The initial hemorrhage causes an elevation of the local hydrostatic pressure and direct trauma to the brain tissue. When critical areas of the brain are affected, even a small amount of bleeding can have a dramatic effect. Trauma to the brainstem and reticular activating system can lead to apnea and sudden cardiovascular collapse. As the hematoma retracts, serum leaks out of the capillaries and causes perihematomal edema. Blood released from the capillaries activates the coagulation cascade, and thrombin is released. The lysis of red blood cells releases hemoglobin and other neurotoxic inflammatory mediators and contributes to secondary brain injury.

Larger hemorrhages can cause an external mass effect by placing pressure on the third or fourth ventricle, causing obstruction and leading to dilation of the lateral ventricles and frontal horns *(Figure 19-1)*. Hydrocephalus also can occur with ICH complicated by IVH *(Figure 19-2)*.

Most of the extravasation of contrast in the angiogram of a patient with an ICH is seen within the first 3 to 6 hours after the onset of ictus.[2] Since the overall volume of the cranial vault cannot change, an increase in volume in one of its components (eg, the brain parenchyma, cerebrospinal fluid [CSF], and blood) leads to the displacement of other structures or an increase in intracranial pressure (ICP).[6-8] The incompressibility of the intracranial compartment is known as the Monro-Kellie doctrine: any increase in volume of one of the components must be compensated by a decrease in volume of another.[6-8] The rise in the ICP that occurs later than 6 hours after ictus is thought to be caused by edema, hydrocephalus, or continued hemorrhage. Within the hemotoma, the actual focus of contrast extravasation, called the "spot sign" when seen on computed tomography angiography, is predictive of further hemorrhagic enlargement. Stroke experts are awaiting the results of ongoing trials designed to identify patients with spot signs who appear to be at greatest risk for hemorrhagic enlargement and might benefit most from early aggressive hemostatic therapy *(Figure 19-3)*.[9]

Strategies used to reduce hemorrhagic enlargement and edema are listed in Table 19-2.

TABLE 19-1. Intracerebral Hemorrhage Score

	Component	Score
GCS score	3–4	2
	5–12	1
	13–15	0
Intracerebral hemorrhage volume (mL)	≥30	1
	<30	0
Intraventricular extension of intracerebral hemorrhage	Yes	1
	No	0
Infratentorial origin of intracerebral hemorrhage	Yes	1
	No	0
Age (years)	≥80	1
	<80	0

Total Score and 30-Day Mortality
0 = 0%
1 = 13%
2 = 26%
3 = 72%
4 = 97%
5 ≤ 100%

From: Hemphill JC 3rd, Bonovich DC, Besmertis L, Manley GT, Johnston SC. The ICH score: a simple, reliable grading scale for intracerebral hemorrhage. *Stroke*. 2001 Apr;32(4):891-7.

FIGURE 19-1. Hypertensive Intraparenchymal Hematoma with Subfalcine Herniation

Nonenhanced axial computed tomography (CT) demonstrates a large right basal ganglionic hypertensive bleed (*) with mass effect and midline shift or a subfalcine herniation to the left *(black arrows)*. The frontal horns are part of the lateral ventricles. The right frontal horn is compressed so severely that it is almost completely obliterated. Dilation of the left frontal horn is the result of obstructive hydrocephalus, a consequence of compression of the third ventricle. Blood has also accumulated in the lateral ventricles *(white arrows)*.

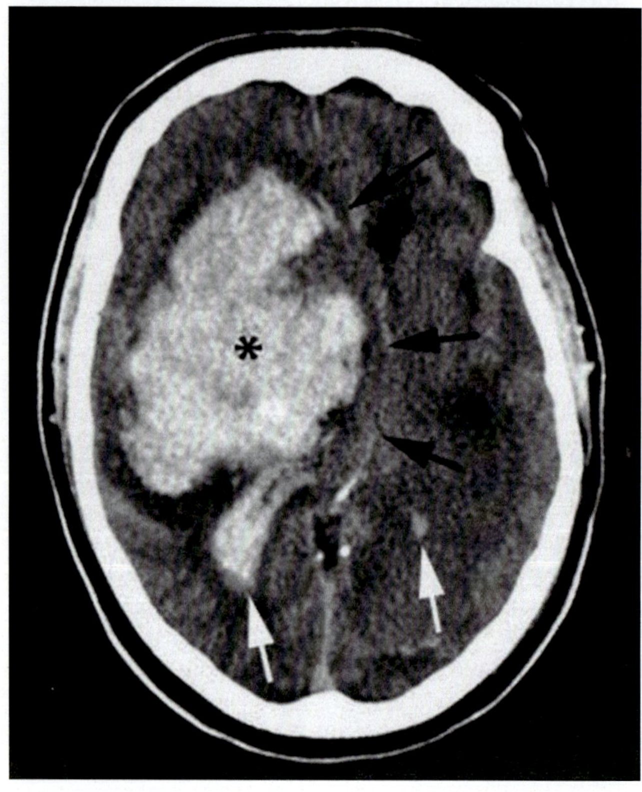

PEARLS

- ✓ After the initial ictus, hematoma enlargement is common in patients with ICH and dramatically increases morbidity and mortality rates.[2]
- ✓ If increasing ICP is left untreated, herniation can occur.

TABLE 19-2. Treatment Strategies to Reduce Hemorrhagic Enlargement and Edema

Blood pressure reduction
Hemostatic therapy
Clot drainage
Decreasing intracranial pressure
Euvolemic resuscitation

TABLE 19-3. Essentials of Acute ICH Management

Airway assessment
Early intubation and mechanical ventilation
Hemostatic therapy
Blood pressure control
ICP monitoring
Supportive care (eg, managing hyperglycemia, hyperthermia, and seizures)

Acute Management

Rapid assessment, stabilization, and anticipation of the next steps in management are all essential to the emergency department evaluation of patients with ICH *(Table 19-3)*. In certain circumstances, rapid consultation with a neurosurgeon

FIGURE 19-2. Massive ICH and IVH

Axial nonenhanced CT scan demonstrates a large bright or hyperattenuating dense hemorrhage throughout the left basal ganglia, extending intraventricularly. Clotted blood blocks the third ventricle, leading to marked hydrocephalus.

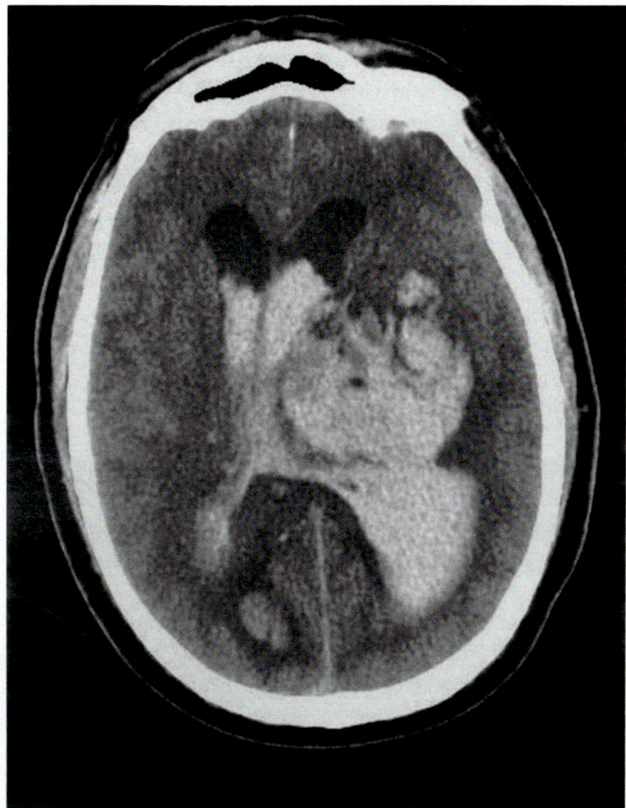

FIGURE 19-3. Spot Sign with ICH

Axial CT shows a large right-sided intracerebral hemorrhage with spot sign *(arrows)*.

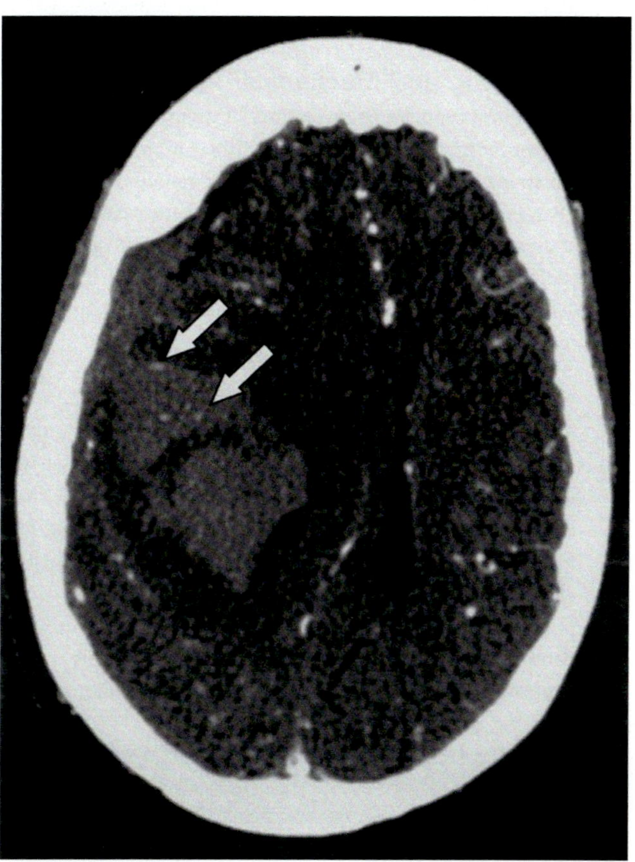

and transfer to an appropriate facility offer the best chance for survival.[3-5] A careful history and physical examination must be performed. Laboratory studies should include a complete blood count, prothrombin and partial thromboplastin time measurements, liver and renal function tests, serum glucose measurements, and a toxicology screen.[2-4] Additional testing includes electrocardiography and chest radiography.

Airway Assessment

Upon arrival, the patient should receive a rapid airway evaluation and be assessed for the potential loss of protective airway reflexes. Complications such as difficulty handling secretions or swallowing, hyperventilation, and hypoventilation warrant immediate intubation. A rapid neurological examination should be performed to gauge responsiveness to vocal or painful stimuli.

It is important to keep the systolic blood pressure well controlled when intubating a patient with an ICH. Etomidate is a good induction agent because it has a rapid onset of action, has minimal hemodynamic effects, and allows a quick recovery. Dexmedetomidine is an alternative induction agent that is hemodynamically stable and does not carry the risk of adrenal suppression.[8]

Neuromuscular-blocking drugs can facilitate airway control and prevent complications during intubation. Because depolarizing neuromuscular blockade can cause muscle contractions and theoretically increase ICP, a nondepolarizing agent such as rocuronium, vecuronium, or cisatracurium is preferred for patients with ICH.[8,10]

Maintaining adequate analgesia and sedation will prevent the patient from hyperventilating, facilitate imaging, and allow continuation of the evaluation, especially if long-acting neuromuscular-blocking agents have been administered.

Propofol, which is an ideal agent for continued sedation, has a rapid onset of action and is easy to titrate and reverse, thereby enabling evaluation of the patient's neurological status. It is essential to carefully titrate propofol to avoid its major side effect, hypotension. Continued sedation with this agent requires attentive monitoring for the signs of propofol infusion syndrome: severe metabolic acidosis, rhabdomyolysis, hyperkalemia, and renal failure along with hypertriglyceridemia and arrhythmias.[8,10] The infusion must be stopped if any signs or symptoms of this complication appear. Simple measures such as elevating the head of the bed and fever control also can be used to reduce ICP.

PEARLS

- ✓ Elevate the head of the bed to 30° to improve venous return and aid in the reduction of ICP.
- ✓ Aggressively treat fever.

Breathing and Mechanical Ventilation

Typical ventilator strategies may be inappropriate for ICH patients because they induce hypercarbia and increase PEEP, which may exacerbate ICP via decreased venous outflow. Therefore, implementation of a neuroprotective ventilatory strategy is important to maintain normocarbia and a target partial pressure of carbon dioxide ($PaCO_2$) between 35 and 40 mm Hg.[3-5,8,10] Initial settings for mechanical ventilation are presented in Table 19-4.

Blood Pressure Control

Blood pressure control remains a critical component in the management of patients with ICH. Unlike ischemic stroke, in which medical complications are the most common cause of death, spontaneous ICH must be managed by identifying the location and extent of the initial bleeding and rapidly initiating efforts to prevent hematoma enlargement.

Blood pressure control and its management are critical determinants of outcome, but the target range remains controversial. It also is unclear if elevations in blood pressure are inciting events for ICH or the body's way of attempting to stabilize cerebral perfusion pressure (CPP). The goal of blood pressure management is to maintain adequate CPP and limit hematoma expansion. The mean arterial pressure (MAP) minus the ICP is equal to the CPP. MAP is calculated as the diastolic blood pressure plus one-third of the difference between the systolic and diastolic blood pressures. For example, a blood pressure of 120/80 mm Hg indicates a MAP of 93.3 (80 + 13.3). The goal for CPP is between 50 and 70 mm Hg.[3-5,8,10]

Cerebral blood flow normally is maintained at a relatively constant level through the autoregulation of cerebrovascular resistance (CVR). This process can become dysfunctional in ICH, so the brain becomes exquisitely sensitive to even minor changes in CPP. An acute reduction in blood pressure can decrease CPP, resulting in ischemia. Conversely, excessive elevations in the blood pressure increase the CPP and can lead to hematoma expansion and injury. IVH can cause a rise in ICP, and therefore diminish the CPP. All treatment efforts are aimed at maintaining this delicate balance and homeostasis.

TABLE 19-4. Initial Mechanical Ventilatory Settings[3,8,10]

Mode: assist control
Tidal volume: 6 mL/kg of ideal body weight
Respiratory rate: 18 to 22 breaths/min
Fio_2: 100%
PEEP: 5–7 cm H_2O

TABLE 19-5. Recommendations for Treating Elevated Blood Pressure in Patients with Spontaneous ICH

1. For ICH patients with SBP between 150 and 220 mm Hg and without contraindication to acute BP treatment, acute lowering of SBP to 140 mm Hg is safe *(Class I; Level of Evidence A)* and can be effective for improving functional outcome *(Class IIa; Level of Evidence B)*. (Revised from the previous guideline).
2. For ICH patients with SBP >220 mm Hg, it may be reasonable to consider aggressive reduction of BP with a continuous intravenous infusion and frequent BP monitoring *(Class IIb; Level of Evidence C)*. (New recommendation).

Recommendations from: Hemphill JC, Greenberg SM, Anderson CS, et al. Guidelines for the Management of Spontaneous Intracerebral Hemorrhage. *Stroke.* 2015;46(7):2032-2060.

PEARL

A CPP between 50 and 70 mm Hg appears to be neuroprotective.

Blood pressure should be adjusted in an effort to maintain adequate CPP *(Tables 19-5* and *19-6)*. The initial reduction of blood pressure should be no more than 15% in the first hour because many patients have acclimated to higher levels and rapid reductions may worsen ischemia.[3-5,8,10] Systolic blood pressures between 150 and 220 can be reasonably and safely lowered to 180 mm Hg, and perhaps as low as 140 mm Hg.[11,12] Systolic blood pressures greater than 220 should be aggressively reduced with continuous intravenous infusions and close monitoring. Clinicians can reduce the risk of hematoma expansion and improve outcomes by avoiding overshoots and fluctuations in pressure. It is important to remember that no clinical guideline recommends allowing the blood pressure to remain extremely elevated without treatment.[13,14]

Isotonic fluids such as normal saline should be used in the initial resuscitation of patients with ICH. They offer the advantage of maintaining homeostasis by exerting little osmotic effect on surrounding tissues.[8,10,13] Dextrose-containing solutions (D5W) and half normal saline introduce free water into the intravascular space, leading to increased capillary leakage and worsening perihematomal edema. These solutions also can contribute to hyperglycemia, which may be detrimental to stroke patients.[4,8,10,13] The goal of fluid resuscitation should be to keep the patient euvolemic (not severely fluid restricted) and normal to hyperosmolar. Adequate resuscitation can be assessed by maintaining a urine output of 0.5 to 1 mL/kg/hr.

Hemostatic Therapy

When a patient who is taking anticoagulant medication, who has a coagulopathy, or who has received tissue plasminogen activator (tPA) presents with an ICH, it is critical to provide

TABLE 19-6. Blood Pressure Medications Used in ICH

Agent	Initial	Infusion
Clevidipine	N/A	1 mg/hr, then double rate every 90 seconds until BP goal achieved (maximum 21 mg/hr)
Esmolol	250 mcg/kg IV push loading dose	25–300 mcg/kg/min
Hydralazine	5–20 mg IV push every 30 min	1.5–5 mcg/kg/min
Labetalol	5–20 mg every 15 min	2 mg/min (maximum 300 mg/day)
Nicardipine	N/A	5–15 mg/hr

[a]Because of the risk of precipitous blood pressure lowering, the first dose of enalapril should be 0.625 mg.

Recommendations from: Andrews CM, Jauch EC, Hemphill JC, et al. Emergency Neurological Life Support: Intracerebral Hemorrhage. *Neurocritical Care.* 2012;17(S1):37-46.

aggressive hemostatic therapy to prevent hematoma enlargement.[15] Importantly, therapy should not be delayed while awaiting the results of coagulation tests. Anticoagulant-related ICH accounts for 9% to 11% of total ICH.[16] An elevated international normalized ratio (INR) places the patient at risk for significant hematoma enlargement and death. The risk of ICH nearly doubles for each 0.5-point increase in the INR above 4.5. Patients who develop this complication while taking warfarin should receive vitamin K (5–10 mg via slow IV infusion over 10 minutes) and therapy to replace vitamin K-dependent factors.[4]

These patients also should receive either fresh frozen plasma (FFP, 4-6 units) or prothrombin complex concentrate (PCC). The American College of Chest Physicians recommends using PCC rather than FFP for the rapid reversal of vitamin-K antagonists in life-threatening bleeding.[17] PCC demonstrates a faster reversal of elevations in INR than vitamin K and FFP. Four-factor PCC contains therapeutic levels of factors II, VII, IX, and X. PCC, which also decreases the incidence of hematoma expansion, offers a therapeutic advantage over FFP because it contains more concentrated factors in smaller volumes and does not have to be blood-type specific or thawed.[18]

A number of new direct oral anticoagulants (DOACs) have come to the market since warfarin and include the Xa inhibitors rivaroxaban (Xarelto) and abixiban (Eliquis) and the direct thrombin inhibitor dabigatran (Pradaxa). These newer agents are popular because of their rapid time to peak action and wide therapeutic window, which obviate the need for frequent therapeutic monitoring.[19] The DOACs directly antagonize the action of normal levels of circulating clotting factors; therefore, the traditional agents used to reverse vitamin K-dependent factors are ineffective in reversing the anticoagulants. While costly, 4-factor PCC can be considered for ICH patients who have been taking rivaroxaban or apixiaban. Dabigatran is a direct thrombin inhibitor that works distal to the other DOACs and is less protein bound. In 2015 the FDA approved idarucizumab (Praxbind), a humanized monoclonal antibody that binds to and reverses the effects of dabigatran. In patients with life-threatening intracerebral hemorrhage, the drug can be given as a 5-mg bolus or infusion *(Table 19-7)*.[19]

For patients who have been given intravenous tPA for ischemic stroke, the risk of ICH is between 3% and 9%. Interestingly, this complication occurs in 0.5% to 0.6% of those treated with thrombolytic agents for other acute arterial and venous occlusions, with higher rates of hemorrhage in the elderly.[2-4] Patients with ICH secondary to thrombolytic therapy should receive cryoprecipitate and platelet transfusions.

Administer protamine sulfate (1 mg/100 units of heparin) to patients in whom ICH develops while they are receiving heparin therapy. Protamine sulfate is given by slow intravenous injection, not to exceed 5 mg/min, with a total dose not to exceed 50 mg. The dose should be adjusted down from the last time heparin was given. Importantly, protamine sulfate can cause hypotension, nausea, vomiting, and anaphylaxis. Any reversal should be

TABLE 19-7. Oral Anticoagulants and Reversal Strategies

Agent	Mechanism	Reversal Strategies
Warfarin	Vitamin K antagonist	Vitamin K (5-10 mg IV) ***PLUS*** FFP (4-6 units) or 4-factor PCC (50 IU/kg)
Dabigatran	Direct thrombin inhibitor	Idarucizumab (5 mg IV) Hemodialysis Possibly PCC (50 IU/kg) (no definite data)
Rivaroxaban **Apixaban**	Factor Xa inhibitor	Activated charcoal (if ingestion <2 hrs) 4-factor PCC (50 IU/kg)

Adapted from Levine M, Goldstein JN. Emergency reversal of anticoagulation: novel agents. *Curr Neurol Neurosci Rep.* 2014; 14 (8); 471.

evaluated with standard coagulation studies performed 30 minutes after infusions, with the target being the normalization of laboratory markers.

ICP Monitoring and Treatment

Increased ICP may directly result from the hematoma or secondarily from the surrounding edema. Patient management begins with elevation of the head of the bed, fluid resuscitation, and sedation and analgesia.[4,5] Further treatment of elevated ICP in the setting of ICH is extrapolated from data on patients with traumatic brain injury and consists of efforts to maintain a normal ICP while retaining adequate CPP.[4,5,8,10] Normal ICP is less than 10 mm Hg; elevated ICP is defined as more than 20 mm Hg.

The Lund protocol assumes disruption of the blood-brain barrier and recommends manipulations to decrease the hydrostatic forces and increase the osmotic forces that favor the maintenance of fluid within the vascular compartment to reduce the ICP. Mannitol and hypertonic saline are two osmotic agents used to manage increased ICP *(Table 19-8)*. Hypertonic saline is increasingly being used in various settings as an alternative to mannitol for the treatment of cerebral edema. Theoretically, hypertonic saline is advantageous over mannitol because the blood-brain barrier is less permeable and it might be a more effective osmotic agent. It is also a volume expander that does not appear to have any nephrotoxicity. It is administered as boluses of 3% to 23% every 3 to 4 hours or as a continuous infusion. The goal is to maintain a serum sodium concentration of 145 to 155 mmol/L.[10]

Another approach to treating increased ICP is CPP-guided therapy, which focuses on augmenting blood pressure to achieve a CPP between 50 and 70 mmHg. Although this therapy can help minimize reflex vasodilation and increase blood flow, the risk of cerebral ischemia and hypoxia remains. There is some concern that elevating blood pressure to maintain CPP can exacerbate intracranial hypertension.[4,8]

For the patient who is rapidly deteriorating, hyperventilation may be concurrently induced with osmolar therapy and neuromuscular blockade. In these cases, the target $PaCO_2$ is 30 to 35 mm Hg.[3,5,8,10] Hyperventilation works through vasoconstriction in the cerebral vasculature, resulting in decreasing cerebral blood volume.[20] The effects of hyperventilation last 24 hours, so the approach is reserved for patients with signs of herniation and for situations in which the ICP needs to be optimized on the way to definitive therapy. Adequate sedation must continue. It is critical to work closely with a neurosurgeon, who might place an intracranial monitoring device to directly measure the ICP *(Table 19-9)*.

TABLE 19-8. Mannitol Therapy for Increased ICP

Initial dose: 1–1.5 g/kg of a 20% solution
Infusion: 0.25–0.5 g/kg every 6 hours
Goal: maintain serum osmolarity of 300–320 mOsm/kg

PEARL

Hyperventilation can be used in the event of active deterioration when the patient is on the way to a definitive surgical intervention.

Direct monitoring allows the accurate measurement of ICP and assessment of the effects of therapy. Most interventions that reduce ICP are effective for only a limited time. An important early goal in the management of a presumed elevated ICP is the placement of a monitoring device.[2-5,8,10]

Drainage of cerebrospinal fluid (CSF) is an effective method of lowering the ICP, particularly in the setting of hydrocephalus. Ventriculostomy is typically performed by a neurosurgeon; the decision to insert an intraventricular catheter must be made by an experienced neurosurgical team that can monitor the device and augment treatment as necessary.

Some devices directly measure ICP (eg, a subarachnoid or subdural bolt, subdural catheter, or intraparenchymal sensor) and are placed into the brain tissue. These devices use microtransducers and fiberoptic transducers, which are easier to insert than standard ventriculostomy catheters. However, they are less accurate for monitoring ICP because they cannot be reset to zero.[2]

PEARL

The decision to operate is based on the patient's clinical presentation and functional anatomy; neurological deficits, GCS score, age, and CT images that demonstrate midline shift and hydrocephalus also should be considered.[2-4,19]

Surgical Intervention

Several factors aid the neurosurgeon in deciding when to operate on a patient with an ICH *(Table 19-10)*. Craniotomy is typically performed when there are signs of increased ICP, such as mass effect or midline shift and the absence of basal cisterns on the CT scan. The patient's age and level of function prior to the event must also be considered.[2-5] Young patients and those

TABLE 19-9. Conditions Warranting ICP Monitoring

Clinical deterioration
Process merits aggressive medical care
Unilateral or bilateral posturing
SBP <90 mm Hg
High risk for increased ICP
Comatose and GCS score <8
Evidence of ICP on CT scan: • Mass lesion • Midline shift • Effacement of the basilar cisterns

functioning at higher levels tend to have better outcomes.

While open craniotomy and drainage by direct visualization remains the gold standard for the evacuation of hematomas, there are other surgical techniques that can be used successfully. A burr hole also can be made in the skull, allowing needle aspiration of the hematoma and insertion of a 3- to 4-mm microsilicone catheter. Because the consistency of each clot is unpredictable, it can be difficult to aspirate blood through a catheter without direct visualization.

Stereotactic surgery is an organized approach in three dimensions. In the past, the procedure was done with a frame; newer techniques are frameless. A special CT or MRI scan is used to perform a computational analysis with a set of markers or fiducials affixed to the skull or scalp. The technique provides a detailed set of coordinates targeting precise sites in the brain that require drainage.[2,8,10] Stereotactic aspiration also has been combined with fibrinolysis and mechanical assist devices such as the Archimedes screw to aid in clot removal. The neuroendoscopic approach uses direct visualization and ultrasound guidance with a dual-channel drain. The hematoma cavity is rinsed with artificial CSF through a second catheter, and hemostasis can be obtained through the use of laser devices.[2,8,10]

There is no general agreement on the best time and indications for surgery in patients with supratentorial ICH. However, early surgical intervention (≤30 hours) offers no benefit over conservative management in patients with spontaneous, nontraumatic supratentorial ICH.[21]

When the ICH is lobar and large and extends into the ventricles, mortality rates approach 80% to 90%.[2,21,22] Figure 19-4 represents a large left-sided intracerebral intraparenchymal hemorrhage in a 70-year-old man who was not taking anticoagulants and who presented obtunded (paralyzed and deeply comatose) as a result of a large bleed in the dominant hemisphere, with midline shift. Despite the fact that the lesion was operatively approachable, it resided near eloquent (essential) regions of the brain. The neurosurgeon and family chose initial conservative management followed by admission and observation; unfortunately, the patient died.

For contained deeper thalamic and putamen intracerebral intraparenchymal hemorrhage, mortality rates are significantly lower (20%–40%).[2] Because these lesions are difficult to reach by standard craniotomy, less invasive methods to evacuate clots and monitor ICP are being explored. Two new alternatives to standard craniotomy are stereotactic catheter placement with CSF drainage and monitoring along with microsurgery and endoscopic clot evacuation. Less aggressive surgical techniques appear to cause fewer insults to eloquent brain while still allowing blood drainage and monitoring of ICP.

TABLE 19-10. Indications for Surgical Intervention[2,3,5,8,10,21,22]

Cerebellar hemorrhage >3 cm
Cerebellar hemorrhage with hydrocephalus
Clinically deteriorating status with signs of increased ICP
Lobar hemorrhages within 1 cm of the cranium

FIGURE 19-4. Large Intraparenchymal Intracerebral Hemorrhage

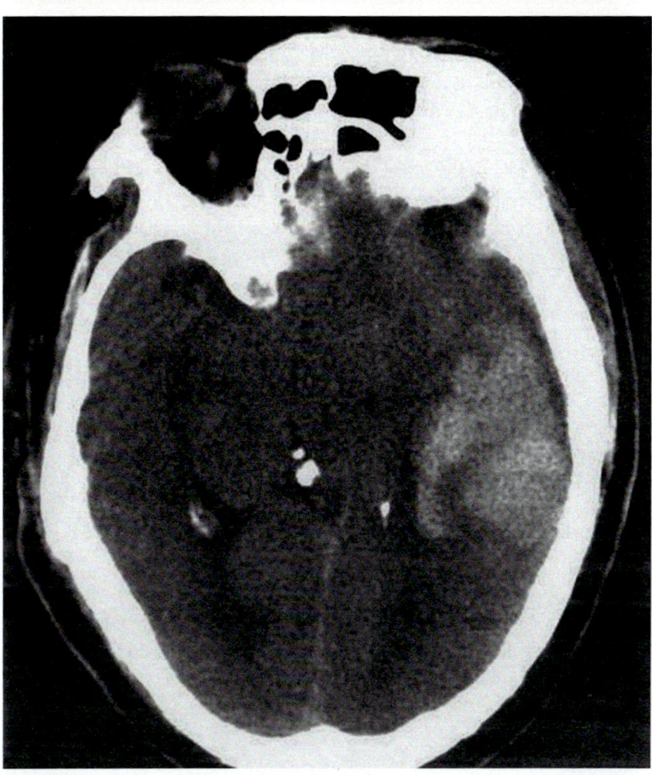

Subcortical lobar ICHs that are located within 1 to 2 cm of the brain's surface and are smaller than 2 to 3 cm produce milder deficits, have the best prognosis, and are survived by 90% of patients.[2] These lesions are easily accessible via standard craniotomy *(Figure 19-5)*.[23]

The indications for surgery in supratentorial and infratentorial cerebral hemorrhage are different. Cerebellar hemorrhages larger than 3 cm that cause brainstem compression or hydrocephalus are almost universally fatal without surgical intervention. Emergent evacuation of the hemorrhage provides the only chance of survival; clinical outcomes depend on prompt access to a qualified and experienced neurosurgeon *(Figure 19-6)*. Patients with smaller cerebellar hemorrhages without brainstem compression can be managed medically and do reasonably well.

Newer techniques are beginning to shape the management of ICH. The use of intraventricular thrombolytics has improved outcomes for hemorrhagic stroke patients who have intraventricular bleeding and hydrocephalus.[24] Small doses of thrombolytics are directly injected into the ventricles, and clotted blood in the ventricles is drained through a ventriculostomy, reducing hydrocephalus and ICP.

Another intervention involves directly injecting tPA into the

FIGURE 19-5. Moderate Subcortical Intracerebral Hemorrhagic Stroke

This moderately sized, right-sided intracerebral hemorrhagic stroke (*) occurred in a 40-year-old man who was awake but confused; there was no midline shift, no intraventricular extension, no hydrocephalus, and no clinical weakness. This bleed in the easily accessible frontal area of the brain in an awake patient was evacuated and treated by standard craniotomy without difficulty by the neurosurgeon.

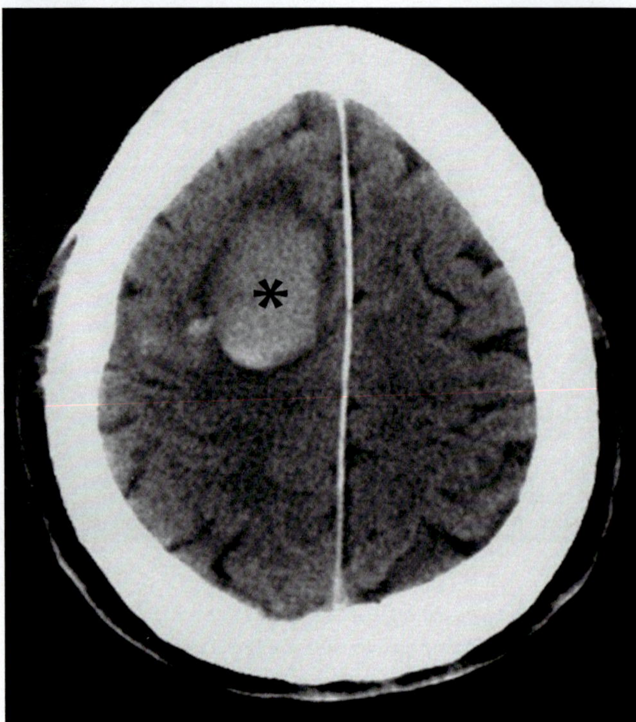

FIGURE 19-6. Cerebellar/Infratentorial Bleed in a Child

Prognosis will be related to timely access to an operating room and an experienced neurosurgeon. Hematoma* has extended extraaxially *(arrow)* and into fourth ventricle *(arrowhead).*

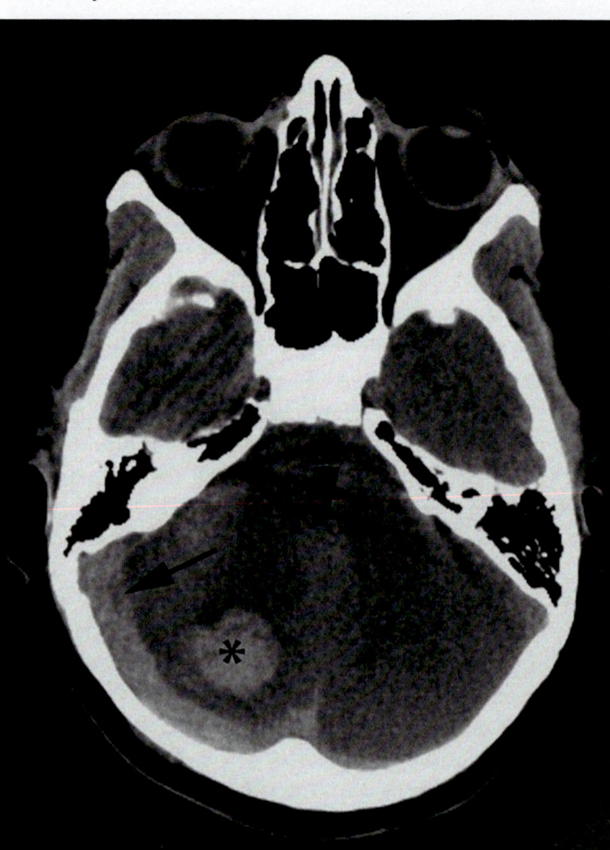

clot using minimally invasive surgery. With this method, which appears to reduce the risk of perihematoma edema, the clot undergoes lysis and then can be removed quickly and safely.[25,26] It is important to note that successful clot removal is intimately related to the expert placement and positioning of the catheter.

Supportive Care

Most if not all patients with ICH are critically ill upon arrival and should be transferred to an intensive care unit, where they can be managed by physicians trained in neurocritical care.[7] Patients who are hyperglycemic upon arrival have worse outcomes than those who aren't, regardless of their diabetic status.[27] Declining glucose levels decrease the risk of hematoma expansion; early glucose control may improve outcomes. Although no specific target range has been established, glucose levels should be kept below 180 mg/dL and hypoglycemia should be avoided.[4,27]

Fever, a common complication of ICH, escalates metabolic demand in the brain and increases cerebral blood flow and volume in the cranial vault, further elevating ICP. Aggressive fever control with acetaminophen and mechanical cooling can reduce the risk of mortality and improve outcomes.[27]

Patients with lobar ICH are at an increased risk of seizures, especially within the first 72 hours. The effect of this complication on outcomes is unclear, but those with clinically significant seizures should be treated with anticonvulsants. The prophylactic administration of antiepileptic medications generally is not recommended for patients with ICH, however, and has been linked to worse outcomes.[27]

ICH also is associated with Cushing (stress) ulcers and gastrointestinal bleeds; prophylactic treatment with an H2 blocker or proton pump inhibitor should be initiated in these patients.

Conclusion

The effective management of ICH in the emergency department relies on rapid patient assessment and stabilization. The emergency physician should consider several therapeutic strategies in such scenarios and consult with neurology, neurosurgery, and interventional radiology teams.

KEY POINTS

1. Maintain vigilance for the need to intubate patients with ICH, who are at high risk for neurological deterioration and loss of protective airway reflexes.
2. Maintain $PaCO_2$ levels between 35 and 45 mm Hg.
3. Maintain plateau pressure <30 cm H_2O.
4. Maintain pH >7.15.
5. Fluctuations in blood pressure can worsen neurological injuries and outcomes.
6. The goal of fluid resuscitation should be to keep the patient euvolemic and normal to hyperosmolar.
7. Provide hemostatic therapy as soon as possible for patients with ICH who have been using an anticoagulant or have a known factor deficiency.
8. Anticipate that the patient may lose the airway.
9. Avoid rapid shifts and fluctuations in blood pressure.
10. Rapidly reverse coagulopathy.
11. Know the indications for surgery.
12. Maintain normoglycemia.
13. Treat fever.
14. Gastric prophylaxis reduces morbidity.
15. Encourage early mobilization and rehabilitation if the patient is stable.
16. Administer anticonvulsant drugs to patients experiencing convulsive seizures.
17. Evacuate cerebellar hemorrhages.

REFERENCES

1. Ropper AH, Samuels MA, Klein JP. *Adam's and Victor's Principles of Neurology.* 10th ed. New York, NY: McGraw-Hill; 2014.
2. Winn RH. *Youmans Neurological Surgery.* 6th ed. Philadelphia, PA: Saunders; 2011.
3. Broderick J, Connolly S, Feldmann E, et al. Guidelines for the management of spontaneous intracerebral hemorrhage in adults: 2007 update: a guideline from the American Heart Association/American Stroke Association Stroke Council, High Blood Pressure Research Council, and the Quality of Care and Outcomes in Research Interdisciplinary Working Group. *Circulation.* 2007;116:e391-e413.
4. Morgenstern LB, Hemphill JC, Anderson C, et al. Guidelines for the management of spontaneous intracerebral hemorrhage: a guideline for healthcare professionals from the American Heart Association/American Stroke Association. *Stroke.* 2010;41:2108-2129.
5. Juvela S, Kase CS. Advances in intracerebral hemorrhage management. *Stroke.* 2006;37:301-304.
6. Mokri B. The Monro-Kellie hypothesis: applications in CSF volume depletion. *Neurology.* 2001;56:1746-1748.
7. Neff S, Subramaniam RP. Monro-Kellie doctrine. *J Neurosurg.* 1996;85:1195.
8. Irwin RS, Rippe JM. *Irwin and Rippe's Intensive Care Medicine.* 7th ed. Philadelphia, PA: Lippincott Williams & Wilkins; 2011.
9. Gonzales NR. Ongoing clinical trials in intracerebral hemorrhage. *Stroke.* 2013;44(6 suppl 1):S70-S73.
10. Gabrielli A, Layon AJ, Yu M. *Civetta, Taylor and Kirby's Critical Care.* 4th ed. Philadelphia, PA: Lippincott Williams & Wilkins; 2009.
11. Qureshi AI, Palesch YY, Barsan WG, et al. Intensive Blood-Pressure Lowering in Patients with Acute Cerebral Hemorrhage. *New England Journal of Medicine.* 2016;375(11):1033-1043.
12. Hemphill JC, Greenberg SM, Anderson CS, et al. Guidelines for the Management of Spontaneous Intracerebral Hemorrhage. *Stroke.* 2015;46(7):2032-2060.
13. Elliott J, Smith M. The acute management of intracerebral hemorrhage: a clinical review. *Anesth Analg.* 2010;110:1419-1427.
14. Hill M, Muir K. INTERACT-2: Should the blood pressure be aggressively lowered acutely after intracerebral hemorrhage? *Stroke.* 2013;44:2951-2952.
15. Aguilar MI, Hart RG, Kase CS, et al. Treatment of warfarin-associated intracerebral hemorrhage: literature review and expert opinion. *Mayo Clin Proc.* 2007;82:82-92.
16. Kase C. Intracerebral hemorrhage. In Daroff RB, ed. *Bradley's Neurology in Clinical Practice.* 6th ed. Philadelphia, PA: Elsevier/Saunders; 2012:1054-1069.
17. Holbrook A, Schulman S, Witt DM, et al. Evidence-based management of anticoagulant therapy: antithrombotic therapy and prevention of thrombosis, 9th ed: American College of Chest Physicians Evidence-Based Clinical Practice Guidelines. *Chest.* 2012;141(2 suppl):e152S-e184S.
18. Huttner HB, Schellinger PD, Hartmann M, et al. Hematoma growth and outcome in treated neurocritical care patients with intracerebral hemorrhage related to oral anticoagulant therapy: comparison of acute treatment strategies using vitamin K, fresh frozen plasma, and prothrombin complex concentrates. *Stroke.* 2006;37:1465-1470.
19. Steiner T, Bohm M, Dichgans M, et al. Recommendations for the emergency management of complications associated with the new direct oral anticoagulants (DOACs), apixaban, dabigatran and rivaroxaban. *Clin Res Cardiol.* 2013;102:399-412.
20. Sadoughi A, Rybinnik I, Cohen R. Measurement and management of increased intracranial pressure. *Open Crit Care Med J.* 2013;6(1):56.
21. Mendelow AD, Gregson BA, Fernandes HM, et al. STICH investigators. Early surgery versus initial conservative treatment in patients with spontaneous supratentorial intracerebral haematomas in the International Surgical Trial in Intracerebral Haemorrhage (STICH): a randomised trial. *Lancet.* 2005;365:387-397.
22. Gregson BA, Mendelow AD. STICH investigators. A tool for predicting outcome after spontaneous supratentorial intracerebral hemorrhage [abstract]. *Stroke.* 2006;37:624.
23. Mendelow AD, Gregson BA, Rowan EN, et al. Early surgery versus initial conservative treatment in patients with spontaneous supratentorial lobar intracerebral haematomas (STICH II): a randomised trial. *Lancet.* 2013;382:397-408.
24. Morgan TA, Awad I, Keyl P. Preliminary report of the clot lysis evaluating accelerated resolution of intraventricular hemorrhage (CLEAR-IVH) clinical trial. *Acta Neurochir Suppl.* 2008;105:217-220.
25. Morgan T, Zuccarello M, Narayan R, et al. Preliminary findings of the minimally-invasive surgery plus rtPA for intracerebral hemorrhage evacuation (MISTIE) clinical trial. *Acta Neurochir Suppl.* 2008;105:147-151.
26. Mould WA, Carhuapoma JR, Muschelli J, et al. Minimally invasive surgery plus recombinant tissue-type plasminogen activator for intracerebral hemorrhage evacuation decreases perihematomal edema. *Stroke.* 2013;44(3):627-634.
27. Caceres JA, Goldstein JN. Intracranial hemorrhage. *Emerg Med Clin North Am.* 2012;30:771-794.

Subarachnoid Hemorrhage

20

IN THIS CHAPTER

- Criteria for intubation
- Circulatory complications
- Neuroimaging
- Hydrocephalus and cerebral edema
- Neurological deterioration

Wan-Tsu W. Chang and Evie G. Marcolini

Subarachnoid hemorrhage (SAH) is a neurological emergency that poses a high risk of sudden decline and death. Approximately 12% to 15% of patients die before reaching the hospital and 50% of survivors suffer from persistent neurological deficits; however, potentially lifesaving interventions during early resuscitation are available.[1,2] As with any other critically ill patient, the initial management of SAH should focus on stabilizing the airway, breathing, and circulation; reducing the risks of rebleeding; and preventing secondary brain injuries.

Airway

Intubation

Endotracheal intubation should be considered for any patient with a Glasgow Coma Scale (GCS) score below 8; however, those who present with minimal neurological deficits can experience a precipitous deterioration due to the development of obstructive hydrocephalus. Therefore, those with or at risk for hydrocephalus should be assessed for airway protection, especially if transport to another facility is planned.

Rapid-Sequence Intubation

In the SAH patient, the reflex sympathetic response to laryngoscopy increases the risk of rebleeding prior to coiling or clipping the "unsecured" aneurysm. Pretreatment with fentanyl can attenuate the effect on the reflex sympathetic response.[4] Evidence to support the use of lidocaine in pretreatment is mixed and limited.[5] The use of antihypertensives should be balanced with the risk of hypotension associated with the concurrent administration of induction agents.

PEARL

Consider using a titratable antihypertensive infusion, especially at the time of intubation, to avoid hypotension associated with the concurrent administration of induction agents.

Breathing

Hypoxia, defined as an arterial partial pressure of oxygen (PaO_2) less than 60 mm Hg or an oxygen saturation less than 90%, is associated with increased morbidity and mortality in patients with brain injuries.[6,7] This is also true for patients with SAH. There is no ideal PaO_2 or oxygen saturation because these targets vary individually and over the course of injury, depending on cerebral metabolism. Cerebral hypoxia can occur despite "normal" systemic oxygenation and perfusion in response to microvascular and cellular metabolic dysfunction; however, excessive oxygen can potentiate secondary brain injury and is associated with worse outcomes.[7-9] The goal is to maintain normoxia.

Hyperventilation, which induces potent cerebral vasoconstriction and decreases cerebral blood flow (CBF), is an effective method of reducing intracranial pressure (ICP). It is important to note that a sustained reduction in CBF can result in cerebral ischemia.[10] Hyperventilation to a partial pressure of carbon dioxide ($PaCO_2$) of 25 to 35 mm Hg should be used only in acutely herniating patients as a temporizing measure, and in concert with more definitive therapies such as osmotic therapy and cerebrospinal fluid drainage to reduce ICP. The target $PaCO_2$ in a patient without suspected intracranial hypertension is 35 to 45 mm Hg.

Mechanical Ventilation

Mechanical ventilation is invariably necessary in critically ill SAH patients with intracranial hypertension, who often have decreased levels of consciousness and require airway protection. Patients with neurological injuries are predisposed to sepsis, acute lung injury, and acute respiratory distress syndrome (ARDS) due to an increased risk of aspiration.[11,12] Neurogenic pulmonary edema can occur and is postulated to be a result of catecholamine surge or pulmonary hypertension secondary to primary brain injury. Lung-protective ventilation strategies such as low tidal volume ventilation can result in hypoventilation and, subsequently, hypercapnia and respiratory acidosis.

Although a pH as low as 7.20 can be tolerated by some ARDS patients, those with a concomitant brain injury such as SAH with intracranial hypertension will be less tolerant given their more tenuous cerebral physiology. Similarly, higher positive end-expiratory pressure (PEEP) is associated with increased ICP.[13] The risks of mechanical ventilation strategies must be weighed against the risks of ARDS, and therapy should be individualized to the SAH patient with intracranial hypertension, likely with adjunctive cerebral monitoring.

PEARL

Hypercapnia and the use of a higher PEEP increase the risk of ICP in SAH patients and should be avoided during acute resuscitation. When these treatments are deemed necessary, they should be used in conjunction with cerebral monitoring.

Circulation

Cerebral autoregulation is a mechanism of normal brain that maintains constant CBF over a range of mean arterial pressure (MAP) through the modulation of cerebral vascular tone. In patients with a brain injury such as SAH, autoregulation is often disrupted and changes in MAP directly affect CBF.[14-17] Optimization of MAP is critically important in maintaining cerebral perfusion; however, cerebral hypoperfusion can occur even with a normal MAP. Induced hypotension has been used in the past during the surgical treatment of ruptured cerebral aneurysms to prevent rerupture; however, data suggest that this practice could increase the risk of cerebral ischemia and neurological deficits.[14,18] No studies have been conducted to determine the optimal systolic blood pressure target for acute resuscitation. In patients with suspected intracranial hypertension, ICP monitoring allows the use of cerebral perfusion pressure (CPP) as a resuscitation target. In SAH, the optimal MAP and CPP are likely patient and time dependent.

Hypertension in patients with unsecured ruptured aneurysms is associated with rebleeding. This risk is highest immediately after the initial ictus but persists each day the ruptured aneurysm goes untreated.[19-21] Consequently, an urgent evaluation of patients with SAH and prompt referral for neurosurgery consultation are essential. Retrospective studies suggest a higher rate of rebleeding with SBP above 160 mm Hg and a severe initial bleed.[22] Therefore, the American Heart Association (AHA), the American Stroke Association (ASA), and the Neurocritical Care Society (NCS) recommend maintaining SBP below 160 mm Hg and MAP below 110 mm Hg before the ruptured aneurysm has been secured.[1,23,24]

Blood Pressure Management

The ideal antihypertensive to use in patients with SAH is a parenteral agent that produces a rapid and predictable dose response while minimizing adverse cerebral effects. The AHA and ASA recommend nicardipine and labetalol as initial options for blood pressure management. Agents such as sodium nitroprusside, hydralazine, and enalaprilat are not recommended as they have adverse effects on CBF and ICP and unpredictable and prolonged antihypertensive effects.[1,23,25]

Neurogenic Cardiomyopathy

Neurogenic stress-induced cardiomyopathy is a syndrome characterized by reversible left ventricular dysfunction, electrocardiographic changes, and elevated myocardial markers in the absence of obstructive coronary artery disease. The disorder is estimated to occur in 0.8% of patients with SAH and is predominantly found in those with poor Hunt and Hess grades *(Table 20-1)*.[26] Patient management primarily is supportive; it also is important to maintain an optimal intravascular volume status to prevent cerebral ischemia in the setting of cerebral vasospasm. Inotropic agents and vasopressors might be necessary to maintain cerebral perfusion. An intraaortic balloon pump can be used in patients who are refractory to medications, but the concomitant requirement for therapeutic anticoagulation precludes this strategy in those with unsecured aneurysms.

PEARLS

- ✓ Patients with suspected intracranial hypertension might be at risk for cerebral hypoperfusion despite a normal MAP.
- ✓ Neurogenic cardiomyopathy is characterized by reversible left ventricular dysfunction, electrocardiographic changes, and elevated myocardial markers in the absence of obstructive coronary artery disease.

Neuroimaging

Once SAH is confirmed, a neurosurgical consultation should be obtained and transfer to a high-volume SAH center with neurosurgical and endovascular specialists should be considered, as patient outcomes are better at high-volume facilities.[27-29] Neurovascular imaging will be requested by neurosurgical consultants to determine the cause of the SAH and for surgical planning. Computed tomography angiography (CTA) is a less invasive imaging modality with a sensitivity similar to that of catheter angiography for aneurysms larger than 3 mm.[30] Operator skill level and experience reading the scans are important factors for detecting cerebral aneurysms using CTA. Magnetic resonance angiography (MRA) has a sensitivity similar to that of CTA, but a lower specificity for detecting aneurysms.[31] Cerebral angiography is the current standard for diagnosing cerebral aneurysms as the cause of SAH.[1,23] The added benefit of cerebral angiography is that it provides an opportunity to perform endovascular interventions as definitive therapy for ruptured aneurysms. The choice of imaging modality largely depends on institutional practices. The treatment of SAH is time sensitive, and decisions regarding when to perform endovascular coiling or surgical clipping rely on many factors, including the stability of the clot.

Other Treatment Considerations

A major component in the management of patients with SAH is the prevention of secondary brain injuries. Hydrocephalus, cerebral edema, intracranial hypertension, seizures, and fever can all contribute to cerebral ischemia. Delayed cerebral ischemia can result from cerebral vasospasm. Neurological deterioration from these insults can be subtle, especially in poor-grade patients.

FIGURE 20-1. Classic Characteristics of Hydrocephalus

This axial (cross-sectional) CT of the head without contrast shows a massive subarachnoid hemorrhage secondary to the rupture of an intracranial aneurysm. Blood *(hyperdensity)* can be seen filling the subarachnoid and ventricular spaces. There is dilation of the fourth ventricle and temporal horns of the lateral ventricle, consistent with hydrocephalus.

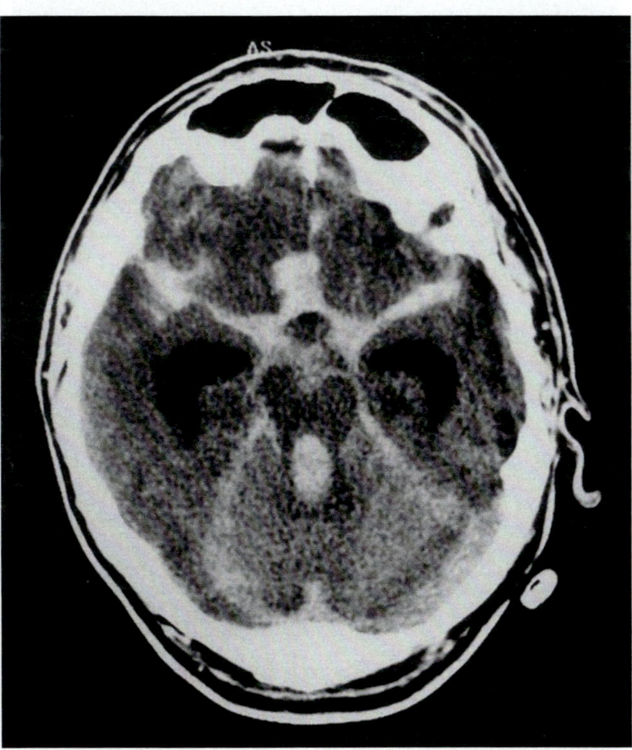

Hydrocephalus

Hydrocephalus, which is common in patients with SAH, is characterized by symptoms that range from headache to coma *(Figure 20-1)*.[32,33] If the symptoms are mild, patients may be observed with frequent neurological examinations. If the patient has a decreased level of consciousness, hydrocephalus can be treated by placing an external ventricular drain, which allows ICP monitoring as well as CSF drainage. If left untreated, the disorder can lead to intracranial hypertension and cerebral ischemia with potential cerebral herniation. Therefore, acute obstructive hydrocephalus caused by SAH is a neurological emergency.

Cerebral Edema

Up to 20% of patients with SAH develop global cerebral edema resulting from ictal intracranial circulatory arrest.[34] An acute rise in ICP at the time of aneurysm rupture causes global cerebral ischemia and loss of consciousness. Delayed global cerebral edema can result from the cytotoxic effects of blood products, microvascular ischemia, and autoregulation dysfunction.[34,35] Computed tomographic evidence of global cerebral edema is an independent predictor of mortality and poor functional outcome after SAH.[34]

Intracranial Hypertension

The management of intracranial hypertension should follow a tiered approach *(Table 20-2)*.[36] Initial treatment includes noninvasive techniques such as elevating the head of the bed, maintaining the neck in neutral position, and avoiding neck constriction. The placement of an external ventricular drain allows ICP monitoring and CSF drainage. Both mannitol and hypertonic saline are effective in decreasing ICP and improving CPP by decreasing brain edema.[37,38] Mannitol and hypertonic saline also increase CBF in regions of hypoperfusion via immediate rheological effects.[39] Refractory intracranial hypertension might require management with pharmacological coma, paralysis, and surgical decompression.[40,41]

TABLE 20-1. Hunt and Hess Grading Scale

Grade 0	Unruptured aneurysm
Grade 1	Asymptomatic or minimal headache and slight nuchal rigidity
Grade 2	Moderate to severe headache, nuchal rigidity, no neurological deficit except cranial nerve palsy
Grade 3	Drowsiness, confusion, or mild neurological deficit
Grade 4	Stupor, moderate to severe hemiparesis
Grade 5	Coma, decerebrate posturing, moribund appearance

Seizure Prophylaxis

In a patient with an unsecured aneurysm, seizures can lead to rebleeding and increased ICP and should be treated with anticonvulsants. The short-term use of prophylactic anticonvulsants is not supported by strong data and should be considered on a case-by-case basis, as recommended by the AHA/ASA and NCS guidelines.[1,23,24] Although phenytoin traditionally has been used for seizure prophylaxis in brain-injured patients, it is associated with worse long-term cognitive outcomes.[42-44] The efficacy of levetiracetam is similar to that of phenytoin and may be better tolerated.[45,46] Patients with SAH and altered mental status are at risk for nonconvulsive status epilepticus, which can increase cerebral metabolic demand and put the brain at risk for ischemia.[47,48] Continuous electroencephalography (EEG) should be considered in such cases to monitor for nonconvulsive status epilepticus.[24]

Temperature Management

Fever, the most common medical complication of SAH, is independently associated with worse cognitive outcomes regardless of the fever's origin.[49-51] The complication also has been linked to symptomatic vasospasm, likely due to the inflammatory response in SAH, and commonly is associated with a decreased level of consciousness.[52]

Antipyretics traditionally are the first-choice therapy for the management of fever. Data support the use of acetaminophen (6 g/day) over ibuprofen (2,400 mg/day) for maintaining normothermia.[53] External cooling techniques such as fanning, evaporative cooling, and ice packs have poor efficacy.[54] Surface cooling devices, including cooling blankets and hydrogel-coated energy transfer pads, are more effective in reducing the fever burden but are associated with a higher incidence of shivering.[55] Intravascular catheter-based heat exchange systems are similarly effective without increasing the risk of infection.[56] An infusion of normal saline (4°C) is a rapid, safe, and effective method of fever control.[57] Although a stepwise, escalating approach to temperature management is conventional, prophylactic normothermia may be most effective in reducing the fever burden and improving outcomes.[58,59]

Under normal conditions, shivering and vasoconstriction work to maintain a core body temperature of 37°C (98.6°F) when the level falls below 36°C (98.8°F). In patients with brain injuries such as SAH, the temperature set point is elevated, triggering a thermoregulatory response. The increased metabolic demand of uncontrolled shivering can lead to catabolism and defeat the benefits of fever control in critically ill SAH patients. Shivering can be managed using skin counterwarming, magnesium, buspirone, meperidine, or sedatives.[54,60]

TABLE 20-2. Tiered ICP Management

Tier	Management
Tier 0	Head of bed >30 degrees Optimize physiological parameters Normothermia goal Adequate sedation and analgesia
Tier 1*	CSF drainage via ventriculostomy Mannitol, bolus of 0.5–1 g/kg Hypertonic saline
Tier 2*	Additional hyperosmolar therapies Propofol bolus and infusion Paralytic infusion
Tier 3*	Decompressive hemicraniectomy Barbiturate coma Decompressive laparotomy or thoracotomy

*Hyperventilation should only be used as a bridge to more definitive therapies.

Antifibrinolytic Therapy

When early definitive treatment of a ruptured aneurysm is not possible because of the patient's instability, administration of an antifibrinolytic agent such as epsilon-aminocaproic acid or tranexamic acid can be considered. Preoperative antifibrinolytic treatment is associated with a reduction in rebleeding but an increase in cerebral ischemia.[19,61,62] The use of antifibrinolytic agents should be discussed with neurosurgical consultants if definitive treatment of the ruptured aneurysm will be delayed.

Neurological Deterioration

Neurological decline in a patient with SAH can be caused by several different processes. Rebleeding can occur before the ruptured aneurysm is secured, with the risk highest in patients with poor Hunt and Hess grades.[21,22] In the first 72 hours after ictus, patients are in danger of developing hydrocephalus, which most commonly presents as decreased level of consciousness. The risk of cerebral vasospasm is highest 3 to 5 days after ictus. Although radiographic vasospasm can be seen in 30% to 70% of patients, about 50% are clinically symptomatic, presenting with focal neurological deficits that can resolve or progress to cerebral infarction.[63] Treating symptomatic cerebral vasospasm reduces cerebral ischemia by improving CBF and decreasing cerebral metabolism. While avoiding hypovolemia is key, there is no evidence that hypervolemia is more beneficial than euvolemia.[64,65]

PEARLS

- ✓ Loss of consciousness at ictus of aneurysm rupture suggests intracranial circulatory arrest and is associated with early global cerebral edema.
- ✓ Brain injuries such as SAH raise the temperature set point; therefore, normalization of temperature can cause shivering as a thermoregulatory response.
- ✓ Routine 30-minute EEGs can miss more than 50% of patients with nonconvulsive status epilepticus.

Hemodynamic augmentation is another strategy for improving CBF; however, this technique increases the risk of rebleeding if a ruptured aneurysm is not yet secured. The endovascular administration of vasodilators and angioplasty can be considered in selected patients in consultation with neurosurgery and interventional neuroradiology. Oral nimodipine reduces morbidity and improves functional outcomes in patients with SAH.[66] The drug is commonly administered as 60 mg every 4 hours, but the dose can be divided (30 mg every 2 hours) if hypotension is evident.

A fluctuating neurological exam or persistent altered mental status might be the result of subclinical seizures. Routine 30-minute EEGs can miss more than 50% of patients with nonconvulsive status epilepticus; continuous EEG monitoring should be established if subclinical seizures are suspected. Monitoring for 24 hours is recommended in noncomatose patients and 48 hours in comatose patients.[67,68]

The management of neurological deterioration in patients with SAH initially should focus on optimizing physiological parameters such as oxygenation, ventilation, cerebral perfusion, intracranial pressure, and temperature. Repeat neuroimaging should be obtained to evaluate for rebleeding, hydrocephalus, and cerebral edema. Advanced neuroimaging and further invasive diagnostics should be discussed with neurosurgical consultants.

Summary

Patients with SAH require intubation for airway protection if the GCS score is below 8 or neurological deterioration is anticipated. The target $PaCO_2$ should be 35 to 45 mm Hg when intracranial hypertension is suspected, and SBP should be maintained above 90 mm Hg and below 160 mm Hg, especially during rapid sequence intubation. When intracranial hypertension is suspected, MAP should be maintained for CPP. Other important management strategies include elevating the head of the bed more than 30 degrees and controlling pain and fever. Seizure prophylaxis can be considered, and neurosurgery should be consulted for definitive treatment of a ruptured aneurysm. Some cases may warrant transfer to a high-volume neurosurgical/endovascular center.

REFERENCES

1. Connolly ES, Rabinstein AA, Carhuapoma JR, et al. Guidelines for the management of aneurysmal subarachnoid hemorrhage: a guideline for healthcare professionals from the American Heart Association/American Stroke Association. *Stroke.* 2012;43(6):1711-1737.
2. Schievink W, Wijdicks E, Parisi J, et al. Sudden death from aneurysmal subarachnoid hemorrhage. *Neurology.* 1995;45(5):871-874.
3. Vermeulen MJ, Schull MJ. Missed diagnosis of subarachnoid hemorrhage in the emergency department. *Stroke.* 2007;38(4):1216-1221.
4. Kim JT, Shim JK, Kim SH, et al. Remifentanil vs. lignocaine for attenuating the haemodynamic response during rapid sequence induction using propofol: double-blind randomised clinical trial. *Anaesth Intensive Care.* 2007;35(1):20-23.
5. Robinson N, Clancy M. In patients with head injury undergoing rapid sequence intubation, does pretreatment with intravenous lignocaine/lidocaine lead to an improved neurological outcome? A review of the literature. *Emerg Med J.* 2001;18(6):453-457.
6. Chesnut RM, Marshall LF, Klauber MR, et al. The role of secondary brain injury in determining outcome from severe head injury. *J Trauma.* 1993;34(2):216-222.
7. Davis DP, Meade W, Sise MJ, et al. Both hypoxemia and extreme hyperoxemia may be detrimental in patients with severe traumatic brain injury. *J Neurotrauma.* 2009;26(12):2217-2223.
8. Ramakrishna R, Stiefel M, Udoteuk J, et al. Brain oxygen tension and outcome in patients with aneurysmal subarachnoid hemorrhage. *J Neurosurg.* 2008;109:1075-1082.
9. Rincon F, Kang J, Maltenfort M, et al. Association between hyperoxia and mortality after stroke: a multicenter cohort study. *Crit Care Med.* 2014;42(2):387-396.
10. Carrera E, Schmidt JM, Fernandez L, et al. Spontaneous hyperventilation and brain tissue hypoxia in patients with severe brain injury. *J Neurol Neurosurg Psychiatry.* 2010;81(7):793-797.
11. Kahn JM, Caldwell EC, Deem S, et al. Acute lung injury in patients with subarachnoid hemorrhage: incidence, risk factors, and outcome. *Crit Care Med.* 2006;34(1):196-202.
12. Bruder N, Rabinstein A. Cardiovascular and pulmonary complications of aneurysmal subarachnoid hemorrhage. *Neurocrit Care.* 2011;15(2):257-269.
13. Nemer SN, Caldeira JB, Azeredo LM, et al. Alveolar recruitment maneuver in patients with subarachnc … approaches. *J Cr* …
14. Farrar JK, Gama … blood flow durin …
15. Bederson JB, Le … hemorrhage. *Ne* …
16. Lang EW, Diehl … subarachnoid h … blood flow veloc …
17. Soehle M, Czos … subarachnoid h …

KEY POINTS

1. Consider intubation for airway protection if the GCS score is <8 or if neurological deterioration is anticipated.
2. Avoid hypoxia and hyperoxia, which can potentiate secondary brain injury and are associated with worse outcomes.
3. The target $PaCO_2$ in a patient without suspected intracranial hypertension is 35 to 45 mm Hg. Hyperventilation should be used only in an acutely herniating patient as a temporizing measure and in concert with more definitive therapies such as osmotic therapy and ventriculostomy drainage.
4. The AHA and ASA recommend maintaining SBP <160 mm Hg and MAP <110 mm Hg in patients with unsecured SAH to reduce the risk of aneurysmal rebleeding. Nicardipine and labetalol are equally efficacious for blood pressure management.
5. Neurogenic c… with supporti… agents and by… intravascular …
6. Patients with … evaluations. T… associated wi…
7. Acute obstru… emergency d… death.
8. The manager… hypertension… maintaining t… neck constric…
9. Fever is inde… outcomes in …
10. Maintaining … improve outc…

18. Hitchcock E, Tsementzis S, Dow A. Short- and long-term prognosis of patients with a subarachnoid haemorrhage in relation to intra-operative period of hypotension. *Acta Neurochir.* 1984;70(3-4):235-242.
19. Adams HP, Kassell NK, Torner JC, et al. Early management of aneurysmal subarachnoid hemorrhage. *J Neurosurg.* 1981;54(2):141-145.
20. Kassell N, Torner J. Aneurysmal rebleeding : a preliminary report from the Cooperative Aneurysm Study. *Neurosurgery.* 1983;13(5):379-481.
21. Naidech AW, Janjua N, Kreiter KT, et al. Predictors and impact of aneurysm rebleeding after subarachnoid hemorrhage. *Arch Neurol.* 2005;62(3):410-416.
22. Ohkuma H, Tsurutani H, Suzuki S. Incidence and significance of early aneurysmal rebleeding before neurosurgical or neurological management. *Stroke.* 2001;32(5):1176-1180.
23. Bederson JB, Connolly ES, Batjer HH, et al. Guidelines for the management of aneurysmal subarachnoid hemorrhage: a statement for healthcare professionals from a special writing group of the Stroke Council, American Heart Association. *Stroke.* 2009;40(3):994-1025.
24. Diringer MN, Bleck TP, Claude Hemphill J, et al. Critical care management of patients following aneurysmal subarachnoid hemorrhage: recommendations from the Neurocritical Care Society's Multidisciplinary Consensus Conference. *Neurocrit Care.* 2011;15(2):211-240.
25. Rose JC, Mayer SA. Optimizing blood pressure in neurological emergencies. *Neurocrit Care.* 2004;1(3):287-299.
26. Abd TT, Hayek S, Cheng J, et al. Incidence and clinical characteristics of takotsubo cardiomyopathy post-aneurysmal subarachnoid hemorrhage. *Int J Cardiol.* 2014;176(3):1362-1364.
27. Johnston SC. Effect of endovascular services and hospital volume on cerebral aneurysm treatment outcomes. *Stroke.* 2000;31(1):111-117.
28. Bardach NS, Zhao S, Gress DR, et al. Association between subarachnoid hemorrhage outcomes and number of cases treated at California hospitals [editorial comment]. *Stroke.* 2002;33(7):1851-1856.
29. Berman MF, Solomon RA, Mayer SA, et al. Impact of hospital-related factors on outcome after treatment of cerebral aneurysms. *Stroke.* 2003;34(9):2200-2207.
30. Donmez H, Serifov E, Kahriman G, et al. Comparison of 16-row multislice CT angiography with conventional angiography for detection and evaluation of intracranial aneurysms. *Eur J Radiol.* 2011;80(2):455-461.
31. Sailer A, Wagemans B, Nelemans P, et al. Diagnosing intracranial aneurysms with MR angiography: systematic review and meta-analysis. *Stroke.* 2014;45(1):119-126.
32. Van Gijn J, Hijdra A, Wijdicks EF, et al. Acute hydrocephalus after aneurysmal subarachnoid hemorrhage. *J Neurosurg.* 1985;63(3):355-362.
33. Graff-Radford NR, Torner J, Adams HP, et al. Factors associated with hydrocephalus after subarachnoid hemorrhage - report of the Cooperative Aneurysm Study. *Arch Neurol.* 2014;46(7):744-752.
34. Claassen J, Carhuapoma JR, Kreiter KT, et al. Global cerebral edema after subarachnoid hemorrhage: frequency, predictors, and impact on outcome. *Stroke.* 2002;33(5):1225-1232.
35. Mocco J, Prickett CS, Komotar RJ, et al. Potential mechanisms and clinical significance of global cerebral edema following aneurysmal subarachnoid hemorrhage. *Neurosurg Focus.* 2007;22(5):1-4.
36. Stevens RD, Huff JS, Duckworth J, et al. Emergency neurological life support: intracranial hypertension and herniation. *Neurocrit Care.* 2012;17(suppl 1):S60-S65.
37. Freshman S, Battistella F, Matteucci M, et al. Hypertonic saline (7.5%) versus mannitol: a comparison for treatment of acute head injuries. *J Trauma.* 1993;35(3):344-348.
38. Wang LC, Papangelou A, Lin C, et al. Comparison of equivolume, equiosmolar solutions of mannitol and hypertonic saline with or without furosemide on brain water content in normal rats. *Anesthesiology.* 2013;118(4):903-913.
39. Scalfani M, Dhar R, Zazulia A, et al. Effect of osmotic agents on regional blood flow in traumatic brain injury. *J Crit Care.* 2012;27(5):526 e7-e12.
40. Eisenberg HM, Frankowski RF, Contant CF, et al. High-dose barbiturate control of elevated intracranial pressure in patients with severe head injury. *J Neurosurg.* 1988;69(1):15-23.
41. Sadaka F, Veremakis C. Therapeutic hypothermia for the management of intracranial hypertension in severe traumatic brain injury: a systematic review. *Brain Inj.* 2012;26(7-8):899-908.
42. Lanzino G, D'Urso PI, Suarez J. Seizures and anticonvulsants after aneurysmal subarachnoid hemorrhage. *Neurocrit Care.* 2011;15(2):247-256.
43. Naidech AM, Kreiter KT, Janjua N, et al. Phenytoin exposure is associated with functional and cognitive disability after subarachnoid hemorrhage. *Stroke.* 2005;36(3):583-587.
44. Tartara A, Galimberti CA, Manni R, et al. Differential effects of valproic acid and enzyme-inducing anticonvulsants on nimodipine pharmacokinetics in epileptic patients. *Br J Clin Pharmacol.* 1991;32(3):335-340.
45. Shah D, Husain AM. Utility of levetiracetam in patients with subarachnoid hemorrhage. *Seizure.* 2009;18(10):676-679.
46. Karamchandani RR, Fletcher JJ, Pandey AS, et al. Incidence of delayed seizures, delayed cerebral ischemia and poor outcome with the use of levetiracetam versus phenytoin after aneurysmal subarachnoid hemorrhage. *J Clin Neurosci.* 2014;21(9):1507-1513.
47. Claassen J, Perotte A, Albers D, et al. Nonconvulsive seizures after subarachnoid hemorrhage: multimodal detection and outcomes. *Ann Neurol.* 2013;74(1):53-64.
48. Claassen J, Albers D, Schmidt JM, et al. Nonconvulsive seizures in subarachnoid hemorrhage link inflammation and outcome. *Ann Neurol.* 2014;75(5):771-781.
49. Kilpatrick MM, Lowry DW, Firlik AD, et al. Hyperthermia in the neurosurgical intensive care unit. *Neurosurgery.* 2000;47(4):850-856.
50. Rabinstein AA, Sandhu K. Non-infectious fever in the neurological intensive care unit: incidence, causes and predictors. *J Neurol Neurosurg Psychiatry.* 2007;78(11):1278-1280.
51. Fernandez A, Schmidt JM, Claassen J, et al. Fever after subarachnoid hemorrhage: risk factors and impact on outcome. *Neurology.* 2007;68(13):1013-1019.
52. Yoshimoto Y, Tanaka Y, Hoya K. Acute systemic inflammatory response syndrome in subarachnoid hemorrhage. *Stroke.* 2001;32(9):1989-1993.
53. Dippel DWJ, van Breda EJ, van der Worp HB, et al. Effect of paracetamol (acetaminophen) and ibuprofen on body temperature in acute ischemic stroke PISA, a phase II double-blind, randomized, placebo-controlled trial. *BMC Cardiovasc Disord.* 2003;8:1-8.
54. Scaravilli V, Tinchero G, Citerio G. Fever management in SAH. *Neurocrit Care.* 2011;15(2):287-294.
55. Mayer SA, Kowalski RG, Presciutti M, et al. Clinical trial of a novel surface cooling system for fever control in neurocritical care patients. *Crit Care Med.* 2004;32(12):2508-2515.
56. Diringer MN. Treatment of fever in the neurological intensive care unit with a catheter-based heat exchange system. *Crit Care Med.* 2004;32(2):559-564.
57. Badjatia N, Bodock M, Guanci M, et al. Rapid infusion of cold saline (4 degrees C) as adjunctive treatment of fever in patients with brain injury. *Neurology.* 2006;66(11):1739-1741.
58. Broessner G, Lackner P, Fischer M, et al. Influence of prophylactic, endovascularly based normothermia on inflammation in patients with severe cerebrovascular disease: a prospective, randomized trial. *Stroke.* 2010;41(12):2969-2972.
59. Badjatia N, Fernandez L, Schmidt JM, et al. Impact of induced normothermia on outcome after subarachnoid hemorrhage: a case-control study. *Neurosurgery.* 2010;66(4):696-701.
60. Badjatia N. Hyperthermia and fever control in brain injury. *Crit Care Med.* 2009;37(7 suppl):S250-S257.
61. Baharoglu M, Germans M, Rinkel G, et al. Antifibrinolytic therapy for aneurysmal subarachnoid haemorrhage. *Cochrane Database Syst Rev.* 2013;(8):CD001245.
62. Hillman J, Fridriksson S, Nilsson O, et al. Immediate administration of tranexamic acid and reduced incidence of early rebleeding after aneurysmal subarachnoid hemorrhage: a prospective randomized study. *J Neurosurg.* 2002;97(4):771-778.
63. Vergouwen MDI, Vermeulen M, van Gijn J, et al. Definition of delayed cerebral ischemia after aneurysmal subarachnoid hemorrhage as an outcome event in clinical trials and observational studies: proposal of a multidisciplinary research group. *Stroke.* 2010;41(10):2391-2395.
64. Lennihan L, Mayer SA, Fink ME, et al. Effect of hypervolemic therapy on cerebral blood flow after subarachnoid hemorrhage. *Stroke.* 2000;31(2):383-391.
65. Egge A, Waterloo K, Sjoholm H, et al. Prophylactic hyperdynamic postoperative fluid therapy after aneurysmal subarachnoid hemorrhage: a clinical, prospective, randomized, controlled study. *Neurosurgery.* 2001;49(3):593-606.
66. Allen G, Preziosi T, Battye R, et al. Cerebral arterial spasm - a controlled trial of nimodipine in patients with subarachnoid hemorrhage. *N Engl J Med.* 1983;308(11):619-624.
67. Claassen J, Mayer SA, Kowalski RG, et al. Detection of electrographic seizures with continuous EEG monitoring in critically ill patients. *Neurology.* 2004;62(10):1743-1748.
68. Pandian JD, Cascino GD, So EL, et al. Digital video-electroencephalographic monitoring in the neurological-neurosurgical intensive care unit. *Arch Neurol.* 2004;61:1090-1094.

The Crashing Anaphylaxis Patient

21

IN THIS CHAPTER

- Airway management
- Epinephrine — which patients, by what route, and when to avoid
- Second-line pharmacotherapy — antihistamines, corticosteroids
- Patient disposition

Jonathan E. Davis and Robert L. Norris

Anaphylaxis is a severe, life-threatening, systemic reaction that has a rapid and often unpredictable onset of potentially lethal symptoms. The disorder, which can affect patients in every age group, must be swiftly and aggressively treated.[1] Anaphylaxis results from the sudden release of active mediators from mast cells, which are located in tissues, and basophils in the bloodstream. The clinical syndrome is variable and can involve multiple targets, including the skin and respiratory, gastrointestinal (GI), cardiovascular, and central nervous systems *(Table 21-1)*.[2] Respiratory and cardiovascular derangements carry the greatest potential for morbidity and mortality.

The signs and symptoms of an acute allergic reaction are best viewed as a continuum *(Figure 21-1)*. It is useful to define a point along this spectrum that distinguishes anaphylaxis from milder allergic phenomena because anaphylaxis necessitates aggressive treatment. A reasonable *working* definition of the disorder involves allergic signs/symptoms with respiratory compromise and/or hemodynamic instability (ranging from presyncope to cardiovascular collapse). Although international experts have proposed clinical criteria for diagnosing anaphylaxis, the accuracy of these guidelines in the emergency department is imperfect; clinical judgment remains paramount *(Table 21-2)*.[3,4]

Pathophysiology

A classic IgE-mediated allergic response (Gell and Coombs type I, immediate hypersensitivity) consists of three phases:

1. **Sensitization:** Allergen exposure leads to the production of IgE antibodies.
2. **Early reaction:** Subsequent allergen exposure causes an IgE-mediated release of preformed substances from mast cells and basophils.
3. **Late reaction:** Immune cells produce additional inflammatory mediators.

Treatment is aimed at halting preformed mediator release and shutting down the intracellular machinery that produces new mediators.

An anaphylactoid reaction (also known as *nonallergic anaphylaxis*) is an immediate systemic reaction resulting

FIGURE 21-1. The Clinical Spectrum of Allergic Manifestations

The arrow denotes the point at which a reaction should be classified as anaphylaxis.

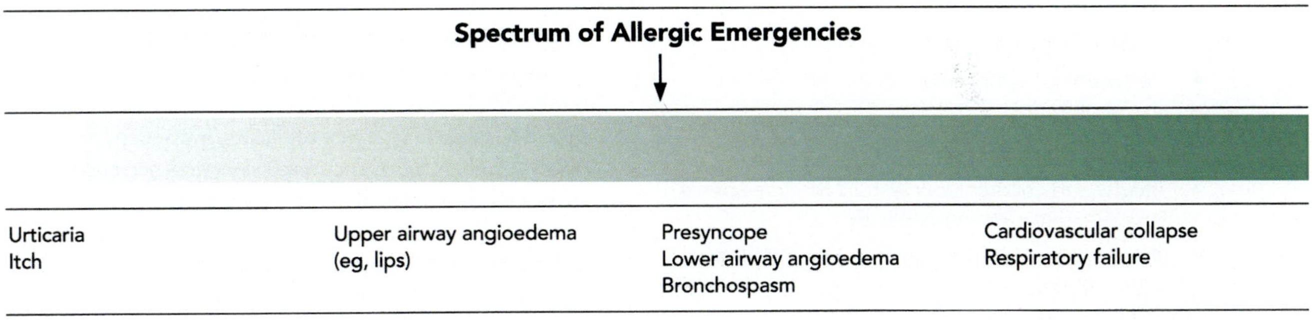

Spectrum of Allergic Emergencies

Urticaria Itch	Upper airway angioedema (eg, lips)	Presyncope Lower airway angioedema Bronchospasm	Cardiovascular collapse Respiratory failure

from directly stimulated release of identical mediators from mast cells and basophils. This reaction differs from allergic anaphylaxis in that it is not IgE mediated, does not require prior sensitization, and can occur on first exposure to the inciting agent.[5] The clinical presentation and management of anaphylactoid reactions are identical to those of allergic anaphylaxis.

TABLE 21-1. Target Organs and Manifestations in Anaphylaxis

Cardiovascular system	Hypotension, lightheadedness, near syncope, syncope, arrhythmias, angina
Central nervous system	Headache, confusion, altered level of consciousness
Gastrointestinal system	Nausea, vomiting, diarrhea, cramping
Respiratory system	**Upper airway:** Oropharyngeal, hypopharyngeal, or laryngeal edema; dysphonia, hoarseness, dysphagia, rhinorrhea, congestion, sneezing **Lower airway:** Bronchospasm
Skin	Flushing, erythema, pruritus, urticaria, angioedema

TABLE 21-2. Clinical Criteria for Diagnosing Anaphylaxis[2]

Anaphylaxis is highly likely when any ONE of the following three criteria is fulfilled:

1. Acute onset of an illness (minutes to several hours) with involvement of the skin, mucosal tissue, or both (eg, generalized hives; pruritus or flushing; swollen lips, tongue, uvula) and at least one of the following:
   - Respiratory compromise
   - Reduced blood pressure (BP) or associated symptoms of end-organ dysfunction
2. Two (or more) of the following, occurring rapidly (minutes to several hours) after exposure to a likely allergen for that patient:
   - Involvement of the skin or mucosal tissue
   - Respiratory compromise
   - Reduced BP or associated symptoms
   - Persistent GI symptoms
3. Reduced BP after exposure to a known allergen for that patient (minutes to several hours):
   - Infants and children: low systolic BP (age specific) or >30% decrease in systolic BP
   - Adults: systolic BP <90 mm Hg or >30% decrease from baseline

Etiology

Anaphylaxis has multiple etiologies, including foods, medications, stinging insects, latex, and exercise *(Table 21-3)*. Food is the most common cause of the disorder in children, whereas medications are the most common culprit in adults.[4,6,7] Many infants outgrow their allergies to eggs, milk, and soy products. On the other hand, food allergies in adults (eg, peanut, tree nuts, fish, and shellfish) can remain problematic throughout life even if they first develop during childhood.

Mortality

Certain factors are associated with severe or fatal anaphylaxis *(Table 21-4)*. In particular, asthma has been shown to be an independent risk factor for death from anaphylaxis.[8,9] Peanuts and tree nuts have also been associated with severe symptoms, accounting for most fatal or near-fatal food reactions in the United States.[10] Adolescents appear to be at increased risk for severe or fatal reactions. Teenagers are more inclined to deny symptoms or engage in risky behaviors despite a known allergy, and are less likely to recognize allergic triggers and carry or use their epinephrine self-administration devices.[11] Concurrent medications such as beta-adrenergic blockers and angiotensin-converting enzyme (ACE) inhibitors also may increase the risk of severe sequelae or even death.[12]

PEARL

In children, anaphylaxis is most commonly food induced; in adults, medications are the likeliest culprits.

Emergency Department Evaluation

Anaphylaxis must be considered in the differential diagnosis for any patient with an acute onset of respiratory distress, bronchospasm, hypotension, or cardiac arrest *(Table 21-5)*. A thorough evaluation begins with rapid triage and stabilization. Patients with rapidly progressing symptoms or abnormal vital signs should be immediately taken to an area fully equipped with advanced airway equipment and critical care capabilities. Anaphylaxis is a dynamic process; frequent reassessments are crucial. It also should be appreciated that even stable patients with initially mild symptoms can deteriorate rapidly. The clinical presentation of anaphylaxis can vary; respiratory symptoms predominate in children, and cardiovascular manifestations predominate in adults.[7,13]

History and Physical Examination

In many cases, the most valuable information comes from those who observed an allergic event from its onset. Time should be taken to interview caretakers, bystanders, friends, family members, emergency medical services personnel, and anyone else who might have witnessed an out-of-hospital episode to elicit specific information regarding the initial signs and symptoms. Although there is great variability, one study in children determined that the mean latency period between allergen exposure and symptom onset was about 15 minutes.[14] The patient's medical history should focus on prior allergies, asthma, and other preexisting atopic conditions. The clinician should remain particularly vigilant when managing asthma or reactive airway disease; if the condition is poorly controlled, fatal anaphylactic reactions are more likely.[15,16]

The signs and symptoms of anaphylaxis and their frequencies (based on a compilation of nearly 1,900 patients representing all ages and reactions resulting from a wide variety of allergens) are presented in Table 21-6.[17] Respiratory failure and cardiovascular collapse are major threats to life. Loss of up to 35% of circulating blood volume, primarily from third spacing, can occur within 10 minutes after the onset of symptoms.[18] Cutaneous findings are entirely absent in up to 10% of cases of anaphylaxis, and severe reactions can occur with no cutaneous manifestations whatsoever.[17,19,20]

Emergency Department Treatment

As with any acute condition, initial attention must focus on the ABCs — airway, breathing, and circulation. Definitive airway management is of paramount importance, as the window for effective intervention can rapidly dwindle if decisions are not made swiftly and decisively. Anticipate challenges with laryngoscopy, and simultaneously prepare initial and contingency airway plans. Avoid sedatives that can depress blood pressure. Exercise extreme caution with paralytics, as mask or supraglottic rescue ventilation can be significantly impaired in patients with upper airway edema. An awake, sedated approach (eg, awake fiberoptic intubation) may be preferable.[4] Optimizing success of the first look/first pass is essential regardless of the approach employed.

Most patients with anaphylaxis should be continuously monitored (cardiac and pulse oximetry) and receive supplemental oxygen and intravenous crystalloid infusions via large-bore lines. Optimally, patients should be placed in the supine position; pregnant women should be placed on their left side. Remain vigilant for early clinical signs of shock. Compensated pediatric shock can present with tachycardia alone; hypotension can be a late finding. The recommended initial pediatric fluid infusion (crystalloid or colloid) is 10 to 20 mL/kg, titrated to response.[1] Fluid administration (≥80–100 mL/kg) may become necessary in some cases. Common medications used in the treatment of anaphylaxis are listed in Table 21-7.

TABLE 21-3. Causes of Anaphylaxis

Category	Example(s)
Foods	**Children:** eggs, milk, soy **Adults:** peanuts, tree nuts, fish, shellfish
Medications	Antimicrobials, NSAIDS, anesthetics, insulin
Hymenoptera	Family Apidae (honeybee, bumblebee), Vespidae (yellow jacket, hornet, wasp), Formicidae (fire ant)
Latex	Proteins in natural rubber latex; additives used in processing latex
Vaccines	Proteins cross-reactive with egg; hydrolyzed gelatin, sorbitol, neomycin
Blood components	Packed red blood cells
Biological fluids	Human seminal fluid
Exercise	Ingestion of certain foods prior to exercise
Idiopathic	Diagnosis of exclusion

PEARL

Be particularly vigilant in patients with a history of bronchospasm (eg, asthma, reactive airway disease) in whom fatal anaphylactic reactions are more likely.

Epinephrine

Epinephrine should be considered a second "A" (adrenaline) in the "ABC" prioritization of anaphylaxis management. Aggressive treatment with appropriate doses and routes of epinephrine is universally recommended as first-line therapy. Poor outcomes most often are associated with failed or delayed administration.[8] Epinephrine has numerous identifiable physiological benefits in the treatment of anaphylaxis (*Table 21-8*), although particular indications and dosing regimens are a frequent source of confusion.[22] Practitioners should err on the side of injecting epinephrine sooner except possibly in patients with clearly mild allergic symptoms that do not appear to be progressing.

Generally, epinephrine is given intramuscularly in the anterolateral thigh. The intramuscular route is preferred over subcutaneous administration regardless of the patient's age.[22] Subcutaneous absorption is highly dependent on cutaneous blood flow, which can be compromised in anaphylaxis and further aggravated by epinephrine's potent local vasoconstrictor activity, leading to slow and erratic absorption.[23,24] The typical dose for intramuscular administration is 0.01 mg/kg, up to a maximum of 0.2 to 0.5 mg (maximum 0.3 mg for children) of a 1:1,000 dilution, repeated every 5 minutes as needed.[25]

Great caution should be exercised when using IV

TABLE 21-4. Risk Factors for Severe, Near-Fatal, and Fatal Anaphylaxis[4]

Peanut or tree nut allergy
Preexisting respiratory or cardiovascular disease
Asthma
Delayed administration of epinephrine
Previous biphasic anaphylactic reactions
Advanced age
Mast cell disorders

epinephrine to manage anaphylaxis. Major adverse events can occur when the drug is administered too rapidly or in excessive dosages.[26-30] Intravenous epinephrine has been associated with the induction of fatal cardiac arrhythmias, myocardial infarction, and intracranial hemorrhage; however, other factors related to the underlying pathophysiological process (eg, hypoxia, acidosis, effects of inflammatory mediators) may be responsible for the observed complications.[27-31] The IV route should be reserved for cases of severe cardiovascular compromise (ie, a profound decrease in peripheral perfusion that would significantly hamper intramuscular absorption) or when repeated intramuscular dosing (eg, 2 or 3 doses) fails to alleviate symptoms.

A firm intravenous dose cannot be recommended; the appropriate quantity depends on the severity of the episode and should be titrated to response. A frequently recommended adult intravenous dosing regimen uses a 1:100,000 epinephrine solution, slowly infusing 100 mcg (0.1 mg) over 5 to 10 minutes *(Table 21-9)*.[17,25,32] During anaphylaxis, 5- to 10-mcg IV bolus doses have been suggested for treating hypotension and 100- to 500-mcg IV boluses have been suggested for adults with severe cardiovascular collapse.[33] A continuous IV epinephrine infusion is a reasonable option (1–10 mcg/min, titrated to response; pediatric patients, 0.1–2 mcg/kg/min).[34] It is paramount to double check the dosage to avoid a medication error catastrophe.

Whenever the intravenous route is required, a continuous low-dose infusion is likely the safest and most effective approach for patients of any age, as the dose can be titrated to desired effect while minimizing the potential for accidental administration of large or concentrated bolus doses.[2] There are, however, very few controlled studies to support these recommendations.[35]

Although there is a paucity of controlled data to adequately address safety concerns, some lessons can be gleaned from experience with the use of epinephrine for asthma.[26,27] These data should not be overly generalized, but they suggest a more favorable safety profile for epinephrine than is routinely acknowledged, particularly when the agent is administered via non-IV routes. Younger patients have an even more attractive risk-benefit profile for the drug in general, as they are likely to tolerate most complications better than adults.

PEARL

For pediatric patients, double-check weight-based dosages of intravenous epinephrine to avoid a medication error catastrophe.

Of concern to many practitioners is the administration of the medication to higher-risk patients, particularly those who

TABLE 21-5. Differential Diagnoses

Category	Example(s)
Anaphylactic and anaphylactoid reactions	Reactions to exogenously administered agents Related to physical factors (exercise, cold, heat, sunlight) Idiopathic
Vasopressor reactions	Neurocardiogenic reaction
Other forms of shock	Hemorrhagic Cardiogenic Endotoxic
"Flush" syndromes	Carcinoid Postmenopausal Medullary carcinoma of the thyroid
"Restaurant" syndromes	Monosodium glutamate (MSG) reaction Scombroid poisoning
Excess endogenous production of histamine syndromes	Systemic mastocytosis Urticaria pigmentosa Basophilic leukemia Acute promyelocytic leukemia
Nonorganic disease	Panic attack Munchausen stridor Vocal cord dysfunction syndrome Globus hystericus
Miscellaneous	Angiotensin-converting enzyme (ACE); inhibitor/angiotensin receptor blocker (ARB)-associated angioedema Hereditary angioedema Pheochromocytoma

Adapted from: Lieberman P. Anaphylaxis and anaphylactoid reactions. In: Adkinson NF Jr, Yunginer JW, Busse WW, et al, eds. *Middleton's Allergic Principles and Practice*. 6th ed. St Louis, MO: Mosby-Yearbook; 2003:1510. Copyright 2003. Used with permission from Elsevier.

TABLE 21-6. Symptom Frequency[17]

	Sign/Symptom	Frequency (%)*
Cutaneous	Overall Urticaria and angioedema Flushing Pruritus without rash	90 85–90 45–55 2–5
Respiratory	Overall Dyspnea, wheeze Upper airway angioedema Rhinitis	40–60 45–50 50–60 15–20
Cardiovascular	Dizziness, syncope, hypotension	30–35
Abdominal	Nausea, vomiting, diarrhea, cramping	25–30
Miscellaneous	Headache Substernal pain Seizure	5–8 4–6 1–2

Data based on a compilation of the records of 1,865 patients.
*Percentages are approximate.

TABLE 21-7. Common Medications Used in the Treatment of Anaphylaxis

Agent	PEDIATRIC Route	Dosage	ADULT Route	Dosage
Epinephrine	IM IV	0.01 mg/kg (maximum 0.3 mg per dose) 0.1–2 mcg/kg/min infusion	IM IV	0.3–0.5 mg every 5 min as needed 100 mcg of 1:100,000 dilution over 5–10 min *OR* Continuous IV infusion of 1–10 mcg/min
H_1 antihistamine	IV/IM	Diphenhydramine, 1 mg/kg (maximum 50 mg)	IV/IM	Diphenhydramine, 25–50 mg
H_2 antihistamine	IV	Ranitidine, 1 mg/kg (maximum 50 mg)	IV	Ranitidine, 50 mg
Corticosteroid	IV	Methylprednisolone, 1–2 mg/kg (maximum 125 mg)	IV	Methylprednisolone, 125 mg
Bronchodilator	Nebulized	Albuterol, 1.25–2.5 mg per dose, repeat as needed	Nebulized	Albuterol, 2.5 mg per dose, repeat as needed

are elderly or have comorbid conditions such as hypertension, coronary artery disease, or cerebrovascular disease. Such decisions must be evaluated on a case-by-case basis, with a rapid weighing of benefits against potential risks. Critical to this equation is the fact that anaphylaxis is a life-threatening emergency and, as such, is associated with morbidity and mortality in these higher-risk cases. The potential risks associated with epinephrine need to be balanced against the danger of withholding the most critical therapy in anaphylaxis management.

Antihistamines

Antihistamines should never be utilized in lieu of epinephrine in the management of anaphylaxis. Although H_1 antihistamines are commonly used in allergic emergencies, there is some debate over their benefit in these scenarios.[36] Less-sedating H_1 antagonists such as cetirizine (Zyrtec) and loratadine (Claritin) may be used as a substitute for oral diphenhydramine in those with milder allergic symptoms; however, these agents have no role in the crashing patient because they are not available for intravenous use in the US.

Although the precise role of H_2 antagonists in the treatment of allergic emergencies has yet to be completely elucidated, they are recommended due to their potential benefits and low propensity for adverse events.[36-38] There is no specific evidence regarding the superiority of one particular H_2 antihistamine, but agents other than cimetidine might be preferable to avoid effects on the cytochrome P450 system.[39]

TABLE 21-8. Physiological Effects of Epinephrine in Anaphylaxis

Receptor	Effect
Alpha	Increased peripheral vascular resistance Reversal of peripheral vasodilation Decreased angioedema and urticaria
$Beta_1$	Positive cardiac inotropic effects Positive cardiac chronotropic effects
$Beta_2$	Bronchodilation Increased intracellular cAMP production (reduces inflammatory mediator production/release from mast cells and basophils)

Corticosteroids

Corticosteroids traditionally have been used as adjuncts in the management of anaphylaxis. Although the effects of these agents have never been validated in controlled trials, their administration is warranted in allergic emergencies (particularly severe cases) because of their known benefits in the treatment of asthma and other allergic diseases.[40] The theoretical objective of corticosteroid therapy is to temper the continued intracellular synthesis and release of potent proinflammatory mediators. This may blunt — although not necessarily prevent — biphasic or multiphasic anaphylaxis. In practice, the intravenous route often is preferred. There is no evidence to support any specific dose, route of administration, or particular formulation.

Inhaled Bronchodilators

Nebulized inhaled bronchodilators (eg, albuterol sulfate) may be continuously or intermittently used for the treatment of anaphylaxis-induced bronchospasm.

PEARL

Ventilator management of intubated anaphylaxis patients can be challenging. It is prudent to employ low respiratory rates and prolonged expiratory times in cases of significant bronchospasm. Barotrauma should be strongly considered, along with other causes, in the ventilated anaphylaxis patient with acute decompensation.

Glucagon; Alternative Vasopressors

Glucagon can have a role in treating anaphylaxis refractory to standard therapy, especially in the case of coexisting beta-adrenergic receptor blockade.[41] Epinephrine stimulates intracellular cyclic AMP (cAMP) production through interactions with beta-adrenergic receptors. Glucagon exerts its intracellular effects by mediating cAMP production independent of the adrenergic system.[42] Despite limited evidence, glucagon might benefit patients who are taking beta blockers when all other treatments have failed.[43] The initial pediatric bolus dose is 20 to 30 mcg/kg (maximum 1 mg).[17] The recommended adult dose is 1 to 5 mg IV over 5 minutes, followed by a continuous infusion of 5 to 15 mcg/min titrated to clinical response.[17] Airway protection should be considered prior to infusion, as glucagon can induce vomiting.

Adjunctive vasopressor agents should be considered in the event that epinephrine and volume expansion fail to maintain adequate blood pressure or perfusion. In such cases, norepinephrine, dopamine, or vasopressin should be considered.

Disposition

One of the greatest challenges in treating patients with allergic emergencies is determining their appropriate disposition *(Table 21-10)*. Patients with severe reactions (eg, hypotension or airway involvement) or a slow response to standard therapies requires admission for continued monitoring. On the other end of the spectrum, those with clearly mild reactions may be safely discharged. Most patients fall somewhere in between, making such decisions more difficult.

TABLE 21-9. Recommended Dilution of Epinephrine for Intravenous Use in Adult Patients with Anaphylaxis[28]

Push-dose Epinephrine
Create 10 mL of a 1:100,000 epinephrine dilution.
Add 0.1 mg (0.1 mL) of a 1:1,000 epinephrine solution to 9.9 mL normal saline or add 0.1 mg (1 mL) of 1:10,000 epinephrine solution to 9 mL normal saline. Resulting solution = 0.1 mg of epinephrine (100 mcg) in 10 mL = 10 mcg/mL
Then administer 10 mL of a 1:100,000 epinephrine solution over 5–10 minutes. 100 mcg over 5–10 minutes = 10–20 mcg/min
Continuous Epinephrine Infusion
Create 1 L of a 1:1,000,000 epinephrine dilution.
Add 1 mg (1 mL) of a 1:1,000 epinephrine solution to 1 L of 5% dextrose in water (or 1 L of normal saline). Resulting solution = 1 mg epinephrine (1,000 mcg) in 1 L = 1 mcg/mL
Then infuse at a rate of 1 mcg/min, titrated to response to a maximum dose of 10 mcg/min.

It is critical to recognize the potential for recurrent (biphasic or multiphasic) anaphylaxis, which is defined as the reappearance of allergic phenomena following the complete resolution of the original reaction, without reexposure to the inciting allergen. Recurrence can involve only nuisance-level symptoms or more ominous physiological derangements, including respiratory compromise and hemodynamic instability. While the rate of recurrence has been reported to be as high as 20%, the actual rate of clinically significant recurrence is likely much lower than this, though manifestations can be severe and can recur as long as 72 hours after the inciting event.[44,45]

Corticosteroid administration does not eliminate the possibility of recurrence. Clinically important biphasic reactions during the index or subsequent emergency department visits are very rare.[46] Protracted (prolonged or refractory) anaphylaxis has also been reported.[47] Patients with this condition can present with refractory hypotension or bronchospasm, posing unique challenges in terms of circulatory support and ventilator management, respectively.

Although there is no firmly established observation time following an episode of anaphylaxis, clinicians should maintain a low threshold for prolonged observation, particularly when high-risk features (eg, asthma, nut allergies) are present. A minimum of several hours following treatment is reasonable for mild episodes, and at least 24 hours of observation is prudent for severe cases or patients with high-risk or otherwise troubling features. Recent consensus statements recommend 4 to 8 hours for most patients, with more prolonged times or admission for those with severe or refractory symptoms or reactive airway disease.[24]

PEARL

Many patients with initially mild symptoms can exhibit life-threatening anaphylaxis after a second exposure to the same allergic trigger.

Postreaction Treatment

There is little disagreement that epinephrine self-administration devices should be prescribed for individuals with a history of anaphylaxis involving respiratory distress or shock and who cannot reliably avoid the triggering allergen.[48] The immediate availability of self-injectable epinephrine is important in the initial 72-hour period for the treatment of recurrent anaphylaxis induced by *any* allergen. A more difficult decision involves patients who experienced only mild symptoms after exposure.[49] An initial episode, no matter how innocuous, does not predict the severity of future events, particularly in the case of food-induced allergy.[50] Approximately 50% of patients with initially mild symptoms exhibit life-threatening anaphylaxis after a second exposure to the same allergic trigger.[51] In a small percentage of patients, the symptoms are more severe than during the initial event.[52]

TABLE 21-10. Considerations for Patient Disposition

Factor	Examples of High-Risk Features
Presenting symptom severity	Initially severe symptoms are an important consideration even if symptoms have improved (or resolved) following the initiation of treatment.
Anaphylaxis history	Any history of severe, protracted, biphasic or recurrent anaphylaxis
Particular allergen	Nut (peanut, tree nuts) reactions are associated with high morbidity and mortality.
Medical comorbidities	Conditions such as asthma (particularly high morbidity and mortality rates in the setting of anaphylaxis), other respiratory diseases, cardiovascular disease, renal disease (at risk for fluid overload with volume resuscitation), or mast cell disorders
Baseline medications	Particularly, use of beta-adrenergic blockers (including ophthalmic preparations)
Access to medical care	Distant from or having reduced access to medical care
Age	Patients at extremes of age have reduced compensatory abilities; adolescents may be at risk for severe/fatal anaphylaxis because of compliance issues.
Home situation	Patients who live alone; barriers to understanding discharge instructions and self-care

Patients, caretakers, and teachers should be instructed regarding the proper use of epinephrine delivery devices; optimally, patients should leave the emergency department with two devices in hand. Epinephrine commonly is formulated in premeasured 0.3-mg or 0.15-mg dosage options *(Table 21-11)*.[11] Great care must be exercised if the decision is made to teach parents how to draw up a dose of the drug for children weighing less than 10 kg. Evidence has demonstrated that caretakers have significant difficulty administering appropriate doses.[53]

Other recommended postreaction treatments include oral H_1/H_2 antihistamines and corticosteroids. Oral medications can be continued for at least 72 hours, although there is no specific evidence to support a firm recommendation.[54]

Conclusion

Anaphylactic reactions can be life-threatening and are almost always unanticipated. Any delay in the recognition of initial signs and symptoms can result in a poor outcome. Even when the symptoms are initially mild, the potential for progression to airway obstruction or vascular collapse must be appreciated and treatment must be swiftly and aggressively initiated. Epinephrine is the cornerstone of therapy; second-line pharmacotherapies include H_1/H_2 antihistamines and corticosteroids. Disposition from the emergency department is fraught with potential dangers. Prolonged observation is prudent following significant reactions and for patients with other high-risk features, particularly asthma or nut (eg, peanut, tree nut) allergies. Ensuring that patients have continuous access to and familiarity with their epinephrine self-administration device is critical to preventing morbidity and mortality.

TABLE 21-11. Weight-Based Epinephrine Self-Administration Device Selection

Weight (kg)	Epinephrine Dose/Device
<10	Ampule/needle/syringe administration
10–25	0.15-mg EpiPen Jr.
>25	0.3-mg EpiPen

REFERENCES

1. Simons FER, Ardusso LRF, Bilo MB, et al. World Allergy Organization guidelines for the assessment and management of anaphylaxis. *World Allergy Organ J.* 2011;4(2):13-37.
2. Sampson HA, Munoz-Furlong A, Campbell RL, et al. Second symposium on the definition and management of anaphylaxis: summary report – Second National Institute of Allergy and Infectious Disease/Food Allergy and Anaphylaxis Network symposium. *J Allergy Clin Immunol.* 2006;117(2):391-397.
3. Campbell RL, Hagan JB, Manivannan V, et al. Evaluation of the National Institute of Allergy and Infectious Disease/Food Allergy & Anaphylaxis Network criteria for the diagnosis of anaphylaxis in emergency department patients. *J Allergy Clin Immunol.* 2012;129(3):748-752.
4. Campbell RL, Li JTC, Nicklas RA, et al. Emergency department diagnosis and treatment of anaphylaxis: a practice parameter. *Ann Allergy Asthma Immunol.* 2014;113:599-608.
5. Johansson SG, Bieber T, Dahl R, et al. Revised nomenclature for allergy for global use: report of the Nomenclature Review Committee of the World Allergy Organization, October 2003. *J Allergy Clin Immunol.* 2004;113(5):832-836.
6. Sampson HA. Anaphylaxis and emergency treatment. *Pediatrics.* 2003;111:1601-1608.
7. Braganza SC, Acworth JP, Mckinnon DRL, et al. Paediatric emergency department anaphylaxis: different patterns from adults. *Arch Dis Child.* 2006;91:159-163.
8. Sampson HA, Mendelson L, Rosen JP. Fatal and near-fatal anaphylactic reactions to food in children and adolescents. *N Engl J Med.* 1992;327:380-384.
9. Roberts G, Patel N, Levi-Schaffer F, et al. Food allergy as a risk factor for life-threatening asthma in childhood: a case-controlled study. *J Allergy Clin Immunol.* 2003;112(1):168-174.
10. American College of Allergy, Asthma & Immunology. Food allergy: a practice parameter. *Ann Allergy Asthma Immunol.* 2006;96:S1-S68.
11. Sicherer SH, Simons FER, Section on Allergy and Immunology, American Academy of Pediatrics. Self-injectable epinephrine for first-aid management of anaphylaxis. *Pediatrics.* 2007;119(3):638-646.
12. Simons KJ, Simons FER. Epinephrine and its use in anaphylaxis: current issues. *Curr Opin Allergy Clin Immunol.* 2010;10(4):354-361.
13. Sampson HA. Anaphylaxis: persistent enigma. *Emerg Med Australas.* 2006;18:101-102.
14. Novembre E, Cianferoni A, Bernardini R, et al. Anaphylaxis in children: clinical and allergologic features. *Pediatrics.* 1998;101:e8.
15. Bock SA, Munoz-Furlong A, Sampson HA. Fatalities due to anaphylactic reactions to foods. *J Allergy Clin Immunol.* 2001;107:191-193.
16. Sampson HA, Munoz-Furlong A, Bock SA, et al. Symposium on the definition and management of anaphylaxis: summary report. *J Allergy Clin Immunol.* 2005;115(3):584-591.
17. Joint Task Force on Practice Parameters for the American Academy of Allergy, Asthma & Immunology; the American College of Allergy, Asthma & Immunology; and the Joint Council of Allergy, Asthma & Immunology. The diagnosis and management of anaphylaxis: an updated practice parameter. *J Allergy Clin Immunol.* 2005;115:S483-S523.
18. Fisher MM. Clinical observations on the pathophysiology and treatment of anaphylactic cardiovascular collapse. *Anaesth Intensive Care.* 1986;14:17-21.
19. Viner NA, Rhamy RK. Anaphylaxis manifested by hypotension alone. *J Urol.* 1975;113:108-110.
20. Soreide E, Buxrud T, Harboe S. Severe anaphylactic reactions outside hospital: etiology, symptoms and treatment. *Acta Anaesthesiol Scand.* 1988;32:339-342.

KEY POINTS

1. Risk factors for fatal anaphylaxis include a history of asthma or bronchospasm, a history of nut allergy (peanut, tree nuts), delayed administration of epinephrine, use of beta-adrenergic blockers or ACE inhibitors, and adolescent age.
2. Patients who initially present with mild symptoms and appear to be stable can deteriorate rapidly.
3. Cutaneous findings (eg, urticaria or flushing) might be entirely absent.
4. Involvement of the respiratory or cardiovascular system distinguishes anaphylaxis from other allergic phenomena.
5. Up to 35% of the circulating blood volume can be lost within 10 minutes after the onset of anaphylaxis, primarily from third spacing.
6. Epinephrine is the single most important and sole first-line pharmacological agent for the treatment of anaphylaxis. It should be promptly administered to any patient with anaphylaxis.
7. Current guidelines recommend intramuscular epinephrine administration into the anterolateral thigh. To save vital time in the management of a rapidly decompensating patient, consider the use of an autoinjector unit (eg, EpiPen or Auvi-Q).
8. Administer IV epinephrine for severe cardiovascular compromise or when repeated intramuscular doses have failed.
9. Anaphylaxis is a life-threatening emergency with inherent morbidity and mortality. Therefore, the risks of epinephrine administration must be balanced against the risks of withholding the most critical pharmacotherapy available.
10. **Epinephrine**
    - Undisputed first-line agent and treatment of choice for anaphylaxis; despite this status, the drug remains underutilized.
    - Intramuscular administration in the anterolateral thigh is preferred. Reserve intravenous administration for patients in extremis and unresponsive to repeated intramuscular dosages and those in profound shock.
    - There are no absolute contraindications; exercise caution in patients taking beta-adrenergic blockers and in pregnant patients.
11. **Antihistamines**
    - Adjunctive therapy for anaphylaxis
    - Should never be used as a substitute for epinephrine
    - Combined H_1 + H_2 blockade is preferable.
12. **Corticosteroids**
    - Adjunctive therapy for anaphylaxis
    - Should never be used as a substitute for epinephrine
    - Possible role in mitigating recurrent anaphylaxis

21. Sheikh A, Shehata A, Brown SGA, et al. Adrenaline for the treatment of anaphylaxis: Cochrane systematic review. *Allergy.* 2009;64:204-212.
22. Lieberman P. Use of epinephrine in the treatment of anaphylaxis. *Curr Opin Allergy Clin Immunol.* 2003;3:313-318.
23. Simons FER, Roberts JR, Gu X, et al. Epinephrine absorption in children with a history of anaphylaxis. *J Allergy Clin Immunol.* 1998;101:33-37.
24. Simons FER, Gu X, Simons KJ. Epinephrine absorption in adults: intramuscular versus subcutaneous injection. *J Allergy Clin Immunol.* 2001;108:871-873.
25. Soar J, Deakin CD, Nolan JP, et al. European Resuscitation Council Guidelines for Resuscitation 2005: Section 7. Cardiac arrest in special circumstances. *Resuscitation.* 2005;67(suppl 1):S135-S170.
26. McLean-Tooke APC, Bethune CA, Fay AC, et al. Adrenaline in the treatment of anaphylaxis: what is the evidence? *BMJ.* 2003;327:1332-1335.
27. Johnston SL, Unsworth J, Gompels MM. Adrenaline given outside the context of life threatening allergic reactions. *BMJ.* 2003;326:589-590.
28. Douglass JA, O'Hehir RE. Adrenaline and non-life threatening allergic reactions. *BMJ.* 2003;327:226-227.
29. Karch SB. Coronary artery spasm induced by intravenous epinephrine overdose. *Ann Emerg Med.* 1989;7:485-488.
30. Ellis AK, Day JH. The role of epinephrine in the treatment of anaphylaxis. *Curr Allergy Asthma Rep.* 2003;3:11-14.
31. Brown AF. Intramuscular or intravenous adrenaline in acute, severe anaphylaxis? *J Accid Emerg Med.* 2000;17:152-155.
32. Barach EM, Nowak RM, Lee TG, et al. Epinephrine for treatment of anaphylactic shock. *JAMA.* 1984;251:2118-2122.
33. Hepner DL, Castells MC. Anaphylaxis during the perioperative period. *Anesth Analg.* 2003;97:1381-1395.
34. Liberman DB, Teach SJ. Management of anaphylaxis in children. *Pediatr Emerg Care.* 2008;24:861-866.
35. Brown SGA, Blackman KE, Stenlake V, et al. Insect sting anaphylaxis; prospective evaluation of treatment with intravenous adrenaline and volume resuscitation. *Emerg Med J.* 2004;21:149-154.
36. Sheikh A, Ten Broek V, Brown SG, et al. H1-antihistamines for the treatment of anaphylaxis: Cochrane systematic review. *Allergy.* 2007;62:830-837.
37. Lin RY, Curry A, Pesola G, et al. Improved outcomes in patients with acute allergic syndromes who are treated with combined H1 and H2 antagonists. *Ann Emerg Med.* 2000;36:462-468.
38. Runge JW, Martinez JC, Caravati EM, et al. Histamine antagonists in the treatment of allergic reactions. *Ann Emerg Med.* 1992;21:237-242.
39. Shannon M. Drug-drug interactions and the cytochrome P450 system: an update. *Pediatr Emerg Care.* 1997;13:350-353.
40. Choo KJ, Simons FE, Sheikh A. Glucocorticoids for the treatment of anaphylaxis. *Cochrane Database Syst Rev.* 2012 Apr 18;4:CD007596.
41. Pollack CV. Utility of glucagon in the emergency department. *J Emerg Med.* 1993;11:195-205.
42. Sherman MS, Lazar EJ, Eichacker P. A bronchodilator action of glucagon. *J Allergy Clin Immunol.* 1988;81:908-911.
43. Thomas M, Crawford I. Best evidence topic reports: glucagon infusion in refractory anaphylactic shock in patients on beta-blockers. *Emerg Med J.* 2005;22:272-276.
44. Lieberman P. Biphasic anaphylaxis. *Ann Allergy Asthma Immunol.* 2005;95:217-226.
45. Lee S, Bellolio F, Hess EP, et al. Time of onset and predictors of biphasic anaphylactic reactions: a systematic review and meta-analysis. *J Allergy Clin Immunol Pract.* 2015;3(3):408-416.el-e2.
46. Grunau BE, Li J, Yi TW, et al. Incidence of clinically important biphasic reactions in emergency department patients with allergic reactions or anaphylaxis. *Ann Emerg Med.* 2014;63:6:736-744.
47. Stark BJ, Sullivan TJ. Biphasic and protracted anaphylaxis. *J Allergy Clin Immunol.* 1986;78(1 Part 1):76-83.
48. Sheikh A, Simons FE, Barbour V, et al. Adrenaline auto-injectors for the treatment of anaphylaxis with and without cardiovascular collapse in the community. *Cochrane Database Syst Rev.* 2012 Aug 15;8:CD008935.
49. Sicherer SH, Simons ER. Quandaries in prescribing an emergency action plan and self-injectable epinephrine for first-aid management of anaphylaxis in the community. *J Allergy Clin Immunol.* 2005;115:575-583.
50. Kumar A, Teuber SS, Gershwin ME. Why do people die of anaphylaxis? A clinical review. *Clin Devel Immunol.* 2005;12:281-287.
51. Vander Leek TK, Liu AH, Stefanski K, et al. The natural history of peanut allergy in young children and its association with serum peanut-specific IgE. *J Pediatr.* 2000;137:749-755.
52. Smit DV, Cameron PA, Rainer TH. Anaphylaxis presentations to an emergency department in Hong Kong: incidence and predictors of biphasic reactions. *J Emerg Med.* 2005;28:381-388.
53. Simons FER, Chan ES, Cu X, et al. Epinephrine for out-of-hospital (first-aid) treatment of anaphylaxis in infants: is the ampule/needle/syringe method practical? *J Allergy Clin Immunol.* 2001;108:1040-1044.
54. Brown AFT. Therapeutic controversies in the management of acute anaphylaxis. *J Accid Emerg Med.* 1998;15:89-95.

Bedside Ultrasonography

22

IN THIS CHAPTER

- Cardiac assessment
- Inferior vena cava evaluation
- Lung examination
- Abdominal aorta examination
- Ultrasound-guided fluid management
- Cardiac arrest evaluation

Justin O. Cook, Lisa D. Mills, and Daniel R. Mantuani

Bedside or point-of-care ultrasonography contributes a wealth of clinical information to the emergency department assessment of the undifferentiated, critically ill patient. Benefits of this imaging modality and focused echocardiography include a shorter time to diagnosis, increased accuracy, and the ability to evaluate a patient's response to resuscitation (when using serial examinations).[1-3]

Several approaches to the assessment of critically ill patients in the emergency department and intensive care unit using ultrasonography have been described. The most notable include the echo-guided life support (EGLS) algorithm, the undifferentiated hypotension protocol (UHP), the CORE scan, the FALLS protocol, the BLEEP protocol, and the rapid ultrasound in shock (RUSH) protocol.[4-9]

Cardiac Examination

Echocardiography, the most technically challenging bedside ultrasound application, can be extremely valuable in the acute setting. The emergency physician's immediate goals should be to detect pericardial tamponade, estimate left ventricular contractility, and evaluate for acute right ventricular strain. The accuracy of these assessments increases with focused training.[10-13]

Echocardiographical Technique

Rapid bedside echocardiography consists of any of three basic views: parasternal, subxiphoid or subcostal (familiar to most as the cardiac view traditionally employed in the focused assessment with sonography for trauma [FAST] exam), and apical. The parasternal views are further divided into long-axis (PSLAX) and short-axis (PSSAX). A single window provides limited information and can be influenced by the clinical scenario; it is optimal to obtain multiple views. All basic echocardiography can be performed with a microconvex or curvilinear transducer. The microconvex transducer is advantageous because it can fit between rib spaces and is supported by cardiac-specific software.

Begin with the patient in a supine position. The PSLAX view is obtained by placing the curvilinear or microconvex transducer in the left parasternal area at approximately the fourth rib interspace, with the transducer marker pointing toward the patient's right shoulder or left hip. (The screen indicator is located on the upper left side of the screen.) These are both common orientations in emergency medicine echocardiography and differ from standard cardiology views, which align probe markers with the patient's left shoulder. Oriented in this manner, the window reveals the left ventricle deep to the smaller right ventricle, with the aortic outflow tract to the left side of the screen and the mitral valve at the center of the image *(Figure 22-1)*. The bright white (hyperechoic) stripe beneath the wall of the left ventricle is the pericardium. The round, dark structure beneath the pericardium is the descending thoracic aorta, a key landmark for determining the location of a fluid collection *(Figures 22-1 and 22-2)*.

From here, the PSSAX view can be obtained by rotating the probe 90 degrees, pointing it toward the patient's left shoulder. This gives a view of the left ventricle in cross-section. The subxiphoid or subcostal view *(Figure 22-3)* uses the liver as an acoustic window to visualize the heart, as in the FAST exam. Although this view is particularly valuable in assessing for pericardial effusion, it has limited utility in estimating ejection fraction.

Although the apical view yields a rather complete and anatomically familiar representation of the heart, it can be the most difficult of the three primary windows to obtain consistently.[14] Place the transducer at the point of maximal impulse (often slightly inferolateral to the left nipple) with the patient in the left lateral decubitus position to obtain the apical four-chamber view *(Figure 22-4)*. Direct the indicator toward the bed, rotating toward the left axilla to sharpen the image.

Angle the entire transducer to about 45 degrees, with the cord tilted toward the patient's feet and aligned with the long axis of the left ventricle.

Pericardial Effusion

The detection of a hemodynamically significant pericardial effusion may be the most important and timely diagnostic appraisal to be made in a critically ill patient. Tamponade can cause sudden cardiac collapse and must be promptly managed. The signs and symptoms of pericardial effusion (and even tamponade) may be clinically occult. The incidence of the abnormality in patients presenting with dyspnea can be as high as 14%; roughly 4% of emergency department patients with dyspnea have symptomatic effusions.[15] The finding of a pericardial effusion in a dyspneic or hemodynamically compromised patient must immediately raise concerns for cardiac tamponade. The physician can synthesize the clinical picture with echocardiographic findings to determine the significance of this abnormality.

FIGURE 22-1. PSLAX Long-Axis View

Probe marker *(PM)* at upper left side of screen. Left ventricle *(LV)*, right ventricle *(RV)*, pericardial stripe *(PS)*, aortic outflow tract *(Ao)*, mitral valve *(MV)*, descending thoracic aorta *(DTA)*.

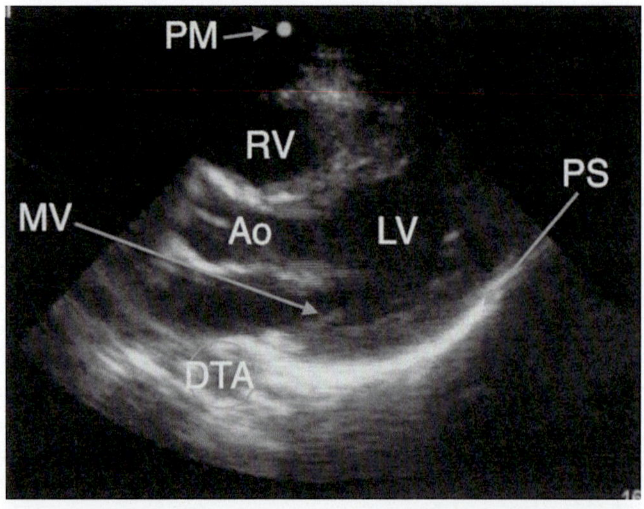

FIGURE 22-2. PSLAX View

The descending thoracic aorta *(arrow)* can be seen in cross-section.

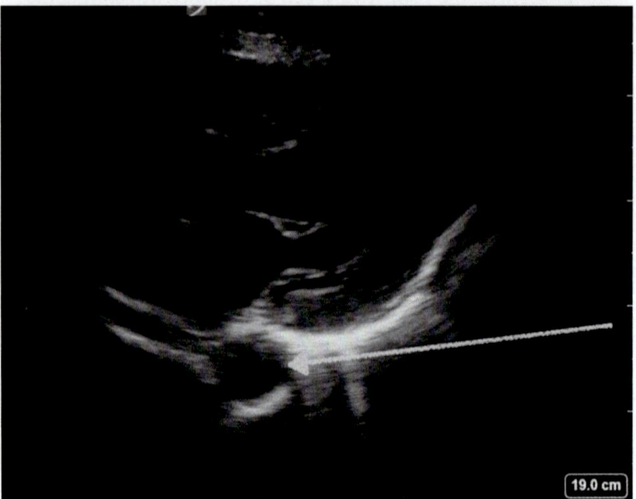

An effusion is likely to be dependent. In the PSLAX view, this abnormality manifests as a black (anechoic) stripe posterior (far field) to the left ventricle but anterior (near field) to the bright, hyperechoic stripe of the pericardium. Such a dark fluid collection *posterior* (far field) to the pericardial stripe indicates a pleural effusion, a "masquerader" of pericardial effusion. In the subxiphoid view, an effusion often appears as an anechoic stripe anterior (near field) between the liver and the right ventricle and is surrounded by the bright white of the pericardium. Larger accumulations can be seen in both the near and far fields surrounding the myocardium in the parasternal *(Figure 22-5)* or subxiphoid views.

PEARL

Beware of potential false-positive results. In both the PSLAX and subxiphoid views, an anterior hazy stripe may be a fat pad (a normal finding). Generally, an effusion is dark (if it is fresh blood) or has a mixed density (if it contains clotted blood).

Tamponade is most readily seen as right ventricular collapse in diastole, often appearing as a "bowing" or inward concavity of the right ventricular free wall; this can be appreciated in the PSLAX view. In other views, right atrial collapse in systole also can indicate tamponade. Impending tamponade is suggested by a "plethoric" inferior vena cava (IVC) (ie, an IVC that shows no change in caliber with spontaneous respiration). This finding is expected in patients with elevated right-sided filling pressures, underscoring the importance of pairing the cardiac and IVC examinations.

Ejection Fraction

Left ventricular function should be assessed in critically ill patients because it can reveal the cause of the illness and provide prognostic information to guide fluid therapy.[2,4,5,9,16] The general trend in emergency medicine is to use qualitative rather than quantitative assessments of left ventricular function with a goal of classifying the ejection as poor, normal, or hyperdynamic.[17] Depressed left ventricular function in a patient with acute decompensated heart failure is easily recognizable on bedside ultrasound. During sepsis, cardiac dysfunction can develop in those who had normal cardiac function at baseline.[18] These patients should be identified early, as they are often more challenging to manage with fluid therapy. Fluid resuscitation guided by echocardiographic findings is endorsed in the *Surviving Sepsis Campaign* protocol.[19] The use of transthoracic echocardiography is appropriate for evaluating hypotension; however, its role in assessing fluid status in the acute setting is uncertain.[20]

The PSLAX view is the most commonly used window for estimating left ventricular function. With real-time visualization of the contracting ventricle in the PSLAX view, the physician can reasonably estimate ejection fraction, categorizing its function among three general appearances — normal, depressed, or hyperdynamic. In addition, ventricular filling can be assessed as a marker of volume status.

Most clinicians prefer to estimate ejection fraction by visually assessing the left ventricle, as opposed to eliciting a more time-consuming series of measurements from static images or "cine" extrapolations.[17] Ejection fraction is normal when the septal and posterior walls (those most readily seen in the PSLAX view) contract at least 50% in systole relative to their position in diastole (ie, the black cavity within the gray walls of the left ventricle decreases by approximately 50%). In a depressed (hypodynamic) heart, the walls of the left ventricle close significantly less than 50% during systole *(Figure 22-6)*. The left ventricle is described as hyperdynamic when its walls appear to nearly touch in systole and are relatively small compared with the chamber itself (indicating poor ventricular filling). Additional information about contractility and specific wall motion abnormalities can be obtained in the PSSAX view.

Optimal views can be hindered by the patient's habitus or the cause of the critical illness. In such instances and if a PSLAX view can be obtained, the movement of the mitral valve during diastole roughly estimates the left ventricular ejection fraction. An anterior mitral valve leaflet that "slaps" up against the septum usually indicates normal left ventricular function. An anterior mitral valve leaflet that does not come closer than 7 mm to the ventricular septum represents significant depression. This measurement can be easily obtained by less-experienced sonographers and correlates well with visual estimates of left ventricular ejection fraction made by those well versed in echocardiography.[21]

Cardiac function should be assessed early in the resuscitation of the hypotensive patient. For a significantly depressed ejection fraction, especially when pulmonary edema is evident, aggressive fluid resuscitation should be limited and applied with close observation. Consider vasopressor therapy and the early addition of inotropic agents to support cardiac and pulmonary function. A cardiology consultation and other interventions (eg, balloon pump or emergent cardiac catheterization) should be considered based on clinical features, laboratory data, the electrocardiogram (ECG), and resource availability. The finding of a hyperdynamic heart is particularly valuable, as it suggests that the patient might benefit from volume resuscitation.

Dynamic measurements of ventricular ejection fraction and cardiac output generally are beyond the limited echocardiographic studies performed in the acute setting; however, they are described in this chapter to provide a complete scope of practice.

FIGURE 22-3. Subxiphoid View of the Heart

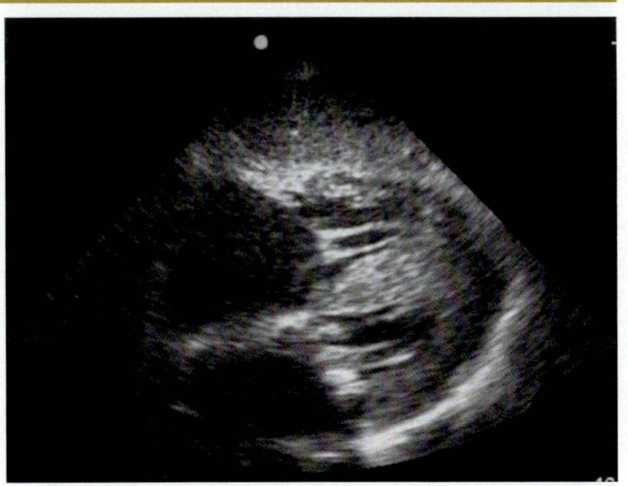

FIGURE 22-4. Apical View of the Heart

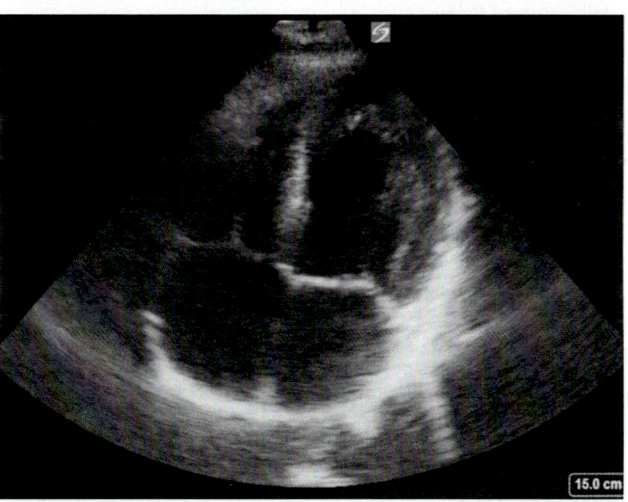

FIGURE 22-5. Pericardial Effusion (PSLAX View)

Note that fluid collects posteriorly in the dependent area, the most common site for effusions in this window. The effusion appears anterior to the unlabeled dark circle (the descending thoracic aorta), a clue that this is a pericardial (rather than pleural) effusion.

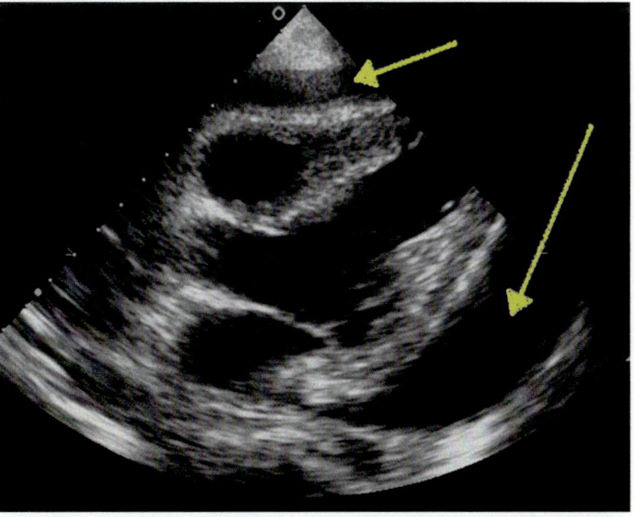

PEARL

Early utilization of bedside echocardiography in cardiovascular collapse can help guide the administration of intravenous fluids, vasopressors, and inotropic agents.

Right Ventricular Strain

Echocardiography is not a substitute for lung imaging in the diagnosis of pulmonary embolism because no sonographic finding is sufficiently specific for the disorder. Definitive imaging is difficult to obtain in an unstable patient. After excluding tamponade and more readily assessed causes of circulatory compromise such as tension pneumothorax, a bedside echocardiogram can provide evidence to suggest a hemodynamically compromising pulmonary embolism. Data suggest that the imaging modality can accurately assess right ventricular strain in the acute setting.[22]

A massive pulmonary embolus can cause right ventricular strain. This manifests in several ways, including increased right ventricular size and wall-motion changes. Normally the right ventricle is about 50% to 60% of the size of the left. In cases of of acute right ventricular strain, the right chamber enlarges and may equal or exceed the size of the left ventricle. The echocardiographic windows most valuable for this comparison are the apical, subxiphoid, and parasternal views. Excessive right ventricular strain causes dilation and hypokinesis of the right ventricle. In the setting of pulmonary embolism, the classic finding of hypokinesis of the right ventricular freewall with sparing of the right ventricle apex (McConnell sign) may be more suggestive of acute pulmonary embolism as distinct from other causes of chronic right ventricular strain.[23]

In the PSSAX view, the "D sign," or flattening of the septum (caused by increased right-sided pressures with concomitant decreased left-sided filling pressures), also can suggest an acute pulmonary embolus *(Figure 22-7)*.[24] A deep venous, right atrial or right ventricular clot can offer additional clues.[25] Bedside ultrasound has additional utility in patients whose clinical presentations strongly suggest pulmonary embolism and whose echocardiographic findings indicate right heart strain. If hemodynamic instability precludes computed tomography (CT) for definitive diagnosis, bedside ultrasound can be used to quickly evaluate the lower extremities for deep vein thrombosis.

The finding of right ventricular strain in a patient with acute pulmonary embolism can be of prognostic value as a mode of risk stratification and in consideration of thrombolytic therapy. Even normotensive patients with these findings have a significantly higher risk of inpatient mortality and shock related to the embolism.[26]

FIGURE 22-6. Massive Pericardial Effusion

PSSAX view of massive pericardial effusion with inward deflection of RV free wall *(arrow)*, suggesting tamponade.

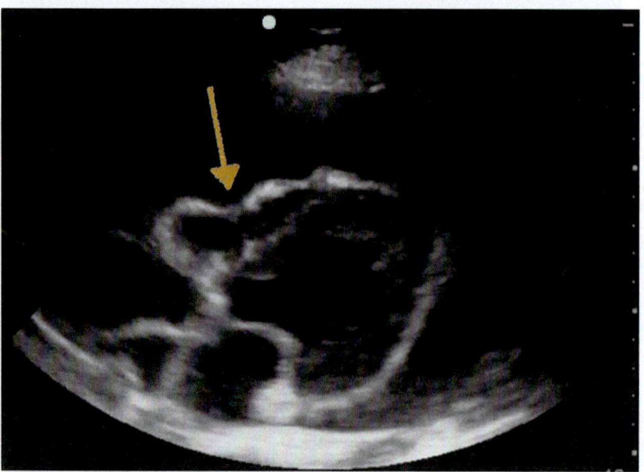

FIGURE 22-7. Septal Bowing

The left ventricle *(arrow)* has bowed in response to the pressure differential between the right and left ventricles, the so-called "D sign." Notice the dilated right ventricle *(RV)* compared with the small and underfilled left ventricle *(LV)*.

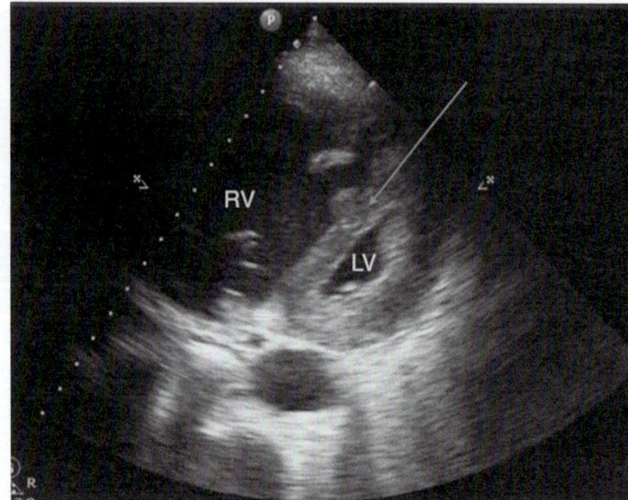

Image courtesy of Michael Stone, ACMC-Highland.

PEARLS

- ✓ These echocardiographic findings suggest PE:
  - Right ventricular size equal to or greater than left ventricular size with right ventricular hypokinesis
  - McConnell sign: right ventricular hypokinesis with sparing of right ventricle apex
  - D sign (flattening of the septum into the left ventricle, as seen in the PSSAX view *[Figure 22-7]*)
- ✓ Caveat: An enlarged, thick-walled right ventricle suggests long-standing rather than acute strain.

Wall-Motion Abnormalities

In patients with acute coronary syndrome, the detection of wall-motion abnormalities on echocardiography illuminates acute cardiac dysfunction and is of value if the ECG is ambiguous or the patient has a left bundle-branch block of unknown age.

To assess these defects, look for thickening within the ventricular muscle. Normally, the myocardium thickens in early systole. An ischemic myocardium can have a variety of appearances, described as hypokinetic (decreased systolic thickening), akinetic (no systolic thickening), or dyskinetic (outward bowing of the wall in systole). These findings can occur globally, as in diffuse cardiomyopathy, or segmentally, as in a singularly compromised vascular territory.

Although the PSLAX view allows a rapid gestalt of left ventricular function, it is limited to the assessment of the interventricular and lateral walls. When imaging the left ventricle for wall-motion abnormalities, the PSSAX view provides the most data by revealing the entire circumference of the left cavity. Sonographers can get their bearings by first locating the interventricular septum, using this landmark to identify other areas of the myocardium. From the septum, the transducer can be scanned toward the right shoulder and then toward the left hip, panning through the entire left ventricle. This allows the entire left chamber to be imaged from apex to aortic valve.[27]

PEARL

In the right clinical setting, the presence of pericardial effusion should prompt the physician to consider aortic dissection; tamponade is often the immediate cause of sudden cardiac collapse in type A dissections. In such cases, pericardiocentesis may offer only transient benefits.

Thoracic Aorta Examination

A thoracic aortic dissection can be identified rapidly with close inspection of the descending artery. Critical bedside diagnoses have been described in an increasing number of case reports.[28-31] Transthoracic echocardiography provides three key views of the thoracic aorta: the aortic root, aortic arch, and a single limited image of the descending aorta. The root can be well visualized via the PSLAX window and captures a single slice of the descending aorta.

The suprasternal window allows imaging of the aortic arch when the transducer is placed in the sternal notch and directed toward the patient's feet. When this view is successfully obtained, the window displays the arch in detail *(Figure 22-8)*. The addition of color flow enables the study of blood flow relative to the dissection flap. Features suggestive of aortic dissection include an intimal flap or dilated aortic root (>3.8 cm in diameter), which can best be identified in the PSLAX view *(Figure 22-9)*.

Inferior Vena Cava Examination

One of the most challenging tasks in any resuscitation is determining a patient's volume status. Recent debate, especially in the sepsis literature, has elaborated on the concept of *fluid responsiveness* — defined as the likelihood that cardiac output (and therefore perfusion) will increase in response to volume infusion. The usefulness of the most widely accepted marker of volume status, central venous pressure (CVP), recently has been called into question despite its history as the centerpiece of early goal-directed therapy and sepsis management.[32]

The case against CVP revolves around its inability to reasonably predict fluid responsiveness. Dynamic markers such as pulse-pressure variation (PPV) and the passive leg raise (PLR) maneuver have gained broader acceptance. In addition to PPV and PLR, sonographic evaluation of the IVC can be a valuable tool for assessing volume status and the "tank.[5]

Ultrasound's ability to predict volume responsiveness is less obvious; however, evidence cited in intensive care literature suggests a useful relationship.[33,34] Ultrasonography of the IVC

FIGURE 22-8. Suprasternal View

The arrow indicates a normal aortic arch.

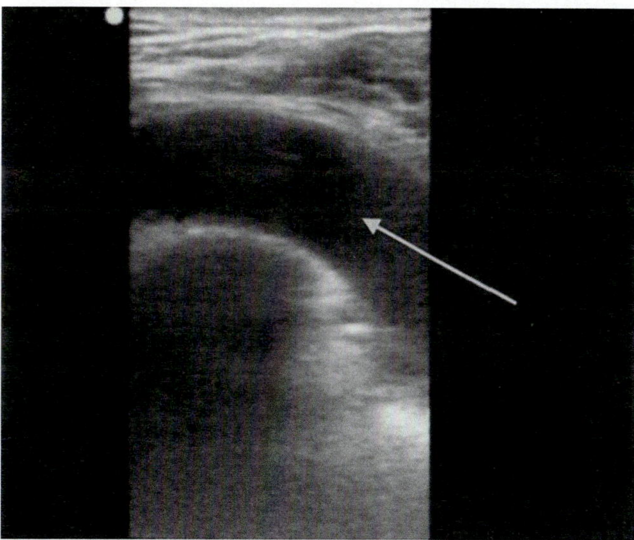

Image courtesy of Arun Nagdev, ACMC-Highland.

FIGURE 22-9. PSLAX View

Descending thoracic aorta; circled hypoechoic area with hyperechoic, mobile, linear dissection flap *(arrow)*. The boxed area includes the aortic outflow tract and somewhat dilated aortic root.

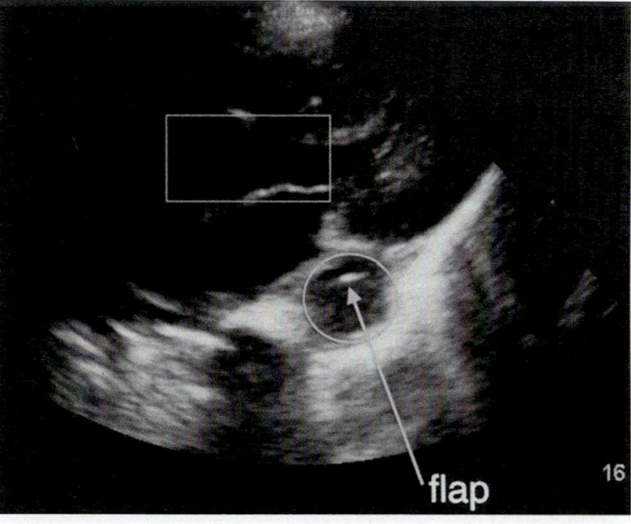

offers clear advantages over invasive measures of CVP because it is noninvasive and easily repeated (serial assessments of response to therapy are the cornerstone of critical care). Bedside sonography (using visual estimation) has been shown to accurately predict low CVP in the emergency department.[35]

To visualize the IVC, place a curvilinear or microconvex transducer in the subxiphoid area, directed perpendicular to the floor. The transducer indicator should point to the patient's right, in alignment with emergency medicine convention. Identify the round, hypoechoic (dark) aorta to the left of the patient's spine, the eccentrically shaped hypoechoic IVC to the right of the spine, and the bright thoracic spine deep relative to those structures in this transverse/axial plane. Next, tilt the cable end of the transducer to the patient's left, centering the vein in the image field, and rotate the transducer clockwise 90 degrees to view the IVC longitudinally. Visualize the right atrium contracting at the cephalic termination of the IVC *(Figure 22-10)*.

From here, the goal is to visually estimate the change in IVC diameter (collapse of the near-field wall toward the far-field wall) with normal respiration (or with positive-pressure ventilation) at a point approximately 3 cm distal to the junction with the right atrium, or at about the level of the right renal vein takeoff.[36] The degree of collapse compared to normal size is believed to correlate with intravascular volume status and is described as the caval index. An IVC collapse of more than 50% (caval index <0.5) suggests a CVP below 8 cm H_2O (ie, a hypovolemic state). Collapse of less than 50% (caval index <0.5) suggests a CVP greater than 10 cm H_2O; this value is less certain given the vagaries of CVP as a marker of intravascular volume status.

A particularly dehydrated patient can show a frankly "flat-appearing" IVC, which is demonstrative of volume depletion *(Figure 22-11)*. Treatment hinges on the patient's presentation and the desired clinical endpoint. In some cases, the IVC appears to not change with the respiratory cycle. A so-called plethoric IVC suggests elevated right atrial pressure. The differential diagnosis includes massive pulmonary embolus, tamponade, significant pulmonary hypertension, volume overload with cardiac dysfunction, restrictive heart disease, intrinsic positive end-expiratory pressure, tension pneumothorax, and any cause of elevated intrathoracic pressure.

The relationship between IVC diameter and inspiration is reversed in patients on positive-pressure ventilation because positive pressure during lung inflation/inspiration results in IVC *distention.* In such cases, chest wall mechanics and changes in intraabdominal pressure make the relationship between IVC diameter and respiration more complex. A patient with an IVC that distends more than 15% with positive-pressure ventilation is more likely to be fluid responsive, while one with no significant increase in vein diameter is less likely to benefit from fluids.[37] Given these small shifts, this time-consuming determination must be measured with screen calipers using static images.

Volume-overloaded patients who have undergone previous treatment with vasodilators or diuretics might demonstrate significant IVC collapse (despite having significant fluid volume), yielding a false-positive interpretation.

FIGURE 22-10. IVC (Longitudinal View)

Note the right atrial border to the left side of the image. Assess the IVC diameter at a point ~3 cm caudal to the right atrial junction.

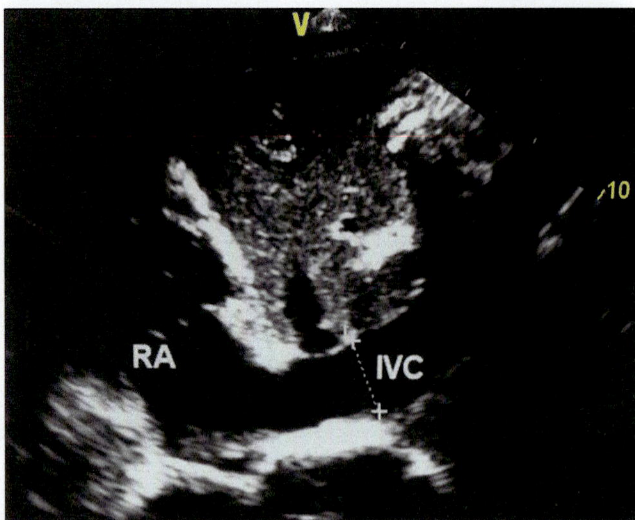

FIGURE 22-11. IVC ("Flat")

Longitudinal view of a very narrow IVC *(yellow lines)*, suggestive of volume depletion.

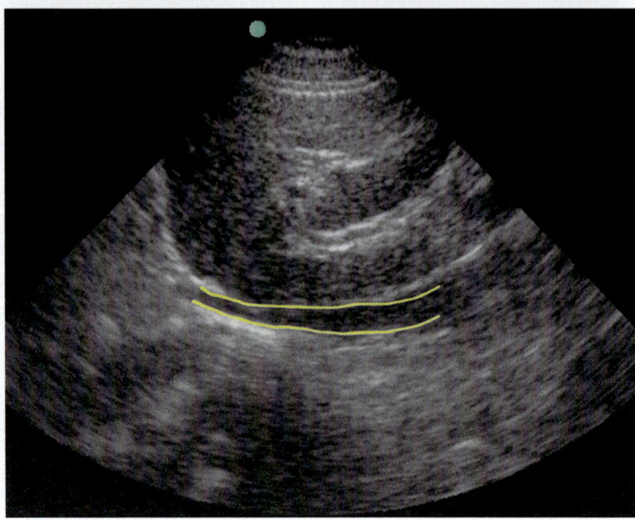

Lung Examination

Emergency and critical care physicians increasingly are using ultrasonography to evaluate lung pathologies. The most established applications include detecting the presence of lung sliding, excluding pneumothorax or an unventilated lung (as with mainstem intubation), and imaging the costophrenic angles to reveal pleural effusion. Parenchymal lung processes such as pulmonary edema (and other causes of interstitial fluid, including pulmonary contusion and acute lung injury) and pneumonia can be readily identified by bedside ultrasound.

Pneumothorax is routinely diagnosed via chest radiograph; however, this approach can be time-consuming and insensitive.

Multiple studies have demonstrated that the sensitivity of ultrasonography for the detection of pneumothorax appears to rival that of chest radiography; CT remains the gold standard.[38,39] Patient positioning (eg, a supine trauma patient) can obfuscate the radiographic findings. Although x-ray remains the best means for confirming pneumothorax size, ultrasonography also can make such predictions when the lung point can be seen.

Pneumothorax

Many providers use a linear transducer to assess lung sliding; however, microconvex, phased-array, and curved transducers at decreased depth also can be used. These lower-frequency tools allow deeper penetration and imaging of lung parenchyma at the expense of detail. A linear transducer may be preferable when performing a focused examination for pneumothorax.

Orient the linear transducer longitudinally on the supine patient. Beginning at the second or third intercostal space, visualize the bright, hyperechoic pleura between the ribs (the ribs appear as bright, semicircular surfaces with shadowing distally). Compare the affected side with the unaffected side. Image the lung in at least three interspaces, bilaterally, while focusing on the location in which a pneumothorax might be expected (ie, the highest-altitude area of the chest, where air would collect), and where the pain is most concentrated. Depending on the clinical situation, this examination also may be performed as part of a more comprehensive lung protocol, employing curvilinear or phased-array transducers.

A normal lung rapidly dissipates echoes and therefore does not provide an image that can be clearly resolved by ultrasound. The pleura are easily appreciated as hyperechoic lines between rib shadows. Once the pleura has been identified, look for lung sliding — the appearance of the visceral pleura sliding back and forth with respiration at the interface of the pleural layers *(Figure 22-12)*. This finding is normal.

Although it is subtle in some patients, an additional finding in the normal lung is the appearance of brightly hyperechoic, round "beads" with linear far-field artifacts that slide horizontally side-to-side with respiration. These expected artifacts are called comet tails *(Figure 22-13)*. Additionally, horizontal, hyperechoic lines that arise at regular intervals from the pleural line are called A-lines. This artifact represents a normal (or excessive) amount of air in the alveolar spaces and suggests normal lung parenchyma *(Figure 22-13a)*. A progressive disappearance of A-lines occurs with increasing lung density, as may be the case with various types of lung pathologies.

The absence of lung sliding (the pleura appearing as a stationary hyperechoic line during respiration) suggests pneumothorax *(Figure 22-14)*. This finding lacks specificity, as sliding also can be noted in nonventilated lungs, areas of obliterated or pathological pleural interface (as in the patient who has had therapeutic pleurodesis for recurrent pneumothorax), and occasionally in cases of severe bullous lung disease. It has been reported in cases of severe infiltrate, pulmonary tuberculosis, and acute respiratory distress syndrome.[40,41]

FIGURE 22-12. B-Lines

Side-to-side movement of the bright pleural interface or lung artifacts, as in B-lines *(arrows)*; rib shadow *(R)*.

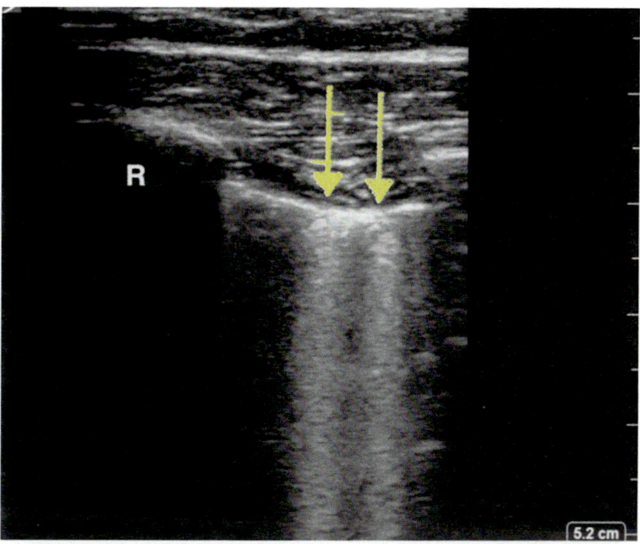

FIGURE 22-13. Comet Tails

A single comet tail *(arrow)* emanating from the pleural line; rib shadow *(R)*.

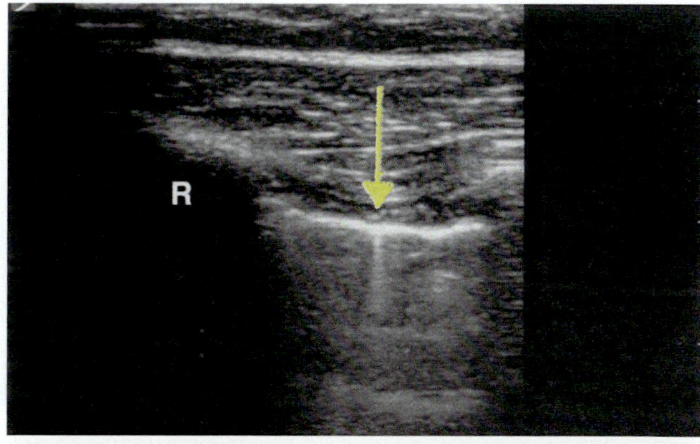

FIGURE 22-13a. A-Lines

Double arrow represents the pleural line, with repeated artifactual lines at roughly the same interval far afield. Anechoic or black areas (in area of lower arrows) represent rib shadows.

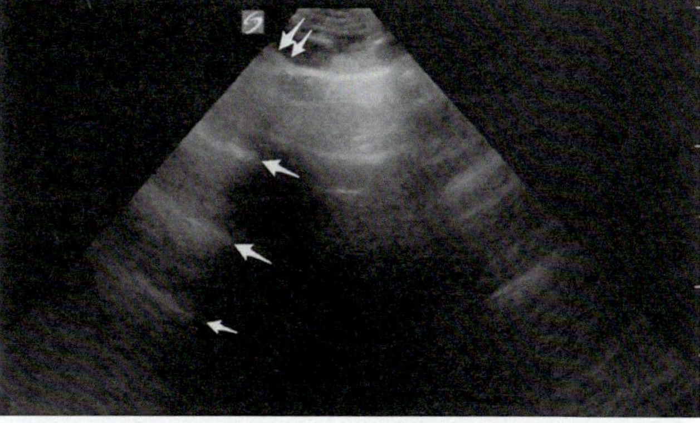

FIGURE 22-14. Absence of Lung Sliding

The ribs *(R)* seen in a transverse section display distal shadowing. The white line indicates the pleura without comet tails.

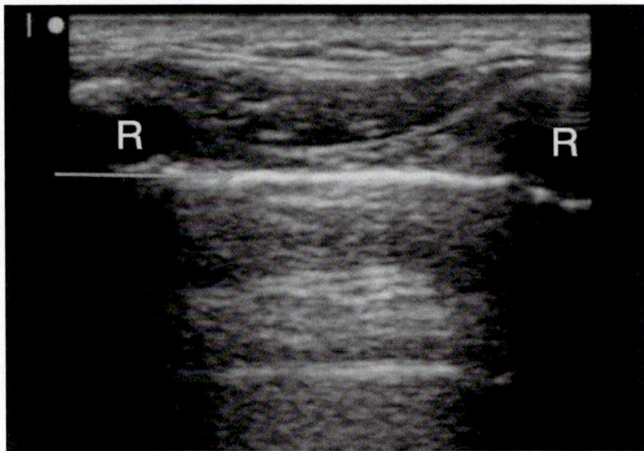

FIGURE 22-15. Seashore Sign

The seashore sign seen on M-mode. Note linearity above the bright, white pleural interface, with granularity deep to this line.

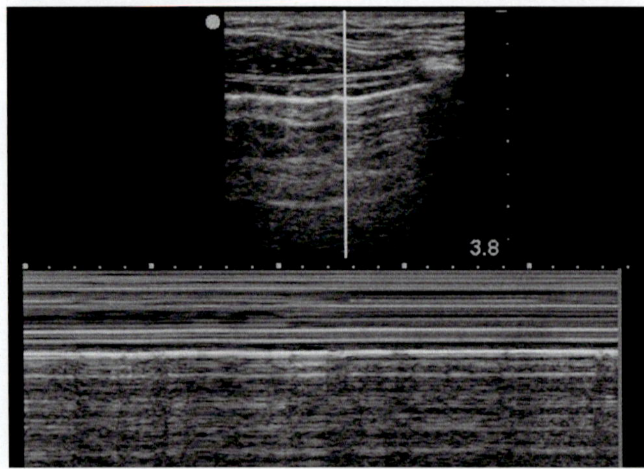

FIGURE 22-16. Stratosphere Sign

The stratosphere sign seen on M-mode. Linearity predominates, giving an appearance of "waves" without any "beach."

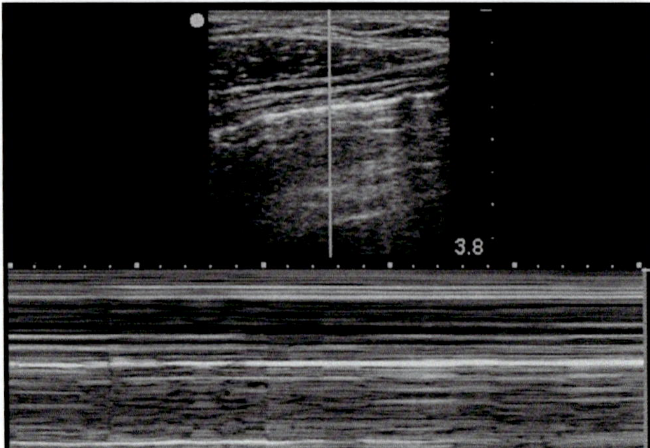

Although lung sliding can be difficult to discern in some cases, employing "movement mode" (M-mode) on the ultrasound machine can increase sensitivity. With this approach, data from a single vertical slice of the image (usually displayed as a vertical green line on first press of the M-mode button) are displayed in the y-axis over time (x-axis = time). Represented in this way, the normal finding is the "beach" or "seashore sign" — a linear appearance in the upper part of the image ("waves") with granularity ("sand") below the level of pleura. Such a linear finding in M-mode represents a structure with no significant movement relative to the y-axis. This is expected with the soft tissues of the chest wall, assuming the operator is holding the transducer immobile against the chest. In a normal lung, side-to-side motion at the pleural interface and below results in a "grainy" artifact deep to the level of the pleura, representing a sand-like appearance *(Figure 22-15)*. The seashore sign is normal.

Conversely, linearity below and above the pleural interface suggests the absence of pleural movement on the side being examined (ie, "waves" but no "sand"). This has been called the "stratosphere sign" or the "barcode sign" and may indicate a pneumothorax *(Figure 22-16)*. These uses of M-mode can also be applied with the curved or phased-array transducer.

Imaging both sides of the chest will increase sensitivity and allow a comparison for discerning subtle or seemingly vague abnormalities. The absence of sliding will only be seen in the interspaces where the pneumothorax is located. Small pneumothoraces — and those in locations difficult to image (apical or medial, in particular) — are poorly detected by ultrasound.[38] The overall sensitivity for pneumothorax approaches 90%.[39]

The lung pulse suggests the direct apposition of parietal and visceral pleura (ie, absence of pneumothorax). This finding can be particularly useful when assessing areas of lung that, by virtue of their close proximity to the heart, might not clearly demonstrate lung sliding.[42] The lung pulse, whch appears as a pulsatile movement of the visceral pleura on the parietal pleura, is subtle and occurs at the rate of cardiac oscillations.

While all of these findings can be used to exclude pneumothorax with great sensitivity, their absence does not necessarily confirm the diagnosis. The visualization of a lung-sliding interface and the absence of sliding in a single rib interspace (the so-called "lung point") is highly indicative of pneumothorax (with specificity as high as 100%).[43] This marker suggests the leading edge of the pneumothorax — the point at which the pleura separates at the chest wall *(Figure 22-17)*.

Pleural Effusion

A pleural effusion or hemothorax also can be readily identified in the critically ill patient. With the patient supine, place the transducer in the midaxillary to posterior axillary line within the 8th to 11th interspaces. Fluid will appear black (hypoechoic) between the white (hyperechoic) pleura. The physician can quickly image the pleural interface to assess for an intrathoracic collection of fluid *(Figure 22-18)*. These windows are often obtained in the right and left upper-quadrant views of the FAST exam.

Comprehensive Lung Examination

Beyond detecting pneumothorax and pleural effusion, a more comprehensive lung examination allows the evaluation of many other lung pathologies. Although debate continues about the optimal type of transducer to employ in these scenarios, microconvex and convex "general purpose" abdominal-type probes may be best in settings that provide minimal ultrasound signal processing. Phased-array probes, which conveniently do not require the operator to change transducers when initiating concomitant "bundled" cardiac imaging, also can be used. Clinical data do not differ significantly between devices.[44]

Several more comprehensive protocols have been suggested, including the Volpicelli method, which divides each anterior lung into four zones bisected by vertical axillary lines. The horizontal line is formed at the level of the nipple, bound anteriorly by the parasternal line and posteriorly by the posterior axillary line. This four-zone-per-side approach allows a rapid, systematic lung evaluation and may be more practical than the proposed 28-zone exam.[45]

Lung Interstitial Syndrome

Interstitial fluid in the lung can be readily identified by the presence and density of B-lines. These vertical reverberation artifacts are believed to be formed by a decreased acoustic mismatch between the lung and the surrounding tissues such that the ultrasound beam is partly reflected as it travels farther afield.[44]

B-lines have been described as "laser-like" and appear as discrete, vertical, hyperechoic artifacts that move with respiration. By definition, they extend brightly without diminution to the far field of the image (distinct from normal comet tails seen with lung sliding, which trail off only after a few centimeters).[42] An area of lung with increased interstitial fluid is defined by the presence of three or more B-lines in a longitudinal plane between two ribs.[42]

The density of lung water appears to directly correlate with the number of B-lines present in a given sonographic window. A heavily populated area suggests marked interstitial fluid. It has been suggested that lung ultrasound is a reliable "densitometer" of lung water.[46] Unlike in conventional radiographs, the appearance of B-lines seems to respond in real time to changes in the presence of extravascular lung water *(Figure 22-18a)*.[47]

Although the presence of these artifacts is nonspecific, their distribution and the appearance of the pleural interface can reveal the underlying lung pathology.[44] B-lines caused by cardiogenic pulmonary edema tend to be bilateral, more dependent, and symmetrical. Acute lung injury or ARDS shows an irregular, patchy pattern of bilateral B-lines, often with adjacent subpleural consolidations and a fragmented pleural interface. Making these distinctions based on ultrasound alone can be difficult. ARDS can be more easily differentiated from acute decompensated heart failure by incorporating results from the bedside echocardiography and ultrasound of the IVC. Focal unilateral artifacts can be

FIGURE 22-17. Lung Point Sign

The long arrow indicates the pleural interface where sliding lung can be seen; this finding is absent to the right of this point. Arrow indicates the edge at which pleura separate.

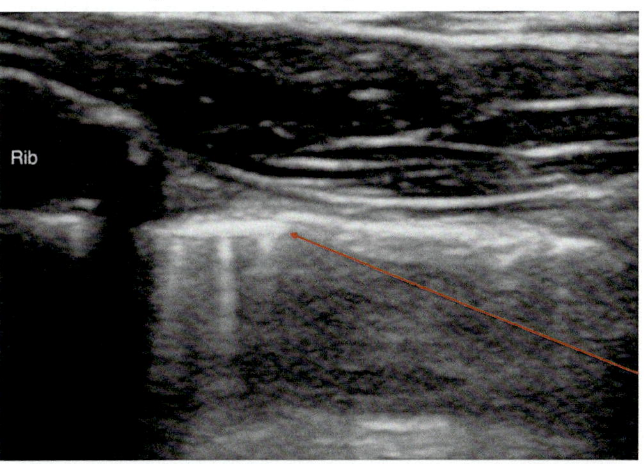

FIGURE 22-18. Right Costophrenic Angle

The superior edge of the liver can be seen on the right with an adjacent anechoic pleural effusion *(arrow)*. Note anechoic pleural effusion compared with adjacent lung segment *(star)*.

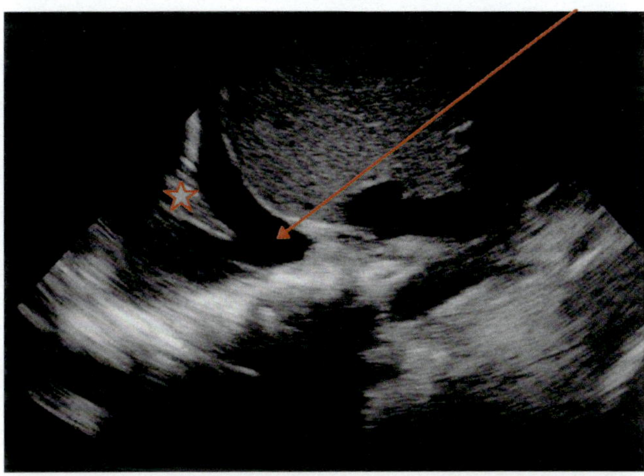

FIGURE 22-18a. B-lines

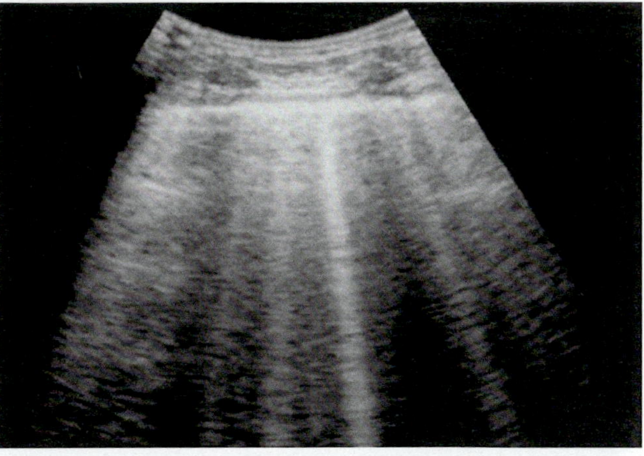

indicative of early or interstitial pneumonia and, in trauma patients, may be the manifestation of a pulmonary contusion. A wedge-shaped area of lung with B-lines might suggest a peripheral pulmonary infarction.

Point-of-care ultrasound has a high sensitivity and specificity (comparable to conventional chest radiography) for the detection of cardiogenic pulmonary edema, as demonstrated by the presence of B-lines.[48] This sign cannot be seen if air is interposed between the chest wall and affected lung (eg, when there is a concomitant pneumothorax in the thoracic area being imaged). The presence of B-lines excludes pneumothorax in the area of the chest deep to the transducer.

FIGURE 22-18b. Subpleural Lesions

Irregularity can be seen on the left side of the screen at the pleural interface. Hypoechoic rib shadowing divides dense hyperechoic areas of lung; note the B-lines and absence of A-lines.

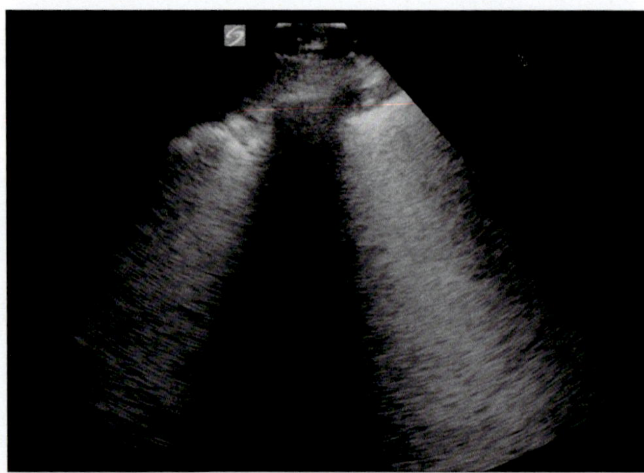

FIGURE 22-18c. Lung Consolidation

Note hepatization of the lung, giving the appearance of organ-like density (with internal hyperechoic air bronchograms) surrounded by hypoechoic pleural fluid.

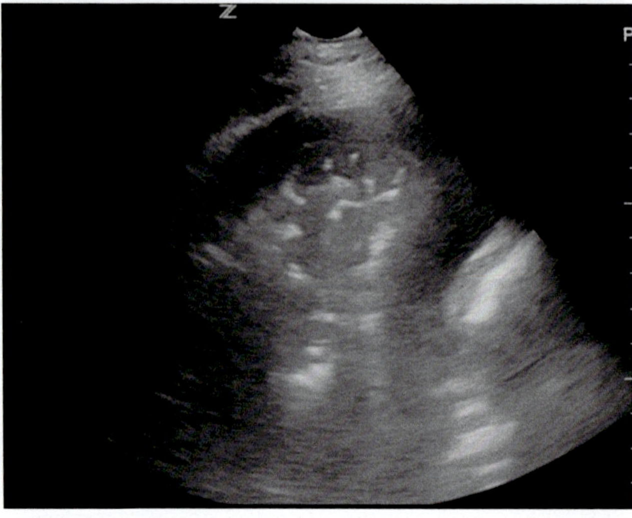

Lung Consolidation

The limited acoustic window of healthy lung offers little to generate a coherent image. The sonographer uses artifacts (eg, A-lines, pleural sliding) to infer the absence of disease. A consolidated portion of lung that is dense with pus or fluid will appear similar to an organ (eg, liver) and devoid of A-lines; it also may demonstrate air bronchograms and subpleural lesions *(Figure 22-18b)*. The sonographic appearance of consolidated lung *(Figure 22-18c)* may represent infiltrate, compressive atelectasis, the infarcted lung of a pulmonary embolism, metastasis, or contusion.[44] Interposed air (pneumothorax) does not allow imaging of any distal lung structures, pathological or not.

Abdominal Aorta Examination

The abdominal aorta should be assessed much like the IVC. With the patient supine, place a curved abdominal-type or microconvex transducer in the epigastric area, aiming perpendicular to the floor. Turn your attention to the aorta at this level, imaging it in the transverse plane. Interposed bowel markedly decreases image quality and can hinder the initial identification of the aorta. Apply steady pressure (this may take some time) to displace bowel from between the transducer and the aorta. Follow the artery down to the level of the aortic bifurcation (near the umbilicus), noting to the size of the artery and its appearance. The transducer should be rotated 90 degrees to view the aorta in its longitudinal plane. When assessing an obese patient, it can be easier to initiate imaging at the umbilicus, where the aorta often is more superficial.

Measure the aorta from outer wall to outer wall. A diameter larger than 3 cm is technically aneurysmal, and a diameter wider than 5 cm should raise immediate concern, especially if the patient is symptomatic *(Figure 22-18d)*. A mural thrombus in the vessel will appear gray, in contrast to black blood. If the aorta is not aneurysmal and clinical suspicion is suggestive, look for an intimal flap. Color-flow technology can elucidate flow on either side of the flap and demonstrate perfusion to branching vessels. This information can contribute to prognostic considerations in the management of a patient with an acute dissection.

Ultrasound-Guided Fluid Management

When treating critically ill, persistently hypotensive patients, it can be challenging to identify those who will benefit from additional intravenous fluid boluses. Clinicians often administer liters of fluid empirically during the initial resuscitation, although only 50% of hemodynamically unstable patients are volume responsive.[49] Insufficient fluid resuscitation results in tissue hypoperfusion and worsening organ dysfunction. Volume expansion in non-preload-dependent patients can lead to iatrogenic pulmonary edema, worsening ARDS, respiratory failure, third spacing of fluid, intraabdominal hypertension, prolonged time on mechanical ventilation, and an increased risk of death.[50]

Point-of-care ultrasound is a noninvasive technique for assessing intravascular volume status and predicting fluid responsiveness. This section addresses specific applications of bedside ultrasound to guide fluid management in the critically ill hypotensive patient and should be considered in conjunction with information in Chapter 4.

Fluid Tolerance

An assessment of left ventricular ejection fraction, lung ultrasound for pulmonary edema, and IVC collapsibility should be performed in all hypotensive patients to determine cardiopulmonary status. These tools can help the emergency physician rapidly identify patients who will benefit from further fluid administration and exclude those who may be harmed secondary to volume overload.

A normal or hyperdynamic left ventricle will tolerate fluids, particularly when there is no evidence of interstitial edema on lung ultrasound and a collapsible or flat IVC. Early signs of poor left ventricular function should alert the clinician that there is likely a narrow therapeutic window for intravenous fluids. In such cases, serial assessments of the IVC for B-lines should be performed if additional fluids are given. When non-cardiogenic pulmonary edema is demonstrated on lung ultrasound with preserved left ventricular systolic function and a collapsing IVC, the decision to administer additional fluids must be made with caution.

The IVC has limited use as a surrogate for assessing right atrial filling pressure to guide fluid management.[51] In spontaneously breathing patients, studies have shown that a caval index of IVC inspiratory collapse greater than 50% correlates with a CVP below 8 mm Hg.[52] The caval index (calculated as IVC expiratory diameter - IVC inspiratory diameter ÷ IVC expiratory diameter) is measured 2 cm proximal to the confluence of the hepatic vein in the subcostal view. For patients receiving positive-pressure ventilation, IVC distensibility (dIVC) can be measured instead of the caval index (calculated as IVC max. - IVC min. ÷ IVC max.) A dIVC greater than 18% may have a high sensitivity and specificity for fluid responsiveness.[53] In practice, most clinicians assess IVC collapse or distensibility using visual gestalt rather than actual measurements.

Cardiogenic shock can be easily diagnosed by visualizing poor left ventricular contractility, diffuse bilateral B-lines, and a plethoric IVC. In these clearcut cases, no fluids are indicated. When there is poor left ventricular contractility and bilateral A-lines on lung ultrasound, the patient may benefit from intravenous fluids, especially in the setting of a collapsing IVC. A plethoric IVC by itself cannot be interpreted to have a maximized preload and does not preclude volume responsiveness.

Fluid Responsiveness

Fluid responsiveness typically is defined as an increase in cardiac output by more than 15% after the administration of a fluid bolus (500-1000 mL). Measurements of stroke volume, cardiac output, or a surrogate marker before and after a fluid challenge can help confirm the benefit of a given bolus. With some training, bedside ultrasound can be used to measure changes in stroke volume, cardiac output, and carotid blood flow to determine if a patient is likely to benefit from additional fluids.

Passive Leg Raise Maneuver

A passive leg raise maneuver accomplishes a reversible fluid challenge of 300 to 500 mL; the technique is performed by laying the patient supine from a semirecumbent position and elevating the legs to 45 degrees. In theory, this practice can identify those who are unlikely to respond to fluids and prevent potentially ineffective or even harmful treatments.

FIGURE 22-18d. Abdominal Aortic Aneurysm

AAA seen in cross-section, with thrombus in the *far field.*

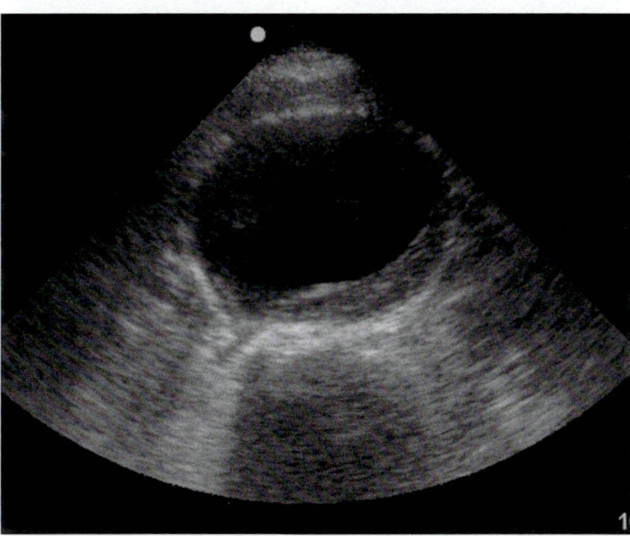

FIGURE 22-19. Measuring LVOT Diameter

Measure in parasternal long view, inner wall to inner wall at the aortic annulus.

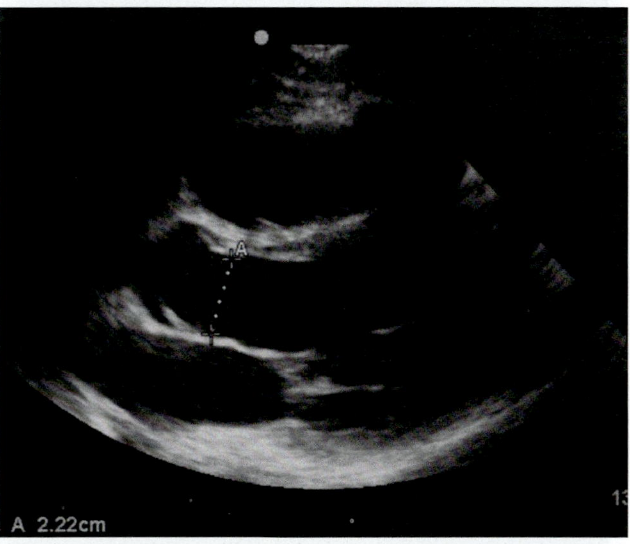

Aortic Outflow Tract Blood Flow

Measuring stroke volume (SV) and cardiac output (CO) requires a more advanced skillset and the ability to navigate the various Doppler settings and recordings particular to each ultrasound machine. The ability to reliably visualize the left ventricular outflow tract (LVOT) with an apical long or five-chamber view is essential.

FIGURE 22-20. Apical 5-Chamber View

This view can be obtained first to measure $LVOT_{VTI}$. Using pulsed wave Doppler, place the gate inside the LVOT proximal to the aortic valve.

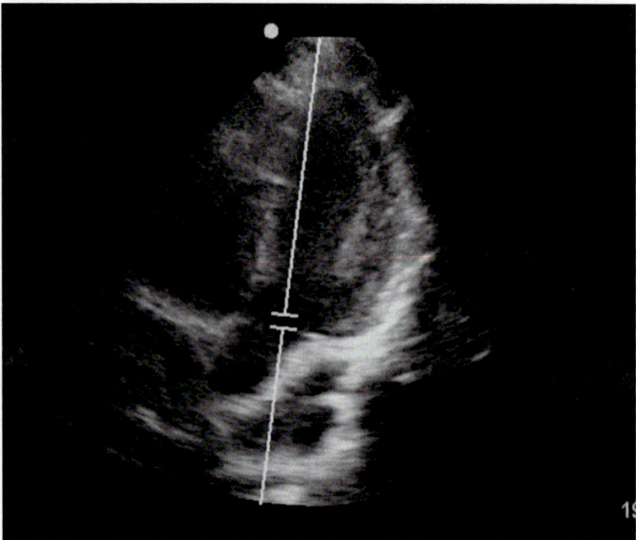

FIGURE 22-21. Measuring LVOT VTI

Using pulsed wave Doppler, the gate is placed in the LVOT proximal to the aortic valve. Trace the negative deflection and record the data.

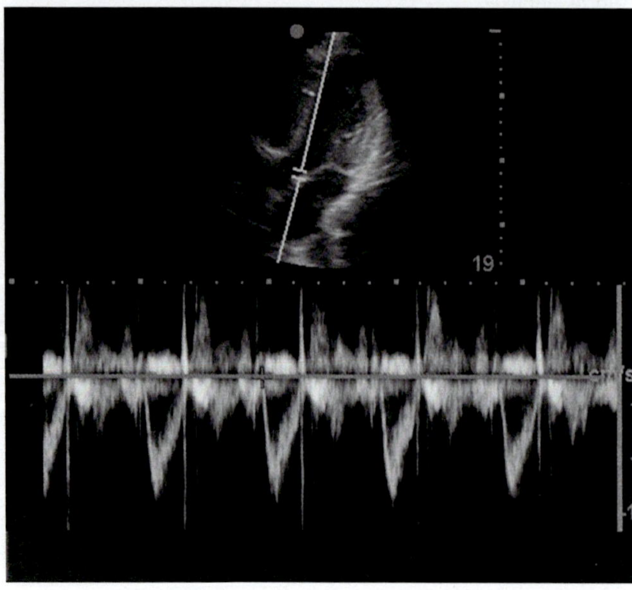

Measuring Stroke Volume/Cardiac Output

In the parasternal long axis, visualize the LVOT and freeze the image. Toggle the image to the midsystolic period (mitral valve is closed, aortic valve is open) when the LVOT diameter is greatest. Measure the LVOT diameter just proximal to the aortic valve leaflets at the aortic annulus, and save the recording *(Figure 22-19)*. Next, measure the LVOT VTI *(LVOT velocity time integral)* in a five-chamber or apical long view (rotate 90° from a four-chamber view). Change the setting to Doppler mode and press the PW (pulse-wave) button. Place the gate in the LVOT proximal to the aortic valve (AV), press the Doppler button, and freeze the image after a few cardiac cycles *(Figure 22-20)*. Trace the downward spike to obtain LVOT VTI and then save the recording *(Figure 22-21)*. Most ultrasound machines should be able to compute SV and CO from this data, which will be found under "Reports." The heart rate (HR) may need to be entered manually to calculate CO from SV using the valve radius. The following equations can be used:

$$CO = SV \times HR$$

$$SV = LVOT\ VTI \times \pi r^2$$

$$CO = LVOT\ VTI \times \pi r^2 \times HR$$

Common Carotid Arterial Blood Flow

If adequate echocardiographic views are difficult to obtain, measurements of the common carotid artery (CCA) blood flow can be used as an alternative to LVOT VTI. Because the common carotid arteries receive 15% of the CO, measuring changes in CCA blood flowafter fluid challenges or passive leg raise maneuvers can help determine fluid responsiveness. An increase in CCA VTI (CCA velocity time integral) of more than 20% after a passive leg raise maneuver (an increase of SV by >10% measured by bioreactance) is an indicator of fluid responsiveness.[54]

$$\textbf{CCA flow} = \pi \times (\text{CCA diameter})^2 / 4 \times \text{CCA VTI} \times \text{HR}$$

To determine CCA blood flow, two sonographic measurements are needed: the CCA diameter and CCA VTI. Using a linear probe in long axis, find the carotid bulb just proximal to the bifurcation of the internal and external carotid arteries. Freeze the image and toggle to find the largest diameter during systole. Approximately 1 cm proximal to the carotid bulb, measure from intima to intima and record the number *(Figure 22-22)*. Change the setting to "Pulse Wave Doppler." Also at 1 cm proximal to the carotid bulb, place the Doppler gate in the center of the vessel and angle it as parallel as possible to the direction of flow. The angle of isonation (the angle between the direction of the transducer and blood flow) should be as close to 60 degrees as possible. Press the Doppler button to allow spectral tracing, and measure the VTI by tracing the downward velocity signal to calculate the area under the curve *(Figure 22-23)*. Save the recording and input HR. The ultrasound machine will then calculate the CCA blood flow.

Cardiac Arrest Evaluation

Echocardiography can suggest a cause of circulatory collapse (eg, pericardial effusion with tamponade or hypovolemia) in patients with and without palpable pulses. Pulses are notoriously difficult to assess during cardiac arrest.[55] Visualization of the contractile function of the heart will identify organized cardiac activity in a pulseless patient, a finding that should prompt aggressive resuscitative efforts. Cardiac standstill, defined as a complete absence of cardiac activity, portends a more dismal prognosis and may reinforce the decision to discontinue resuscitative measures.[56] M-mode can be used to better discern subtle cardiac movements when cardiac windows are somewhat limited.

The examination can be performed using the parasternal or subxiphoid view during pulse checks in CPR.[57] All efforts should be made to minimize any interruptions in chest compressions, and the timing of sonography should be limited to the duration of the rhythm check. Preparation is essential; gel should be applied to the transducer and the settings must be optimized on the machine prior to taking a "quick look." The subxiphoid view can be useful (particularly for detecting pericardial effusion) during chest compressions. An algorithm for bedside ultrasonography in patients with non-arrhythmogenic cardiac arrest has been proposed.[58]

KEY POINTS

1. The echocardiographic evaluation of critically ill patients, especially those who are hypotensive or dyspneic, should immediately aim to exclude pericardial effusion.
2. Use multiple cardiac views to increase the sensitivity of the examination.
3. The finding of a pericardial effusion in a dyspneic or hemodynamically impaired patient should raise immediate suspicion for cardiac tamponade.
4. Combination views of the IVC and lungs on cardiac ultrasound can provide complementary information.
5. The ejection fraction can be estimated reliably and sufficiently with a visual assessment.
6. In a spontaneously breathing patient, the relatively negative intrathoracic pressure of inspiration draws blood from the IVC into the thorax, resulting in a transient decrease in the caliber of the IVC.
7. Reassess the IVC after interventions to assess response to therapy.
8. Lung ultrasound is often bundled with cardiac ultrasound for greatest clinical utility.
9. Point-of-care ultrasound demonstrates high sensitivity for the detection of pneumothorax and interstitial lung water.
10. A frequent misconception is that aortic rupture can be detected by ultrasonography. In fact, most ruptures occur into the retroperitoneum, an area that cannot be visualized with this modality.

FIGURE 22-22. Measuring Arterial Blood Flow

Determine common carotid arterial blood flow by measuring the diameter of the artery during systole, inner wall to inner wall, approximately 1 cm proximal to the carotid bulb.

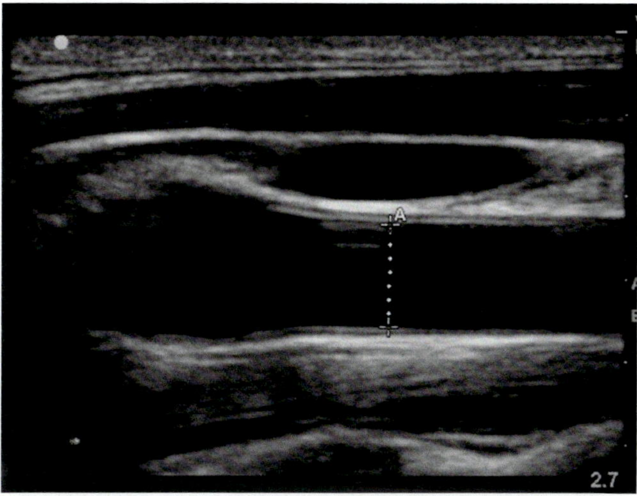

FIGURE 22-23. Measuring CCA VTI

Using pulsed wave Doppler, place the gate at the same level as the measurement for the CCA diameter.

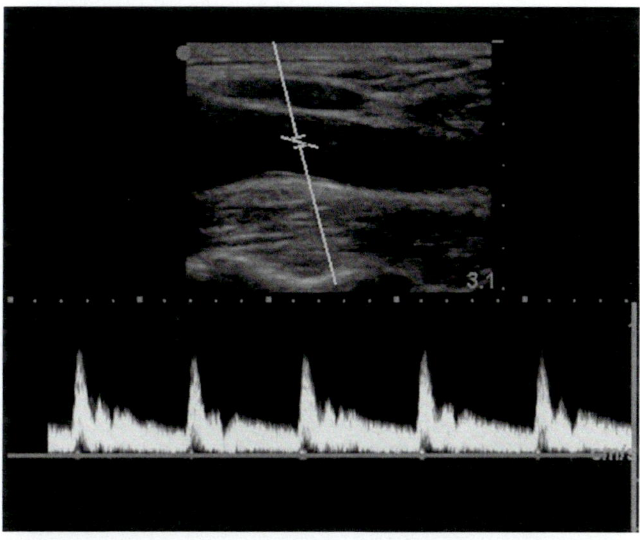

Conclusion

Ultrasonography enables the rapid identification of pathologies and provides a means of reassessment after therapeutic interventions in critically ill patients. Applications for critical care ultrasonography continue to be discovered and investigated. As skill with this imaging modality in the emergency department increases, so will the sophistication of our studies and the quality of our instruments.

Acknowledgment

The authors would like to thank Arun Nagdev, Michael Stone, and Ralph Wang for their teaching contributions in the creation of this chapter.

REFERENCES

1. Hothi SS, Sprigings D, Chambers J. Point-of-care cardiac ultrasound in acute medicine — the quick scan. *Clin Med.* 2014;14:608-611.
2. Jones AE, Tayal VS, Sullivan DM, et al. Randomized, controlled trial of immediate versus delayed goal-directed ultrasound to identify the cause of nontraumatic hypotension in emergency department patients. *Crit Care Med.* 2004;32:1703-1708.
3. Au S-M, Vieillard-Baron A. Bedside echocardiography in critically ill patients: a true hemodynamic monitoring tool. *J Clin Monit Comput.* 2012;26:355-360.
4. Rose J, Bair A, Mandavia D, et al. The UHP ultrasound protocol: a novel ultrasound approach to the empiric evaluation of the undifferentiated hypotensive patient. *Am J Emerg Med.* 2001;19:299-302.
5. Perera P, Mailhot T, Riley D, et al. The RUSH exam: Rapid Ultrasound in SHock in the evaluation of the critically ill. *Emerg Med Clin North Am.* 2010;28:29-56.
6. Wu T. The CORE scan: concentrated overview of resuscitative efforts. *Crit Care Clin.* 2014;30:151-175.
7. Lanctot YF, Valois M, Bealieu Y. EGLS: echo guided life support. An algorithmic approach to undifferentiated shock. *Crit Ultrasound J.* 2011;3:129.
8. Lichtenstein DA, Karakitsos D. Integrating ultrasound in the hemodynamic evaluation of acute circulatory failure (FALLS — the fluid administration limited by lung sonography protocol). *J Crit Care.* 2012;27:533.e11-9.
9. Pershad J, Myers S, Plouman C, et al. Bedside limited echocardiography by the emergency physician is accurate during evaluation of the critically ill patient. *Pediatrics.* 2004;114:e667–e671.
10. Randazzo MR, Snoey ER, Levitt MA, et al. Accuracy of emergency physician assessment of left ventricular ejection fraction and central venous pressure using echocardiography. *Acad Emerg Med.* 2003;10:973-977.
11. Moore CL, Rose GA, Tayal VS, et al. Determination of left ventricular function by emergency physician echocardiography of hypotensive patients. *Acad Emerg Med.* 2002;9:186-193.
12. Jones AE, Craddock PA, Tayal VS, et al. Diagnostic accuracy of identification of left ventricular function among emergency department patients with nontraumatic symptomatic undifferentiated hypotension. *Shock.* 2005;24:513-517.
13. Mandavia DP, Hoffner RJ, Mahaney K, et al. Bedside echocardiography by emergency physicians. *Ann Emerg Med.* 2001;38:377-382.
14. Moore CM. Current issues with emergency cardiac ultrasound probe and image conventions. *Acad Emerg Med.* 2008;15:278-284.
15. Blaivas M. Incidence of pericardial effusions in patients presenting to the emergency department with unexplained dyspnea. *Acad Emerg Med.* 2001;8:1143-1146.
16. Ferrada P, Vanguri P, Anand RJ, et al. A, B, C, D, echo: limited transthoracic echocardiogram is a useful tool to guide therapy for hypotension in the trauma bay — a pilot study. *J Trauma Acute Care Surg.* 2013;74:220-223.
17. Pinsky MR, Payen D. Functional hemodynamic monitoring. *Crit Care.* 2005;9:566-572.
18. Vieillard-Baron A, Caille V, Charron C, et al. Actual incidence of global left ventricular hypokinesia in adult septic shock. *Crit Care Med.* 2008;36:1701-1706.
19. Bouferrache K, Amiel JB, Chimot L, et al. Initial resuscitation guided by the Surviving Sepsis Campaign recommendations and early echocardiographic assessment of hemodynamics in intensive care unit septic patients: a pilot study. *Crit Care Med.* 2012;40:2821-2827.
20. Douglas PS, Garcia MJ, Haines DE, et al. ACCF/ASE/AHA/ ASNC/HFSA/HRS/SCAI/ SCCM/SCCT/SCMR 2011 Appropriate Use Criteria for Echocardiography. A Report of the American College of Cardiology Foundation Appropriate Use Criteria Task Force, American Society of Echocardiography, American Heart Association, American Society of Nuclear Cardiology, Heart Failure Society of America, Heart Rhythm Society, Society for Cardiovascular Angiography and Interventions, Society of Critical Care Medicine, Society of Cardiovascular Computed Tomography, Society for Cardiovascular Magnetic Resonance American College of Chest Physicians. *J Am Soc Echocardiogr.* 2011;24:229-267.
21. Secko MA, Lazar JM, Salciccioli LA, et al. Can junior emergency physicians use E-point septal separation to accurately estimate left ventricular function in acutely dyspneic patients? *Acad Emerg Med.* 2011;18:1223-1226.
22. Taylor RA, Moore CL. Accuracy of emergency physician-performed limited echocardiography for right ventricular strain. *Am J Emerg Med.* 2014;32:371-374.
23. McConnell MV, Solomon SD, Rayan ME, et al. Regional right ventricular dysfunction detected by echocardiography in acute pulmonary embolism. *Am J Cardiol.* 1996;78:469-473.
24. Come PC. Echocardiographic evaluation of pulmonary embolism and its response to therapeutic interventions. *Chest.* 1992;101:151S-162S.
25. Goldhaber SZ. Echocardiography in the management of pulmonary embolism. *Ann Intern Med.* 2002;136:691-700.
26. Grifoni S, Olivotto I, Cecchini P, et al. Short-term clinical outcome of patients with acute pulmonary embolism, normal blood pressure, and echocardiographic right ventricular dysfunction. *Circulation.* 2000;101:2817-2822.
27. Frenkel O, Riguzzi C, Nagdev A. Identification of high-risk patients with acute coronary syndrome using point-of-care echocardiography in the ED. *Am J Emerg Med.* 2014;32:670-672.
28. Budhram G, Reardon R. Diagnosis of ascending aortic dissection using emergency department bedside echocardiogram. *Acad Emerg Med.* 2008;15:584.
29. Fojtik JP, Costantino TG, Dean AJ. The diagnosis of aortic dissection by emergency medicine ultrasound. *J Emerg Med.* 2007;32:191-196.
30. Blaivas M, Sierzenski PR. Dissection of the proximal thoracic aorta: a new ultrasonographic sign in the subxiphoid view. *Am J Emerg Med.* 2002;20:344-348.
31. Barrett C, Stone MB. Emergency ultrasound diagnosis of type A aortic dissection and apical pleural cap. *Acad Emerg Med.* 2010;17:e23-e24.
32. Marik PE, Baram M, Vahid B. Does central venous pressure predict fluid responsiveness? A systematic review of the literature and the tale of seven mares. *Chest.* 2008;134:172-178.
33. Feissel M, Michard F. The respiratory variation in inferior vena cava diameter as a guide to fluid therapy. *Intensive Care Med.* 2004;30:1834-1837.
34. Vignon P. Evaluation of fluid responsiveness in ventilated septic patients: back to venous return. *Intensive Care Med.* 2004;30:1699-1701.
35. Nagdev AD, Merchant RC, Tirado-Gonzalez A, et al. Emergency department bedside ultrasonographic measurement of caval index for non-invasive determination of low central venous pressure. *Ann Emerg Med.* 2010;55:290-295.
36. Wallace DJ, Allison M, Stone MB. Inferior vena cava percentage collapse during respiration is affected by the sampling location: an ultrasound study in healthy volunteers. *Acad Emerg Med.* 2010;17:96-99.
37. Barbier C, Loubieres Y, Schmit C, et al. Respiratory changes in inferior vena cava diameter are helpful in predicting fluid responsiveness in ventilated septic patients. *Intensive Care Med.* 2004;30:1740-1746.
38. Wilkerson RG, Stone MB. Sensitivity of bedside ultrasound and supine anteroposterior chest radiographs for the identification of pneumothorax after blunt trauma. *Acad Emerg Med.* 2010;17:11-17.
39. Raja AS, Jacobus CH. Systematic review snapshot: how accurate is ultrasonography for the detection of pneumothorax? *Ann Emerg Med.* 2013;61:207-208.
40. Lichtenstein DA, Menu Y. A bedside ultrasound sign ruling out pneumothorax in the critically ill: lung sliding. *Chest.* 1995;108:1345-1348.
41. Simon BC, Paolinetti L. Two cases where bedside ultrasound was able to distinguish pulmonary bleb from pneumothorax. *J Emerg Med.* 2005;29:201-205.
42. Volpicelli G, Elbarbary M, Blaivas M, et al. International evidence-based recommendations for point-of-care lung ultrasound. *Intensive Care Med.* 2012;38:577-591.
43. Lichtenstein D, Meziere G, Biderman P, et al. The "lung point": an ultrasound sign specific to pneumothorax. *Intensive Care Med.* 2000;26:1434-1440.
44. Gargani L, Volpicelli G. How I do it: lung ultrasound. *Cardiovasc Ultrasound.* 2014;12:25-35.
45. Volpicelli G, Mussa A et al. Bedside lung ultrasound in the assessment of alveolar-insteritial syndrome. *Am J Emerg Med* 2006;24:689-96.
46. Gargani L, Picano E, et al. Lung water assessment by lung ultrasonography in critical care: a pilot study. *Intensive Care Med* 2013; 39:74-84.
47. Noble VE, Murray AF, Capp R, et al. Ultrasound assessment for extravascular lung water in patients undergoing hemodialysis: time course for resolution. *Chest.* 2009;135:1433-1439.
48. Al Deeb M, Barbic S, Featherstone R, et al. Point-of-care ultrasonography for the diagnosis of acute cardiogenic pulmonary edema in patients presenting with acute dyspnea: a systematic review and meta-analysis. *Acad Emerg Med.* 2014;21:843-852.
49. Marik PE, Baram M, Vahid B. Does central venous pressure predict fluid analysis? A systematic review of the literature and the tale of seven mares. *Chest.*2008;134:172-178.
50. Thiel SW, Kollef MH, Isakow W. Non-invasive stroke volume measurement and passive leg raising predict volume responsiveness in medical ICU patients: an observational cohort study. *Crit Care.* 2009;13:R111.
51. Dipti A, Soucy Z, Surana A, et al. Role of inferior vena cava diameter in assessment of volume status: a meta-analysis. *Am J Emerg Med.* 2012;30:1414-1419.
52. Nagdev AD, Merchant RC, Tirado-Gonzalez A, et al. Emergency department bedside ultrasonographic measurement of the caval index for noninvasive determination of low central venous pressure. *Ann Emerg Med.* 2010;55:290-295.
53. Barbier C, Loubieres Y, Schmit C, et al. Respiratory changes in inferior vena cava diameter are helpful in predicting fluid responsiveness in ventilated septic patients. *Intensive Care Med.* 2004;30:1740-1746.
54. Marik PE, Levitov A, Young A, Andrews L. The use of bioreactance and carotid Doppler to determine volume responsiveness and blood flow redistribution following passive leg raising in hemodynamically unstable patients. *Chest.* 2013;143:364-370.
55. Andrew H, Travers, Thomas D, et al. Part 4: CPR overview: 2010 American Heart Association Guidelines for Cardiopulmonary Resuscitation and Emergency Cardiovascular Care. *Circulation.* 2010;122(suppl 3):S676-S684.
56. Salen P, Melniker L, Chooljian C, et al. Does the presence or absence of sonographically identified cardiac activity predict resuscitation outcomes of cardiac arrest patients? *Am J Emerg Med.* 2005;23:459-462.
57. Tsung JW, Blaivas M. Feasibility of correlating the pulse check with focused point-of-care echocardiography during pediatric cardiac arrest: a case series. *Resuscitation.* 2008;77:264-269.
58. Hernandez C, Shuler K, Hannan H, et al. C.A.U.S.E.: cardiac arrest ultra-sound exam — a better approach to managing patients in primary non-arrhythmogenic cardiac arrest. *Resuscitation.* 2008;76:198-206.

The Difficult Emergency Delivery

23

IN THIS CHAPTER

- Assessment of the laboring patient
- Preparing for precipitous delivery
- Management of delivery complications
- Cardiac arrest in pregnancy
- Perimortem cesarean delivery

Sarah K. Sommerkamp and Carrie D. Tibbles

The arrival of a woman in labor is an anxiety-provoking event for all involved. Many of these patients have had little or no prenatal care, increasing the risk of complications for both mother and fetus.[1,2]

Triage

Any patient who presents to the emergency department is entitled to medical screening, as stipulated by the Emergency Medical Treatment and Labor Act (EMTALA). If that examination indicates an emergency medical condition in a pregnant woman in labor, stabilization does not necessarily require delivery, as the acute setting is suboptimal for childbirth. Interhospital and intrahospital transfers of patients in labor must be carefully considered, and the physician must ensure that the benefits of transport outweigh its risks. Furthermore, clinicians must be aware of hospital policies regarding laboring patients and the resources available for them.

PEARLS

- ✓ Under EMTALA guidelines, the stabilization of a pregnant woman who is having contractions does not automatically mean that the baby must be delivered in the emergency department.
- ✓ The physician who initiates an interhospital transfer must ensure that the benefits of transport outweigh the risks.

Assessment

After 20 weeks' gestation, any woman with complaints of abdominal pain, back pain, or vaginal bleeding or discharge should be assessed for active labor *(Figure 23-1)*.[3,4] A focused history and physical examination should be performed, and information should be gathered about gestational age and parity. If the gestational age is unknown, it can be estimated based on the date of the patient's last menstrual period (Nägele rule), fundal height, or ultrasonography.[5]

PEARLS

- ✓ Nägele rule: Date of delivery = first day of last menstrual period + 9 months + 7 days
- ✓ Measure the fundal height with a tape measure from the pubic symphysis to the top of the fundus. The measurement in centimeters roughly estimates the gestational age in weeks. Fundal height at the umbilicus represents about 20 weeks' gestation.

Specific questions about potential membrane rupture, vaginal bleeding, loss of mucus plug, timing of contractions, and the urge to push can help differentiate between true and false labor *(Figure 23-2)*. In the brief review of systems, it also is important to ask about fevers, headache, visual changes, significant edema, and right upper quadrant pain to assess for potential complications such as infection or preeclampsia. Details also should be obtained about prior surgeries, medications, and allergies.

The physical examination should start with an assessment of vital signs, airway, breathing, and circulation; the fundal height and position of the fetus also must be evaluated. It is estimated that the frequency of malpresentation at 32 weeks is as high as 15% and decreases to 4% at term.[6] If time permits, Leopold maneuvers may be attempted to determine fetal lie. This approach *(Figure 23-3)* is sensitive and specific when performed by an experienced clinician.[6] For emergency physicians who are unfamiliar with such maneuvers, ultrasonography is a more useful tool for determining the position of the head, location of the placenta, presence of amniotic fluid, and fetal heart rate.

FIGURE 23-1. Assessment of the Pregnant Patient in Labor

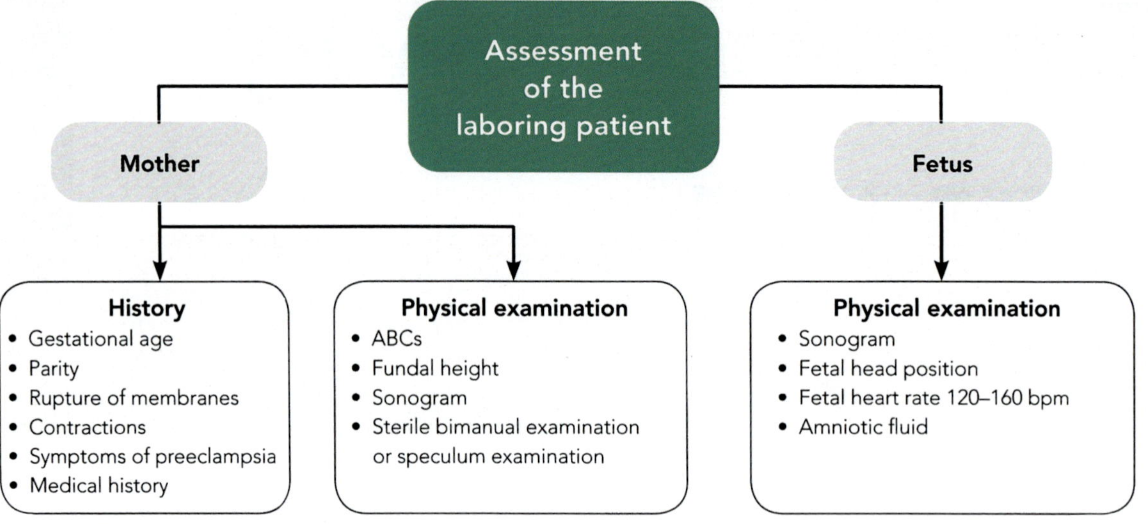

FIGURE 23-2. Triage of the Pregnant Patient in Labor

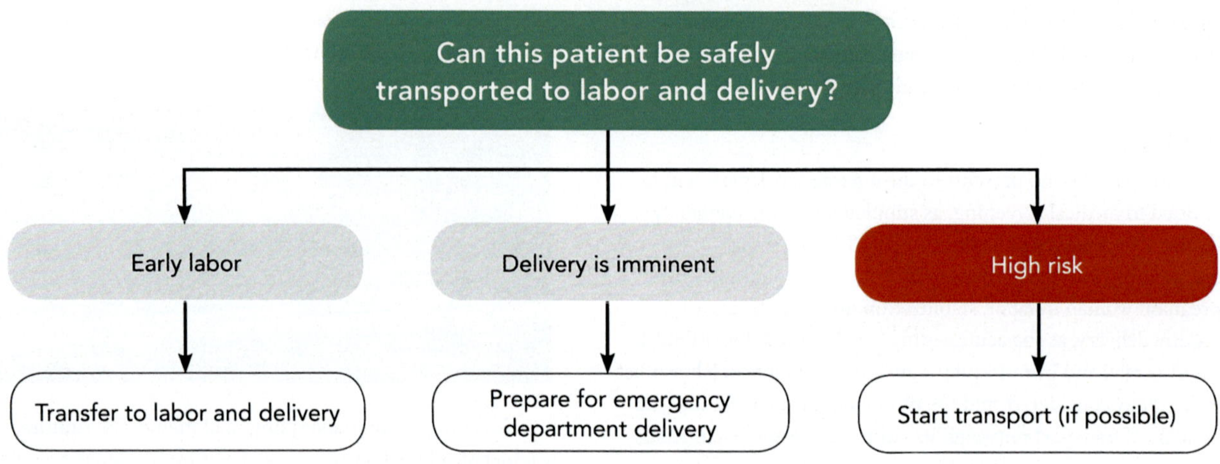

If there is no significant vaginal bleeding and the patient appears to be in active labor, a sterile bimanual examination should be performed to determine cervical dilation, effacement, and fetal station. Cervical dilation refers to the diameter of the cervix. Cervical effacement, or thinning of the cervix, is described as a percentage (0% to 100%) of normal cervical length (about 2 cm). Fetal station refers to the level of the presenting part compared with the maternal ischial spine. Presentation above the ischial spine is referred to as −1 station; presentation at the ischial spine is 0 station. If the presenting part is below the ischial spine, the scenario is a +1, +2, or +3 station.[7] A patient who is 10-cm dilated, 100% effaced, and at +3 station has an impending delivery. A bimanual examination should not be performed if there is significant vaginal bleeding; hemorrhage can indicate placenta previa or abruption. If either disorder is suspected, the patient should be transferred immediately to labor and delivery for a possible cesarean delivery.[3]

A sterile speculum examination can be used to visualize the cervix and determine if amniotic fluid is leaking. Amniotic fluid will turn nitrazine paper yellow to blue and, when smeared on a

TABLE 23-1. Equipment for Emergency Delivery
Sterile gloves and gown
Cleaning solution
Two hemostat clamps
Scissors
Bulb syringe
Red-topped blood collection tube (cord blood)
Infant warmer
Neonatal resuscitation equipment

glass slide, will form crystals in a fern-like pattern.[3] If amniotic fluid is detected, it is important to note the presence or absence of brown staining. Meconium contamination occurs in 20% of vaginal deliveries, and fetal aspiration of meconium can cause severe neonatal distress.[3,8]

PEARLS

- ✓ Recognize that the cervix can lie inferior to the fetal head when the head is engaged, making the assessment more challenging. The clinician can run a hand along the contour of the head until the cervix is reached.
- ✓ If meconium is present, prepare for potential respiratory distress in the newborn.

Preparation for Delivery

Emergency physicians should know where their department's delivery kit is located *(Table 23-1)*. A neonatal warmer and resuscitation equipment should be available. If the hospital has an obstetrical and neonatal team, it should be immediately contacted if there is notification from prehospital personnel of a precipitous delivery.

Normal Delivery

Normal labor is divided into three stages: 1) the start of regular contractions to full cervical dilation, 2) delivery of the infant, and 3) delivery of the placenta.[9] This chapter focuses on the second and third stages. During the second stage of labor, the patient should be placed in the dorsal lithotomy position. Physicians must know the cardinal movements of labor

FIGURE 23-3. Leopold Maneuver

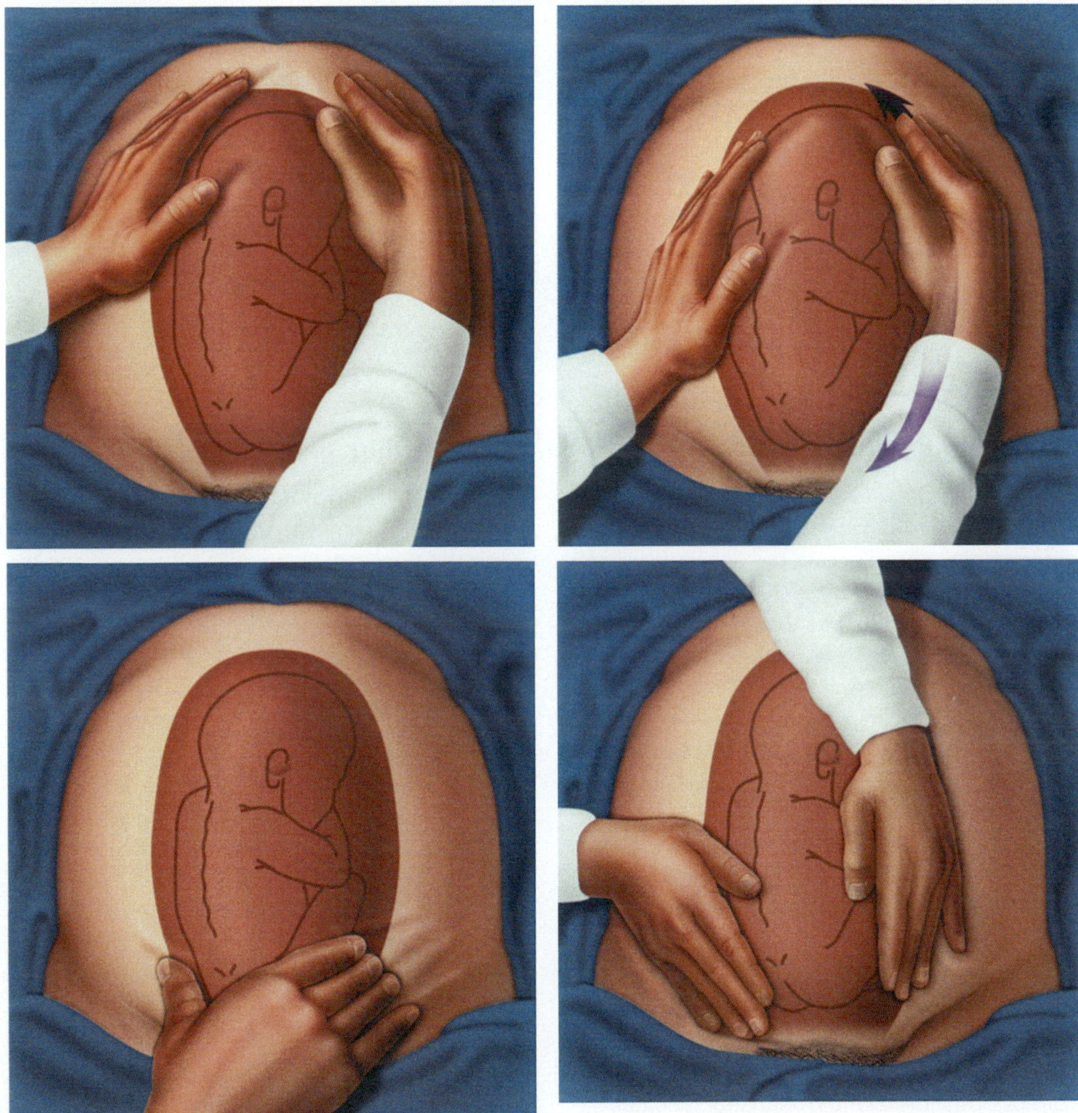

FIGURE 23-4. Sequence of Normal Delivery

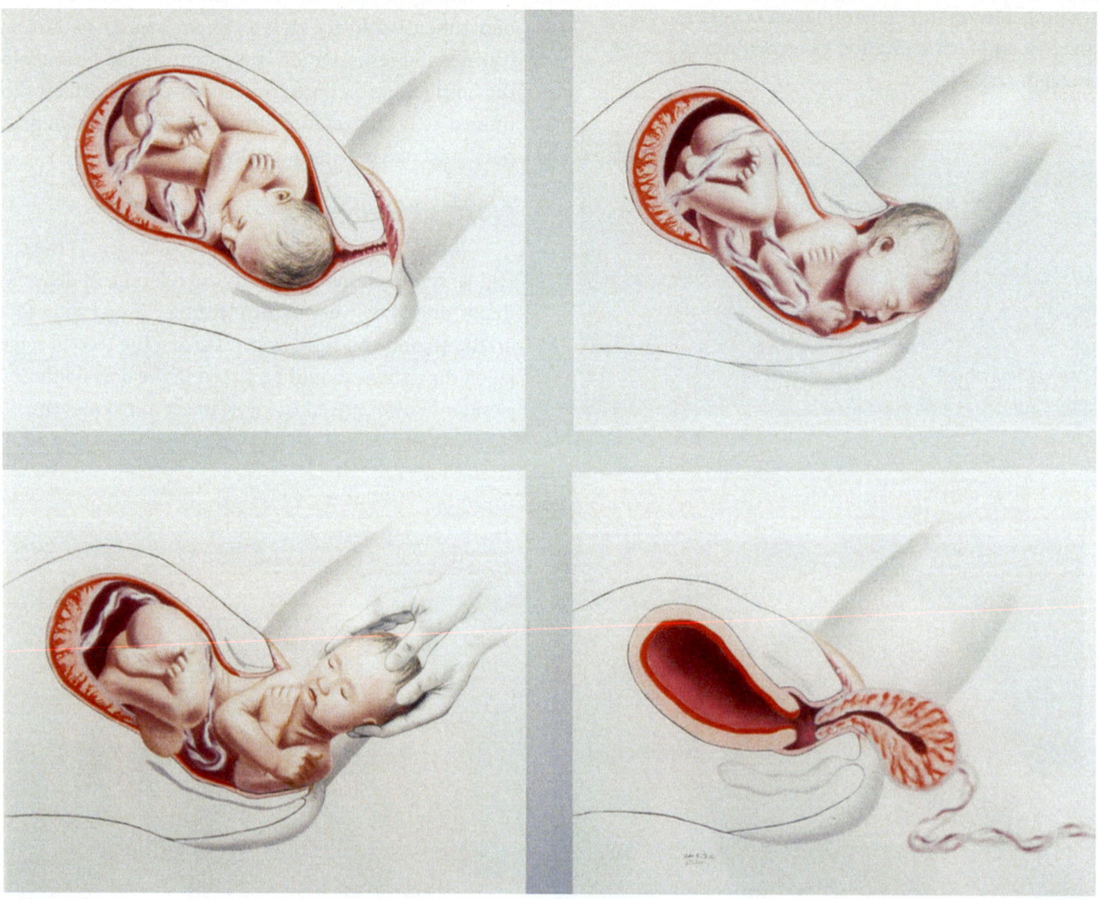

When managing a patient in the second stage, the following approach can be used:

1. If time permits, the perineal area should be cleaned and draped with sterile towels.
2. As extension of the head occurs, the perineum will start to bulge and crowning will be seen.
3. Most women will have the urge to push. If necessary, a mediolateral episiotomy can be performed at this time, but only if absolutely necessary. The procedure is associated with increased maternal blood loss, risk of disruption of the anal sphincter, and a delayed return to sexual activity.[9]
4. To minimize injury to the perineum, gentle pressure can be applied on the draped perineum with one hand while placing the other hand on the presenting head to minimize uncontrolled movements, which can tear the perineum.[3,4]
5. The neck should be swept with an index finger to check for a nuchal cord, which should be gently slipped over the infant's head. If the cord cannot be repositioned, the clinician can attempt to deliver the infant through the cord by pushing it over the neonate's shoulders. The third option is to somersault the infant out, with the cord remaining around the neck but the head and neck in close proximity to the mother's perineum.[10] If the cord is too tight, two clamps can be applied and the cord can be cut between them to escalate delivery.[4,9]
6. With the next contraction, external rotation of the head occurs; the shoulder should follow the path of the head. Gentle downward traction should be applied to deliver the anterior shoulder, which rotates under the pubic arch.
7. The posterior shoulder should be delivered while gentle upward traction is applied to the head.
8. Finally, the body and legs should be delivered.
9. A bulb syringe can be used to clear the infant's airway.
10. Two clamps can be placed on the cord 3 or 4 cm from the infant and cut between them. The cord blood should be placed in a sterile vacuum blood-collection tube.[3]
11. The newborn can be stimulated and warmed by being placed in the mother's arms or a warmer.
12. Apgar scores should be obtained at 1, 5, and 10 minutes.

(*Figure 23-4*) to guide the delivery. The head engages at the end of pregnancy (during the first stage of labor). Flexion, descent, and internal rotation result in the sagittal suture (crown) moving into the anterior/posterior diameter of the pelvis.[9]

PEARL

When delivery is imminent, the neonatal warmer should be prepared.

The third stage involves delivery of the placenta, which can take 2 to 30 minutes. Signs of placental separation include a gush of fresh blood, cord lengthening, and a firming of the uterus.[9] It is acceptable to apply gentle traction on the cord while applying counter pressure just above the symphysis to prevent uterine inversion.[9] Once the placenta is delivered, it should be inspected to ensure complete removal. To decrease the risk of postpartum hemorrhage from uterine atony, transabdominally massage the uterus and start 20 units of oxytocin in 1 liter of normal saline at 200 mL/hr.[9,11] Ten units of oxytocin can be intramuscularly administered prior to delivery of the placenta if intravenous access was not obtained. It is essential to ensure that no twin is present before administering oxytocin; in such cases, the uterus will contract down on the twin, creating potentially life-threatening conditions. Finally, the perineum, vagina, and cervix should be inspected for lacerations requiring repair.

Complications of Delivery

Shoulder Dystocia

Shoulder dystocia, an obstetrical emergency that occurs in up to 2% of vaginal deliveries, often is signaled by the fetal head recoiling back toward the perineum (the turtle sign).[12] This complication occurs when the infant's shoulder girdle is in the anteroposterior rather than the oblique position, causing it to become lodged behind the pubic symphysis.[12] Risk factors include macrosomia, maternal obesity, and prolonged second-stage labor.[12] Shoulder dystocia is associated with complications such as neonatal brachial plexus injury, clavicle and humerus fracture, and neonatal asphyxia.[13]

As soon as dystocia is identified, the mother should be stopped from pushing and help should be enlisted. The bladder can be drained to create more room anteriorly, and an episiotomy might be warranted.[4] The clinician should attempt to turn the neonate's shoulder to the oblique and deliver. If no experienced care provider is present or if there is no room to adjust fetal presentation, proceed with changing the mother's position.[14,15] Two assistants should flex the mother's thighs back to her chest (McRoberts maneuver) to rotate the pubic symphysis cephalad and dislodge the anterior shoulder (*Figure 23-5*). If unsuccessful, an assistant can stand on a stool and apply significant suprapubic pressure to dislodge the anterior shoulder from behind the symphysis. Success rates of these two procedures have been reported between 54% and 90%.[12,16] These maneuvers can be combined and should only be attempted once, as additional trials can prolong the birth process.

If the shoulders are still not deliverable but there is room to manipulate the infant's position, a Woods corkscrew maneuver can be performed by pushing the posterior shoulder 180 degrees clockwise to make it the anterior shoulder (*Figure 23-6*). The anterior shoulder can be moved by placing two fingers behind the scapula and using posterior pressure to rotate the body and adduct the shoulder.[17] If this is not successful, the clinician should attempt to deliver the posterior arm by inserting a hand posteriorly and applying gentle pressure at the antecubital fossa to flex the arm and sweep it over the chest. If there is no room for shoulder movement, the mother can be placed on her

FIGURE 23-5. McRoberts Maneuver

The technique consists of removing the legs from the stirrups and sharply flexing the thighs up onto the abdomen. The assistant is simultaneously providing suprapubic pressure (*vertical arrow*).

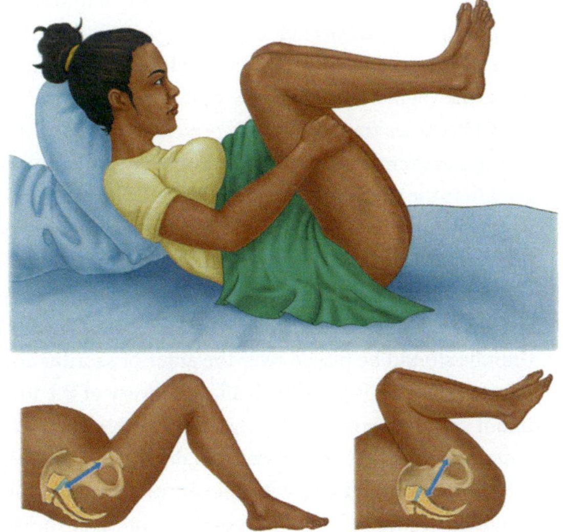

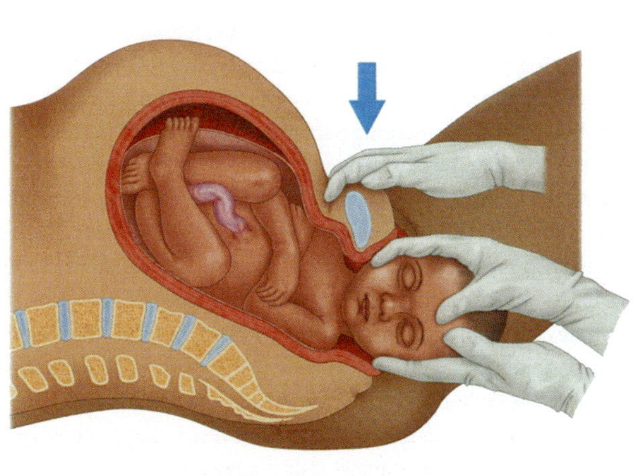

FIGURE 23-6. Woods Corkscrew Maneuver

The hand is placed behind the posterior shoulder of the fetus. The shoulder is then rotated progressively 180 degrees in a corkscrew manner to release the impacted anterior shoulder.

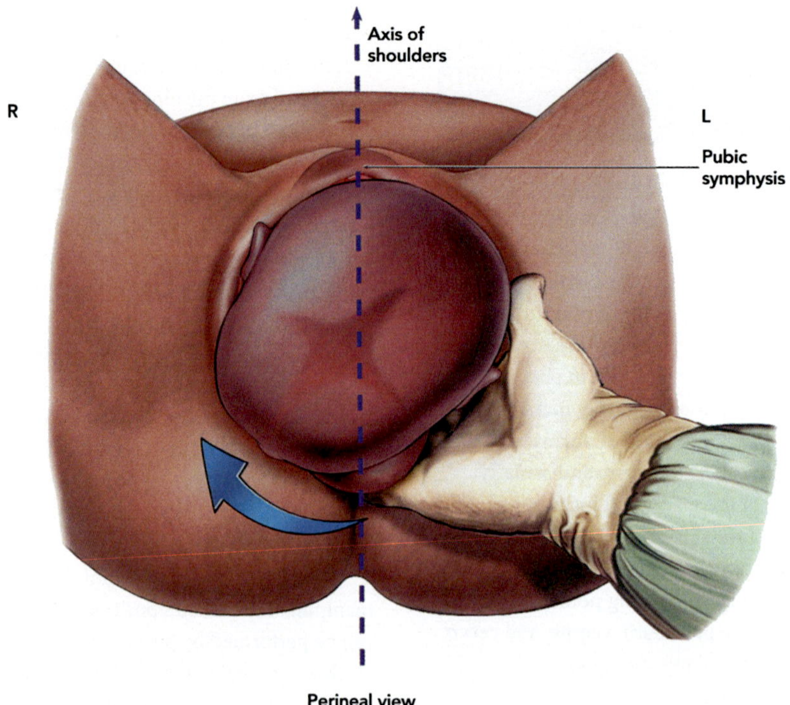

hands and knees (the Gaskins all-fours maneuver). This position uses the force of gravity to help dislodge the shoulder. If these approaches fail, the clavicle can be fractured to diminish the width of the shoulder girdle and deliver the infant.[16]

Umbilical Cord Prolapse

Umbilical cord prolapse occurs when the cord passes through the cervix with or without the presenting part. The incidence of overt prolapse (displacement of the cord into the vagina after rupture of the membranes) in cephalic presentations is about 0.5%, a rate that is higher in cases of malpresentation.[16] This is a life-threatening emergency for the fetus since the presenting part compresses the cord and restricts blood flow and oxygen. If a cord is felt or seen, the mother should be told to stop pushing, and the presenting part should be lifted off the cord. The cord should be placed back into the vagina for warmth. If obstetrical support is available, an immediate cesarean section should be requested. If transport to the operating suite is necessary, pressure may be relieved by placing the patient in the Trendelenburg position or manually lifting the presenting part off the cord. Filling the bladder with 500 mL of saline to elevate the presenting part has also been described.[16] If a prolonged time to cesarean section delivery is anticipated, a tocolytic agent (eg, terbutaline, 0.25 mg) can be administered subcutaneously.[18]

When obstetrical support is unavailable and delivery is imminent, the cord should be manually reduced into the vagina and vaginal delivery should be completed rapidly.[3,16] Perinatal mortality rates from umbilical cord prolapse are lower than 10% as a result of a growing number of cesarean sections and improved neonatal resuscitation skills.[19]

Breech Presentation

Breech presentation, which complicates 3% to 4% of all pregnancies, carries a high rate of perinatal morbidity and mortality caused by congenital abnormalities and complications such as cord prolapse and birth trauma.[12,16] Three types of breech presentation occur: complete breech (thighs and knees flexed), footling breech (one or both legs extended), and frank breech (thighs flexed and knees extended) *(Figure 23-7)*.[12] The difficulty with these scenarios is that delivery of the legs and torso does not dilate the vaginal canal enough for the passage of the fetal head, which becomes trapped. Breech presentation can be identified by vaginal examination or ultrasonography. Although cesarean section is the preferred method of delivery in such cases, it is not always feasible. It is best to avoid applying traction on the legs or body until the infant is delivered to the level of the umbilicus.

If delivery is imminent with a breech presentation, one leg should be delivered followed by the other leg. The clinician's thumbs should be placed over the anterior sacrum and the fingers over the iliac crests to allow delivery of the torso. The infant should be rotated 90 degrees to enable delivery of the anterior arm, and then rotated 180 degrees for delivery of the second arm. Finally, with the sacrum anterior, a second provider should apply suprapubic pressure over the head while the clinician's fingers remain over the maxillary process to keep the infant's head flexed. The fingers of the clinician's other hand should be hooked over the shoulder while gentle downward traction is applied.[12,16] If the head cannot be delivered through the cervix, incisions can be made at the 6-o'clock or the 2- and 10-o'clock positions of the cervix, but this causes significant maternal hemorrhage.[12,16]

Postpartum Hemorrhage

Postpartum hemorrhage is the second most common cause of pregnancy-related death in the United States.[20] It is classified as immediate (ie, within the first 24 hours) or delayed (ie, after the first 24 hours and up to 6 weeks).[11] Causes of immediate postpartum hemorrhage, defined as blood loss greater than 500 mL during a vaginal delivery, are listed in Table 23-2. Although the management of delayed postpartum hemorrhage is beyond the scope of this chapter, it is well-described in emergency medicine textbooks. The astute emergency physician must not wait for changes in the vital signs to consider the possibility of bleeding (tachycardia could be the mother's response to pain, and hypotension is a late finding).

Uterine atony, the most common cause of postpartum hemorrhage, most frequently occurs when the uterus has been overextended (macrosomia) or fatigued from prolonged labor, and in cases of precipitous delivery.[11] Management consists of manual massage, with one hand placed externally on the

TABLE 23-2. Causes of Immediate Postpartum Hemorrhage

Tone	Atony
Trauma	Genital or cervical lacerations, hematoma
Tissue	Retained products or twins
Thrombin	Disseminated intravascular coagulation, coagulopathy
Twisted	Uterine inversion or rupture

FIGURE 23-7. Management of the Vaginal Frank Breech Delivery (Pinard Maneuver)

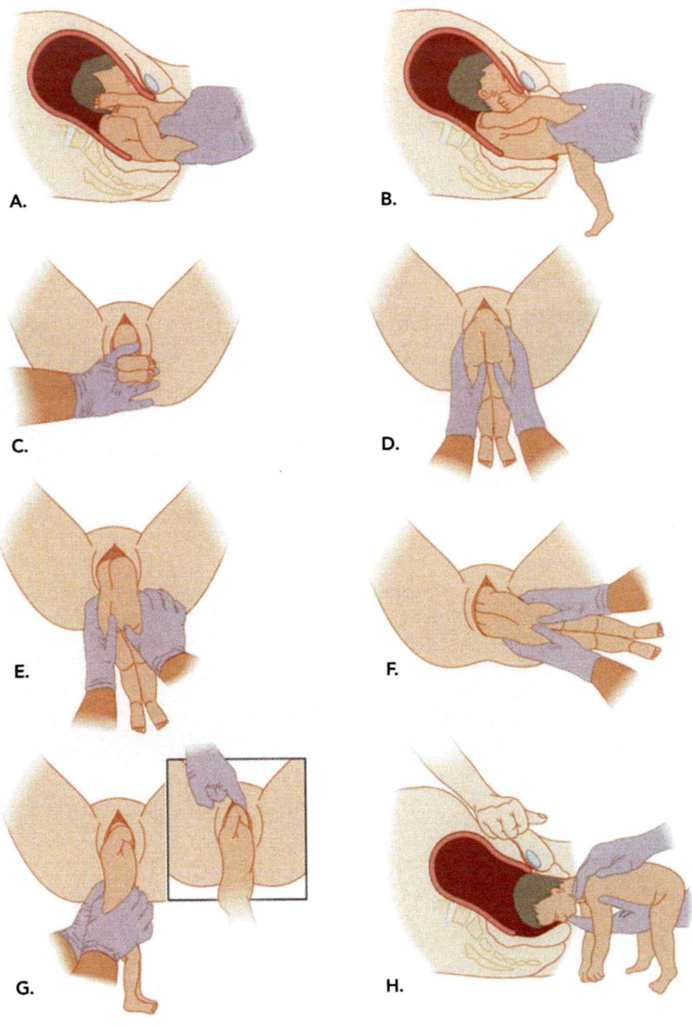

A. The operator's hand is placed behind the fetal thigh, putting gentle pressure at the knee and allowing delivery of the leg.

B. A similar maneuver of the opposite leg.

C. Grasp the feet with the thumb and third finger over the lateral malleolus, and place the second finger between the two ankles.

D. With maternal expulsive efforts, deliver the breech to the level of the umbilicus. Keep the sacrum anterior.

E. Again, with maternal expulsive efforts, deliver the infant to the level of the clavicles, keeping the sacrum anterior.

F. Rotate the fetus 90 degrees, which allows visualization of the now anterior right arm.

G. The arm is well visualized. Use a single digit to deliver it. Deliver the opposite arm by rotating the fetus 180 degrees in a clockwise direction and repeating the maneuver.

H. Deliver the fetal vertex by placing your fingers over the maxillary processes of the fetus, with the body kept parallel to the floor. The body should never be lifted above parallel to prevent hyperextension of the neck. An assistant applies suprapubic pressure, aiding flexion of the fetal head and accomplishing delivery.

From: Tintinalli J, Stapczynski J, Ma OJ, et al, eds. *Tintinalli's Emergency Medicine: A Comprehensive Study Guide*. 7th ed. New York, NY: McGraw-Hill; 2010:710. Copyright McGraw-Hill, 2010. Used with permission.

FIGURE 23-8. Procedure for Perimortem Cesarean Section

A. Make a midline vertical abdominal incision just below the umbilicus to the symphysis pubis. **B.** Some clinicians recommend incising from the xiphoid to the symphysis pubis. **C.** Make a vertical uterine incision. **D.** Deliver the fetus.

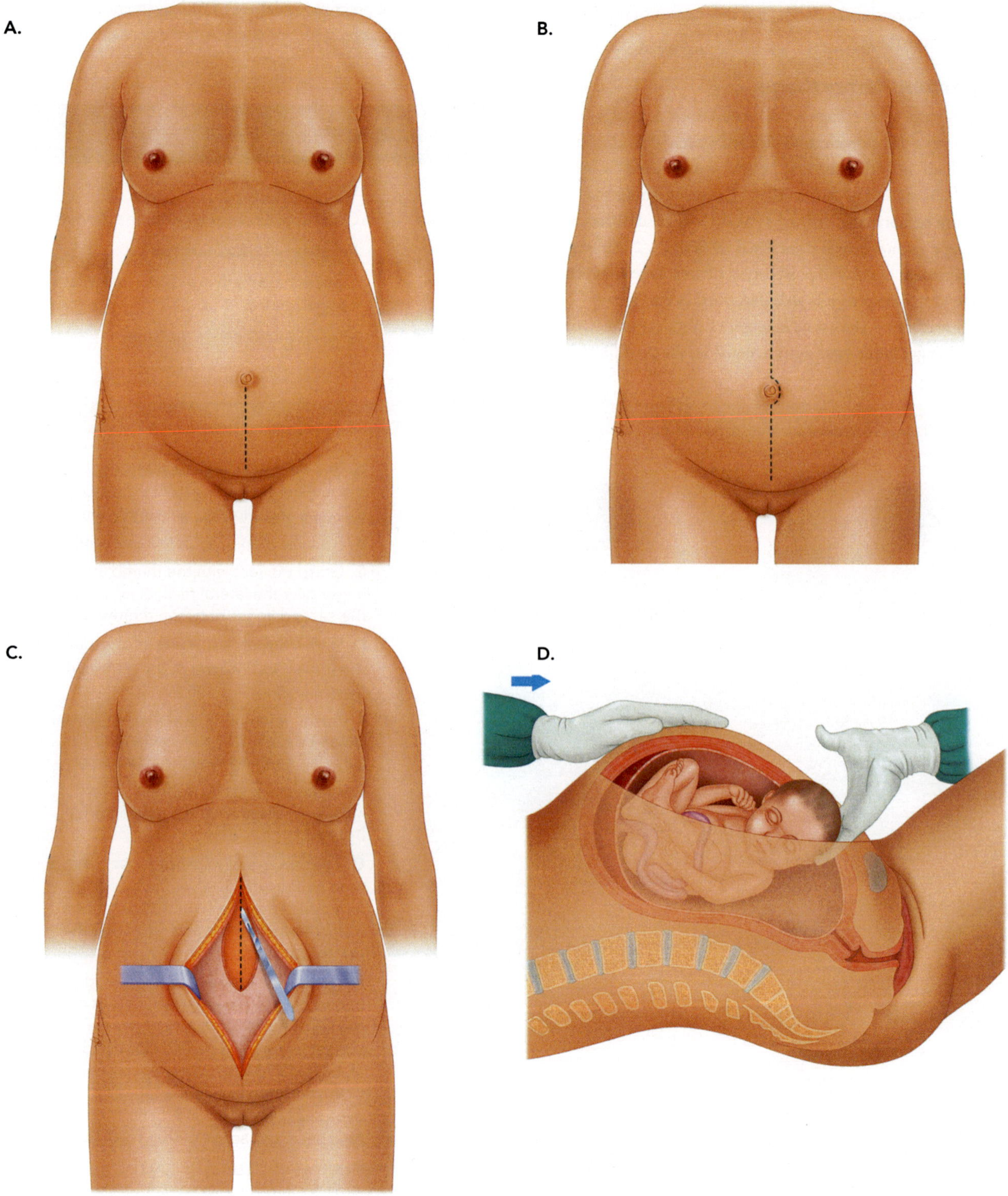

A.

B.

C.

D.

abdomen and the other placed internally, massaging the uterus upward.[11] Simultaneously, medications may be started to increase uterine muscle tone *(Table 23-3)*.[21] If this fails, the birth canal should be inspected for lacerations or hematomas of the perineum, vagina, or cervix. Cervical lacerations may require surgical intervention, but bleeding can be staunched with ring forceps prior to moving the patient to the operating room. Retained placental parts, which also can precipitate bleeding, may be found by digital examination of the uterus. If they cannot be removed easily, wait for obstetrical backup and consider packing the uterus if hemorrhage is significant.[11]

Uterine Inversion/Uterine Rupture

The incidence of uterine inversion is about 1 in 2,500 pregnancies. Although its cause is unclear, the complication is often described in association with cord traction and excessive fundal pressure.[22] Recognition and immediate action are crucial. All uterotonic medications should be stopped immediately, and the uterus should be manually reduced by applying pressure on the fundus with a hand directed inward toward the umbilicus.[22] If the placenta remains attached, it should not be removed before the uterus has been reduced. Pharmacological relaxation of the uterus with terbutaline, magnesium, or nitroglycerin may be required for reduction.[22] Once the uterus is reduced, uterotonic medications can be restarted.

PEARL

Oxytocin should not be given as an intravenous push because it causes hypotension. The uterus has limited receptors for oxytocin, so it cannot respond to increased doses. Additional medications should be trialed if bleeding persists.

Uterine rupture is a rare but life-threatening obstetrical emergency.[22] Risk factors include previous cesarean delivery, use of labor-induction medications, and trauma.[22] Clinical presentations can vary from uterine tenderness to maternal shock.[22] Surgical intervention is required if this condition is suspected; the clinician should continue standard hypovolemic resuscitation practices until surgical support is available.

Cardiac Arrest During Pregnancy

The 2010 update of the advanced cardiac life support (ACLS) protocols published by the American Heart Association contains no change in medications or indications for defibrillation in pregnant women experiencing cardiac arrest; however, other adjustments are recommended.[23]

The gravid uterus causes significant aortocaval compression; therefore, the revised ACLS recommendations call for the use of a backboard supported by blankets, a wedge, or even a chair during cardiopulmonary resuscitation (CPR) to achieve 15 to 30 degrees of left lateral tilt to facilitate venous return. Manual displacement of the uterus by pulling to the maternal left or pushing from the maternal right has been shown to be equal or superior to the tilt approach in increasing venous return. Drug delivery can be limited by the uterus, so placement of an upper body line should be considered. Because of the enlarged uterus and the resulting upward shift of the internal organs, heart, and diaphragm, hand placement for CPR of a pregnant patient should be slightly higher on the chest than for a nonpregnant patient.

Tocodynamometer and fetal heart monitors, if present, should be removed to eliminate the theoretical risk of arcing if shocks are required. The emergency physician should be prepared for a difficult airway caused by airway edema, secretions, decreased functional residual capacity, increased oxygen demand, and heightened aspiration risk. Patients in cardiac arrest who have received magnesium should immediately receive calcium. Possible causes of cardiac arrest during pregnancy include pulmonary and amniotic fluid embolism.

Perimortem Cesarean Section

Perimortem cesarean section should be considered in any pregnant patient in cardiac arrest with a viable fetus of more than 24 weeks' gestation.[23,24] Based on limited data, the procedure *(Figure 23-8)* should be initiated within 4 minutes after maternal cardiac arrest.[25] Although most surviving infants are delivered within 5 to 15 minutes after the death of the mother, one case report describes a child who was delivered 30 minutes after maternal cardiac arrest and was developing normally 4 years later.[26,27] Another case report describes the management of a woman in cardiac arrest and pregnant with

TABLE 23-3. Medical Management of Uterine Atony

Medication	Dose	Side Effects
Oxytocin	20 units in 500 mL normal saline at 10 mL/min until uterus is firm *OR* 10 units IM	Hypotension, nausea, vomiting
Methylergonovine maleate	0.2 mg IM; may repeat every 2–4 hours	Hypertension, nausea, vomiting
Carboprost tromethamine	250 mcg IM	Nausea, vomiting, diarrhea
Dinoprostone	20 mg suppository vaginally or rectally	Abdominal pain, nausea, vomiting

twins, who regained spontaneous circulation after 18 minutes of CPR; cesarean section was performed 2 hours after the mother's revival.[28]

PERIMORTEM CESAREAN SECTION STEPS

1. CPR should be continued throughout the procedure.
2. If gestational age is unknown, fundal height can be measured while CPR is ongoing.
3. Make a midline vertical incision from the epigastric area to the pubic symphysis.
4. Penetrate all abdominal layers and find the uterus.
5. Use retractors or assistants to hold back the abdominal wall. Drain the bladder if time permits.
6. Make an incision at the fundus of the uterus. Insert two fingers to lift the uterine wall away from the fetus.
7. Using a scalpel or scissors, incise from the fundus to the bladder reflection.[3]
8. Remove the infant, suction the mouth, and clamp the cord.
9. The incision made on the mother should be closed based on the projected course of resuscitation efforts and in conjunction with a surgical team.

Perimortem cesarean section has been shown to improve both maternal and fetal survival rates. The recommendation for starting the procedure within 4 minutes after arrest is based on the timing of cerebral ischemia; however, even under the best circumstances, it is difficult to perform a perimortem cesarean section in an emergency department in less than 5 minutes.[29]

The decision to undertake a perimortem cesarean section is a particularly difficult one. Emergency physicians must be aware of the indications for this procedure and its sequence. Time to delivery is a crucial factor. In some cases, cesarean section improves the mother's hemodynamics to the extent that resuscitation might be successful.[26] Multiple factors must be considered, including the age of the infant, duration of the cardiac arrest and whether it was witnessed, ability of the hospital to care for the infant, and availability of surgical and obstetrical backup.

Conclusion

Although emergency deliveries are rare, they do occur. Clinicians must be aware of hospital policies and the availability of resources to support such events. A woman who presents in labor should be assessed with a focused history and physical examination. If time permits, sonography should be used to

KEY POINTS

1. Perform a focused history and physical examination.
   - Assess fetal position and heartbeat.
   - Look for the presence of amniotic fluid.
   - Perform a sterile bimanual examination or sterile speculum examination.
2. Steps in normal delivery:
   - Clean the perineum.
   - Apply gentle pressure to the perineum with one hand, and control delivery of the head with the other hand.
   - Sweep the neck to check for a nuchal cord.
   - Deliver the anterior shoulder.
   - Deliver the posterior shoulder.
   - Deliver the body.
   - Suction the airway.
   - Clamp and cut the cord.
   - Document the Apgar score at 1, 5, and 10 minutes.
3. For shoulder dystocia:
   - Step 1: Stop pushing. Consider draining the bladder and performing an episiotomy.
   - Step 2a: If an experienced practitioner is present, check for room to move the fetal shoulders.
   - Step 2b: If an experienced practitioner is not present or if there is no room to adjust the fetus, perform a McRoberts maneuver and apply suprapubic pressure.
   - Step 3: Attempt a Woods maneuver, depending on the room available to rotate.
   - Step 4: Roll the mother into the Gaskins all-fours position.
   - Step 5: Deliver the posterior arm.
   - Step 6: As a last resort, fracture the clavicle.
4. For umbilical cord prolapse:
   - Place patient in the Trendelenburg position.
   - Lift the presenting part off the cord.
   - Fill the bladder with 500 mL of saline to elevate the presenting part.
   - Await obstetrical support to perform a cesarean section.
5. For a breech presentation:
   - Deliver the legs.
   - Keep the sacrum anterior.
   - Deliver the torso.
   - With the sacrum anterior, keep the infant's head flexed, and apply downward traction over the shoulders.
   - Clamp and cut the cord.
6. Uterine atony is the most common cause of postpartum hemorrhage. Treatment includes manual massage of the uterus and administration of uterotonic medications.
7. Start perimortem cesarean section within 4 minutes after maternal cardiac arrest (sooner if possible).
   - Most experts believe that informed consent for this procedure is not necessary.

assess the fetal position in preparation for a normal vaginal or breech delivery. Complications should be anticipated, including shoulder dystocia, umbilical cord prolapse, nuchal cord, and postpartum hemorrhage. If a pregnant woman goes into cardiac arrest, the physician should remember the ABCs, assess fundal height, and prepare for a cesarean section.

REFERENCES

1. Brunette DD, Sterner SP. Prehospital and emergency department delivery: a review of eight years' experience. *Ann Emerg Med.* 1989;18:1116-1118.
2. Elixhauser A, Machlin SR, Zodet MW, et al. Health care for children and youth in the United States: 2001 annual report on access, utilization, quality, and expenditures. *Ambul Pediatr.* 2002;2:419-437.
3. Stallard TC, Burns B. Emergency delivery and perimortem C-section. *Emerg Med Clin North Am.* 2003;21:679-693.
4. Burg MD. Emergency delivery. In: Wolfson AB, ed. *Harwood-Nuss' Clinical Practice of Emergency Medicine.* 6th ed. Philadelphia, PA: Lippincott Williams & Wilkins; 2015:691-694.
5. VanRooyen MJ, Scott JA. Emergency delivery. In: Tintinalli JE, Stapczynski JS, Ma OJ, eds. *Emergency Medicine: A Comprehensive Guide.* 7th ed. New York, NY: McGraw-Hill; 2011:703-711.
6. Lydon-Rochelle M, Albers L, Gorwoda J, et al. Accuracy of Leopold maneuvers in screening for malpresentation: a prospective study. *Birth.* 1993;20:132-135.
7. Lund KJ, McManaman J. Normal labor, delivery, newborn care, and puerperium. In: Gibbs RS, Karlan BY, Haney AF, Nygaard IE, eds. *Danforth's Obstetrics and Gynecology.* 10th ed. Philadelphia, PA: Lippincott Williams & Wilkins; 2008:22-42.
8. Gianopoulos JG. Emergency complications of labor and delivery. *Emerg Med Clin North Am.* 1994;12:201-217.
9. Archie CL, Roman AS. Normal & abnormal labor & delivery. In: DeCherney AH, Nathan L, Laufer N, et al, eds. *Current Diagnosis and Treatment: Obstetrics & Gynecology.* 11th ed. New York, NY: Lange Medical Books/McGraw-Hill; 2013:154-162.
10. Melvin C, Downe S. Management of the nuchal cord: a summary of the evidence. *Br J Midwifery.* 2007;15:617-620.
11. Mendelson MH, Lang JP. Postpartum emergencies. In: Wolfson AB, ed. *Harwood-Nuss' Clinical Practice of Emergency Medicine.* 6th ed. Philadelphia, PA: Lippincott Williams & Wilkins; 2015:695-698.
12. Brost BC, VanDorsten JP. Emergency vaginal delivery. In: Pearlman MD, Tintinalli JE, eds. *Emergency Care of the Woman.* New York, NY: McGraw-Hill; 1998:119-136.
13. Rahman J, Bhattee G, Rahman MS. Shoulder dystocia in a 16-year experience in a teaching hospital. *J Reprod Med.* 2009;54:378-384.
14. Inglis SR, Feier N, Chetiyaar JB, et al. Effects of shoulder dystocia training on the incidence of brachial plexus injury. *Am J Obstet Gynecol.* 2011;204:322.e1-6.
15. Stitely ML, Gherman RB. Shoulder dystocia: management and documentation. *Semin Perinatol.* 2014;38:194-200.
16. Kish K. Malpresentation & cord prolapse. In: DeCherney AH, Nathan L, Laufer N, et al, eds. *Current Diagnosis and Treatment: Obstetrics & Gynecology.* 11th ed. New York, NY: Lange Medical Books/McGraw-Hill; 2013:317-333.
17. Silver DW, Sabatino F. Precipitous and difficult deliveries. *Emerg Med Clin North Am.* 2012;30:961-975.
18. Phelan ST, Holbrook BD. Umbilical cord prolapse: a plan for an ob emergency. *Contemp Ob Gynecol.* 2013;58: 28-36.
19. Lin MG. Umbilical cord prolapse. *Obstet Gynecol Surv.* 2006;61:269-277.
20. Kung HC, Hoyert DL, Xu J, et al. Deaths: final data for 2005. *Natl Vital Stat Rep.* 2008;56(10):1-120.
21. Postpartum hemorrhage — acute. In: DISEASEDEX™ Emergency Medicine Summary in Micromedex 1.0. Greenwood Village, CO: Thomson Reuters (Healthcare) Inc; 2009.
22. Mirza FG, Gaddipati S. Obstetric emergencies. *Semin Perinatol.* 2009;33:97-103.
23. Vanden Hoek TL, Morrison LJ, Shuster M, et al. Part 12: Cardiac arrest in special situations: 2010 American Heart Association guidelines for cardiopulmonary resuscitation and emergency cardiovascular care. *Circulation.* 2010;122:S829-S861.
24. Montufar-Rueda C, Gei A. Cardiac arrest during pregnancy. *Clin Obstet Gynecol.* 2014;57:871-881.
25. Katz VL, Dotters DJ, Droegemueller W. Perimortem cesarean delivery. *Obstet Gynecol.* 1986;68:571-576.
26. Katz V, Balderston K, DeFreest M. Perimortem cesarean delivery: were our assumptions correct? *Am J Obstet Gynecol.* 2005;192:1916-1921.
27. Capobianco G, Balata A, Mannazzu MC, et al. Perimortem cesarean delivery 30 minutes after a laboring patient jumped from a fourth-floor window: baby survives and is normal at age 4 years. *Am J Obstet Gynecol.* 2008;198:e15-e16.
28. Matsuoka A, Tanaka M, Satoshi D, et al. What enabled mother and twins to survive 18 minute maternal cardiac arrest? *Case Rep Perinatal Med.* 2014;3:103-106.
29. Katz VL. Perimortem cesarean delivery: its role in maternal mortality. *Semin Perinatol* 2012;36:68-72.
30. Holbrook BD, Phelan ST. Umbilical cord prolapse. *Obstet Gynecol Clin North Am.* 2013;40:1-14.

Neonatal Resuscitation

24

IN THIS CHAPTER

- Identifying the critically ill newborn
- Managing the airway
- Postresuscitation care
- Managing congenital anomalies and heart disease
- Withholding/discontinuing resuscitation

Lisa Greenfield and **Aaron Leetch**

Few things are as terrifying to an emergency physician as a cyanotic neonate after a precipitous delivery. Although most infants need little more than supportive care, the emergency department often selects for those in need of more intervention. Several maternal and fetal conditions can alert clinicians to the potential need for resuscitation (*Table 24-1*).[1] Because these scenarios are not commonplace in the acute setting, this chapter focuses on only the most important aspects of the American Heart Association (AHA) guidelines, and provides additional tips for successfully managing these fragile cases (*Figure 24-1*).[2]

The resuscitation of a newborn differs from that of adults, children, and even slightly older infants for one main reason: a neonatal resuscitation is almost exclusively focused on *respiration* as the key component of transition from fetal circulation. Even in neonatal intensive care units (NICUs) and delivery rooms, chest compressions and drugs are used very infrequently.[3]

TABLE 24-1. Maternal and Fetal Conditions Predicting the Need for Resuscitation

Maternal
Preeclampsia/eclampsia
Diabetes mellitus
Placental abruption
Trauma
Fever
No prenatal care
Illicit drug use
Fetal
Meconium-stained amniotic fluid
Early gestational age
Known congenital anomalies
Oligo/polyhydramnios
Prolonged rupture of membranes

The first breath is the catalyst for an infant's transition from intrauterine to extrauterine life. This vital automatic response prompts amniotic fluid in the lungs to absorb, umbilical vessels to constrict, and pulmonary arterioles to dilate.[4] As pulmonary arterial pressure decreases, blood preferentially flows to the lungs, enabling oxygenation and normal systemic circulation (*Figure 24-2*). For this reason, clearing the infant's airway and lungs to stimulate that first breath is crucial to survival. The 2015 AHA guidelines also suggest that a 30- to 60-second delay in cord clamping and cutting may help reduce morbidity; however, this is a weak recommendation and may complicate an already stressful resuscitation with a precipitous emergency department delivery.

Most of the mainstays of adult resuscitation are not recommended for neonates by the AHA or the American Academy of Pediatrics. For example, the *only* drug recommended for infant resuscitation is epinephrine; there is no place for atropine, lidocaine, or cardioversion for a newborn in respiratory depression.[2] Neonates who cannot be resuscitated with epinephrine simply cannot be resuscitated. Likewise, rapid-sequence intubation is inappropriate for a newly delivered critically ill infant; nearly all will tolerate endotracheal intubation without sedation. Once cardiorespiratory physiology has been stabilized (often in several days), the patient can be treated according to the pediatric advanced life support (PALS) algorithm.

Specialized Equipment

Aside from typical advanced airway tools, suction, intravenous lines, and monitors, neonatal resuscitation requires several other specialized pieces of equipment (*Table 24-2*).[3] If a delivery is anticipated, an overhead warmer should be powered on and cleared of everything except blankets and a bulb suction

FIGURE 24-1. Neonatal Resuscitation Algorithm

Intubation may be considered at any point in the algorithm. Adhere as closely as possible to the "golden minute" to address airway, warmth, breathing, and circulation.[2]

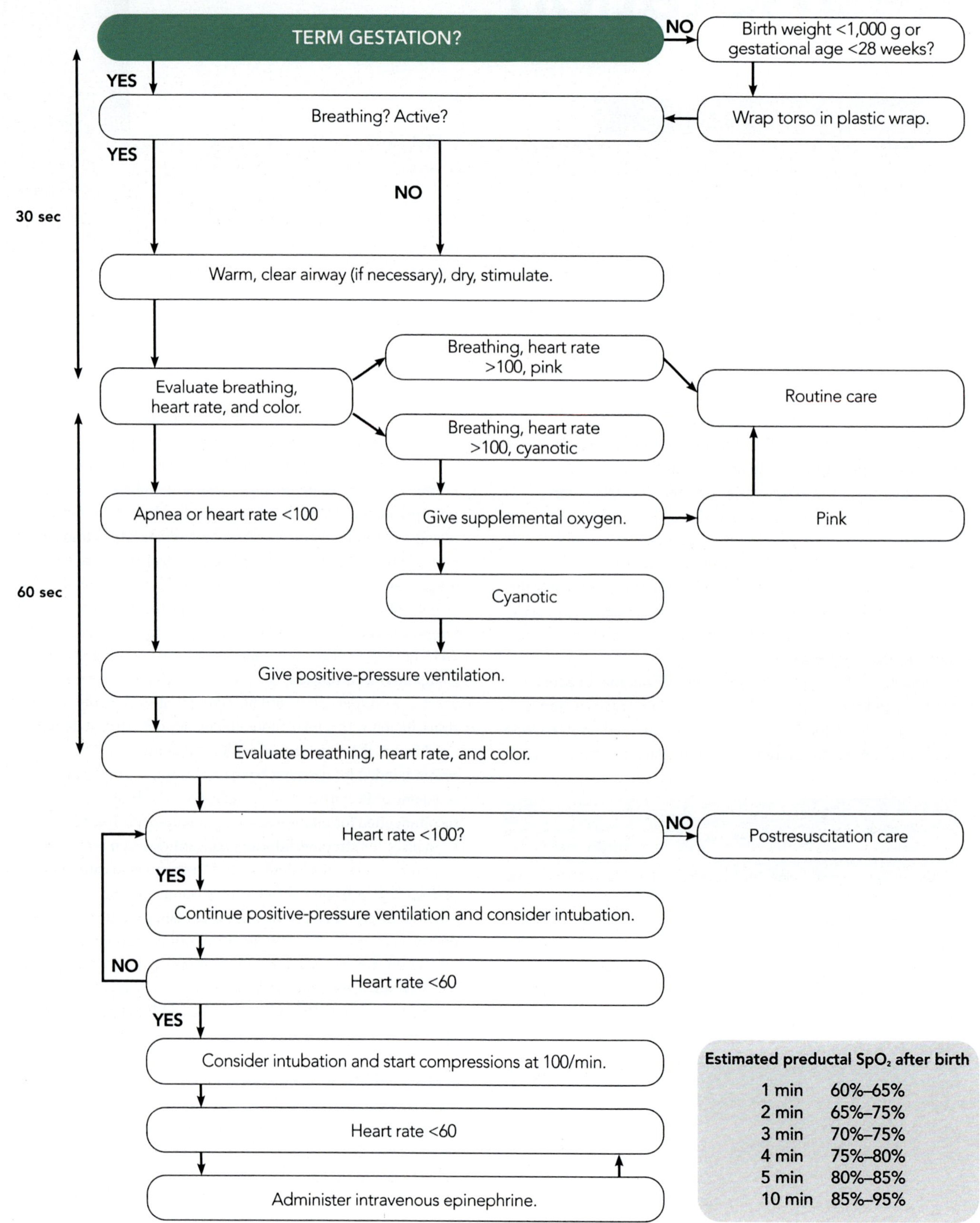

FIGURE 24-2. Intrauterine and Extrauterine Cardiac Flow

A. In utero, pulmonary arterial pressure is elevated and blood flows preferentially to the systemic circulation via right-to-left shunts.
B. After the first breath, pulmonary arterial pressure decreases and the foramen ovale and ductus arteriosus close, allowing normal pulmonary and systemic flow.

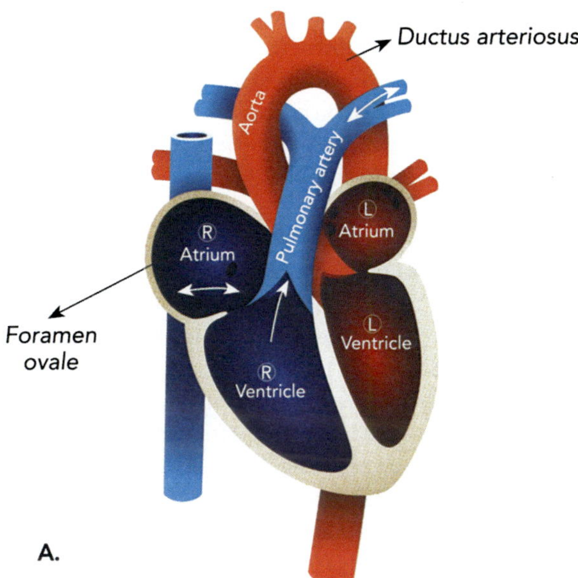

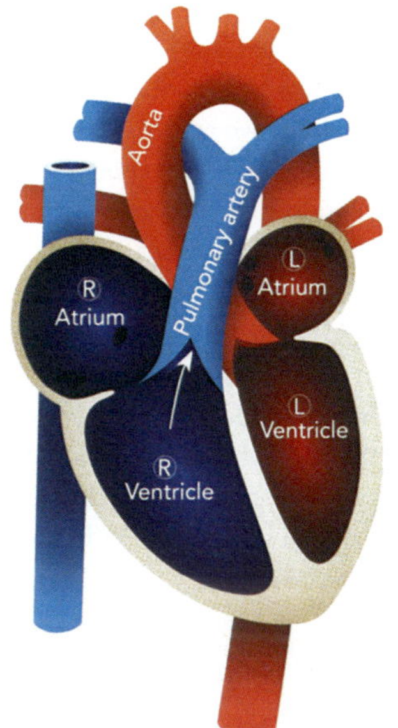

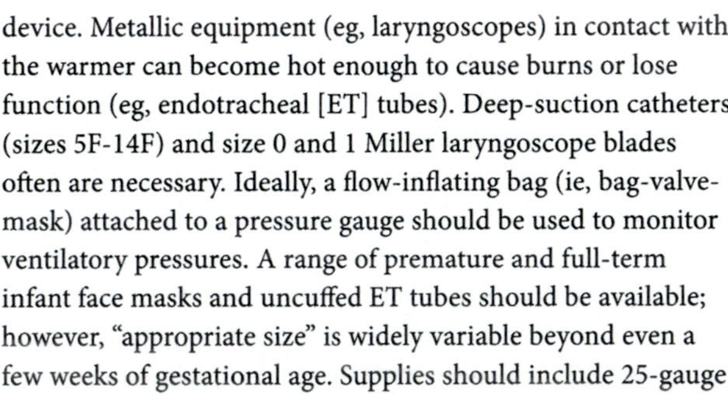

device. Metallic equipment (eg, laryngoscopes) in contact with the warmer can become hot enough to cause burns or lose function (eg, endotracheal [ET] tubes). Deep-suction catheters (sizes 5F-14F) and size 0 and 1 Miller laryngoscope blades often are necessary. Ideally, a flow-inflating bag (ie, bag-valve-mask) attached to a pressure gauge should be used to monitor ventilatory pressures. A range of premature and full-term infant face masks and uncuffed ET tubes should be available; however, "appropriate size" is widely variable beyond even a few weeks of gestational age. Supplies should include 25-gauge catheters for peripheral access and umbilical catheters for central access. Scalp veins and intraosseous lines also are options for obtaining vascular access in infants. Evidence suggests that an intraosseous line should be considered if rapid access is required and when a health care professional familiar with rapid umbilical line placement is not available.[5]

TABLE 24-2. Important Neonatal Resuscitation Equipment
Warm, clean blankets
Plastic wrap or bag
Bulb syringe
Suction catheters (10F or 12F)
Bag-valve-mask
Full-term and preterm face masks
Laryngeal mask airway (size 1)
Laryngoscope with Miller size 0 and 1 blades
Endotracheal tubes (sizes 2.5, 3.0, 3.5, 4.0)
End-tidal carbon dioxide detector
25-gauge catheters
Umbilical line kit
Normal saline
Access to 1:10,000 epinephrine

Ultrasonography has become a readily available and well-used imaging modality in the emergency department setting. Birth weight and gestational age can be estimated using crown-to-rump length and biparietal measurements. Many ultrasound machines are programmed to convert these measurements into age and weight, and can be useful when anticipating a difficult or premature delivery.

Identifying the Critically Ill Neonate

Immediately after birth, most neonates show some degree of cyanosis, pallor, poor muscle tone, or weak respiratory effort. It is what an infant does in the first 60 seconds that differentiates a healthy patient from one who is seriously ill. Newborns can be categorized as stable, purely cyanotic, or critical (*Table 24-3*).[4] Constant reevaluation of respiratory effort, heart rate, and color will aid in resuscitation. AHA guidelines allot 60 seconds for initial interventions, reevaluation, and the initiation of positive-pressure ventilation (PPV), if indicated.[2]

If there is no change in color, tone, or respiratory effort or if a child is bradycardic after this "golden minute," critical illness if more likely. Recent research suggests that the recommended 60-second interval may be too short, as most newborns cannot be managed within this time frame.

Contrary to popular belief, the Apgar score (*Table 24-4*) cannot be used to determine whether resuscitation is needed, although it is a good determinant of how the infant is responding to resuscitation efforts.

Airway/Temperature

After an infant is delivered, start a timer to keep the resuscitation on pace. Providing warmth is as important as clearing the airway, and the two can be done simultaneously. Newborns are highly susceptible to evaporative heat losses and will quickly decompensate if allowed to become hypothermic. Place the child under a radiant warmer and/or dry vigorously with warm blankets to maintain a temperature between 36.5°C and 37.5°C (97.7°F–99.5°F). Interventions such as maintaining ambient temperatures above 26°C (78.8°F), reducing maternal hypothermia, and using warm resuscitation gases can decrease the risk of hypothermia and thus improve survival.[7] Extremely premature infants (<28 weeks' gestation or weighing ≤1,000 g) should be wrapped in food-grade plastic wrap to prevent radiant heat loss.[8,9]

PEARL

When managing a neonate, providing warmth is as important as clearing the airway.

Place the infant in the sniffing position, being careful not to hyperextend the neck *(Figure 24-2)*. If nasal or oral secretions are obvious, clear the mouth and then the nose with bulb suction or a deep-suction catheter attached to wall suction. Infants are obligate nose breathers and must have a patent nasopharynx. If the patient is breathing spontaneously and there is no obvious airway obstruction, suctioning should not be performed because it can cause reflex bradycardia that further complicates resuscitation. If the neonate has not yet begun to cry or grimace, continue to dry the infant vigorously and stimulate by rubbing the back or flicking/slapping the feet.

Infants with meconium-stained amniotic fluid at delivery are at risk for aspiration and the complications of aspiration pneumonia and respiratory compromise. Suctioning of the perineum or trachea are no longer recommended for infants who present with meconium, as these techniques do not appear to decrease the incidence of aspiration.[6,10,11] Previous versions of the AHA guidelines have recommended endotracheal intubation and suctioning for meconium-stained infants who are not vigorous and who are making no respiratory effort. However, new guidelines caution against this tactic, as there is no known benefit, and it likely will delay the more important step of positive-pressure ventilation.

TABLE 24-3. Clinical Classification of Neonates

Stable	Breathing Heart rate >100 beats/min No central cyanosis (pink oral mucous membranes)
Purely cyanotic	Breathing Heart rate >100 beats/min Central cyanosis (blue mucous membranes)
Critical	Apnea *OR* Heart rate <100 beats/min Central cyanosis

Neonatal Airways

Miller blades are recommended for neonates because their airways are more anterior and the epiglottis is more malleable and difficult to control. Size 0 blades are used for premature infants (<36 weeks) and size 1 for term infants (>36 weeks). Size 00 blades are available for extremely low-birth-weight patients (<28 weeks), but they can occlude the oropharynx and might be too short to reach the airway. All ET tubes used for neonatal resuscitation should be uncuffed, according to AHA guidelines. Because the airway size varies so much, depending on gestational age, the standard shorthand of (age + 16)/4 for size and 3 x ET tube length for depth of insertion is unreliable. The correct size and depth can be estimated using weight or gestational age (*Table 24-5*).[3]

To reiterate, rapid-sequence intubation is never indicated immediately after delivery. Newborns should be directly intubated without medications. Placing a small towel under the shoulders can aid in airway alignment. Infants' vocal cords lack the pearly appearance seen in adults and older children; the color more nearly matches that of the surrounding tissue. Weak respiratory effort can cause some movement of the cords, allowing distinction from the esophagus. Vocal cords can be identified by their physical proximity to the epiglottis. Once intubation is successful and confirmed (using examination and capnometry), the ET tube should be secured by bracing it against the patient's gum and lip with one finger while an assistant tapes the tube in place.

PEARL

Rapid-sequence intubation is never indicated immediately after delivery.

The neonatal airway is very short, so tracheal intubation can result in right mainstem bronchus placement; in addition, the tube can be dislodged with small flexion or extension of the neck. A cervical collar or towel rolls placed on either side of the head can prevent movement. Obtain a chest radiograph to confirm the position after securing the ET tube. After the infant is intubated, be careful not to ventilate too vigorously, so as to avoid barotrauma or pneumothorax. All intubated infants should be reevaluated frequently for adverse sequelae of positive-pressure ventilation.

TABLE 24-4. Apgar Mnemonic and Scoring System

	0	1	2
Appearance (color)	Central cyanosis	Peripheral cyanosis	Pink
Pulse	Absent	<100 beats/min	>100 beats/min
Grimace (cry)	Absent	Grimace, no cry	Strong cry, cough
Activity (tone)	Limp	Some flexion	Active motion
Respiratory effort	Apneic	Weak respirations	Strong respirations

Breathing

After the initial steps, continue to evaluate respiratory effort, heart rate, and color.[3] Stable infants can simply be observed. Cyanotic patients with a heart rate faster than 100 beats/min and active respiratory effort (purely cyanotic infants) might require only supplemental oxygen. Acrocyanosis (cyanosis limited to the hands and feet) can persist for hours and is not necessarily a sign of poor perfusion or oxygenation. Central cyanosis (of the trunk, oral mucosa, or lips) always indicates poor perfusion or oxygenation and must be addressed immediately. Remember that a pulse oximeter placed on an acrocyanotic extremity can provide falsely low readings of oxygen level. The AHA recommends placing a pulse oximeter on the right hand (preductal saturation) and aiming for normal oxygen saturation after 10 minutes.[2] The neonate's clinical appearance is just as important as pulse oximetry for assessing respiratory status.[12]

PEARL

A pulse oximeter placed on an acrocyanotic extremity can provide falsely low oxygen levels. Only central cyanosis (blue mucous membranes) requires intervention.

Oxygen can be delivered via any free-flowing mechanism (eg, face mask or tubing held in a cupped hand). Self-inflating devices such as a bag-valve-mask must be squeezed and are not ideal for blow-by oxygenation. After receiving oxygen, infants should show color change within several seconds. There is a concern among neonatologists that resuscitation on 100% oxygen can be detrimental to premature infants because of high levels of free oxygen radicals. Prolonged use has been associated with complications such as retinopathy of prematurity and bronchopulmonary dysplasia, especially in infants born at less than 28 weeks' gestational age.

An initial fraction of inspired oxygen (FiO_2) of 21% to 30% oxygen has been shown to be safer than 65% to 100%.[13] This method has been correlated with less oxidative stress and improved morbidity rates compared with high-flow oxygen; however, it is likely to require an upward titration of oxygen content in order to maintain appropriate saturation levels.[6,13,14] Many neonatologists start resuscitation on room air (21% oxygen) using an oxygen blender and then titrate it as clinically indicated. If this tool is not available, flow rate can be adjusted to deliver various oxygen concentrations via self-inflating bags with reservoirs. A flow rate of 0.25 L/min delivers an oxygen concentration of 30% to 35%, while 1 L/min delivers 40% to 60%.[15] If available, continuous positive airway pressure devices can be used for patients who are spontaneously breathing but showing signs of distress.

Infants with apnea or a heart rate slower than 100 beats/min and those who do not improve after blow-by oxygenation should receive positive-pressure ventilation via a bag-valve-mask (BVM) device, aiming for a respiratory rate of 40 to 60 breaths/min.[2] Infants are far more susceptible to barotrauma and pneumothorax than adults are because of their lower lung volumes. Therefore, a pressure gauge should be used with a flow-inflating bag to keep peak inspiratory pressures below 30 to 40 cm H_2O in term infants, and between 20 and 25 cm H_2O in preterm infants.[16] If a pressure gauge is unavailable, gently squeeze the bag only enough to provide symmetrical chest rise. Laryngeal mask airways can be used if BVM ventilation is ineffective and endotracheal intubation fails; however, research into this method is limited to case studies.[17]

High airway pressures are easy to generate in newborns. Pneumothorax is not an uncommon event if peak inspiratory pressures are not monitored carefully on a manometer. Dislodgement of the ET tube, obstruction with secretions, and mechanical failure of equipment are more common than pneumothorax, however, and should be evaluated prior to decompression. Congenital diaphragmatic hernia can cause

TABLE 24-5. Neonatal ET Tube Size and Depth of Insertion[3]

Gestational Age	Weight (g)	ET Tube Size	ET Tube Depth (at the lip)
<28 weeks	<1,000	2.5	6–7
28–34 weeks	1,000–2,000	3.0	7
34–38 weeks	2,000–3,000	3.5	8
>38 weeks	3,000–4,000	3.5	9
>38 weeks	>4,000	3.5–4.0 (rarely)	10

unilateral absent breath sounds and tracheal deviation, and disastrous consequences can result from needle decompression or thoracostomy in these cases. Be aware of this condition and, if possible, obtain a chest film prior to initiating the procedure.

PEARLS

BVM ventilation of infants at 40–60 breaths/min:
- ✓ With manometer, aim for peak airway pressures <30–40 cm H_2O.
- ✓ Without manometer, aim for a gentle symmetrical chest rise.

If pneumothorax is suspected either clinically or on chest radiography, needle decompression should be performed.[2] The AHA guidelines recommend placing an 18- or 20-gauge angiocatheter into the fourth intercostal space in the midaxillary line. A rush of air or fluid should occur, and the needle should be withdrawn while leaving the catheter in place. Attach the catheter to a three-way stopcock, and aspirate the fluid or air with a 20-mL syringe. Secure the catheter prior to transport. A chest tube can be placed at the tertiary center.

Circulation

The heart rate of an infant who does not respond to positive-pressure ventilation eventually will drop. This vital sign is best measured by auscultation or by palpating the umbilicus or the brachial artery. Any patient with a heart rate less than 60 beats/min requires chest compressions to ensure circulation and oxygen delivery to vital organs.[2] If a definitive airway has not yet been established, intubate and start chest compressions simultaneously. Perform compressions with two fingers over the middle of the chest or by encircling the chest with both hands and compressing with the thumbs. The two-thumb encircling-hands technique, which appears to achieve greater systolic blood pressure and coronary perfusion, is recommended over the two-finger technique.[18,19] Perform chest compressions at a rate of 100 beats/min, alternating three compressions to one breath.[4] Heart rate and respiratory status should be reassessed frequently.

TABLE 24-6. Drugs Commonly Used in Neonatal Resuscitation[14]

Resuscitation
Epinephrine (1:10,000), 0.1–0.3 mL/kg IV or 0.3–1 mL/kg ET tube
D10W, 2 mL/kg
Crystalloid/blood products, 10–20 mL/kg
Naloxone, 0.01 mg/kg*
Sodium bicarbonate, 4 mg/kg*
Postresuscitation
Vitamin K, 0.5–1 mg IM
Cardiac
Prostaglandin E_1, 0.05–0.1 mcg/kg/min
Dopamine, 2 mcg/kg/min, starting dose
Milrinone, 0.5–0.75 mcg/kg/min
Furosemide, 1–2 mg/kg
Antibiotics/antivirals
Ampicillin, 50–100 mg/kg
Gentamicin, 3 mg/kg
Acyclovir, 20–30 mg/kg*

*Discuss with neonatologist prior to use.

PEARL

The pulse in an infant is best palpated at the umbilical artery.

If vascular access has not yet been established, an umbilical central line should be placed (*Figure 24-3*).[3] As when placing any other central line, the site should be prepared using sterile technique and an antiseptic wash such as chlorhexidine or povidone-iodine. Place a sterile string or tie at the base of the umbilicus to control bleeding. Using a scalpel, incise the umbilicus and identify two umbilical arteries (smaller) and one umbilical vein (larger). Use fine forceps to gently dilate the vein as needed, and place an umbilical catheter into the vein. For emergency purposes, most catheters can be inserted to a depth of 5 cm and used immediately as a "low umbilical line." Suture the line into the skin, being careful to avoid the Wharton jelly (the gelatinous substance of which the umbilical cord is made), in a manner similar to that used for chest tubes. An abdominal radiograph should be ordered to confirm placement; umbilical lines that are placed too deeply can extend into the liver.

Drugs, Dextrose, and Diagnostics: Postresuscitation Care

If the heart rate remains below 60 beats/min after an airway has been established, adequate ventilation has been given, and 30 seconds of chest compressions have been performed, epinephrine should be the drug of choice.[2] Again, without adequate ventilation, cardiac resuscitation in newborns is futile. Once intravenous access has been established, use 1:10,000-strength epinephrine at 0.1 to 0.3 mL/kg rapid push (equal to 0.01-0.03 mg/kg).[20] This and other resuscitation drugs are listed with doses in Table 24-6. If the neonate's actual weight is unknown, use estimated weights from Table 24-5.

Previous AHA guidelines recommended 0.3 to 1 mL/kg (0.03-0.1 mg/kg) of endotracheal epinephrine if intravenous access could not be obtained. However, recent research shows endotracheal epinephrine to be unsatisfactory; current guidelines indicate intravenous administration of the drug.[6,21] Continue chest compressions and reassess the heart rate after 30 seconds.[2]

Naloxone traditionally has been used at a dose of 0.1 mg/kg, but its role has never been studied. The medication has been known to precipitate seizures in infants with

TABLE 24-7. Common Congenital Heart Diseases

Persistently Cyanotic	Low Cardiac Output	
Blue baby	Gray baby	
Tetralogy of Fallot	*Think sepsis first!*	Ventricular septal defect
Pulmonary stenosis/atresia	Coarctation of the aorta	Atrial septal defect
Tricuspid atresia	Interrupted aorta	Patent ductus arteriosus
Transposition of great arteries	Hypoplastic left heart syndrome	
Truncus arteriosus	Aortic stenosis	
Total anomalous pulmonary venous return	Arrhythmias	

respiratory depression born to opioid-addicted mothers.[22] In general, newborns thought to have respiratory depression from maternal opiate use should be given positive-pressure ventilation until the drugs have been metabolized.

PEARL

Naloxone has been known to precipitate seizures in infants with respiratory depression born to opiate-addicted mothers.[16]

There also is precedent and a theoretical basis for the use of sodium bicarbonate, but its effectiveness has not been well studied. Infants can develop severe acidosis during prolonged resuscitation. The agent is thought to improve the effectiveness of medications such as epinephrine and prevent encephalopathy or death. Doses of 4 mL/kg of 5% sodium bicarbonate are given over several minutes in cases of confirmed acidosis on arterial or venous blood gas sampling; however, limited research suggests no change in morbidity or mortality.[23]

Infants with evidence of blood loss (ie, known abruption, pallor, poor response to resuscitation) might require intravascular repletion. Isotonic crystalloids such as normal saline or Ringer's lactate should be used cautiously at a dose of 10 to 20 mL/kg. Neonates are highly susceptible to fluid shifts and subsequent intraventricular hemorrhage and edema from the rapid infusion of volume expanders, so crystalloids should be given slowly over 5 to 10 minutes.[3,24]

Transfusion of blood products during the initial resuscitation is poorly studied and is neither recommended nor discouraged by AHA guidelines. In emergent cases, irradiated packed red blood cells free of cytomegalovirus can be transfused at 10 mL/kg; however, consultation with a neonatologist is recommended prior to initiating the procedure.

Infants who are unresponsive to volume replacement might need inotropic or vasoactive pressor support. No one specific pressor has been shown to be superior in neonatal shock, but the appropriate agent should be selected based on the cause of the hypotension. Dopamine started at 2 mcg/kg/min traditionally is the agent of choice in noncardiogenic shock, and milrinone started at 0.5 to 0.75 mcg/kg/min is recommended for the management of cardiogenic shock.[12,14,25]

PEARL

If D10W is unavailable, dilute one ampule of D50W in 200 mL of sterile water to make D10W.

TABLE 24-8. Common Congenital Anomalies Requiring Immediate Intervention

Disorder	Examination Findings	Interventions
Congenital diaphragmatic hernia	Respiratory distress Scaphoid abdomen Bowel above the diaphragm on chest film	Immediate intubation Nasogastric tube placement for decompression
Gastroschisis	Evisceration of the bowel through abdominal wall defect without a protective sac	Cover bowel in wet, sterile saline gauze then in a plastic cellophane bag. Avoid touching or twisting bowel as much as possible. Nasogastric tube placement for decompression Ampicillin/gentamicin
Omphalocele	Evisceration of bowel through abdominal wall defect with a protective sac	Cover bowel in wet, sterile saline gauze then in plastic cellophane. Avoid touching or twisting bowel as much as possible. Nasogastric tube placement for decompression
Choanal atresia	Respiratory distress Inability to pass nasogastric tube	Immediate endotracheal intubation

PEARLS

Start intravenous maintenance fluids and give intramuscular vitamin K prior to transfer.

- ✓ Term infants: D10¼ NS at 4 mL/kg/hr; vitamin K, 1 mg
- ✓ Preterm infants: D10¼ NS at 5 mL/kg/hr; vitamin K, 0.5 mg

Once an infant has been stabilized with a heart rate above 100 beats/min and stable respirations, the blood glucose concentration must be measured. Hypoglycemia is associated with a heightened risk of brain injury; the glucose concentration should be checked as quickly as possible.[27] A heelstick blood sugar concentration greater than 40 mg/dL is acceptable in an infant; anything less should be treated with a 2-mL/kg bolus of D10W infused over several minutes.[14] If D10W is unavailable, an ampule of D50W can be diluted in 200 mL of sterile water to yield D10W (undiluted D50W should not be used, as the osmotic load is too high). D10¼ NS should be used as maintenance fluid at a rate of 4 mL/kg/hr in term infants (based on 80-100 mL/kg/day) and 5 mL/kg/hr in preterm neonates (based on 100-120 mL/kg/day). Smaller infants have a higher body surface-to-volume ratio and will lose fluids more quickly.

All newborns — even those who are healthy — require vitamin K within an hour of birth to prevent hemorrhagic disease. Vitamin K should be administered in a dose of 0.5 to 1 mg IM; give 1 mg to larger infants and 0.5 mg to premature neonates.[14] If the patient will be transferred to a tertiary NICU, vitamin K should be given prior to transfer. Erythromycin ophthalmic ointment should be placed on both eyes to prevent gonococcal and chlamydial infections. This, however, is not emergent and can be delayed in a critically ill infant until a tertiary center is reached.

FIGURE 24-3. Placement of an Umbilical Central Line

A. Prep and drape the umbilicus in sterile manner and place an umbilical tie at the base to control bleeding. **B.** Cut the umbilicus to expose the umbilical arteries and vein. The vein will be thin-walled compared with the thicker-walled arteries. **C.** Carefully dilate the umbilical vein with hooked forceps, and cannulate it with an umbilical catheter. **D.** Attach a three-way stopcock and syringe and aspirate until blood flows easily. Pass the umbilical catheter to 5 cm for a low umbilical line.

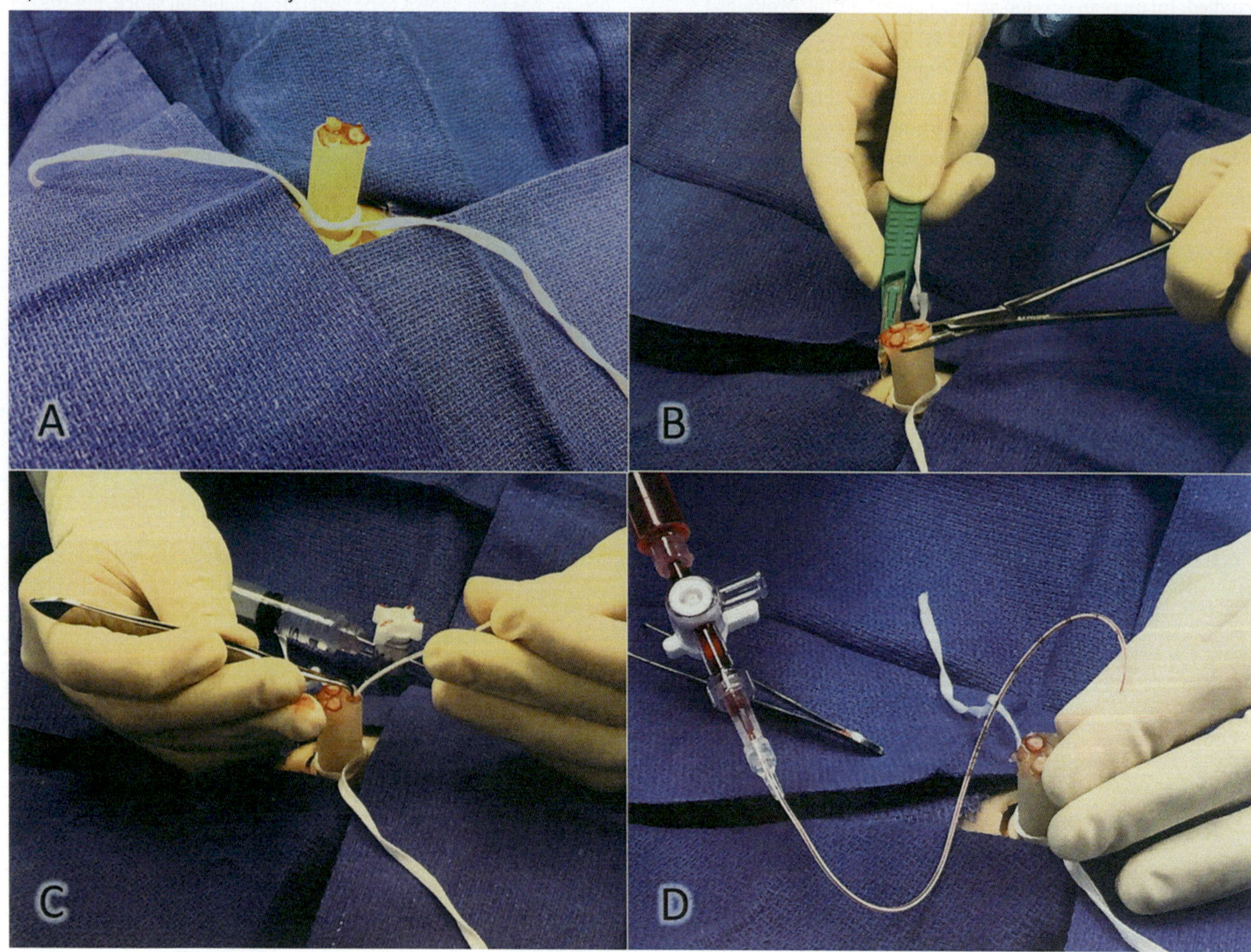

PEARL

Vitamin K should be given to all infants within an hour of birth regardless of clinical condition.

Prostaglandin E_1 (PGE_1) is given as a drip at 0.05 to 0.1 mcg/kg/min to newborns with ductal-dependent congenital heart disease; the indications are discussed later in this chapter.[14] The well-known adverse effect of this agent is apnea, which is rare except with high doses. Infants receiving this treatment do not necessarily need to be intubated empirically or for transport.[26] They should instead be monitored closely for signs of respiratory distress or cardiovascular compromise, and the drip should be decreased to the lowest effective dose possible to achieve adequate oxygenation.

Herpes simplex virus, although uncommon, can be deadly in infants. Signs and symptoms suggestive of herpetic infection include vesicular skin lesions and seizures. The neonate is at risk if the mother has active genital (not oral) lesions at the time of delivery. The virus should be treated initially with acyclovir (20 mg/kg for newborns <35 weeks' gestation, and 30 mg/kg for those born after 35 weeks' gestation).[14] Consultation with a neonatologist is recommended prior to treatment.

Important urgent laboratory studies following resuscitation include a complete blood count (CBC) with differential and platelets, electrolytes, blood cultures, and an arterial blood gas (ABG) measurement. The NICU also will want a blood type and Coombs test to check for ABO incompatibility, as well as total and direct bilirubin levels to monitor for jaundice. A chest film should be obtained to evaluate for aspiration, pneumonia, and ET tube placement if necessary.

PEARL

Grunting, retractions, and a sustained respiratory rate >70 breaths/min can be indicators of impending respiratory compromise.

Respiratory status remains the chief concern after resuscitation. Serious causes of respiratory compromise include sepsis (the most common), meconium aspiration, neonatal respiratory distress syndrome (due to lack of surfactant in premature infants), congenital diaphragmatic hernia, and a myriad of genetic disorders. Intubated infants should be monitored for signs of pneumothorax, including hypoxia and high peak inspiratory pressures. Nonintubated infants should be monitored for work of breathing. Grunting, retractions, and a sustained respiratory rate above 70 breaths/min can indicate impending respiratory compromise.

Any infant with a difficult resuscitation, history of maternal fever, or evidence of respiratory distress after delivery should be assumed to be septic until proven otherwise. Ampicillin (50–100 mg/kg per dose) and gentamicin (3 mg/kg per dose) should be initiated empirically after blood cultures are drawn.[14]

Newborns should be kept warm using an overhead warmer, blankets, or maternal skin-to-skin contact. However, new studies propose a role for induced hypothermia in infants with suspected intrauterine asphyxia and profound metabolic acidosis.[27,28] Although infants with moderate encephalopathy showed increased survival when cooled to 33.5°C (92.3°F), this strategy should not be used routinely and should be discussed with a neonatologist prior to initiation. As a general rule, normothermia should be the goal for this patient population.

PEARLS

Postresuscitation laboratory tests

- ✓ CBC with differential and platelets
- ✓ Electrolytes, blood urea nitrogen, creatinine, and total and direct bilirubin
- ✓ ABG, blood cultures
- ✓ Type and screen with direct/indirect Coombs test

Congenital Heart Disease

Undiagnosed congenital heart disease is a pressing concern in precipitous deliveries, but identifying the underlying structural defect is not nearly as important as finding and treating the pathophysiology behind it. Critical cardiac lesions will present in three ways: persistent cyanosis, low cardiac output, and congestive heart failure (*Table 24-7*).[29] Any infant with these signs and symptoms necessitates a chest radiograph and an electrocardiogram (ECG). Early echocardiography and consultation with a pediatric cardiologist should be considered.

Persistent cyanosis in an infant *without respiratory distress* can be a manifestation of cardiac lesions, persistent pulmonary hypertension, or lung disease.[23] These patients often appear "comfortably blue" and usually have a loud murmur on examination. In most cases, parenchymal lung disease easily can be identified on a chest film; however, a hyperoxia test also should be used to improve diagnostic accuracy. This test involves comparing arterial oxygen saturation on room air with saturation on 100% oxygen. Measure partial pressure of oxygen (Po_2) using preoxygenation and postoxygenation ABG values. A Po_2 below 100 mm Hg suggests congenital heart disease with significant right-to-left shunting.

Importantly, an infant with persistent pulmonary hypertension can have a negative hyperoxia test. Any neonate with a failed hyperoxia test should receive both a therapeutic and diagnostic trial of PGE_1. It can be difficult to establish arterial access in a neonate, so pulse oximetry can be used as a surrogate for the ABG measurement when needed. Total anomalous pulmonary venous return (TAPVR) is the one cardiac abnormality that will produce a normal hyperoxia test and will not respond to PGE_1. The quickest way to diagnose this condition is with an echocardiogram, and emergent surgical intervention is the only treatment. Classic radiographic findings in persistently cyanotic infants include a boot-shaped heart in those with tetralogy of Fallot, a "snowman" in those with TAPVR, and an "egg-on-a-string" sign in those with transposition of the great arteries.

Poor cardiac output causes a patient to appear pale gray, with poor peripheral pulses and often no murmur.[23] These neonates appear septic and should be treated initially with intravenous fluid resuscitation and antibiotics. Sepsis is far more common than congenital heart disease, but the latter diagnosis should be considered in patients who do not respond to initial sepsis treatment.

PEARLS

The Hyperoxia Test

- ✓ Obtain ABG measurements with the patient on room air and 100% oxygen.
- ✓ Po_2 >100 mm Hg = Primary pulmonary disease = No PGE_1
- ✓ Po_2 <100 mm Hg = Congenital heart disease with right-to-left shunting or persistent pulmonary hypertension = Trial of PGE_1

Pitfalls

- ✓ Pulse oximetry is not an acceptable substitute for Po_2.
- ✓ Neonates with TAPVR can have a Po_2 >100 mm Hg and no response to PGE_1.

Comparing pulse oximetry on a preductal extremity (right arm) and postductal extremity (left leg) can identify aortic lesions such as coarctation or an interrupted aortic arch. The four extremities might show higher preductal than postductal blood pressures. An early echocardiogram will reveal lesions such as hypoplastic left heart disease or aortic stenosis, which are ductal dependent but not readily identifiable on examination. If an echocardiogram cannot be obtained, a trial of PGE_1 is warranted, and early consultation with a pediatric cardiologist is essential. Tachyarrhythmias and congenital heart block are exceedingly rare, but can be identified quickly from the heart rate and cardiac monitor reading and confirmed on an ECG. In supraventricular tachycardia, adenosine is dosed at 0.05 to 0.1 mg/kg in stable patients, and synchronized cardioversion is used at 0.5 J/kg in unstable patients. Congenital complete heart block warrants emergent pacemaker placement.

Congestive heart failure does not manifest immediately at birth; it takes several weeks to months for the right ventricle to fail as left-to-right shunts become right-to-left shunts.[23] Infants will have symptoms of lethargy, poor feeding, or sweating or cyanosis with feeds. Tachypnea, hepatomegaly, failure to thrive, and murmurs are common findings. These infants will appear septic but will worsen with the administration of intravenous fluids. A chest film likely will show cardiomegaly with pulmonary congestion, and an echocardiogram can confirm the diagnosis. Diuretics such as furosemide (0.5 to 1 mg/kg) can help improve oxygenation, and inotropes such as milrinone (0.5 to 0.75 mcg/kg/min) can improve cardiac output.[14]

Specific Congenital Anomalies

Several congenital anomalies are common to NICU settings but are rarely encountered in emergency departments. After stabilization, patients with these abnormalities should be transferred to a tertiary care NICU for further management. Specific emergent interventions are presented in Table 24-8.[30]

Withholding or Discontinuing Resuscitation

A neonatal resuscitation is difficult enough without having to consider the withdrawal of care; however, there are appropriate times to halt resuscitative efforts.[31,32,33] Infants born earlier than 23 weeks' gestation or with a birth weight less than 500 grams have high mortality and even higher morbidity rates. Similarly, infants without respiratory effort or pulse after 10 minutes of resuscitation are at increased risk of death and severe neurological deficits. Severe congenital abnormalities such as anencephaly and trisomy 13 also are considered to be incompatible with life, and resuscitation may be withheld.

In these circumstances, the decision to cease or withhold

KEY POINTS

1. Neonatal resuscitation is almost exclusively a *respiratory* issue.
2. The *only* drug used in neonatal resuscitation after delivery is epinephrine.
3. The Apgar score is not used to determine the need for resuscitation.
4. Newborns are highly susceptible to evaporative heat losses and will decompensate quickly if allowed to become hypothermic.
5. Infants are obligate nose breathers and must have a patent nasopharynx. If the patient is breathing spontaneously and there is no obvious airway obstruction, suctioning should not be performed because it can cause a reflex bradycardia that further complicates resuscitation.
6. Infants are far more susceptible to barotrauma and pneumothorax than adults.
7. Any neonate with a heart rate <60 beats/min requires chest compressions to ensure circulation and oxygen delivery to vital organs.[2]
8. A heelstick blood sugar concentration >40 mg/dL is acceptable in a neonate; anything less should be treated with a 2-mL/kg bolus of D10W infused over several minutes.[14]
9. Any infant with a difficult resuscitation, history of maternal fever, or evidence of respiratory distress after delivery should be assumed to be septic until proven otherwise.

resuscitative measures should be discussed with the parents. Emergency physicians are not expected to be experts on such disorders, however, and should always err on the side of resuscitation if they are unsure of an infant's prognosis.

Conclusion

Few things are as stressful for the emergency physician as resuscitating a critically ill neonate following a precipitous emergency department delivery. Respiratory causes are the most common culprits of distress in these patients; therefore, the airway should be assessed and ventilation should be supplied within the first 60 seconds of evaluation. It is equally important to keep the neonate warm and dry. Patients who remain bradycardiac despite supplemental oxygen and positive-pressure ventilation require compressions and possibly epinephrine.

Once resuscitated, critically ill infants should receive intravenous fluids containing dextrose, intramuscular vitamin K, and broad-spectrum antibiotics. Congenital heart disease should be suspected in those who are unresponsive to these therapies. Emergency physicians can reduce the rate of morbidity and mortality in these vulnerable patients by employing a systematic clinical approach.

REFERENCES

1. Sutton L, Sayer GP, Bajuk B, et al. Do very sick neonates born at term have antenatal risks? 2. Infants ventilated primarily for problems of adaptation to extra-uterine life. *Acta Obstet Gynecol Scand.* 2001;80:905-916.
2. Wyllie J, Perlman JM, Kattwinkel J, et al. Part 7: Neonatal resuscitation: 2015 International consensus on cardiopulmonary resuscitation and emergency cardiovascular care science with treatment recommendations. *Resuscitation* 95 (2015): e171-203.
3. Kattwinkel J, ed. *Textbook of Neonatal Resuscitation.* 6th ed. Oak Grove Village, IL: American Academy of Pediatrics and American Heart Association; 2011.
4. Clyman R. Mechanisms regulating closure of ductus arteriosus. In: Polin RA, Fox WW, Abman S, eds. *Fetal and Neonatal Physiology.* 4th ed. Philadelphia, PA: WB Saunders; 2010:821-827.
5. Rajani AK, Chitkara R, Oehlert J, Halamek LP. Comparison of umbilical venous and intraosseous access during simulated neonatal resuscitation. *Pediatrics.* 2011;128;e954.
6. McCarthy L, Morley C, Davis P, et al. Timing of interventions in the delivery room: does reality compare with neonatal resuscitation guidelines? *J Pediatr.* 2013;163:1553-1557.
7. Branco de Almeida M, Guinsburg R, Sancho G, et al. Hypothermia and early neonatal mortality in preterm infants. *J Pediatr.* 2014;164:271-275.
8. Vohra S, Frent G, Campbell V, et al. Effect of polyethylene occlusive skin wrapping on heat loss in very low birth weight infants at delivery: a randomized trial. *J Pediatr.* 1999;134:547-551.
9. Saugstad OD. New guidelines for newborn resuscitation. *Acta Paediatr.* 2007;96:333-337.
10. Vain NE, Szyld EG, Prudent LM, et al. Oropharyngeal and nasopharyngeal suctioning of meconium-stained neonates before delivery of their shoulders: multicentre, randomised controlled trial. *Lancet.* 2004;364:597-602.
11. Wiswell TE, Gannon CM, Jacob J, et al. Delivery room management of the apparently vigorous meconium-stained neonate: results of the multicenter, international collaborative trial. *Pediatrics.* 2000;105:1-7.
12. Toth B, Becker A, Seelbach-Gobel B. Oxygen saturation in healthy newborn infants immediately after birth measured by pulse oximetry. *Arch Gynecol Obstet.* 2002;266:105-107.
13. Rook D, Schierbeek H, Vento M, et al. Resuscitation of preterm infants with different inspired oxygen fractions. *J Pediatr.* 2014;164:1322-1326.
14. Kapadia VS, Chalak LF, Sparks JE, et al. Resuscitation of preterm neonates with limited versus high oxygen strategy. *Pediatrics.* 2013;132:e1488–e1496.
15. Thio M, Kempen L, Rafferty A, et al. Neonatal resuscitation in resource-limited settings: titrating oxygen delivery without an oxygen blender. *J Pediatr.* 2014;165:256-260.
16. Vyas H, Milner AD, Hopkin IE, Boon AW. Physiologic responses to prolonged and slow-rise inflation in the resuscitation of the asphyxiated newborn infant. *J Pediatr.* 1981;99:635-639.
17. Paterson SJ, Byrne PJ, Molesky MG, et al. Neonatal resuscitation using the laryngeal mask airway. *Anesthesiology.* 1994;80:1248-1253.
18. Houri PK, Frank LR, Menegazzi JJ, Taylor R. A randomized, controlled trial of two-thumb vs two-finger chest compression in a swine infant model of cardiac arrest. *Prehosp Emerg Care.* 1997;1:65-67.
19. Huynh TK, Hemway RJ, Perlman JM. The two-thumb technique using an elevated surface is preferable for teaching infant cardiopulmonary resuscitation. *J Pediatr.* 2012;161:658-661.
20. Lee C, Custer J, Rau R. Drug doses. In: Custer J, Rau R, eds. *The Harriet Lane Handbook: A Manual for Pediatric House Officers.* 18th ed. Philadelphia, PA: Mosby; 2009.
21. Barber CA, Wyckoff MH. Use and efficacy of endotracheal versus intravenous epinephrine during neonatal cardiopulmonary resuscitation in the delivery room. *Pediatrics.* 2006;118:1028-1034.
22. Gibbs J, Newson T, Williams J, Davidson DC. Naloxone hazard in infant of opioid abuser. *Lancet.* 1989;2(8655):159-160.
23. Lokesh L, Kumar P, Murki S, Narang A. A randomized controlled trial of sodium bicarbonate in neonatal resuscitation — effect on immediate outcome. *Resuscitation.* 2004;60:219-223.
24. So KW, Fok TF, Ng PC, et al. Randomised controlled trial of colloid or crystalloid in hypotensive preterm infants. *Arch Dis Child Fetal Neonatal Ed.* 1997;76:F43-F46.
25. Noori S, Friedlich PS, Seri I. Pathophysiology of shock in the fetus and neonate. In: Polin RA, Fox WW, Abman SH, eds. *Fetal and Neonatal Physiology.* 4th ed. Philadelphia, PA: WB Saunders; 2011:772-782.
26. Meckler GD, Lowe C. To intubate or not to intubate? Transporting infants on prostaglandin E1. *Pediatrics.* 2009;123:e25-e30.
27. Gluckman PD, Wyatt JS, Azzopardi D, et al. Selective head cooling with mild systemic hypothermia after neonatal encephalopathy: multicentre randomised trial. *Lancet.* 2005;365:663-670.
28. Donovan EF, Fanaroff AA, Poole WK, et al. Whole-body hypothermia for neonates with hypoxic-ischemic encephalopathy. *N Engl J Med.* 2005;353:1574-1584.
29. Brooks PA, Penny DJ. Management of the sick neonate with suspected heart disease. *Early Hum Dev.* 2008;84:155-159.
30. Stoll B, Adams-Chapman I. Delivery room emergencies. In: Behrman R, Kliegman R, Jenson HB, Stanton BF, eds. *Nelson Textbook of Pediatrics.* 18th ed. Philadelphia, PA: Saunders Elsevier; 2007:1532.
31. Draper ES, Manktelow B, Field DJ, James D. Tables for predicting survival for preterm births are updated. *BMJ.* 2003;327:872.
32. Jain L, Ferre C, Vidyasagar D, et al. Cardiopulmonary resuscitation of apparently stillborn infants: survival and long-term outcome. *J Pediatr.* 1991;118:778-782.
33. Haddad B, Mercer BM, Livingston JC, et al. Outcome after successful resuscitation of babies born with Apgar scores of 0 at both 1 and 5 minutes. *Am J Obstet Gynecol.* 2000;182:1210-1214.

Pediatric Resuscitation

25

IN THIS CHAPTER

- General approach to the unstable pediatric patient
- Airway and ventilator management
- Cardiac arrest and arrhythmia algorithms
- Recognizing shock and obtaining vascular access

Jenny S. Mendelson and Chad D. Viscusi

More than 25 million children are seen in US emergency departments every year, the vast majority of whom (96%) are treated and released.[1] Despite the frequency of pediatric visits, many emergency physicians confess to feeling unprepared to handle this vulnerable population — a discomfort that is magnified when faced with a critically ill or crashing child.[2] Most clinicians see relatively few of these cases, and thus have limited opportunities to refine paramount skills in advanced pediatric lifesaving techniques and algorithms.

Initial Assessment

An adept emergency physician must be able to make a rapid global clinical assessment when managing a critically ill child. One initial approach is the pediatric assessment triangle (PAT), a widely published and recognized tool used to assess children of all ages with all levels of illness and injury. The PAT focuses on three components — appearance, work of breathing, and circulation — to facilitate a rapid assessment and triage of patients into categories of "sick" or "not sick." The tool does not require a stethoscope or monitoring equipment and can be completed in fewer than 30 seconds.[3]

To evaluate the general appearance of the child, the TICLS (tickles) mnemonic can be used to assess **t**one (moving and resisting examination versus being limp and listless), **i**nteractiveness (alert and attentive versus uninterested or unresponsive), **c**onsolability (comforted by caregiver versus agitated and crying), **l**ook/gaze (fixing on faces or toys versus staring aimlessly and unfocused), and **s**peech/cry (cry is loud and strong versus weak and hoarse). The TICLS assessment can identify more subtle abnormalities than the traditional AVPU (alert, voice, pain, unresponsive) scale. For instance, a child can be on the verge of respiratory failure and still remain "alert."

After the patient's general appearance is assessed, work of breathing should be evaluated. Unlike in adults, work of breathing in a child often is a better indication of oxygenation and ventilation status than breath sounds and respiratory rate. The child should be evaluated for abnormal audible airway sounds, abnormal positioning, retractions, and flaring. The predominant signs of respiratory distress are outlined in Table 25-1; however, these signs may become less apparent once a child tires. Slowing of the respiratory rate and shallow breathing can signal impending respiratory failure.

PEARL

Slowing of the respiratory rate and shallow breathing can signal impending respiratory failure.

The final component of the PAT is an assessment of the circulation to the skin, looking for pallor, mottling, and cyanosis. Cyanosis, while certainly a clear and dramatic sign, has significant limitations as a diagnostic tool. This finding depends on the amount of hemoglobin in the blood and the status of the

TABLE 25-1. Signs of Respiratory Distress in Children
Abdominal breathing
Accessory muscle use
Diaphoresis
Grunting
Nasal flaring
Retractions
Tachypnea
Tripod positioning

FIGURE 25-1. Anatomical Differences

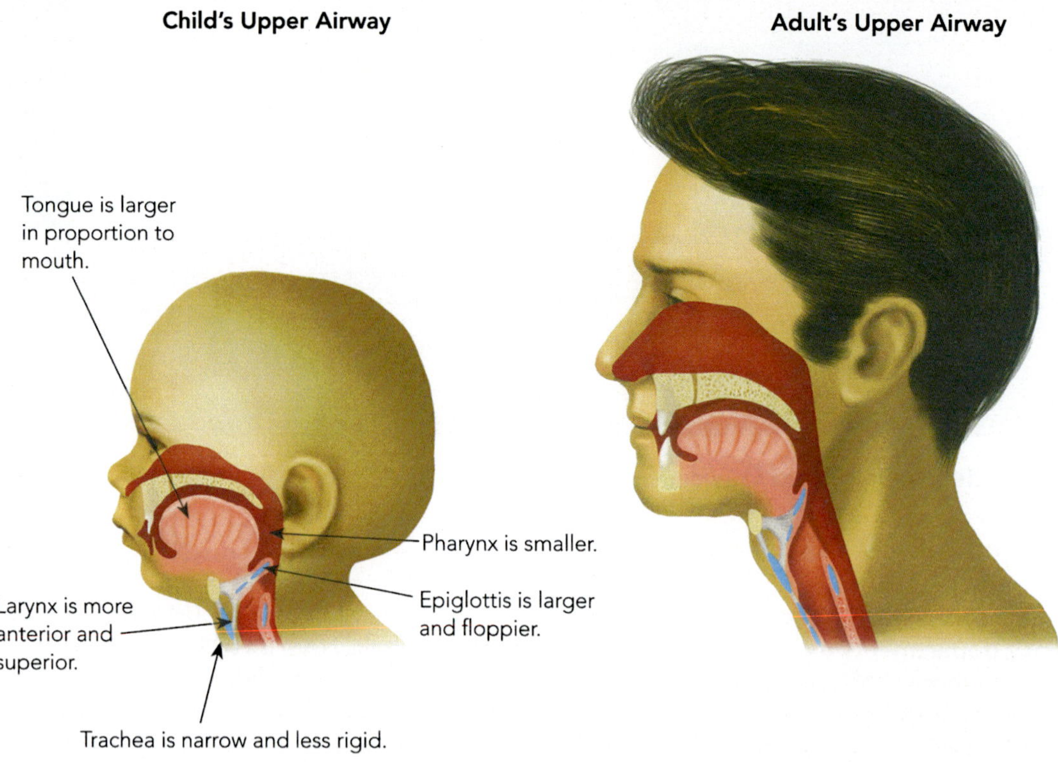

FIGURE 25-2. Pediatric Airway Positioning

Correct

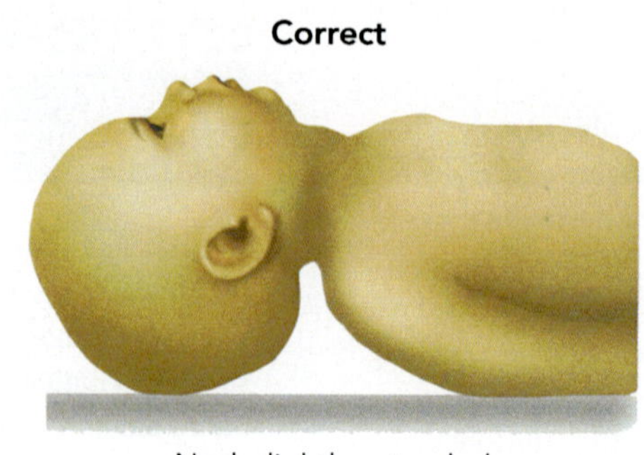

Neck slightly extended

Incorrect

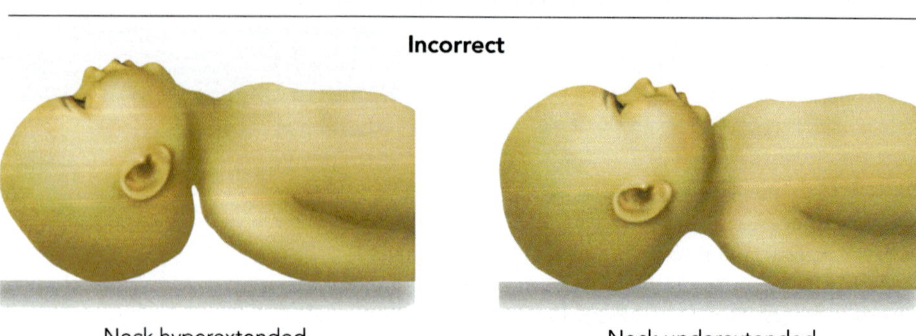

Neck hyperextended

Neck underextended

peripheral circulation. A child with severe anemia, for example, can have significant hypoxia without any visible cyanosis. Conversely, a very young infant whose hemoglobin has not yet fallen from the high levels found at birth may have peripheral cyanosis despite a normal central blood oxygen concentration.

The PAT provides a quick reflection of the adequacy of oxygenation, ventilation, and central nervous system function, subsequently assisting with early recognition and the prioritization of problems. When combined, the three elements of the PAT can establish severity. A child with a normal appearance and increased work of breathing is in respiratory distress. Abnormal appearance and increased work of breathing can be signs of early respiratory failure. Abnormal appearance and abnormally decreased work of breathing are seen in late respiratory failure. Abnormal appearance and decreased circulation indicate shock and should prompt rapid progression through the pediatric primary survey to initiate resuscitation.

Along with the primary assessment, measuring weight should be one of the first steps in the evaluation of a critically ill child. If the weight is unknown or cannot be determined immediately, it can be estimated using the formula: weight (kg) = 2 x age (years) + 10. It is preferable to use a length-based resuscitation tape (eg, Broselow tape), however, which includes recommendations about equipment sizes and drug doses. This eliminates the need to estimate the patient's age and weight and reduces the risk of calculation errors during times of high stress.[4]

Pediatric Primary Survey: the ABCs

In contrast to the PAT, which can be performed in any order, the pediatric primary survey is an ordered, comprehensive hands-on evaluation of cardiopulmonary status. The sequence of interventions is crucial. First and foremost, the airway must be evaluated and secured; breathing must be supported or controlled; and circulation and perfusion must be reestablished or enhanced. The primary survey provides a specific, regimented approach for identifying and mitigating threats before moving to the next step.

Airway

The primary reasons for airway management in patients of any age include inadequate oxygenation, inadequate ventilation, and inadequate airway protection; however, not every critically ill child needs to be intubated. Well-performed noninvasive ventilation usually is sufficient, and several studies have shown that it is safer and equally as effective as endotracheal (ET) intubation, especially in the prehospital setting.[5-7] Effective bag-valve-mask (BVM) ventilation is one of the most critical resuscitation skills to master. Consideration should be given to several anatomical and physiological differences *(Figure 25-1)* between pediatric and adult airways when managing a child in respiratory distress or respiratory failure. As children grow, their anatomies and physiologies become more similar to those of adults; by age 8, the airway is thought to approximate the adult form.

Pediatric anatomical features that affect airway management include a more prominent occiput, a relatively large tongue, small nasal passages, hypertrophied lymphoid tissue, short trachea, long epiglottis, and a larynx that is more anterior and cephalad than that of an adult's.[8] When the child is lying on a flat surface, the size of the occiput causes neck flexion and potential airway compromise. This can be overcome by placing a towel roll behind the infant's shoulders; however, overextension of the neck also can result in airway obstruction.

Infants are obligate nose breathers until age 3 to 6 months, during which time even minor congestion can lead to obstruction. The infant's tongue is larger in proportion to the oral cavity and can easily obstruct the airway. The epiglottis is longer and omega shaped and is positioned in a short neck close to prominent adenoid and tonsillar tissue. The long epiglottis can obscure the laryngoscopic view of the cords, a complication that can be overcome by direct elevation using a straight blade (Miller) rather than indirect elevation using a curved blade (Macintosh) placed in the vallecula.

The glottic opening lies at approximately the level of C2 or C3 in an infant or child, as opposed to C3 or C4 in the adolescent or adult. This superior (cephalad) and anterior placement can make the airway difficult to see behind the tongue on laryngoscopy. Because the cricoid ring is the narrowest portion of the pediatric airway, as opposed to the vocal cords in adults, the tube is able to pass through the cords (but no farther).[9] Finally, the diameter of the pediatric airway is much smaller than the adult airway, making it far more vulnerable to obstruction by foreign objects

TABLE 25-2. Endotracheal Tube and Laryngoscope Blade Sizes

Size of uncuffed ET tube = (age in years/4) + 4
Size of cuffed ET tube (after age 2) = (age in years/4) + 3.5
Suggested laryngoscope blades: • Premature infant: #0 Miller blade (straight) • Term infant to small child: #1 Miller blade (straight) • Child <8 years old: #2 Macintosh blade (curved) • Adolescent/adult: #3 Macintosh blade (curved)

TABLE 25-3. Using the LEMON Mnemonic

L: Look externally (short neck, large tongue, micrognathia).
E: Evaluate the 3-3-2 rule (incisor distance <3 fingerbreadths, hyoid/mentum distance <3 fingerbreadths, thyroid-to-mouth distance <2 fingerbreadths).
M: Mallampati (score ≥3)
O: Obstruction and obesity (presence of any condition that could cause an obstructed airway)
N: Neck mobility (limited neck mobility)

Adapted with permission from "The Difficult Airway Course: Emergency," Airway Management Education Center, www.theairwaysite.com, and from Walls RM, Murphy MF. Identification of the difficult and failed airway. In: Walls RM, Murphy MF, eds. *Manual of Emergency Airway Management.* 4th ed. Philadelphia, PA: Lippincott Williams & Wilkins; 2012:8-21.

and edema. Minor narrowing from respiratory infection or bronchospasm can result in profound airway compromise.

Physiological differences between children and adults that complicate airway management include increased oxygen consumption and metabolic rate and a decreased pulmonary reserve. Infants have 40% the functional residual capacity (FRC) of adults while awake and only 10% while asleep. This decreased FRC means infants have less oxygen available for gas exchange during exhalation or apnea. Infants also have a higher metabolic rate, consuming at least 6 mL of oxygen per minute (versus 3 mL of oxygen per minute in adults).

These factors cause pediatric patients to desaturate much more rapidly than adults during periods of apnea, despite adequate preoxygenation, and conspire to give the intubator less time for direct laryngoscopy.[9] Infants and small children are at further risk of respiratory problems because of their immature physiological responses. The infant may become apneic and bradycardic in response to a hypoxic challenge instead of increasing the respiratory effort and heart rate.[10]

Adequate positioning and airway clearance might be all that is needed to relieve obstruction. The first step should be to place the child in the "sniffing position," with neck extended and chin lifted *(Figure 25-2)*. If there is concern about cervical spinal injury, a jaw thrust should be used instead. If the jaw thrust is ineffective, it is necessary to use the head-tilt/chin-lift technique to establish a patent airway. Supplemental oxygen should be supplied and secretions cleared by suctioning. Placement of a nasal or oral airway can relieve obstruction caused by a large tongue.

Oral airways should be used only in patients without a gag reflex. The appropriate size can be determined by holding the oral airway next to the child's face; with the flange held at the corner of the mouth, the tip of the airway will reach the angle of the mandible. It is crucial to use the correct size; an airway that is too small can push the tongue down and worsen obstruction, whereas an airway that is too large can cause pharyngeal trauma.

Nasal airways can be used in awake patients but cannot be used if a basilar skull fracture or coagulopathy might be present. These tools should be used cautiously in infants, in whom hypertrophied adenoids and tonsils can be traumatized by airway insertion, resulting in bleeding. Inserting the bevel away from the nasal septum can minimize this risk. The appropriately sized nasal airway should reach from the nostril to the tragus of the ear when held against the face, and its width should be less than that of the nostril's. Although BVM ventilation should be considered the gold standard for initial airway management, tracheal intubation offers the advantage of long-term airway maintenance and some protection from aspiration of gastric contents.[11]

Determining the appropriate size of airway equipment can be challenging in pediatric patients. If a length-based resuscitation tape is not available, an age-based formula can be used to estimate endotracheal (ET) tube size (*Table 25-2*). This is more accurate than estimates based on the width of the patient's fifth finger.[12] When preparing for intubation, ensure that tubes half a size smaller and half a size larger are available. The depth of insertion should be approximately 3 times the uncuffed ET tube size in centimeters.

TABLE 25-4. Equipment Needed for Intubation (the SOAP ME Mnemonic)

S: Suction (catheters and Yankauer tips)
O: Oxygen (nasal cannula, oxygen flow, masks, and appropriate bag)
A: Airway (appropriate ET tube, oral/nasal airway, stylets, laryngoscope with functioning light and appropriate blades)
P: Pharmacology (RSI medications)
ME: Monitoring equipment (end-tidal carbon dioxide detector, stethoscope, monitors)

TABLE 25-5. Pediatric RSI Drugs

Pretreatment
Atropine: (0.02 mg/kg IV/ET tube); minimum, 0.1 mg; use to decrease bradycardia from vagal stimulation; always use in patients <5 years and before second dose of succinylcholine.
Induction
Etomidate: (0.2–0.6 mg/kg IV); causes less hypotension than some sedatives.
Fentanyl: (2–5 mcg/kg IV); can cause chest wall rigidity if given rapidly.
Ketamine: (1–2 mg/kg IV); preferred in the presence of bronchospasm; avoid if increased ICP is suspected.
Thiopental: (3-5 mg/kg IV); preferred if increased ICP is suspected; use ½ dose in the presence of hypotension.
Midazolam: (0.2-0.3 mg/kg IV); causes low blood pressure, heart rate, and respiratory rate.
Paralysis
Succinylcholine: (1–2 mg/kg IV); pretreat with atropine in patients <5 years and before all subsequent doses; avoid if hyperkalemia or renal failure is suspected or if the patient has a history of malignant hyperthermia or neuromuscular disease.
Rocuronium: (0.6–1.2 mg/kg IV); onset in 1 min; lasts 30 min.
Delayed-onset paralytics (not suited for RSI)
Pancuronium: (0.04-0.1 mg/kg IV); avoid in asthmatic patients (histamine release) and those with renal failure.
Vecuronium: (0.08-0.1 mg/kg IV); onset in 1–3 min; lasts 90 min.
Cisatracurium: (0.1-0.3 mg/kg IV); onset in 1–3 min; lasts 30–60 min.

From: *EMRA Pediatric Qwic Card*. Dallas, TX: Emergency Medicine Residents Association; 2008. Used with permission.

TABLE 25-6. Comparison of Sizes of Supraglottic Devices and ET Tubes			
Weight (kg)	Laryngeal Mask Airway	King Laryngeal Tube	
<5	1	n/a	3.5
5–10	1.5	n/a	4
10–20	2	2	4.5
20–30	2.5	2.5	5
30–50	3	3	5.5–6
50–70	4	4	6–7
>70	5	4–5	7–8

The use of cuffed tubes in children younger than 8 years previously was discouraged due to a concern for subglottic stenosis caused by ischemic damage to the tracheal mucosa. In recent years, however, this practice has become increasingly common — even preferred. Newer ET tubes are designed to be high volume and low pressure, resulting in a seal at lower pressure. When used in controlled settings with frequent monitoring (typically in a pediatric intensive care unit), cuffed tubes do not appear to increase the risk of postextubation stridor or reintubation rates.[13-15] Cuffed ET tubes also minimize the risk of air leakage (enabling optimized and more consistent ventilation with higher pressures) and decrease the need to exchange inappropriately sized ET tubes.[9]

The key to successful intubation is using a standard procedure every time. Every patient in the emergency department generally is presumed to have a full stomach; therefore, rapid-sequence intubation (RSI) should be the norm, but risks should be considered. As in adult patients, the LEMON mnemonic (*Table 25-3*) can be used to predict difficult airways, although this technique has not been validated for use in children. Another mnemonic that may be helpful is SOAP ME (*Table 25-4*). Gather appropriately sized equipment, including alternative airway management devices and medications. Preoxygenate the patient, keeping in mind that even when appropriately oxygenated, a child will desaturate much more rapidly than an adult. Deliver RSI medications (*Table 25-5*) only when you are confident that BVM ventilation will be successful. The Sellick maneuver (cricoid pressure) is not routinely recommended during rapid-sequence or emergency tracheal intubation in infants and children. Although it has been shown to reduce the risk of gastric insufflation during bagging, there is no evidence that it prevents aspiration. Additionally, excess pressure can collapse or distort the pliable airways of small children, making intubation more difficult.[16,17]

Once the ET tube has been passed, confirm placement using clinical evaluation (gentle symmetrical chest rise, equal bilateral breath sounds, condensation in the tube) as well as an end-tidal carbon dioxide detector. If breath sounds are heard over the stomach, do not remove the tube immediately (breath sounds are easily transmitted in infants and small children). Gurgling sounds suggest esophageal intubation, necessitating tube removal.

Pediatric end-tidal carbon dioxide detectors should be used in patients weighing less than 15 kg and adult end-tidal carbon dioxide detectors in patients weighing more than 15 kg. These tools may not reliably confirm placement in instances of low pulmonary blood flow (eg, cardiac arrest or massive pulmonary embolism).[18] If any uncertainty remains, perform careful direct laryngoscopy to verify that the ET tube passes through the vocal cords. Finally, obtain a chest radiograph to confirm proper tube positioning in the midtrachea.

If a child develops problems with oxygenation or ventilation after intubation, use the DOPE mnemonic when considering potential reasons for this decompensation: **d**islodgement, **o**bstruction, **p**neumothorax, or **e**quipment malfunction/failure. Dislodgement is a frequent problem in small children because of their short trachea length, and small pediatric ET tubes are more easily obstructed than larger adult-sized tubes. When a problem arises, take the patient off the ventilator and bag to ventilate manually. This will eliminate ventilator malfunction as a source of the problem and allow the clinician to use the ease of bagging to assess lung compliance as well as possible tube obstruction.

Auscultate to check for tube position or dislodgement, and use a suction catheter to clear secretions from the tube. Consider an underlying pneumothorax if equipment malfunction, obstruction, and displacement have been eliminated as causes. Needle decompression can be performed if the patient is in extremis. In the stable patient, use a chest radiograph to evaluate tube placement and assess for pneumothorax.[9]

Difficult Airway

When traditional intubation techniques fail, alternative methods must be employed. It is critical to recognize the difficult airway before giving induction agents and paralytics. Findings that predict a difficult airway include a limited mouth opening, cervical spine immobility, small mouth, prominent central incisors, short neck, large tongue, obesity, laryngeal edema, and mandibular or midface dysmorphology or trauma.[8] Consider using the LEMON mnemonic, as discussed previously. In the absence of these findings, an unanticipated difficult pediatric airway is unlikely.

Video laryngoscopy is a viable and increasingly common alternative to a difficult airway; several devices are available in pediatric and neonatal sizes. Research shows mixed results regarding the speed and rate of successful pediatric intubation using video laryngoscopy compared with standard direct laryngoscopy techniques in the hands of novice and experienced intubators.[19-23]

If the child cannot be intubated using standard techniques, effective BVM ventilation should be provided. If this is successful, the clinician has time to optimize further attempts by repositioning the patient and having the most skilled provider repeat the laryngoscopy. If ventilation is still not achieved, a supraglottic airway device can be employed as a rescue tool. The most commonly used supraglottic airway device in pediatrics is the laryngeal mask airway (LMA); however, the King laryngeal tube (KLT) also is available in a range of pediatric sizes, and limited early studies show high success rates.[24,25] (See *Table 25-6* for sizing of supraglottic devices and ET tubes.)

The most recent American Heart Association (AHA) recommendations for pediatric advanced life support state, "When BVM ventilation is unsuccessful and when endotracheal intubation is not possible, the LMA is an acceptable adjunct when used by experienced providers."[26] However, the guidelines warn that complications associated with LMA insertion occur more frequently in young children than in adults.

PEARL

For children younger than 5 years, needle cricothyrotomy with bag ventilation is preferred; for patients between 5 and 10 years, bag ventilation or transtracheal jet ventilation can be used. Children older than 10 years should be of adequate size to allow placement of a larger-bore cricothyroid tube using the Seldinger technique.

If endotracheal intubation fails and ventilation is unsuccessful with alternative airway devices, an invasive airway technique should be used. Options include needle cricothyrotomy and surgical cricothyrotomy. Needle cricothyrotomy is the easier and safer method of the two for temporary ventilatory support in the emergency department. This is only a short-term solution, however; although oxygenation can be preserved, ventilation is often marginal. Insert a 14-gauge catheter over a needle into the cricothyroid membrane while aspirating back. When free flow of air into the syringe is obtained, the position is correct. Consider placing a small amount of sterile saline in the syringe to assist in the detection of aspirated air.

Once cannulated, the catheter can be connected directly to an adapter device or attached to the barrel of a 3-mL syringe and then to a resuscitation bag via the hub of a 7.0 ET tube. For children younger than 5 years, needle cricothyrotomy with bag ventilation is preferred. For patients 5 to 10 years of age, bag ventilation or transtracheal jet ventilation can be used. Children older than 10 years should be of adequate size to allow placement of a larger bore cricothyroid tube using the Seldinger technique.

Breathing

When a child shows evidence of respiratory distress, the first step after airway positioning and clearance simply is to provide supplemental oxygen. Although oxygen delivered by nasal cannula or face mask is preferred and provides a higher inspired FiO_2, blow-by oxygen is an effective alternative for an agitated child who cannot tolerate having something on his or her face.

If inadequate oxygenation and ventilation persist, assisted ventilation might be necessary. As previously mentioned, BVM ventilation is the technique of choice during the initial phase of resuscitation. Although simple and effective, the technique — like everything else in pediatrics — requires appropriately sized equipment. A mask that fits properly covers the child's chin, mouth, and nose. A mask that is too large covers the eyes and extends over the tip of the chin, and one that is too small fails to cover the nose and mouth effectively and cannot make a seal.

In the emergency department, a self-inflating resuscitation bag most commonly is used. This device does not need to be attached to high-flow oxygen to function, although this is a common practice. When using BVM ventilation, take care not to compress the soft tissues of the neck in a young child. Hold the mask using the E-C clamp, using the thumb and index finger on the left hand to form a C that holds the mask onto the child's face, and the other three fingers to form an E along the angle of the jaw. Pull the patient's jaw up to the mask rather than pushing the mask down on the face. Squeeze the bag only until chest rise is seen. Normal tidal volume is 6 to 8 mL/kg, but with the dead space of the device, one can estimate the volume needed as 10 mL/kg.[9] Avoid overventilation, which can lead to gastric distention and an elevated hemidiaphragm.[27]

Hyperventilation is not recommended and can actually be harmful. Increased respiratory rates elevate intrathoracic pressure, thereby decreasing venous return and coronary

TABLE 25-7. Initial Pediatric Ventilator Settings

Pressure control (weight <10 kg)	Volume control (weight >10 kg)
Peak inspiratory pressure = 20–30 cm H_2O *(titrate for TV 8–10 ml/kg)*	**Tidal volume** = 8–10 mL/kg
PEEP = 5 cm H_2O	**PEEP** = 5 cm H_2O
FiO_2 = 100%	FiO_2 = 100%
Respiratory rate = Age appropriate	**Respiratory rate** = Age appropriate

After initial stabilization, titrate FiO_2 for saturations >92%.

perfusion pressure and thus the survival rate.[28] Hyperventilation also drives down the PCO_2, resulting in cerebral vasoconstriction and hypoperfusion. Mild hyperventilation to a goal PCO_2 of 30 to 35 mm Hg should be reserved for patients with signs of impending cerebral herniation and suspected pulmonary hypertension. Once an advanced airway is in place, respirations should be administered simultaneously with chest compressions at a rate of 8 to 10 breaths/min.[26]

Initial ventilator settings for the critically ill child are based on normal physiological parameters for a healthy child of similar weight and age. A positive end-expiratory pressure (PEEP) of 5 cm H_2O is a good starting point. Many ventilators are designed to deliver both pressure and volume control modes of ventilation. Either can be used, but consider pressure mode in infants and smaller children weighing less than 10 kg (*Table 25-7*). In either mode, the goal should be gentle chest rise, good air exchange, and delivery of a tidal volume of about 8 to 10 mL/kg.

PEARL

Avoid plateau pressures >30 cm H_2O to minimize barotrauma.

The target respiratory rate varies with the patient's age. A good starting point is a rate of 30 breaths/min for newborns, 24 for infants, 20 for small children, and 16 for older children and teenagers. The inspiratory time should be set between 0.5 and 1 second to target an inspiratory-to-expiratory ratio of 1:3 and allow adequate time in the exhalation phase of the respiratory cycle for carbon dioxide elimination. In patients demonstrating obstruction (eg, asthmatics), a larger ratio of 1:5 may be required. Avoid plateau pressures greater than 30 cm H_2O to minimize barotrauma. Obtain a blood gas measurement shortly after placing the patient on the ventilator to assess the effectiveness of ventilation.

Circulation

Rapidly assess the circulation to determine the adequacy of cardiac output and perfusion. Add to the PAT assessment of skin perfusion with a hands-on assessment of heart rate, pulse quality, level of consciousness, capillary refill, extremity temperature, skin color, urine output, and blood pressure.[3]

Cardiac Arrest

Although pediatric cardiac arrest is a relatively rare event, occurring in about 16,000 kids per year in the United States, morbidity and mortality after arrest are significant (50%–60%, depending on whether the arrest occurs in or out of the hospital). Many survivors have severe neurological injuries, with good outcomes reported in only 15% to 25% of patients with in-hospital arrest and 2% to 5% of those with out-of-hospital arrest.[29,30]

If a child is unresponsive and not breathing, take up to 10 seconds to check for a carotid, femoral, or brachial pulse. If no pulse is present, begin cardiopulmonary resuscitation (CPR) along with assisted ventilation. The 2010 AHA guidelines reflect a change in the recommended universal sequence: a shift from ABC to CAB, emphasizing the importance of initiating chest compressions immediately after cardiopulmonary arrest. The goal is to perform high-quality CPR with minimal interruptions.[31]

To perform chest compressions for children (approximately 1 year of age to puberty), use the heel of one or two hands to depress the lower half of the sternum to a depth of at least one-third of the anteroposterior (AP) chest diameter (about 5 cm).[32] For children, the compression-to-ventilation ratio is 30:2 for lone rescuers and 15:2 for two rescuers. For infants younger than 1 year, the AHA recommends that lone rescuers use two fingers to depress the sternum at least one-third the depth of the chest (about 4 cm). The two-thumb/encircling hands technique is recommended when two or more health care providers are present. One rescuer's thumbs should forcefully compress the lower third of the sternum, but there are no data to support

TABLE 25-8. Average Vital Signs by Age

Age	Weight (kg)	Heart Rate (bpm)	Respiratory Rate (breaths per minute)	Systolic Blood Pressure (mm Hg)
Newborn	3.5	130-150	40	70
3 months	6	140	30	90
6 months	8	130	30	90
1 year	10	120	26	90
2 years	12	115	26	90
3 years	15	110	24	90
4 years	17	100	24	90
6 years	20	100	20	95
8 years	25	90	20	95
10–12 years	30–40	85	20	100

From: *EMRA Pediatric Qwic Card. 2nd Ed.* Dallas, TX: Emergency Medicine Residents Association; 2013. Used with permission of Dale Woolridge, MD, PhD.

FIGURE 25-3. Algorithm for Bradycardia in Pediatric Patients[26]

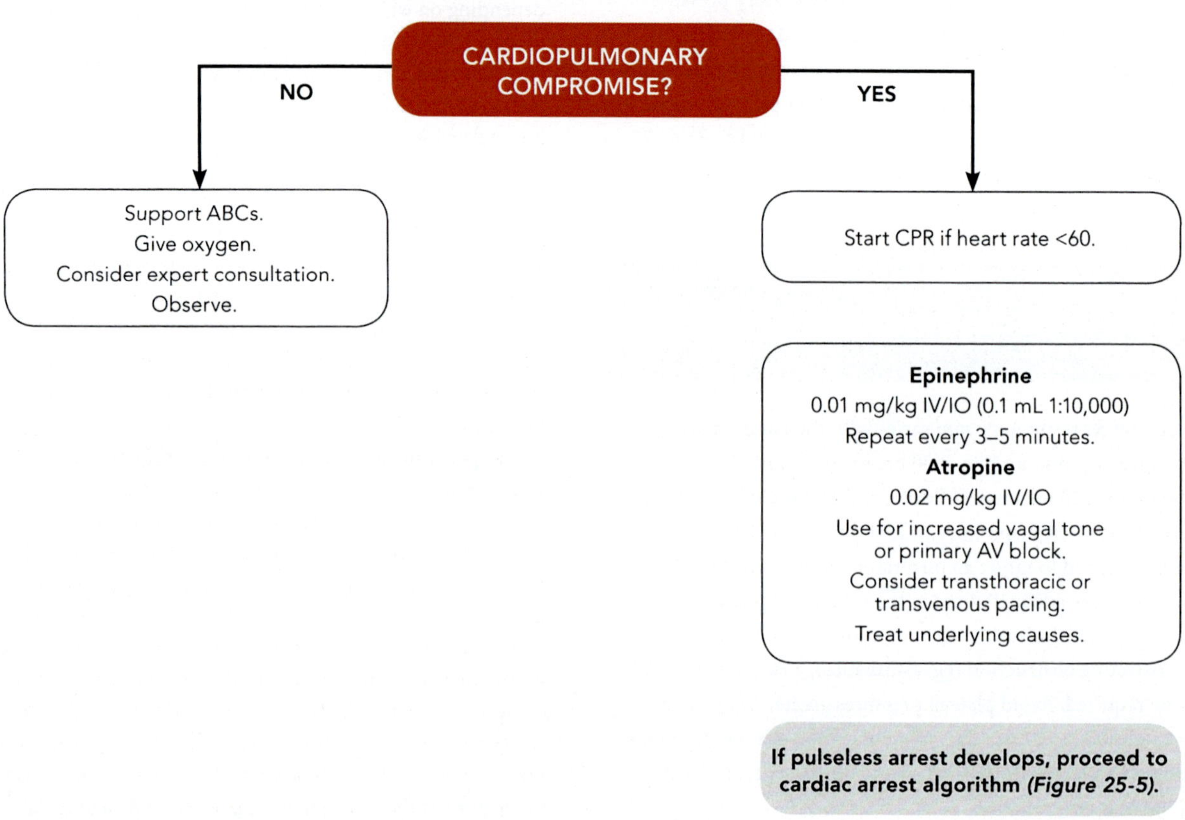

Adapted from the American Heart Association, Inc.

circumferential squeezing of the thorax.[25] The two-thumbs technique is preferred because it improves coronary artery perfusion pressure and may generate higher systolic and diastolic blood pressures.

When performing chest compressions, aim for a rate of at least 100 compressions/min, allowing full chest recoil at the end of each compression. The initial rescuer should be relieved by an alternate after 2 minutes to decrease fatigue; this switch should be performed in less than 5 seconds to minimize interruptions in CPR. In neonates, compressions and ventilations should be given in a 3:1 ratio of compressions to ventilations, with 90 compressions and 30 breaths in 1 minute, for a total of 120 events per minute. When compressions are given continuously, the rate should be 120 compressions per minute.[33]

Because pediatric cardiac arrest most commonly is caused by respiratory failure or shock, return of spontaneous circulation (ROSC) can be achieved in up to 50% of cases with chest compressions and ventilation alone.[34,35] When CPR is performed, however, it often is suboptimal, with compressions that are too few, too shallow, and too weak. Ventilations often are excessive, with too many interruptions in chest compressions.[36,37] Recent guidelines emphasize the importance of high-quality CPR to maximize the likelihood of recovery by improving myocardial, cerebral, and systemic perfusion.

The AHA stresses the need to "push hard and push fast"

FIGURE 25-4. Algorithm for Tachycardia in Pediatric Patients[26]

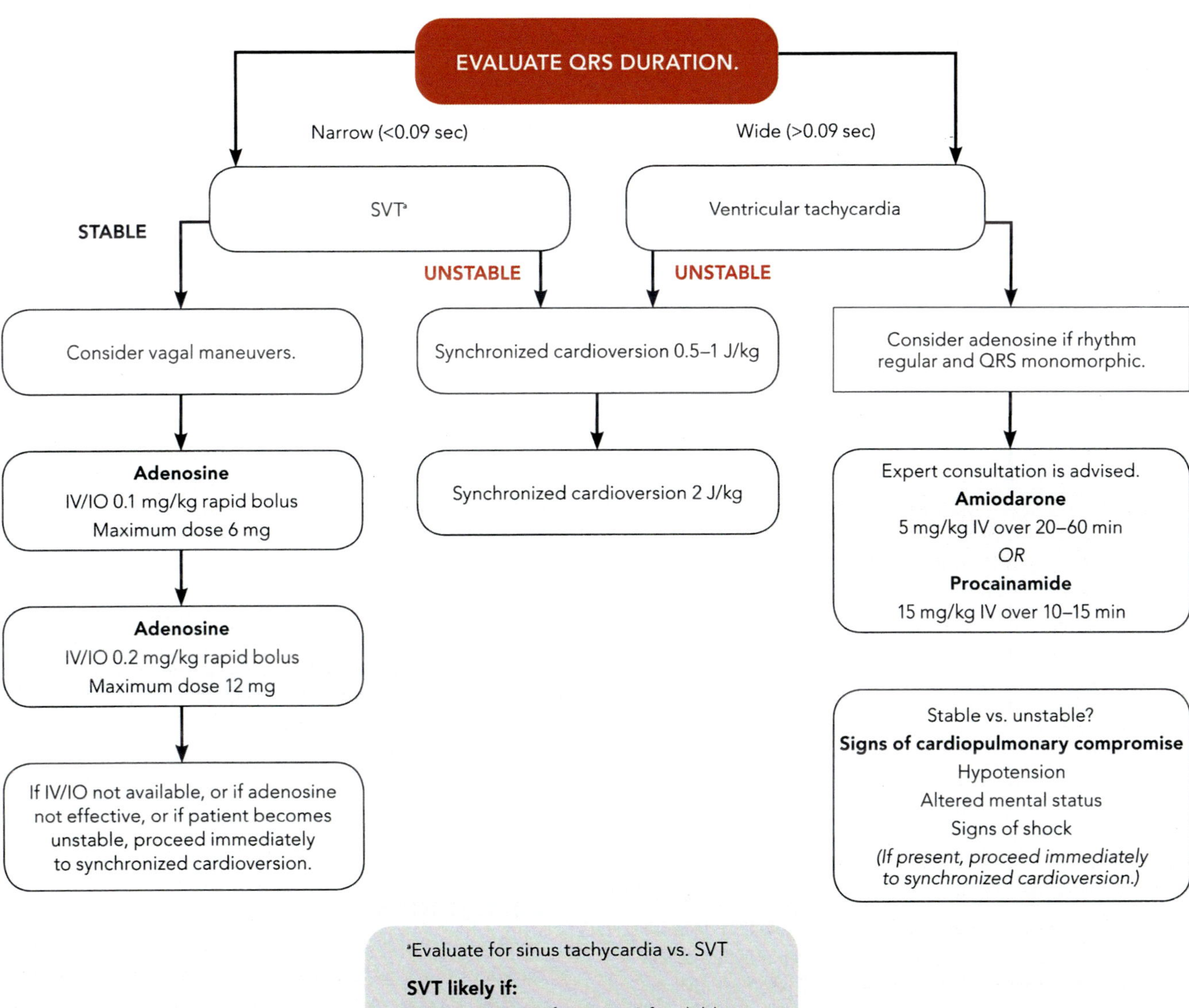

[a]Evaluate for sinus tachycardia vs. SVT

SVT likely if:

- Rate >220 in infants, >180 for children
- P waves absent or abnormal
- Heart rate not variable

Adapted from the American Heart Association, Inc.

FIGURE 25-5. Algorithm for Cardiac Arrest in Pediatric Patients[26]

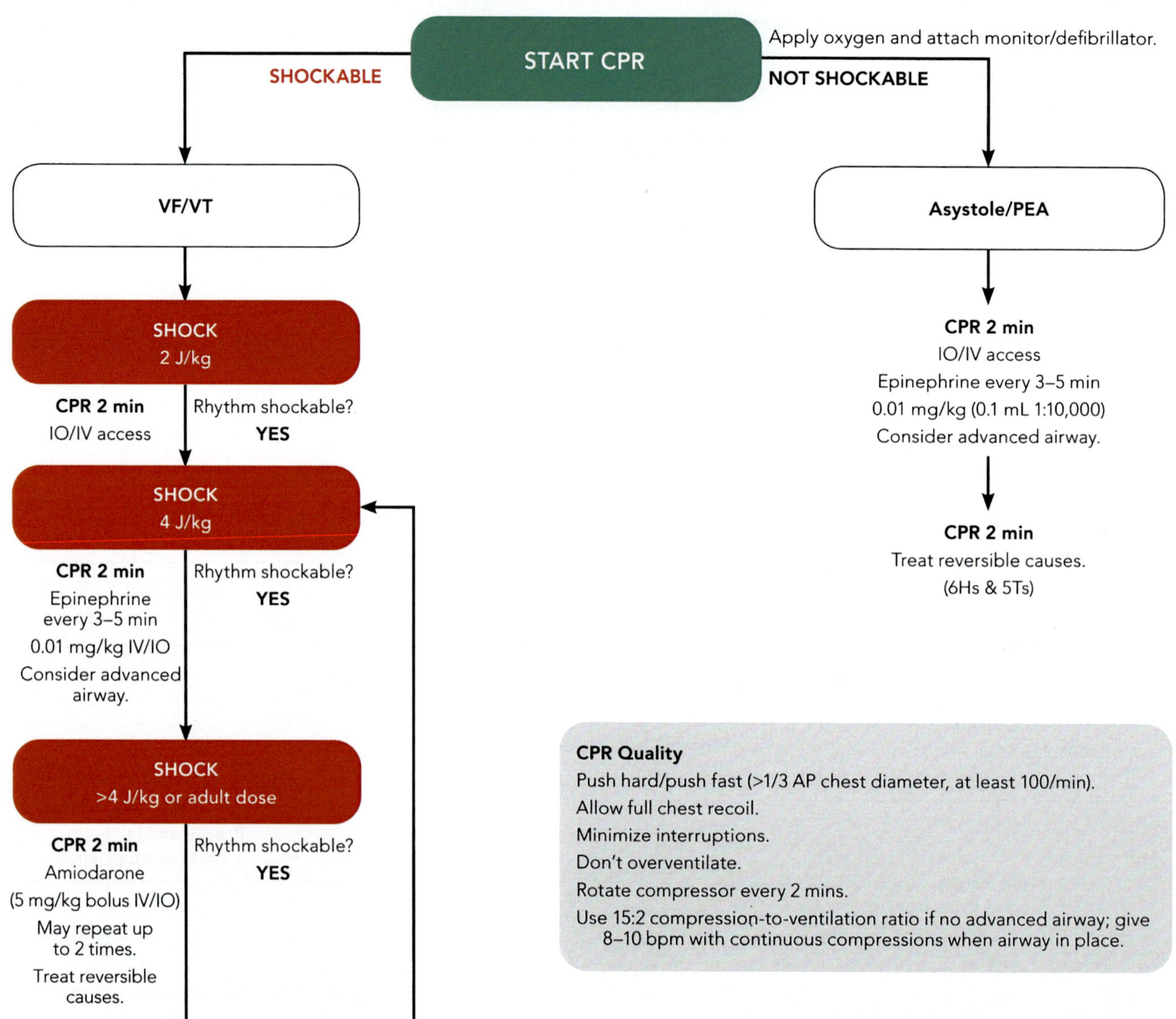

Adapted from the American Heart Association, Inc.

to maximize the effectiveness of compressions. Interruptions in compressions should be minimized because they decrease the rate of return to spontaneous circulation. Rhythm checks should be performed every 2 minutes and result in only brief interruptions in chest compressions. Once an advanced airway is in place, compressions and breaths should be performed continuously without interruption. Continuous end-tidal CO_2 ($ETCO_2$) detection may be useful to gauge the effectiveness of CPR. If the $ETCO_2$ is less than 10 to 15 mm Hg, efforts should focus on improving the quality of chest compressions and avoiding excessive ventilation. An abrupt and sustained increase in $ETCO_2$ might indicate that ROSC has occurred.[26]

Arrhythmias

Rhythm disturbances can be organized into three general categories: fast, slow, and pulseless. The clinical presentation of arrhythmia ranges widely from nonspecific signs and symptoms in a stable child to profound respiratory distress, shock, or arrest. Remember, vital signs are indeed vital (*Table 25-8*).

The most likely cause of bradyarrhythmia in children is hypoxia. First and foremost, supply oxygen and support respirations (*Figure 25-3*). Chest compressions should be started when the heart rate is below 60 beats/min and the child shows signs of poor perfusion, including hypotension, altered mental state, or signs of shock. If bradycardia persists despite good CPR, give epinephrine at a dose of 0.01 mg/kg (0.1 mL/kg of 1:10,000), IV/IO. This dose may be repeated every 3 to 5 minutes. If vagal stimulation or cholinergic drug toxicity is suspected, consider atropine, 0.02 mg/kg IV/IO (minimum dose 0.1 mg; maximum single dose 0.5 mg in a child and 1 mg in an adolescent). This dose can be repeated to a maximum total dose of 1 mg in a child and 2 mg in an adolescent.

Consider cardiac pacing if the bradycardia is caused by complete heart block or sinus node dysfunction, especially if it is associated with congenital or acquired heart disease. If the child progresses to pulseless electrical activity (PEA), switch to the PEA algorithm.[26,38]

When tachycardia is present and the patient is stable with a palpable pulse and adequate perfusion, administer oxygen, support ventilation, establish intravenous access, and obtain an ECG to evaluate the QRS duration (*Figure 25-4*). Narrow complex (<0.09 sec) tachycardia most likely is sinus or supraventricular tachycardia (SVT). Rapid heart rates in children most frequently are due to sinus tachycardia. Although the dysrhythmia itself usually is harmless, its underlying cause should be identified and corrected. Common causes include hypoxemia, hypovolemia, hyperthermia, fever, toxins, pain, and anxiety.

SVT, the most common pediatric tachyarrhythmia, typically presents with a heart rate faster than 180 beats/min in children and above 220 beats/min in infants (but the rate can reach as high as 300 beats/min). If the child is stable, the treatment of choice is vagal stimulation (unless it will significantly delay chemical or electrical cardioversion). In infants and young children, apply a bag of ice/water slurry to the face firmly (but do not occlude the airway). Carotid massage or Valsalva maneuvers such as blowing through a straw or bearing down can be effective in older children. Do not apply ocular pressure, which can damage the retina.

If vagal maneuvers fail to break the rhythm, adenosine should be given as a rapid intravenous bolus of 0.1 mg/kg (maximum initial dose 6 mg). This dose can be doubled on the second attempt to 0.2 mg/kg, with a maximum dose of 12 mg. Remember to administer adenosine fast, followed by an immediate flush of 5 to 10 mL of normal saline. Rapid infusion is necessary because of the very short half-life of the medication. It is best achieved by using two syringes attached to a stopcock to allow rapid administration.

If adenosine fails, consider electrical cardioversion (with sedation), amiodarone, or procainamide. These antiarrhythmic agents prolong the QT interval, must be infused slowly, and should not be used concurrently without expert consultation because they can precipitate torsade de pointes. Verapamil should not be used in infants because it has caused shock and

TABLE 25-9. Reversible Causes of Dysrhythmia, Shock, and Cardiorespiratory Arrest

Six Hs
Hydrogen ion (acidosis)
Hypoglycemia
Hypothermia
Hypo/Hyperkalemia
Hypoxia
Hypovolemia
Five Ts
Tamponade
Tension pneumothorax
Thrombosis (coronary or pulmonary)
Toxins
Trauma

TABLE 25-10. Signs and Symptoms of Shock States in Children

Hypovolemic	Cardiogenic	Distributive
Weak, pale, lethargic	Weak, pale, lethargic	Weak, pale lethargic
Tachypnea (to compensate for metabolic acidosis)	Tachypnea, retractions	Apnea, respiratory distress
Pale, mottled skin	Pale, mottled skin	Pale, mottled skin
Sunken eyes	Cool extremities	Cool or warm extremities
Dry mucous membranes	Hepatomegaly	Tachycardia
Poor skin turgor	Pulmonary edema	Hypotension
Delayed capillary refill	Tachycardia	History of source (allergen trigger, spinal cord injury, infection, etc.)
Cool extremities	Arrhythmia	
Tachycardia	Heart murmur	
Hypotension (late finding)	Hypotension	
History of source (vomiting, diarrhea, hemorrhage, etc.)	History of source (congenital heart disease, etc.)	

cardiac arrest in this population.[39] If the patient becomes unstable or perfusion is poor, proceed immediately to synchronized cardioversion with 0.5 to 1 J/kg. This can be repeated at 2 J/kg if the initial attempt is unsuccessful. Record a rhythm strip continuously during all chemical and electrical rhythm conversion attempts.[26,38]

PEARL

SVT is the most common tachyarrhythmia in children and typically presents with a heart rate >180 beats/min in children, and >220 beats/min in infants (but the rate can reach as high as 300 beats/min).

Wide complex (>0.09 sec) tachycardia usually is ventricular, but it can be supraventricular with aberrant conduction. If perfusion is poor or the child is unstable, proceed directly to synchronized cardioversion (0.5–1 J/kg then 2 J/kg if unsuccessful). If perfusion is adequate, consider giving a dose of adenosine to determine if the rhythm is SVT with aberrant conduction. If the patient is in stable ventricular tachycardia, consider expert consultation for guidance regarding pharmacological conversion with amiodarone, lidocaine, or procainamide. These drugs must be given slowly while carefully monitoring the patient for electrocardiographic and blood pressure changes. Slow or stop drug infusion if the QRS interval widens or the blood pressure falls during drug administration.[26]

The ECG rhythm of a patient in pulseless cardiopulmonary arrest (*Figure 25-5*) can fall into one of two categories: ventricular

TABLE 25-11. Infusion Rates for Vasoactive Medications

Dobutamine: 2–20 mcg/kg/min
Dopamine: 2–20 mcg/kg/min
Epinephrine: 0.1–1 mcg/kg/min
Norepinephrine: 0.1–2 mcg/kg/min
Vasopressin: 0.5 mU/kg/hr

KEY POINTS

1. Briefly assess the child's appearance, work of breathing, and circulation, which will help determine the severity of the patient's condition and direct further management. Use a length-based resuscitation tape (eg, Broselow tape) to determine equipment sizes and drug doses.
2. Physiological differences between children and adults that complicate airway management include increased oxygen consumption and metabolic rate and decreased pulmonary reserve.
3. Consider a cuffed ET tube in all patients beyond the neonatal period. Use a minimal amount of air in the cuff to eliminate air leak. The cuff can be deflated if high airway pressures are not needed.
4. When managing a difficult airway, do not continue to do the same thing and expect a different result. Move on to adjunctive airway devices.
5. Effective bag-mask ventilation might obviate the need for intubation.
   - Prolonged delivery of unnecessarily high oxygen concentrations should be avoided.
   - Do not hyperventilate the patient.
   - Use an age-appropriate rate and a tidal volume of 8 to 10 mL/kg.
6. When CPR is necessary, push hard and push fast, minimize interruptions, allow time for chest recoil, and check rhythm quickly every 2 minutes.
7. The universal compression-to-ventilation ratio is 30:2 for a lone rescuer and 15:2 for two rescuers.
8. Once an advanced airway is in place, deliver simultaneous ventilations and compressions with a ventilation rate of 8 to 10 breaths/min.
9. Defibrillate using a single shock of 2 J/kg followed by immediate resumption of 2 minutes of CPR. If a shockable rhythm persists, deliver 4 J/kg, epinephrine, and another 2 minutes of high-quality CPR. A third shock with more than 4 J/kg, with a maximum of 10 J/kg or the adult dose, and administration of amiodarone or lidocaine are recommended if attempts at defibrillation fail to restore a perfusing rhythm.
10. It is necessary to recognize and treat shock before hypotension occurs in children. Signs of shock that may precede hypotension include delayed capillary refill, cold extremities, weak peripheral pulses, low urine output (<1 mL/kg/hr), and altered mental status.
11. Rapid fluid resuscitation is crucial when managing patients with shock. Give 20 mL/kg x 3 boluses within the first 15 to 20 minutes. If shock persists, consider packed red blood cells and vasopressor medications, and continue resuscitation until vital signs, perfusion, and mental status improve.
12. Provide peripheral vasopressor support until central venous access can be attained in children who are not responsive to fluid resuscitation.
13. Give medications intravenously or intraosseously during resuscitation, and use endotracheal delivery as a last resort (the absorption is inconsistent).
14. After ROSC, optimize cerebral perfusion and cardiac output, avoid hyperthermia and hypoxia, and maintain normotension, normoglycemia, and normocarbia.

tachycardia (VT)/ventricular fibrillation (VF) or PEA/asystole. This distinction is critical, as survival is much more likely after arrests presenting with VT/VF.[40,41] If VF or VT is present or there is a sudden witnessed collapse (which is presumed to be VF), proceed immediately to defibrillation. The defibrillation success rate decreases 5% to 10% with every minute of delay.[42]

Resume CPR after one shock of 2 J/kg unsynchronized. After 2 minutes of CPR, check the rhythm and defibrillate again using 4 J/kg. Make every attempt to minimize the interruption of chest compressions. Give epinephrine, 0.01 mg/kg (0.1 mL/kg of 1:10,000) IV/IO, and repeat every 3 to 5 minutes. Perform another 2 minutes of CPR. If a shockable rhythm persists, deliver a third shock of more than 4 J/kg (maximum dose not to exceed 10 J/kg).

If cardioversion remains unsuccessful after the third defibrillation attempt, continue CPR and consider administering an antiarrhythmic drug. The AHA's 2010 guidelines recommend amiodarone (5 mg/kg IV/IO) and reserve lidocaine (1 mg/kg IV/IO) for situations in which amiodarone is not available. Lidocaine — when used alone — has been associated with improved ROSC and 24-hour survival in children in pulseless VF or VT.[43]

Magnesium sulfate (25-50 mg/kg IV/IO; maximum 2 g) should be given by rapid infusion for polymorphic VT or torsade de pointes. PEA and asystole rhythms are not amenable to electrical cardioversion or defibrillation. Give epinephrine as above, repeating every 3 to 5 minutes, followed each time by 2 minutes of high-quality CPR. Search for contributing and potentially reversible factors (think of the 6 Hs and 5 Ts [*Table 25-9*]), and rapidly correct any identified irregularities. Although the routine use of calcium and sodium bicarbonate is no longer recommended, these agents can be beneficial in specific resuscitation circumstances, including cases of severe acidosis or hyperkalemia.[26] If spontaneous circulation returns, proceed to meticulous post cardiac arrest care.

Shock

Shock is a state of inadequate perfusion resulting in inadequate substrate (oxygen, glucose) delivery to the vital organs. Early recognition is the key to preventing tissue damage and progression to cardiopulmonary arrest. The underlying etiologies of shock can be divided into three main categories: hypovolemic, cardiogenic, and distributive (*Table 25-10*). Hypovolemic shock, the most common culprit in pediatric patients, is characterized by an inadequate circulating intravascular volume that often results from dehydration or hemorrhage.

Distributive shock is characterized by an inadequate distribution of fluid volume, which usually is caused by systemic vasodilation leading to functional hypovolemia. Septic and anaphylactic shock are types of distributive shock that lead to this fluid shifting. Cardiogenic shock is characterized by myocardial dysfunction. Fluid volume can be normal or even slightly increased, but the diminished pump function of the myocardium impairs cardiac output.

Although shock is associated with hypotension, do not over rely on blood pressure measurements. Because of strong compensatory responses, children are able to maintain cardiac output and blood pressure through significant increases in heart rate and systemic vascular resistance. Many children have normal or even slightly elevated blood pressures during the early stages of shock. With acute hemorrhage, blood pressure can be maintained in a normal range until approximately 30% of the circulating blood volume has been lost. Once uncompensated shock ensues, it can progress rapidly to terminal shock that is unresponsive to therapy. Hypotension is a late and ominous sign of shock in children. Every effort should be made to recognize and treat these states before decompensation occurs.[44,45]

PEARL

Many children have normal or even slightly elevated blood pressures during the early stages of shock. With acute hemorrhage, normal blood pressure can be maintained until approximately 30% of the circulating blood volume has been lost.

Resuscitation options for the treatment of shock vary widely depending on the etiology. Regardless of the cause, the initial goal is to rapidly restore tissue perfusion. Administer supplemental oxygen, place cardiopulmonary monitors, and expediently obtain intravenous or intraosseous access. Initial therapeutic endpoints of resuscitation of septic shock include capillary refill of 2 seconds or less, normal blood pressure for age, normal pulses with no differential between peripheral and central pulses, warm extremities, urine output greater than 1 mL/kg/hr, and normal mental status. In advanced care settings, SvO_2 saturation 70% or below and cardiac index between 3.3 and 6.0 L/min/m^2 should be targeted.[46]

Give volume-expanding isotonic crystalloids (normal saline or lactated Ringer's solution) in a bolus of 20 mL/kg *as fast as possible*. Reassess the child after each bolus, and repeat if there is still evidence of poor perfusion. To deliver boluses this rapidly, consider a manual push-pull technique or delivery via pressure bag. Infusion by gravity is not rapid enough.[47] The resuscitation fluid of choice for volume expansion is packed red blood cells (given in 10-mL/kg aliquots), especially when signs of shock persist after 60 mL/kg crystalloid has been administered.

The Society of Critical Care Medicine recommends maintaining a hemoglobin concentration between 8 and 10 g/dL to improve oxygen-carrying capacity and tissue perfusion.[48] If there is a concern for cardiogenic shock, give smaller volumes more slowly while watching carefully for signs of worsening cardiac function and volume overload.[38]

If fluid resuscitation is insufficient to restore perfusion, add vasopressor support (*Table 25-11*). The vasoactive agent should be tailored to the patient and the clinical situation. Dopamine often is the initial vasopressor of choice. Start at 5 mcg/kg/min and titrate up by 2.5 mcg/kg/min every few minutes until perfusion improves and/or the target blood pressure is achieved (usually a mean arterial blood pressure of 65 mm Hg). Dopamine-resistant shock is diagnosed if inadequate perfusion persists after titration to 20 mcg/kg/min. In cases of dopamine-resistant shock, consider norepinephrine (start at 0.05 mcg/kg/min and then titrate by 0.05-0.1 mcg/ kg/min every 3-5 min to a maximum dose of 2 mcg/kg/min) or epinephrine (start at 0.05 mcg/kg/min and then titrate by 0.05-0.1 mcg/kg/ min every 3-5 min to a maximum dose of 1 mcg/kg/min).

In cases of myocardial dysfunction, dobutamine might benefit cardiac output by improving contractility, rate, and myocardial relaxation (start at 2.5 mcg/kg/min and then titrate by 2.5 mcg/kg/min every 3-5 min). Do not delay the initiation of vasopressors while attempting to obtain central venous access; vasoactive medications can be infused temporarily via a peripheral IV line. In cases of fluid-refractory, catecholamine-resistant shock, consider adrenal insufficiency and administer stress-dose hydrocortisone (2 mg/kg, maximum 100 mg).[46,49]

PEARL

When managing a child with septic shock, the vasoactive agent should be tailored to the patient and the clinical situation. Dopamine often is the initial vasopressor of choice.

Hypoglycemia can develop rapidly in shock states in response to high glucose utilization and low glycogen stores. Monitor for this and other electrolyte abnormalities and correct if necessary. In cases of sepsis, promptly administer broad-spectrum antibiotics after appropriate cultures have been obtained.

Vascular Access

Even with adequate CPR, resuscitation drugs may be required to restore a perfusing rhythm. Additionally, rapid fluid resuscitation can prevent shock from progressing to cardiorespiratory failure. Pediatric intravenous placement can be difficult in the hands of an inexperienced clinician, and further complicated by the stress of a code situation. When responding to a crashing or coding child, do not waste time attempting to place a central line; if peripheral intravenous access cannot be secured rapidly (ie, after three attempts), move immediately to intraosseous placement.

Intraosseous lines are a rapid, safe, effective option for resuscitation in all age groups (from premature infants to adults).[50] Newer devices, including spring-loaded needles and powered drills, can facilitate proper placement. Complications are similar to those associated with traditional intraosseous needles, including needle displacement, fracture, infection, and compartment syndrome. Nevertheless, the ease and rapidity of placement, as well as the effectiveness of drug delivery, make it an ideal technique for pediatric resuscitation. The AHA recommends intraosseous access over endotracheal drug delivery, noting that it can be used for the administration of fluids (including blood products) and medications (including pressors) and for initial blood sampling.[26] Equipment for intraosseous access should be made readily available, and caregivers should be familiar with its use.

If attempts at intravenous and intraosseous line placement fail, some medications may be given via the endotracheal route. Certain lipid-soluble drugs such as lidocaine, epinephrine, atropine, and naloxone (LEAN) can be delivered endotracheally. Although optimal endotracheal doses are unknown, most experts recommend double or triple the typical intravenous dose for lidocaine, atropine, and naloxone, and 10 times the typical dose for epinephrine (0.1 mg/kg or 0.1 mL/kg of a 1:1,000 concentration) when given endotracheally.

If using this route, follow the drug dose with a 5-mL normal saline flush. In neonates, this may be too large a volume; instead, dilute the drug to 1 to 2 mL with normal saline and give directly, or use a 5F feeding catheter inserted down the ET tube, followed by 0.5 mL saline. In both cases, immediately give several assisted bag ventilations to help distribute the drug deep into the bronchial tree. Overall, the endotracheal route is discouraged because of erratic and inconsistent drug absorption and potential toxicity.

Postresuscitation Care

When reperfusion is achieved, the immediate postresuscitation phase is critical. During this period, patients are at high risk for brain injury, seizures, ventricular arrhythmias, and extension of reperfusion injuries; interventions should focus on minimizing reperfusion injury and supporting cellular recovery. During the immediate postcardiac arrest period, it is important to avoid hyperthermia and hypoxia and maintain normotension, normoglycemia, and normocarbia. Fever, which is common after pediatric cardiac arrest, is associated with a decreased rate of survival and unfavorable neurological outcomes.[51,52] Therapeutic hypothermia (to 32°C–34°C) (89.6°F–93.2°F)might be beneficial for adolescents who remain comatose following resuscitation from a sudden witnessed out-of-hospital VF cardiac arrest, and may be considered for infants and children who remain comatose following resuscitation.[53]

Conclusion

Unstable pediatric patients present special challenges in the emergency department. Clinicians can deliver focused, effective care by understanding the unique anatomy and physiology of this patient population and by being prepared to employ targeted pediatric procedures.

REFERENCES

1. National Center for Health Statistics, Centers for Disease Control and Prevention, U.S. Department of Health and Human Services. Health, United States, 2013 (Tables 86 and 87). Available at www.cdc.gov/nchs/data/hus/hus13.pdf. Accessed August 25, 2015.
2. Langham M, Keshavarz R, Richardson L. How comfortable are emergency physicians with pediatric patients? *J Emerg Med.* 2004;26:465-469.
3. Dieckmann RA, Brownstein D, Gausche-Hill M. The pediatric assessment triangle: a novel approach for the rapid evaluation of children. *Pediatr Emerg Care.* 2010;26:312-315.
4. Luten R, Wears RF, Broselow J, et al. Managing the unique size-related issues of pediatric resuscitation: reducing cognitive load with resuscitation aids. *Acad Emerg Med.* 2002;9:840-847.

5. Gausche M, Lewis RJ, Stratton SJ, et al. Effect of out-of-hospital pediatric endotracheal intubation on survival and neurological outcome: a controlled clinical trial. *JAMA.* 2000;283:783-790.
6. Stockinger ZT, McSwain NE Jr. Prehospital endotracheal intubation for trauma does not improve survival over bag-valve-mask ventilation. *J Trauma.* 2004;56:531-536.
7. Pitetti R, Glustein JZ, Bhende MS. Prehospital care and outcome of pediatric out-of-hospital cardiac arrest. *Prehosp Emerg Care.* 2002;6:283-290.
8. Sullivan KJ, Kissoon N. Securing the child's airway in the emergency department. *Pediatr Emerg Care.* 2002;18:108-124.
9. Santillanes G, Gausche-Hill M. Pediatric airway management. *Emerg Med Clin North Am.* 2008;26:961-975.
10. Stewart C. Managing the pediatric airway in the ED. *Pediatr Emerg Med Pract.* 2006;3:1-24.
11. Bingham RM, Proctor LT. Airway management. *Pediatr Clin North Am.* 2008;55:873-886.
12. King BB, Baker MD, Braitman LE, et al. Endotracheal tube selection in children: a comparison of four methods. *Ann Emerg Med.* 1993;22:530-534.
13. Khine HH, Corddry DH, Kettrick RG, et al. Comparison of cuffed and uncuffed endotracheal tubes in young children in general anesthesia. *Anesthesiology.* 1997;86:627-631.
14. Newth CJ, Rachman B, Patel N, et al. The use of cuffed versus uncuffed endotracheal tubes in pediatric intensive care. *J Pediatr.* 2004;144:333-337.
15. Deakers TW, Reynolds G, Stretton M, et al. Cuffed endotracheal tubes in pediatric intensive care. *J Pediatr.* 1994;125:57-62.
16. Moynihan RJ, Brock-Utne JG, Archer JH, et al. The effect of cricoid pressure on preventing gastric insufflation in infants and children. *Anesthesiology.* 1993;78:652-656.
17. Walker RW, Ravi R, Haylett K. Effect of cricoid force on airway caliber in children: a bronchoscopic assessment. *Br J Anaesth.* 2010;104:71-74.
18. Li J. Capnography alone is imperfect for endotracheal tube placement confirmation during emergency intubation. *J Emerg Med.* 2001;20:223-229.
19. Kim JT, Na HS, Bae JY, et al. GlideScope video laryngoscope: a randomized clinical trial in 203 paediatric patients. *Br J Anaesth.* 2008;101:531-534.
20. Nouruzi-Sedeh P, Schurmann M, Groeben H. Laryngoscopy via Macintosh blade versus GlideScope success rate and time for endotracheal intubation in untrained medical personnel. *Anesthesiology.* 2009;110:32-37.
21. Sylvia MJ, Maranda L, Harris KL, et al. Comparison of success rates using video laryngoscopy versus direct laryngoscopy by residents during a simulated pediatric emergency. *Simul Healthc.* 2013;8:155-161.
22. Fonte M, Oulego-Erroz I, Nadkarni L, et al. A randomized comparison of the GlideScope videolaryngoscope to the standard laryngoscopy for intubation by pediatric residents in simulated easy and difficult infant airway scenarios. *Pediatr Emerg Care.* 2011;27:398-402.
23. Donoghue AJ, Ades AM, Nishisaki A, et al. Videolaryngoscopy versus direct laryngoscopy in simulated pediatric intubation. *Ann Emerg Med.* 2013;61:271-277.
24. Byars DV, Brodsky RA, Evans D, et al. Comparison of direct laryngoscopy to Pediatric King LT-D in simulated airways. *Pediatr Emerg Care.* 2012;28:750-752.
25. Mitchell MD, Lee White M, King WD, et al. Paramedic King Laryngeal Tube airway insertion versus endotracheal intubation in simulated pediatric respiratory arrest. *Prehosp Emerg Care.* 2012;16:284-288.
26. Kleinman ME, Chameides L, Schexnayder SM, et al. Part 14: Pediatric Advanced Life Support: 2010 American Heart Association Guidelines for Cardiopulmonary Resuscitation and Emergency Cardiovascular Care. *Circulation.* 2010;122(suppl 3):S876-S908.
27. Berg MD, Ahamed IH, Berg RA. Severe ventilatory compromise due to gastric distension during pediatric cardiopulmonary resuscitation. *Resuscitation.* 1998;36:71-73.
28. Aufderheide T, Lurie K. Death by hyperventilation: a common and life-threatening problem during cardiopulmonary resuscitation. *Crit Care Med.* 2004;32(9 suppl):S345-S351.
29. Moler FW, Meert K, Donaldson AE, et al. In-hospital versus out-of-hospital pediatric cardiac arrest: a multicenter cohort study. *Crit Care Med.* 2009;37:2259-2267.
30. Atkins DL, Everson-Stewart S, Sears GK, et al. Epidemiology and outcomes from out-of-hospital cardiac arrest in children: the Resuscitation Outcomes Consortium Epistry-Cardiac Arrest. *Circulation.* 2009;119:1484-1491.
31. Berg MD, Schexnayder SM, Chameides L, et al. Part 13: Pediatric Basic Life Support: 2010 American Heart Association Guidelines for Cardiopulmonary Resuscitation and Emergency Cardiovascular Care. *Circulation.* 2010;122[suppl 3]:S862-S875.
32. Stevenson A, McGowan J, Evans A, et al. CPR for children: one hand or two? *Resuscitation.* 2005;64:205-208.
33. Kattwinkel J, Perlman JM, Aziz K, et al. Part 15: neonatal resuscitation: 2010 American Heart Association Guidelines for Cardiopulmonary Resuscitation and Emergency Cardiovascular Care. *Circulation.* 2010;122(18 suppl 3):S909-S919.
34. Young KD, Gausche-Hill M, McClung CD, et al. A prospective, population-based study of the epidemiology and outcome of out-of-hospital pediatric cardiopulmonary arrest. *Pediatrics.* 2004;114:157-164.
35. Berg MD, Nadkarni VM, Berg RA. Cardiopulmonary resuscitation in children. *Curr Opin Crit Care.* 2008;14:254-260.
36. Donoghue AJ, Nadkarni VM, Berg RA, et al. Out-of-hospital pediatric cardiac arrest: an epidemiologic review and assessment of current knowledge. *Ann Emerg Med.* 2005;46:512-522.
37. Abella BS, Alvarado JP, Myklebust H, et al. Quality of cardiopulmonary resuscitation during in-hospital cardiac arrest. *JAMA.* 2005;293:363-365.
38. Fitzmaurice L, Gerardi MJ. Cardiovascular system. In: Gausche-Hill M, Fuchs S, Yamamoto L, eds. *APLS: The Pediatric Emergency Medicine Resource.* 4th ed. Sudbury, MA: American Academy of Pediatrics and American College of Emergency Physicians; 2007:106-145.
39. Samson RA, Atkins DL. Tachyarrhythmias and defibrillation. *Pediatr Clin North Am.* 2008;55:887-907.
40. Atkins DL, Everson-Stewart S, Sears GK, et al. Epidemiology and outcomes from out-of-hospital cardiac arrest in children: the Resuscitation Outcomes Consortium Epistry-Cardiac arrest. *Circulation.* 2009;119:1484-1491.
41. Samson RA, Nadkarni VM, Meaney PA, et al. Outcomes of in-hospital ventricular fibrillation in children. *N Engl J Med.* 2006;354:2328-2339.
42. Larsen MP, Eisenberg MS, Cummins RO, et al. Predicting survival from out-of-hospital cardiac arrest: a graphic model. *Ann Emerg Med.* 1993;22:1652-1658.
43. Valdes SO, Donoghue AJ, Hoyme DB, et al. Outcomes associated with amiodarone and lidocaine in the treatment of in-hospital pediatric cardiac arrest with pulseless ventricular tachycardia or ventricular fibrillation. *Resuscitation.* 2014;85:381-386.
44. American College of Surgeons. *Advanced Trauma Life Support for Doctors.* 9th ed. Chicago, IL: American College of Surgeons; 2012.
45. Carcillo JA, Fields AI. Clinical practice parameters for hemodynamic support of pediatric and neonatal patients in septic shock. *Crit Care Med.* 2002;30:1365-1378.
46. Dellinger RP, Levy MM, Rhodes A, et al. for the Surviving Sepsis Campaign Guidelines Committee including the Pediatric Subgroup. Surviving Sepsis Campaign: International Guidelines for Management of Severe Sepsis and Septic Shock: 2012. *Crit Care Med.* 2013;41:580-637.
47. Stoner MJ, Goodman DG, Cohen DM, et al. Rapid fluid resuscitation in pediatrics: testing the American College of Critical Care Medicine guideline. *Ann Emerg Med.* 2007;50:601-607.
48. Melendez E, Bachur R. Advances in the emergency management of pediatric sepsis. *Curr Opin Pediatr.* 2006;18:245-253.
49. Turner DA and Kleinman ME. The use of vasoactive agents via peripheral intravenous access during transport of critically ill infants and children. *Pediatr Emer Care.* 2010;26:563-566.
50. De Caen RA, Reis A, Bhutta A. Vascular access and drug therapy in pediatric resuscitation. *Pediatr Clin North Am.* 2008;55:909-927.
51. Laptook A, Tyson J, Shankaran S, et al. Elevated temperature after hypoxic-ischemic encephalopathy: risk factor for adverse outcomes. *Pediatrics.* 2008;122:491-9.
52. Bembea M, Nadkarni V, Diener-West M, et al. Temperature patterns in the early post-resuscitation period after pediatric in-hospital cardiac arrest. *Pediatr Crit Care Med.* 2010;11:723-730.
53. Kleinman ME, de Caen AR, Chameides L, et al. on behalf of the Pediatric Basic and Advanced Life Support Chapter Collaborators. Part 10: pediatric basic and advanced life support: 2010 International Consensus on Cardiopulmonary Resuscitation and Emergency Cardiovascular Care Science with Treatment Recommendations. *Circulation.* 2010;122(suppl 2):S466–S515.

Index

t=table
f=figture

D

E

F

Q

R

S

T

U

V

W